Praise From the Experts

"For the nonstatistician, the array of statistical issues in design and analysis of clinical trials can be overwhelming. Drawing on their years of experience dealing with data analysis plans and the regulatory environment, the authors of *Analysis of Clinical Trials Using SAS: A Practical Guide* have done a great job in organizing the statistical issues one needs to consider both in the design phase and in the analysis and reporting phase. As the authors demonstrate, SAS provides excellent tools for designing, analyzing and reporting results of comparative trials, making this book very attractive for the nonstatistician.

This book will also be very useful for statisticians who wish to learn the most current statistical methodologies in clinical trials. The authors make use of recent developments in SAS - including stratification, multiple imputation, mixed models, nonparametrics, and multiple comparisons procedures - to provide cutting-edge tools that are either difficult to find or unavailable in other software packages. Statisticians will also appreciate the fact that sufficient technical details are provided.

Because clinical trials are so highly regulated, some of the most rigorous and highly respected statistical tools are used in this arena. The methodologies covered in this book have applicability to the design and analysis of experiments well beyond clinical trials; researchers in all fields who carry out comparative studies would do well to have it on their bookshelves."

Peter Westfall, Texas Tech University

"This is a very impressive book. Although it doesn't pretend to cover all types of analyses used in clinical trials, it does provide unique coverage of five extremely important areas. Each chapter combines a detailed literature review and theoretical discussion with a useful how-to guide for practitioners. This will be a valuable book for clinical biostatisticians in the pharmaceutical industry."

Steve Snapinn, Amgen

"Chapter 1 ("Analysis of Stratified Data") will make a very fine and useful addition to the literature on analyzing clinical trials using SAS."

Stephen Senn, University of Glasgow

"Chapter 2 ("Multiple Comparisons and Multiple Endpoints") provides an excellent single-source overview of the statistical methods available to address the critically important aspect of multiplicity in clinical trial evaluation. The treatment is comprehensive, and the authors compare and contrast methods in specific applications. Newly developed gatekeeping methods are included, and the available software makes the approach accessible. The graphical displays are particularly useful in understanding the concept of adjusted p-values."

Joe Heyse, Merck

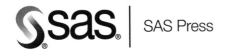
SAS Press

Analysis of Clinical Trials Using SAS®

A Practical Guide

Alex Dmitrienko
Geert Molenberghs
Christy Chuang-Stein
Walter Offen

The Power to Know.

The correct bibliographic citation for this manual is as follows: Dmitrienko, Alex, Geert Molenberghs, Christy Chuang-Stein, and Walter Offen. 2005. *Analysis of Clinical Trials Using SAS®: A Practical Guide*. Cary, NC: SAS Institute Inc.

Analysis of Clinical Trials Using SAS®: A Practical Guide

Contents

Preface

Introduction

Clinical trials have long been one of the most important tools in the arsenal of clinicians and scientists who help develop pharmaceuticals, biologics, and medical devices. It is reported that nearly 10,000 clinical studies are conducted every year around the world. One can find many excellent books that address fundamental statistical and general scientific principles underlying the design and analysis of clinical trials, such as those by Pocock (1983), Fleiss (1986), Meinert (1986), Friedman, Furberg and DeMets (1996), Piantadosi (1997) and Senn (1997). Numerous references can be found in these fine books.

The aim of this book is unique in that we focus in great detail on a set of selected and practical problems facing statisticians and biomedical scientists conducting clinical research. We discuss solutions to these problems based on modern statistical methods and review computer-intensive techniques that help clinical researchers efficiently and rapidly implement these methods in the powerful SAS environment.

It is a challenge to select the few topics that are most important and relevant to the design and analysis of clinical trials. Our choice of topics for this book was guided by the International Conference on Harmonization (ICH) guideline for the pharmaceutical industry entitled "Structure and Content of Clinical Study Reports" (this document is commonly referred to as ICH E3). The document states that

> Important features of the analysis, including the particular methods used, adjustments made for demographic or baseline measurements or concomitant therapy, handling of dropouts and missing data, adjustments for multiple comparisons, special analyses of multicenter studies, and adjustments for interim analyses, should be discussed [in the study report].

Following the ICH recommendations, we decided to focus in this book on the analysis of stratified data, incomplete data, multiple inferences, and issues arising in safety and efficacy monitoring. We also address other statistical problems that are very important in a clinical trial setting, such as reference intervals for safety and diagnostic measurements.

One special feature of the book is the inclusion of numerous SAS macros to help readers implement the new methodology in the SAS environment. The availability of the programs and the detailed discussion of the output from the macros help make the application of new procedures a reality. The authors are planning to make the SAS macros compatible with new SAS products such as SAS Enterprise Guide. Enterprise Guide tasks that implement the statistical methods discussed in the book will be published on the SAS Enterprise Guide Users Group Web site at http://www.segus.org.

The book is aimed at clinical statisticians and other scientists who are involved in the design and analysis of clinical trials conducted by the pharmaceutical industry, academic institutions, or governmental institutions such as the National Institutes of Health (NIH). Graduate students specializing in biostatistics will also find the material in this book useful because of its applied nature.

Because the book is written for practitioners, it concentrates primarily on solutions rather than theory. Although most of the chapters include some tutorial material, this book was not intended to provide a comprehensive coverage of the selected topics. Nevertheless, each chapter gives a high-level description of the theoretical aspects of the statistical problem at hand and includes references to publications that contain more advanced material. In addition, each chapter gives a detailed overview of the underlying statistical principles.

There are some exceptions to the presentation of minimum theory in the book. For example, Chapter 5 discusses the analysis of incomplete data and covers comparatively complex statistical concepts such as multiple imputation. Although the theoretical part is written at a higher statistical level, examples and applications are prepared in such a way that they can be easily understood.

Examples from real trials are used throughout the book to illustrate the concepts being discussed and to help the reader understand their relevance in a clinical trial setting. Most of the data come from real clinical trials. In several cases, because of confidentiality concerns, we relied on simulated data that are representative of real clinical trial data. Although simulated data might lack authenticity, using them does afford us the opportunity to see how close to the truth we can get using the proposed methodology. In this regard, we echo Hastie and Tibshirani's (1990, page 239) statement that "an advantage of using simulated examples is that you know the truth."

Outline of the book

Chapter 1: Analysis of Stratified Data. This chapter discusses the analysis of clinical outcomes in the presence of influential covariates. It reviews stratified analyses of continuous, categorical, and time-to-event endpoints. The chapter also introduces statistical methods for studying treatment-by-stratum interactions.

Chapter 2: Multiple Comparisons and Multiple Endpoints. This chapter reviews statistical strategies for handling multiplicity issues arising in clinical trials. It covers basic single-step multiple tests as well as more advanced closed, fixed-sequence and resampling-based multiple testing procedures. The chapter also describes strategies for handling multiple objectives and dose-finding studies.

Chapter 3: Analysis of Safety and Diagnostic Data. This chapter describes methods for constructing reference intervals for safety and diagnostic measures with various clinical trials applications, such as computation of reference limits based on sample quantiles and tolerance limits. The second part of the chapter reviews statistical methods for the analysis of shift tables produced after reference intervals have been applied to safety and diagnostic data.

Chapter 4: Interim Data Monitoring. The first part of this chapter reviews the popular approaches for designing and monitoring group sequential trials, such as repeated significance tests and the error spending function approach. The second part introduces stochastic curtailment methods, including frequentist, mixed Bayesian-frequentist, and fully Bayesian methods.

Chapter 5: Analysis of Incomplete Data. This chapter discusses basic and more advanced statistical methods for the analysis of incomplete longitudinal data. These methods include complete case analysis, last observation carried forward, likelihood-based methods, and multiple imputation.

Acknowledgments

We would like to thank the following individuals (listed alphabetically) for their valuable comments:

Caroline Beunckens (Limburgs Universitair Centrum)

Prof. Raymond Carroll (Texas A&M University)

Dr. Brenda Gaydos (Lilly)

Dr. Jeffrey Helterbrand (Genentech)

Dr. Joseph Heyse (Merck)

Prof. Jason Hsu (Ohio State University)

Ivy Jansen (Limburgs Universitair Centrum)

Prof. Michael Kenward (London School of Hygiene and Tropical Medicine)

Prof. Richard Kryscio (University of Kentucky)

Dr. Gordon Lan (Aventis)

Dr. Ilya Lipkovich (Lilly)

Dr. Nuwan Nanayakkara (Amylin)

Dr. Gerhardt Pohl (Lilly)

Dr. Andreas Sashegyi (Lilly)

Prof. Stephen Senn (Glasgow University)

Dr. Herbert Thijs (Limburgs Universitair Centrum)

Prof. Geert Verbeke (Katholieke Universiteit Leuven)

Prof. Peter Westfall (Texas Tech University)

Dr. Ilker Yalcin (Lilly)

We are grateful to Grace Ying Li (Lilly) who has carefully tested most of the SAS programs in this book and helped us optimize some of the complicated SAS macros.

Alex Dmitrienko and Walt Offen would like to sincerely thank Lilly Global Statistical Science senior management, in particular Drs. Carlos Alatorre, Todd Sanger and Mike Wilson, for their enthusiastic and continual support of this endeavor.

Geert Molenberghs would like to thank his colleagues for their support.

Christy Chuang-Stein wishes to thank Drs. Mohan Beltangady and Debra Gmerek for their support and encouragement.

We also thank Donna Faircloth, our editor at SAS Books by Users Press, for her support and assistance in preparing this book.

Analysis of Stratified Data

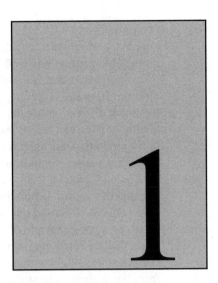

This chapter discusses the analysis of clinical outcomes in the presence of influential covariates such as investigational center or patient demographics. The following analysis methods are reviewed:

- Stratified analyses of continuous endpoints using parametric methods based on fixed and random effects models as well as nonparametric methods.
- Simple randomization-based methods as well as more advanced exact and model-based methods for analyzing stratified categorical outcomes.
- Analysis of stratified time-to-event data using randomization-based tests and the Cox proportional hazards model.

The chapter also introduces statistical methods for studying the nature of treatment-by-stratum interactions in clinical trials.

1.1   Introduction

This chapter addresses issues related to adjustment for important covariates in clinical applications. The goal of an adjusted analysis is to provide an overall test of treatment effect in the presence of factors that have a significant effect on the outcome variable. Two different types of factors known to influence the outcome are commonly encountered in clinical trials: *prognostic* and *non-prognostic* factors (Mehrotra, 2001). Prognostic factors are known to influence the outcome variables in a systematic way. For instance, the analysis of survival data is always adjusted for prognostic factors such as a patient's age and disease severity because these patient characteristics are strongly correlated with mortality. By contrast, non-prognostic factors are likely to impact the trial's outcome but their effects do not exhibit a predictable pattern. It is well known that treatment differences vary, sometimes dramatically, across investigational centers in multicenter clinical trials. However, the nature of center-to-center variability is different from the variability associated with a patient's age or disease severity. Center-specific treatment differences are dependent on a large number of factors, e.g., geographical location, general quality of care, etc. As a consequence, individual centers influence the overall treatment difference in a fairly random manner and it is natural to classify the center as a non-prognostic factor.

Adjustments for important covariates are carried out using randomization- and model-based methods (Koch and Edwards, 1988; Lachin, 2000, Chapter 4). The idea behind randomization-based analyses is to explicitly control factors influencing the outcome variable while assessing the relationship between the treatment effect and outcome. The popular Cochran-Mantel-Haenszel method for categorical data serves as a good example of this approach. In order to adjust for a covariate, the sample is divided into strata that are relatively homogeneous with respect to the selected covariate. The treatment effect is examined separately within each stratum and thus the confounding effect of the covariate is eliminated from the analysis. The stratum-specific treatment differences are then combined to carry out an aggregate significance test of the treatment effect across the strata.

Model-based methods present an alternative to the randomization-based approach. In general, inferences based on linear or non-linear models are closely related (and often asymptotically equivalent) to corresponding randomization-based inferences. Roughly speaking, one performs regression inferences by embedding randomization-based methods into a modeling framework that links the outcome variable to treatment effect and important covariates. Once a model has been specified, an inferential method (most commonly the method of maximum likelihood) is applied to estimate relevant parameters and test relevant hypotheses. Looking at the differences between the two approaches to adjusting for covariates in clinical trials, it is worth noting that model-based methods are more flexible than randomization-based methods. For example, within a model-based framework, one can directly adjust for continuous covariates without having to go through an artificial and possibly inefficient process of creating strata.[1] Further, as pointed out by Koch et al. (1982), randomization- and model-based methods have been historically motivated by two different sampling schemes. As a result, randomization-based inferences are generally restricted to a particular study, whereas model-based inferences can be generalized to a larger population of patients.

There are two important advantages of adjusted analysis over a simplistic pooled approach that ignores the influence of prognostic and non-prognostic factors. First of all, adjusted analyses are performed to improve the power of statistical inferences (Beach and Meier, 1989; Robinson and Jewell, 1991; Ford, Norrie and Ahmadi, 1995). It is well known that, by adjusting for a covariate in a linear model, one gains *precision* which is proportional to the correlation between the covariate and outcome variable. The same is true for categorical and time-to-event data. Lagakos and Schoenfeld (1984) demonstrated that omitting an important covariate with a large hazard ratio dramatically reduces the efficiency of the score test in Cox proportional hazards models.

Further, failure to adjust for important covariates may introduce *bias*. Following the work of Cochran (1983), Lachin (2000, Section 4.4.3) demonstrated that the use of marginal unadjusted methods in the analysis of stratified binary data leads to biased estimates. The magnitude of the bias is proportional to the degree of treatment group imbalance within each stratum and the difference in event rates across the strata. Along the same line, Gail, Wieand and Piantadosi (1984) and Gail, Tan and Piantadosi (1988) showed that parameter estimates in many generalized linear and survival models become biased when relevant covariates are omitted from the regression.

Overview

Section 1.2 reviews popular ANOVA models with applications to the analysis of stratified clinical trials. Parametric stratified analyses in the continuous case are easily implemented using PROC GLM or PROC MIXED. The section also considers a popular nonparametric test for the analysis of stratified

---

[1] However, in fairness, it is important to note that modeling may require more assumptions; e.g., we may need to assume that the outcome variable and covariate are linearly related.

data in a non-normal setting. Linear regression models have been the focus of numerous monographs and research papers. The classical monographs of Rao (1973) and Searle (1971) provided an excellent discussion of the general theory of linear models. Milliken and Johnson (1984, Chapter 10), Goldberg and Koury (1990) and Littell, Freund and Spector (1991, Chapter 7) discussed the analysis of stratified data in an unbalanced ANOVA setting and its implementation in SAS.

Section 1.3 reviews randomization-based (Cochran-Mantel-Haenszel and related methods) and model-based approaches to the analysis of stratified categorical data. It covers both asymptotic and exact inferences that can be implemented in PROC FREQ, PROC LOGISTIC and PROC GENMOD. See Breslow and Day (1980), Koch and Edwards (1988), Lachin (2000), Stokes, Davis and Koch (2000) and Agresti (2002) for a thorough overview of categorical analysis methods with clinical trial applications.

Section 1.4 discusses statistical methods used in the analysis of stratified time-to-event data. The section covers both randomization-based tests available in PROC LIFETEST and model-based tests based on the Cox proportional hazards regression implemented in PROC PHREG. Kalbfleisch and Prentice (1980), Cox and Oakes (1984) and Collett (1994) gave a detailed review of classical survival analysis methods. Allison (1995), Cantor (1997) and Lachin (2000, Chapter 9) provided an introduction to survival analysis with clinical applications and examples of SAS code.

Section 1.5 introduces two popular tests for qualitative interaction developed by Gail and Simon (1985) and Ciminera et al. (1993). The tests for qualitative interaction help clarify the nature of the treatment-by-stratum interaction and identify patient populations that benefit the most from an experimental therapy. They can also be used in sensitivity analyses.

1.2 Continuous Endpoints

This section reviews parametric and nonparametric analysis methods with applications to clinical trials in which the primary analysis is adjusted for important covariates, e.g., multicenter clinical trials. Within the parametric framework, we will focus on fixed and random effects models in a frequentist setting. The reader interested in alternative approaches based on conventional and empirical Bayesian methods is referred to Gould (1998).

EXAMPLE: Multicenter Depression Trial

The following data will be used throughout this section to illustrate parametric analysis methods based on fixed and random effects models. Consider a clinical trial comparing an experimental drug with a placebo in patients with major depressive disorder. The primary efficacy measure was the change from baseline to the end of the 9-week acute treatment phase in the 17-item Hamilton depression rating scale total score (HAMD17 score). Patient randomization was stratified by center.

A subset of the data collected in the depression trial is displayed below. Program 1.1 produces a summary of HAMD17 change scores and mean treatment differences observed at five centers.

Program 1.1 Depression trial data

```
data hamd17;
    input center drug $ change @@;
    datalines;
100 P 18 100 P 14 100 D 23 100 D 18 100 P 10 100 P 17 100 D 18 100 D 22
100 P 13 100 P 12 100 D 28 100 D 21 100 P 11 100 P  6 100 D 11 100 D 25
100 P  7 100 P 10 100 D 29 100 P 12 100 P 12 100 P 10 100 D 18 100 D 14
101 P 18 101 P 15 101 D 12 101 D 17 101 P 17 101 P 13 101 D 14 101 D  7
101 P 18 101 P 19 101 D 11 101 D  9 101 P 12 101 D 11 102 P 18 102 P 15
102 P 12 102 P 18 102 D 20 102 D 18 102 P 14 102 P 12 102 D 23 102 D 19
102 P 11 102 P 10 102 D 22 102 D 22 102 P 19 102 P 13 102 D 18 102 D 24
102 P 13 102 P  6 102 D 18 102 D 26 102 P 11 102 P 16 102 D 16 102 D 17
```

```
102 D  7 102 D 19 102 D 23 102 D 12 103 P 16 103 P 11 103 D 11 103 D 25
103 P  8 103 P 15 103 D 28 103 D 22 103 P 16 103 P 17 103 D 23 103 D 18
103 P 11 103 P -2 103 D 15 103 D 28 103 P 19 103 P 21 103 D 17 104 D 13
104 P 12 104 P  6 104 D 19 104 D 23 104 P 11 104 P 20 104 D 21 104 D 25
104 P  9 104 P  4 104 D 25 104 D 19
;
proc sort data=hamd17;
    by drug center;
proc means data=hamd17 noprint;
    by drug center;
    var change;
    output out=summary n=n  mean=mean std=std;
data summary;
    set summary;
    format mean std 4.1;
    label drug="Drug"
    center="Center"
    n="Number of patients"
    mean="Mean HAMD17 change"
    std="Standard deviation";
proc print data=summary noobs label;
    var drug center n mean std;
data plac(rename=(mean=mp)) drug(rename=(mean=md));
    set summary;
    if drug="D" then output drug; else output plac;
data comb;
    merge plac drug;
    by center;
    delta=md-mp;
axis1 minor=none label=(angle=90 "Treatment difference")
    order=(-8 to 12 by 4);
axis2 minor=none label=("Center") order=(100 to 104 by 1);
symbol1 value=dot color=black i=none height=10;
proc gplot data=comb;
    plot delta*center/frame haxis=axis2 vaxis=axis1 vref=0 lvref=34;
    run;
```

Output from Program 1.1

Drug	Center	Number of patients	Mean HAMD17 change	Standard deviation
D	100	11	20.6	5.6
D	101	7	11.6	3.3
D	102	16	19.0	4.7
D	103	9	20.8	5.9
D	104	7	20.7	4.2
P	100	13	11.7	3.4
P	101	7	16.0	2.7
P	102	14	13.4	3.6
P	103	10	13.2	6.6
P	104	6	10.3	5.6

Figure 1.1 The mean treatment differences in HAMD17 changes from baseline at the selected centers in the depression trial example

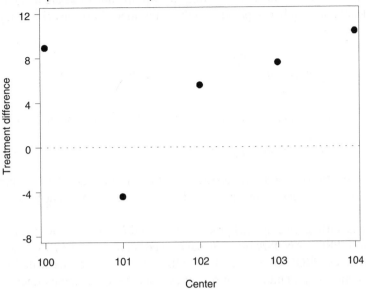

Output 1.1 lists the center-specific mean and standard deviation of the HAMD17 change scores in the two treatment groups. Further, Figure 1.1 displays the mean treatment differences observed at the five centers. Note that the mean treatment differences are fairly consistent at Centers 100, 102, 103 and 104. However, the data from Center 101 appears to be markedly different from the rest of the data.

As an aside note, it is helpful to remember that the likelihood of observing a similar treatment effect reversal by chance increases very quickly with the number of strata, and it is too early to conclude that Center 101 represents a true outlier (Senn, 1997, Chapter 14). We will discuss the problem of testing for *qualitative* treatment-by-stratum interactions in Section 1.5.

1.2.1   Fixed Effects Models

To introduce fixed effects models used in the analysis of stratified data, consider a study with a continuous endpoint comparing an experimental drug to a placebo across m strata (see Table 1.1). Suppose that the normally distributed outcome y_{ijk} observed on the kth patient in the jth stratum in the ith treatment group follows a two-way cell-means model

$$y_{ijk} = \mu_{ij} + \varepsilon_{ijk}. \tag{1.1}$$

In the depression trial example, the term y_{ijk} denotes the reduction in the HAMD17 score in individual patients and μ_{ij} represents the mean reduction in the 10 cells defined by unique combinations of the treatment and stratum levels.

Table 1.1 A two-arm clinical trial with m strata

Stratum 1				Stratum m		
Treatment	Number of patients	Mean		Treatment	Number of patients	Mean
Drug	n_{11}	μ_{11}	$\ldots$	Drug	n_{1m}	μ_{1m}
Placebo	n_{21}	μ_{21}		Placebo	n_{2m}	μ_{2m}

The cell-means model goes back to Scheffe (1959) and has been discussed in numerous publications, including Speed, Hocking and Hackney (1978) and Milliken and Johnson (1984). Let n_{1j} and n_{2j}

denote the sizes of the jth stratum in the experimental and placebo groups, respectively. Since it is uncommon to encounter empty strata in a clinical trial setting, we will assume there are no empty cells, i.e., $n_{ij} > 0$. Let n_1 and n_2 denote the number of patients in the experimental and placebo groups, and let n denote the total sample size, i.e.,

$$n_1 = \sum_{j=1}^{m} n_{1j}, \quad n_2 = \sum_{j=1}^{m} n_{2j}, \quad n = n_1 + n_2.$$

A special case of the cell-means model (1.1) is the familiar main-effects model with an interaction

$$y_{ijk} = \mu + \alpha_i + \beta_j + (\alpha\beta)_{ij} + \varepsilon_{ijk}, \tag{1.2}$$

where μ denotes the overall mean, the α parameters represent the treatment effects, the β parameters represent the stratum effects, and the $\alpha\beta$ parameters are introduced to capture treatment-by-stratum variability.

Stratified data can be analyzed using several SAS procedures, including PROC ANOVA, PROC GLM and PROC MIXED. Since PROC ANOVA supports balanced designs only, we will focus in this section on the other two procedures. PROC GLM and PROC MIXED provide the user with several analysis options for testing the most important types of hypotheses about the treatment effect in the main-effects model (1.2). This section reviews hypotheses tested by the Type I, Type II and Type III analysis methods. The Type IV analysis will not be discussed here because it is different from the Type III analysis only in the rare case of empty cells. The reader can find more information about Type IV analyses in Milliken and Johnson (1984) and Littell, Freund and Spector (1991).

Type I Analysis

The Type I analysis is commonly introduced using the so-called $R()$ notation proposed by Searle (1971, Chapter 6). Specifically, let $R(\mu)$ denote the reduction in the error sum of squares due to fitting the mean μ, i.e., fitting the reduced model

$$y_{ijk} = \mu + \varepsilon_{ijk}.$$

Similarly, $R(\mu, \alpha)$ is the reduction in the error sum of squares associated with the model with the mean μ and treatment effect α, i.e.,

$$y_{ijk} = \mu + \alpha_i + \varepsilon_{ijk}.$$

The difference $R(\mu, \alpha) - R(\mu)$, denoted by $R(\alpha|\mu)$, represents the additional reduction due to fitting the treatment effect after fitting the mean and helps assess the amount of variability explained by the treatment accounting for the mean μ. This notation is easy to extend to define other quantities such as $R(\beta|\mu, \alpha)$. It is important to note that $R(\alpha|\mu)$, $R(\beta|\mu, \alpha)$ and other similar quantities are independent of restrictions imposed on parameters when they are computed from the normal equations. Therefore, $R(\alpha|\mu)$, $R(\beta|\mu, \alpha)$ and the like are uniquely defined in any two-way classification model.

The Type I analysis is based on testing the α, β and $\alpha\beta$ factors in the main-effects model (1.2) in a sequential manner using $R(\alpha|\mu)$, $R(\beta|\mu, \alpha)$ and $R(\alpha\beta|\mu, \alpha, \beta)$, respectively. Program 1.2 computes the F statistic and associated p-value for testing the difference between the experimental drug and placebo in the depression trial example.

Program 1.2 Type I analysis of the HAMD17 changes in the depression trial example

```
proc glm data=hamd17;
    class drug center;
    model change=drug|center/ss1;
    run;
```

Output from Program 1.2

Source	DF	Type I SS	Mean Square	F Value	Pr > F
drug	1	888.0400000	888.0400000	40.07	<.0001
center	4	87.1392433	21.7848108	0.98	0.4209
drug*center	4	507.4457539	126.8614385	5.72	0.0004

Output 1.2 lists the F statistics associated with the DRUG and CENTER effects as well as their interaction (recall that drug|center is equivalent to drug center drug*center). Since the Type I analysis depends on the order of terms, it is important to make sure that the DRUG term is fitted first. The F statistic for the treatment comparison, represented by the DRUG term, is very large ($F = 40.07$), which means that administration of the experimental drug results in a significant reduction of the HAMD17 score compared to the placebo. Note that this *unadjusted analysis* ignores the effect of centers on the outcome variable.

The $R()$ notation helps clarify the structure and computational aspects of the inferences; however, as stressed by Speed and Hocking (1976), the notation may be confusing, and precise specification of the hypotheses being tested is clearly more helpful. As shown by Searle (1971, Chapter 7), the Type I F statistic for the treatment effect corresponds to the following hypothesis:

$$H_I : \quad \frac{1}{n_1} \sum_{j=1}^{m} n_{1j} \mu_{1j} = \frac{1}{n_2} \sum_{j=1}^{m} n_{2j} \mu_{2j}.$$

It is clear that the Type I hypothesis of no treatment effect depends both on the true within-stratum means and the number of patients in each stratum.

Speed and Hocking (1980) presented an interesting characterization of the Type I, II and III analyses that facilitates the interpretation of the underlying hypotheses. Speed and Hocking showed that the Type I analysis tests the simple hypothesis of no treatment effect

$$H : \quad \frac{1}{m} \sum_{j=1}^{m} \mu_{1j} = \frac{1}{m} \sum_{j=1}^{m} \mu_{2j}$$

under the condition that the β and $\alpha\beta$ factors are both equal to 0. This characterization implies that the Type I analysis ignores center effects and it is prudent to perform it when the stratum and treatment-by-stratum interaction terms are known to be negligible.

The standard ANOVA approach outlined above emphasizes hypothesis testing and it is helpful to supplement the computed p-value for the treatment comparison with an estimate of the average treatment difference and a 95% confidence interval. The estimation procedure is closely related to the Type I hypothesis of no treatment effect. Specifically, the "average treatment difference" is estimated in the Type I framework by

$$\frac{1}{n_1} \sum_{j=1}^{m} n_{1j} \bar{y}_{1j.} - \frac{1}{n_2} \sum_{j=1}^{m} n_{2j} \bar{y}_{2j..}$$

It is easy to verify from Output 1.1 and Model (1.2) that the Type I estimate of the average treatment difference in the depression trial example is equal to

$$\widehat{\delta} = \widehat{\alpha}_1 - \widehat{\alpha}_2 + \left(\frac{11}{50} - \frac{13}{50} \right) \widehat{\beta}_1 + \left(\frac{7}{50} - \frac{7}{50} \right) \widehat{\beta}_2$$

$$+ \left(\frac{16}{50} - \frac{14}{50} \right) \widehat{\beta}_3 + \left(\frac{9}{50} - \frac{10}{50} \right) \widehat{\beta}_4 + \left(\frac{7}{50} - \frac{6}{50} \right) \widehat{\beta}_5$$

$$+ \frac{11}{50}\widehat{(\alpha\beta)}_{11} + \frac{7}{50}\widehat{(\alpha\beta)}_{12} + \frac{16}{50}\widehat{(\alpha\beta)}_{13} + \frac{9}{50}\widehat{(\alpha\beta)}_{14} + \frac{7}{50}\widehat{(\alpha\beta)}_{15}$$

$$- \frac{13}{50}\widehat{(\alpha\beta)}_{21} - \frac{7}{50}\widehat{(\alpha\beta)}_{22} - \frac{14}{50}\widehat{(\alpha\beta)}_{23} - \frac{10}{50}\widehat{(\alpha\beta)}_{24} - \frac{6}{50}\widehat{(\alpha\beta)}_{25}$$

$$= \widehat{\alpha}_1 - \widehat{\alpha}_2 - 0.04\widehat{\beta}_1 + 0\widehat{\beta}_2 + 0.04\widehat{\beta}_3 - 0.02\widehat{\beta}_4 + 0.02\widehat{\beta}_5$$

$$+ 0.22\widehat{(\alpha\beta)}_{11} + 0.14\widehat{(\alpha\beta)}_{12} + 0.32\widehat{(\alpha\beta)}_{13} + 0.18\widehat{(\alpha\beta)}_{14} + 0.14\widehat{(\alpha\beta)}_{15}$$

$$- 0.26\widehat{(\alpha\beta)}_{21} - 0.14\widehat{(\alpha\beta)}_{22} - 0.28\widehat{(\alpha\beta)}_{23} - 0.2\widehat{(\alpha\beta)}_{24} - 0.12\widehat{(\alpha\beta)}_{25}.$$

To compute this estimate and its associated standard error, we can use the ESTIMATE statement in PROC GLM as shown in Program 1.3.

Program 1.3 Type I estimate of the average treatment difference in the depression trial example

```
proc glm data=hamd17;
    class drug center;
    model change=drug|center/ss1;
    estimate "Trt diff"
        drug 1 -1
        center -0.04 0 0.04 -0.02 0.02
        drug*center 0.22 0.14 0.32 0.18 0.14 -0.26 -0.14 -0.28 -0.2 -0.12;
    run;
```

Output from Program 1.3

Parameter	Estimate	Standard Error	t Value	Pr > |t|
Trt diff	5.96000000	0.94148228	6.33	<.0001

Output 1.3 displays an estimate of the average treatment difference along with its standard error, which can be used to construct a 95% confidence interval associated with the obtained estimate. The t test for the equality of the treatment difference to 0 is identical to the F test for the DRUG term in Output 1.2. One can check that the t statistic in Output 1.3 is equal to the square root of the corresponding F statistic in Output 1.2. It is also easy to verify that the average treatment difference is simply the difference between the mean changes in the HAMD17 score observed in the experimental and placebo groups without any adjustment for center effects.

Type II Analysis

In the Type II analysis, each term in the main-effects model (1.2) is adjusted for all other terms with the exception of higher-order terms that contain the term in question. Using the $R()$ notation, the significance of the α, β and $\alpha\beta$ factors is tested in the Type II framework using $R(\alpha|\mu, \beta)$, $R(\beta|\mu, \alpha)$ and $R(\alpha\beta|\mu, \alpha, \beta)$, respectively.

Program 1.4 computes the Type II F statistic to test the significance of the treatment effect on changes in the HAMD17 score.

Program 1.4 Type II analysis of the HAMD17 changes in the depression trial example

```
proc glm data=hamd17;
    class drug center;
    model change=drug|center/ss2;
    run;
```

Output from Program 1.4

Source	DF	Type II SS	Mean Square	F Value	Pr > F
drug	1	889.7756912	889.7756912	40.15	<.0001
center	4	87.1392433	21.7848108	0.98	0.4209
drug*center	4	507.4457539	126.8614385	5.72	0.0004

We see from Output 1.4 that the F statistic corresponding to the DRUG term is highly significant ($F = 40.15$), which indicates that the experimental drug significantly reduces the HAMD17 score after an adjustment for the center effect. Note that, by the definition of the Type II analysis, the presence of the interaction term in the model or the order in which the terms are included in the model do not affect the inferences with respect to the treatment effect. Thus, dropping the DRUG*CENTER term from the model generally has little impact on the F statistic for the treatment effect (to be precise, excluding the DRUG*CENTER term from the model has no effect on the numerator of the F statistic but affects its denominator due to the change in the error sum of squares).

Searle (1971, Chapter 7) demonstrated that the hypothesis of no treatment effect tested in the Type II framework has the following form:

$$H_{II}: \quad \sum_{j=1}^{m} \frac{n_{1j}n_{2j}}{n_{1j}+n_{2j}}\mu_{1j} = \sum_{j=1}^{m} \frac{n_{1j}n_{2j}}{n_{1j}+n_{2j}}\mu_{2j}.$$

Again, as in the case of Type I analyses, the Type II hypothesis of no treatment effect depends on the number of patients in each stratum. It is interesting to note that the variance of the estimated treatment difference in the jth stratum, i.e., Var $(\bar{y}_{1j.} - \bar{y}_{2j.})$, is inversely proportional to $n_{1j}n_{2j}/(n_{1j}+n_{2j})$. This means that the Type II method averages stratum-specific estimates of the treatment difference with weights proportional to the precision of the estimates.

The Type II estimate of the average treatment difference is given by

$$\left(\sum_{j=1}^{m} \frac{n_{1j}n_{2j}}{n_{1j}+n_{2j}}\right)^{-1} \sum_{j=1}^{m} \frac{n_{1j}n_{2j}}{n_{1j}+n_{2j}}(\bar{y}_{1j.} - \bar{y}_{2j.}). \tag{1.3}$$

For example, we can see from Output 1.1 and Model (1.2) that the Type II estimate of the average treatment difference in the depression trial example equals

$$\hat{\delta} = \hat{\alpha}_1 - \hat{\alpha}_2 + \left(\frac{11 \times 13}{11+13} + \frac{7 \times 7}{7+7} + \frac{16 \times 14}{16+14} + \frac{9 \times 10}{9+10} + \frac{7 \times 6}{7+6}\right)^{-1}$$

$$\times \left(\frac{11 \times 13}{11+13}\widehat{(\alpha\beta)}_{11} + \frac{7 \times 7}{7+7}\widehat{(\alpha\beta)}_{12} + \frac{16 \times 14}{16+14}\widehat{(\alpha\beta)}_{13} + \frac{9 \times 10}{9+10}\widehat{(\alpha\beta)}_{14} + \frac{7 \times 6}{7+6}\widehat{(\alpha\beta)}_{15}\right.$$

$$\left. -\frac{11 \times 13}{11+13}\widehat{(\alpha\beta)}_{21} - \frac{7 \times 7}{7+7}\widehat{(\alpha\beta)}_{22} - \frac{16 \times 14}{16+14}\widehat{(\alpha\beta)}_{23} - \frac{9 \times 10}{9+10}\widehat{(\alpha\beta)}_{24} - \frac{7 \times 6}{7+6}\widehat{(\alpha\beta)}_{25}\right)$$

$$= \hat{\alpha}_1 - \hat{\alpha}_2 + 0.23936\widehat{(\alpha\beta)}_{11} + 0.14060\widehat{(\alpha\beta)}_{12} + 0.29996\widehat{(\alpha\beta)}_{13} + 0.19029\widehat{(\alpha\beta)}_{14}$$

$$+ 0.12979\widehat{(\alpha\beta)}_{15} - 0.23936\widehat{(\alpha\beta)}_{21} - 0.14060\widehat{(\alpha\beta)}_{22} - 0.29996\widehat{(\alpha\beta)}_{23}$$

$$- 0.19029\widehat{(\alpha\beta)}_{24} - 0.12979\widehat{(\alpha\beta)}_{25}.$$

Program 1.5 computes the Type II estimate and its standard error using the ESTIMATE statement in PROC GLM.

Program 1.5 Type II estimate of the average treatment difference in the depression trial example

```
proc glm data=hamd17;
    class drug center;
    model change=drug|center/ss2;
    estimate "Trt diff"
        drug 1 -1
        drug*center 0.23936 0.14060 0.29996 0.19029 0.12979
            -0.23936 -0.14060 -0.29996 -0.19029 -0.12979;
    run;
```

Output from Program 1.5

Parameter	Estimate	Standard Error	t Value	Pr > |t|
Trt diff	5.97871695	0.94351091	6.34	<.0001

Output 1.5 shows the Type II estimate of the average treatment difference and its standard error. As in the Type I framework, the t statistic in Output 1.5 equals the square root of the corresponding F statistic in Output 1.4, which implies that the two tests are equivalent. Note also that the t statistics for the treatment comparison produced by the Type I and II analysis methods are very close in magnitude, $t = 6.33$ in Output 1.3 and $t = 6.34$ in Output 1.5. This similarity is not a coincidence and is explained by the fact that patient randomization was stratified by center in this trial. As a consequence, n_{1j} is close to n_{2j} for any $j = 1, \ldots, 5$ and thus $n_{1j}n_{2j}/(n_{1j} + n_{2j})$ is proportional to n_{1j}. The weighting schemes underlying the Type I and II tests are almost identical to each other, which causes the two methods to yield similar results. Since the Type II method becomes virtually identical to the simple Type I method when patient randomization is stratified by the covariate used in the analysis, one does not gain much from using the randomization factor as a covariate in a Type II analysis. In general, however, the standard error of the Type II estimate of the treatment difference is considerably smaller than that of the Type I estimate and therefore the Type II method has more power to detect a treatment effect compared to the Type I method.

As demonstrated by Speed and Hocking (1980), the Type II method tests the simple hypothesis

$$H: \quad \frac{1}{m}\sum_{j=1}^{m}\mu_{1j} = \frac{1}{m}\sum_{j=1}^{m}\mu_{2j}$$

when the $\alpha\beta$ factor is assumed to equal 0 (Speed and Hocking, 1980). In other words, the Type II analysis method arises naturally in trials where the treatment difference does not vary substantially from stratum to stratum.

Type III Analysis

The Type III analysis is based on a generalization of the concepts underlying the Type I and Type II analyses. Unlike these two analysis methods, the Type III methodology relies on a reparametrization of the main-effects model (1.2). The reparametrization is performed by imposing certain restrictions on the parameters in (1.2) in order to achieve a full-rank model. For example, it is common to assume that

$$\sum_{i=1}^{2}\alpha_i = 0, \quad \sum_{j=1}^{m}\beta_j = 0,$$

$$\sum_{i=1}^{2}(\alpha\beta)_{ij} = 0, \quad j = 1, \ldots, m, \quad \sum_{j=1}^{m}(\alpha\beta)_{ij} = 0, \quad i = 1, 2. \tag{1.4}$$

Once the restrictions have been imposed, one can test the α, β and $\alpha\beta$ factors using the R quantities associated with the obtained reparametrized model (these quantities are commonly denoted by R^*).

The introduced analysis method is more flexible than the Type I and II analyses and allows one to test hypotheses that cannot be tested using the original R quantities (Searle, 1976; Speed and Hocking, 1976). For example, as shown by Searle (1971, Chapter 7), $R(\alpha|\mu, \beta, \alpha\beta)$ and $R(\beta|\mu, \alpha, \alpha\beta)$ are not meaningful when computed from the main-effects model (1.2) because they are identically equal to 0. This means that the Type I/II framework precludes one from fitting an interaction term before the main effects. By contrast, $R^*(\alpha|\mu, \beta, \alpha\beta)$ and $R^*(\beta|\mu, \alpha, \alpha\beta)$ associated with the full-rank reparametrized model can assume non-zero values depending on the constraints imposed on the model parameters. Thus, each term in (1.2) can be tested in the Type III framework using an adjustment for all other terms in the model.

The Type III analysis in PROC GLM and PROC MIXED assesses the significance of the α, β and $\alpha\beta$ factors using $R^*(\alpha|\mu, \beta, \alpha\beta)$, $R^*(\beta|\mu, \alpha, \alpha\beta)$ and $R^*(\alpha\beta|\mu, \alpha, \beta)$ with the parameter restrictions given by (1.4). As an illustration, Program 1.6 tests the significance of the treatment effect on HAMD17 changes using the Type III approach.

Program 1.6 Type III analysis of the HAMD17 changes in the depression trial example

```
proc glm data=hamd17;
    class drug center;
    model change=drug|center/ss3;
    run;
```

Output from Program 1.6

Source	DF	Type III SS	Mean Square	F Value	Pr > F
drug	1	709.8195519	709.8195519	32.03	<.0001
center	4	91.4580063	22.8645016	1.03	0.3953
drug*center	4	507.4457539	126.8614385	5.72	0.0004

Output 1.6 indicates that the results of the Type III analysis are consistent with the Type I and II inferences for the treatment comparison. The treatment effect is highly significant after an adjustment for the center effect and treatment-by-center interaction ($F = 32.03$).

The advantage of making inferences from the reparametrized full-rank model is that the Type III hypothesis of no treatment effect has the following simple form (Speed, Hocking and Hackney, 1978):

$$H_{III}: \quad \frac{1}{m}\sum_{j=1}^{m}\mu_{1j} = \frac{1}{m}\sum_{j=1}^{m}\mu_{2j}.$$

The Type III hypothesis states that the simple average of the true stratum-specific HAMD17 change scores is identical in the two treatment groups. The corresponding Type III estimate of the average treatment difference is equal to

$$\frac{1}{m}\sum_{j=1}^{m}(\overline{y}_{1j.} - \overline{y}_{2j.}).$$

It is instructive to contrast this estimate with the Type I estimate of the average treatment difference. As was explained earlier, the idea behind the Type I approach is that individual observations are weighted equally. By contrast, the Type III method is based on weighting observations according to the size of each stratum. As a result, the Type III hypothesis involves a direct comparison of stratum means and is not affected by the number of patients in each individual stratum. To make an analogy, the Type I analysis corresponds to the U.S. House of Representatives, where the number of representatives from each state is a function of the state's population. The Type III analysis can be thought of as a statistical equivalent of the U.S. Senate, where each state sends along two Senators.

Since the Type III estimate of the average treatment difference in the depression trial example is given by

$$\widehat{\delta} = \widehat{\alpha}_1 - \widehat{\alpha}_2 + \frac{1}{5}\left[\widehat{(\alpha\beta)}_{11} + \widehat{(\alpha\beta)}_{12} + \widehat{(\alpha\beta)}_{13} + \widehat{(\alpha\beta)}_{14} + \widehat{(\alpha\beta)}_{15}\right.$$
$$\left. - \widehat{(\alpha\beta)}_{21} - \widehat{(\alpha\beta)}_{22} - \widehat{(\alpha\beta)}_{23} - \widehat{(\alpha\beta)}_{24} - \widehat{(\alpha\beta)}_{25}\right],$$

we can compute the estimate and its standard error using the following ESTIMATE statement in PROC GLM.

Program 1.7 Type III estimate of the average treatment difference in the depression trial example

```
proc glm data=hamd17;
    class drug center;
    model change=drug|center/ss3;
    estimate "Trt diff"
        drug 1 -1
        drug*center 0.2 0.2 0.2 0.2 0.2 -0.2 -0.2 -0.2 -0.2 -0.2;
    run;
```

Output from Program 1.7

Parameter	Estimate	Standard Error	t Value	Pr > |t|
Trt diff	5.60912865	0.99106828	5.66	<.0001

Output 1.7 lists the Type III estimate of the treatment difference and its standard error. Again, the significance of the treatment effect can be assessed using the t statistic shown in Output 1.7 since the associated test is equivalent to the F test for the DRUG term in Output 1.6.

Comparison of Type I, Type II and Type III Analyses

The three analysis methods introduced in this section produce identical results in any balanced data set. The situation, however, becomes much more complicated and confusing in an unbalanced setting and one needs to carefully examine the available options to choose the most appropriate analysis method. The following comparison of the Type I, II and III analyses in PROC GLM and PROC MIXED will help the reader make more educated choices in clinical trial applications.

Type I Analysis

The Type I analysis method averages stratum-specific treatment differences with each observation receiving the same weight, and thus the Type I approach ignores the effects of individual strata on the outcome variable. It is clear that this approach can be used only if one is not interested in adjusting for the stratum effects.

Type II Analysis

The Type II approach amounts to comparing weighted averages of within-stratum estimates among the treatment groups. The weights are inversely proportional to the variances of stratum-specific estimates of the treatment effect, which implies that the Type II analysis is based on an optimal weighting scheme when there is no treatment-by-stratum interaction. When the treatment difference does vary across strata, the Type II test statistic can be viewed as a weighted average of stratum-specific treatment differences with the weights equal to sample estimates of certain population parameters. For this reason, it is commonly accepted that the Type II method is the preferred way of analyzing continuous outcome variables adjusted for prognostic factors (Fleiss, 1986; Mehrotra, 2001).

Attempts to apply the Type II method to stratification schemes based on nonprognostic factors (e.g., centers) have created much controversy in the clinical trial literature. Advocates of the Type II approach maintain that centers play the same role as prognostic factors, and thus it is appropriate to carry out Type II tests in trials stratified by center as shown in Program 1.4 (Senn, 1998; Lin, 1999). Note that the outcome of the Type II analysis is unaffected by the significance of the interaction term. The interaction analysis is run separately as part of routine sensitivity analyses such as the assessment of treatment effects in various subsets and the identification of outliers (Kallen, 1997; Phillips et al., 2000).

Type III Analysis

The opponents of the Type II approach argue that centers are intrinsically different from prognostic factors. Since investigative sites actively recruit patients, the number of patients enrolled at any given center is a rather arbitrary figure, and inferences driven by the sizes of individual centers are generally difficult to interpret (Fleiss, 1986). As an alternative, one can follow Yates (1934) and Cochran (1954a), who proposed to perform an analysis based on a simple average of center-specific estimates in the presence of a pronounced interaction. This unweighted analysis is equivalent to the Type III analysis of the model with an interaction term (see Program 1.6).

It is worth drawing the reader's attention to the fact that the described alternative approach based on the Type III analysis has a number of limitations:

- The Type II F statistic is generally larger than the Type III F statistic (compare Output 1.4 and Output 1.6) and thus the Type III analysis is less powerful than the Type II analysis when the treatment difference does not vary much from center to center.

- The Type III method violates the marginality principle formulated by Nelder (1977). The principle states that meaningful inferences in a two-way classification setting are to be based on the main effects α and β adjusted for each other and on their interaction adjusted for the main effects. When one fits an interaction term before the main effects (as in the Type III analysis), the resulting test statistics depend on a totally arbitrary choice of parameter constraints. The marginality principle implies that the Type III inferences yield uninterpretable results in unbalanced cases. See Nelder (1994) and Rodriguez, Tobias and Wolfinger (1995) for a further discussion of pros and cons of this argument.

- Weighting small and large strata equally is completely different from how one would normally perform a meta-analysis of the results observed in the strata (Senn, 2000).

- Lastly, as pointed out in several publications, sample size calculations are almost always done within the Type II framework; i.e., patients rather than centers are assumed equally weighted. As a consequence, the use of the Type III analysis invalidates the sample size calculation method. For a detailed power comparison of the weighted and unweighted approaches, see Jones et al. (1998) and Gallo (2000).

Type III Analysis with Pretesting

The described weighted and unweighted analysis methods are often combined to increase the power of the treatment comparison. As proposed by Fleiss (1986), the significance of the interaction term is assessed first and the Type III analysis with an interaction is performed if the preliminary test has yielded a significant outcome. Otherwise, the interaction term is removed from the model and thus the treatment effect is analyzed using the Type II approach. The sequential testing procedure recognizes the power advantage of the weighted analysis when the treatment-by-center interaction appears to be negligible.

Most commonly, the treatment-by-center variation is evaluated using an F test based on the interaction mean square; see the F test for the DRUG*CENTER term in Output 1.6. This test is typically carried out at the 0.1 significance level (Fleiss, 1986). Several alternative approaches have been suggested in the literature. Bancroft (1968) proposed to test the interaction term at the 0.25 level before including it in the model. Chinchilli and Bortey (1991) described a test for consistency of treatment differences across strata based on the noncentrality parameter of an *F* distribution. Ciminera et al. (1993) stressed that tests based on the interaction mean square are aimed at detecting *quantitative interactions* that may be caused by a variety of factors such as measurement scale artifacts. To alleviate the problems associated with the traditional pretesting approach, Ciminera et al. outlined an alternative method that relies on *qualitative interactions*; see Section 1.5 for more details.

When applying the pretesting strategy, one needs to be aware of the fact that pretesting leads to more frequent false-positive outcomes, which may become an issue in pivotal clinical trials. To stress this point, Jones et al. (1998) compared the described pretesting approach with the controversial practice of pretesting the significance of the carryover effect in crossover trials, a practice that is known to inflate the false-positive rate.

1.2.2   Random Effects Models

A popular alternative to the fixed effects modeling approach described in Section 1.2.1 is to explicitly incorporate random variation among strata in the analysis. Even though most of the discussion on center effects in the ICH guidance document "Statistical principles for clinical trials" (ICH E9) treats center as a fixed effect, the guidance also encourages trialists to explore the heterogeneity of the treatment effect across centers using mixed models. The latter can be accomplished by employing models with random stratum and treatment-by-stratum interaction terms. While one can argue that the selection of centers is not necessarily a random process, treating centers as a random effect could at times help statisticians better account for between-center variability.

Random effects modeling is based on the following mixed model for the continuous outcome y_{ijk} observed on the kth patient in the jth stratum in the ith treatment group:

$$y_{ijk} = \mu + \alpha_i + b_j + g_{ij} + \varepsilon_{ijk}, \tag{1.5}$$

where μ denotes the overall mean, α_i is the fixed effect of the ith treatment, b_j and g_{ij} denote the random stratum and treatment-by-stratum interaction effects, and ε_{ijk} is a residual term. The random and residual terms are assumed to be normally distributed and independent of each other. We can see from Model (1.5) that, unlike fixed effects models, random effects models account for the variability across strata in judging the significance of the treatment effect.

Applications of mixed effects models to stratified analyses in a clinical trial context were described by several authors, including Fleiss (1986), Senn (1998) and Gallo (2000). Chakravorti and Grizzle (1975) provided a theoretical foundation for random effects modeling in stratified trials based on the familiar randomized block design framework and the work of Hartley and Rao (1967). For a detailed overview of issues related to the analysis of mixed effects models, see Searle (1992, Chapter 3). Littell et al. (1996, Chapter 2) demonstrated how to use PROC MIXED in order to fit random effects models in multicenter trials.

Program 1.8 fits a random effects model to the HAMD17 data set using PROC MIXED and computes an estimate of the average treatment difference. The DDFM=SATTERTH option in Program 1.8 requests that the degrees of freedom for the *F* test be computed using the Satterthwaite formula. The Satterthwaite method provides a more accurate approximation to the distribution of the *F* statistic in random effects models than the standard ANOVA method (it is achieved by increasing the number of degrees of freedom for the *F* statistic).

Program 1.8 Analysis of the HAMD17 changes in the depression trial example using a random effects model

```
proc mixed data=hamd17;
    class drug center;
    model change=drug/ddfm=satterth;
    random center drug*center;
    estimate "Trt eff" drug 1 -1;
    run;
```

Output from Program 1.8

```
          Type 3 Tests of Fixed Effects

               Num     Den
Effect          DF      DF     F Value    Pr > F

drug             1     6.77       9.30     0.0194


                      Estimates

                      Standard
Label        Estimate    Error      DF    t Value    Pr > |t|

Trt eff        5.7072    1.8718    6.77       3.05      0.0194
```

Output 1.8 displays the F statistic ($F = 9.30$) and p-value ($p = 0.0194$) associated with the DRUG term in the random effects model as well as an estimate of the average treatment difference. The estimated treatment difference equals 5.7072 and is close to the estimates computed from fixed effects models. The standard error of the estimate (1.8718) is substantially greater than the standard error of the estimates obtained in fixed effects models (see Output 1.6). This is a penalty one has to pay for treating the stratum and interaction effects as random, and it reflects lack of homogeneity across the five strata in the depression data. Note, for example, that dropping Center 101 creates more homogeneous strata and, as a consequence, reduces the standard error to 1.0442. Similarly, removing the DRUG*CENTER term from the RANDOM statement leads to a more precise estimate of the treatment effect with the standard error of 1.0280.

In general, as shown by Senn (2000), fitting main effects as random leads to lower standard errors; however, assuming a random interaction term increases the standard error of the estimated treatment difference. Due to the lower precision of treatment effect estimates, analysis of stratified data based on models with random stratum and treatment-by-stratum effects has lower power compared to a fixed effects analysis (Gould, 1998; Jones et al., 1998).

1.2.3 Nonparametric Tests

This section briefly describes a nonparametric test for stratified continuous data proposed by van Elteren (1960). To introduce the van Elteren test, consider a clinical trial with a continuous endpoint measured in m strata. Let w_j denote the Wilcoxon rank-sum statistic for testing the null hypothesis of no treatment effect in the jth stratum (Hollander and Wolfe, 1999, Chapter 4). Van Elteren (1960) proposed to combine stratum-specific Wilcoxon rank-sum statistics with weights inversely proportional to stratum sizes. The van Elteren statistic is given by

$$u = \sum_{j=1}^{m} \frac{w_j}{n_{1j} + n_{2j} + 1},$$

where $n_{1j} + n_{2j}$ is the total number of patients in the jth stratum. To justify this weighting scheme, van Elteren demonstrated that the resulting test has asymptotically the maximum power against a broad range of alternative hypotheses. Van Elteren also studied the asymptotic properties of the testing procedure and showed that, under the null hypothesis of no treatment effect in the m strata, the test statistic is asymptotically normal.

As shown by Koch et al. (1982, Section 2.3), the van Elteren test is a member of a general family of Mantel-Haenszel mean score tests. This family also includes the Cochran-Mantel-Haenszel test for categorical outcomes discussed later in Section 1.3.1. Like other testing procedures in this family, the van Elteren test possesses an interesting and useful property that its asymptotic distribution is not directly affected by the size of individual strata. As a consequence, one can rely on asymptotic p-values even in sparse stratifications as long as the total sample size is large enough. For more information about the van Elteren test and related testing procedures, see Lehmann (1975), Koch et al. (1990) and Hosmane, Shu and Morris (1994).

EXAMPLE: Urinary Incontinence Trial

The van Elteren test is an alternative method of analyzing stratified continuous data when one cannot rely on standard ANOVA techniques because the underlying normality assumption is not met. As an illustration, consider a subset of the data collected in a urinary incontinence trial comparing an experimental drug to a placebo over an 8-week period. The primary endpoint in the trial was a percent change from baseline to the end of the study in the number of incontinence episodes per week. Patients were allocated to three strata according to the baseline frequency of incontinence episodes.[2]

Program 1.9 displays a subset of the data collected in the urinary incontinence trial and plots the probability distribution of the primary endpoint in the three strata.

Program 1.9 Distribution of percent changes in the frequency of incontinence episodes in the urinary incontinence trial example

```
data urininc;
    input therapy $ stratum @@;
    do i=1 to 10;
        input change @@;
        if (change^=.) then output;
    end;
    drop i;
    datalines;
Placebo  1   -86  -38   43 -100  289    0  -78   38  -80  -25
Placebo  1 -100 -100  -50   25 -100 -100  -67    0  400 -100
Placebo  1  -63  -70  -83  -67  -33    0  -13 -100    0   -3
Placebo  1  -62  -29  -50 -100    0 -100  -60  -40  -44  -14
Placebo  2  -36  -77   -6  -85   29  -17  -53   18  -62  -93
Placebo  2   64  -29  100   31   -6 -100  -30   11  -52  -55
Placebo  2 -100  -82  -85  -36  -75   -8  -75  -42  122  -30
Placebo  2   22  -82    .    .    .    .    .    .    .    .
Placebo  3   12  -68 -100   95  -43  -17  -87  -66   -8   64
Placebo  3   61  -41  -73  -42  -32   12  -69   81    0   87
Drug     1   50 -100  -80  -57  -44  340 -100 -100  -25  -74
Drug     1    0   43 -100 -100 -100 -100  -63 -100 -100 -100
Drug     1 -100 -100    0 -100  -50    0    0  -83  369  -50
Drug     1  -33  -50  -33  -67   25  390  -50    0 -100    .
Drug     2  -93  -55  -73  -25   31    8  -92  -91  -89  -67
Drug     2  -25  -61  -47  -75  -94 -100  -69  -92 -100  -35
Drug     2 -100  -82  -31  -29 -100  -14  -55   31  -40 -100
Drug     2  -82  131  -60    .    .    .    .    .    .    .
Drug     3  -17  -13  -55  -85  -68  -87  -42   36  -44  -98
Drug     3  -75  -35    7  -57  -92  -78  -69  -21  -14    .
;
```

---

[2]This clinical trial example will be used here to illustrate a method for the analysis of non-normally distributed endpoints in the presence of a categorical stratification variable. One can think of other ways of analyzing the urinary incontinence data that may be more appropriate in this setting. For example, one can consider redefining the primary outcome variable since a variable based on percent change from baseline makes an inefficient use of data. Further, categorizing continuous data leads to loss of power and thus the analysis described above will be inferior to an analysis which uses the baseline frequency of incontinence episodes as a continuous covariate. Yet another sensible approach is based on fitting a model that accounts for the discrete nature of incontinence episodes, e.g., a Poisson regression model for counts.

```
proc sort data=urininc;
    by stratum therapy;
proc kde data=urininc out=density;
    by stratum therapy;
    var change;
proc sort data=density;
    by stratum;
* Plot the distribution of the primary endpoint in each stratum;
%macro PlotDist(stratum,label);
axis1 minor=none major=none value=none label=(angle=90 "Density")
    order=(0 to 0.012 by 0.002);
axis2 minor=none order=(-100 to 150 by 50)
    label=("&label");
symbol1 value=none color=black i=join line=34;
symbol2 value=none color=black i=join line=1;
data annotate;
    xsys="1"; ysys="1"; hsys="4"; x=50; y=90; position="5";
    size=1; text="Stratum &stratum"; function="label";
proc gplot data=density anno=annotate;
    where stratum=&stratum;
    plot density*change=therapy/frame haxis=axis2 vaxis=axis1 nolegend;
    run;
    quit;
%mend PlotDist;
%PlotDist(1,);
%PlotDist(2,);
%PlotDist(3,Percent change in the frequency of incontinence episodes);
```

The output of Program 1.9 is shown in Figure 1.2. We can see from Figure 1.2 that the distribution of the primary outcome variable is consistently skewed to the right across the three strata. Since the normality assumption is clearly violated in this data set, the analysis methods described earlier in this section may perform poorly. The magnitude of treatment effect on the frequency of incontinence episodes can be assessed more reliably using a nonparametric procedure. Program 1.10 computes the van Elteren statistic to test the null hypothesis of no treatment effect in the urinary incontinence trial using PROC FREQ. The statistic is requested by including the CMH2 and SCORES=MODRIDIT options in the TABLE statement.

Program 1.10 Analysis of percent changes in the frequency of incontinence episodes using the van Elteren test

```
proc freq data=urininc;
    ods select cmh;
    table stratum*therapy*change/cmh2 scores=modridit;
    run;
```

Output from Program 1.10

```
Summary Statistics for therapy by change
Controlling for stratum
  Cochran-Mantel-Haenszel Statistics (Modified Ridit Scores)

Statistic    Alternative Hypothesis    DF      Value     Prob
---------------------------------------------------------------
    1        Nonzero Correlation        1      6.2505    0.0124
    2        Row Mean Scores Differ     1      6.2766    0.0122
```

Figure 1.2 The distribution of percent changes in the frequency of incontinence episodes in the experimental ($\cdots$) and placebo (—) groups by stratum in the urinary incontinence trial

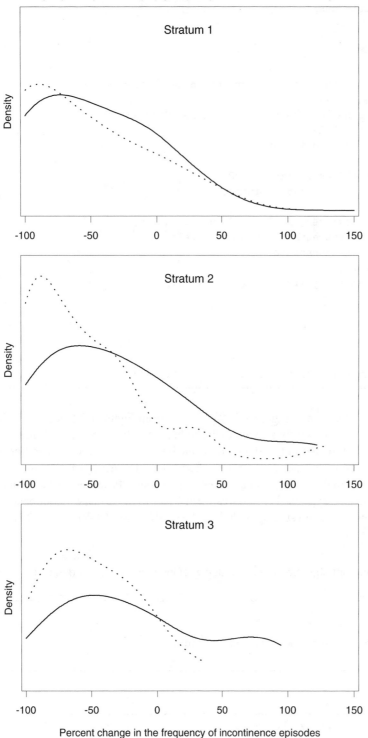

Percent change in the frequency of incontinence episodes

Output 1.10 lists two statistics produced by PROC FREQ (note that extraneous information has been deleted from the output using the ODS statement). The van Elteren statistic corresponds to the row mean scores statistic labeled "Row Mean Scores Differ" and is equal to 6.2766. Since the asymptotic p-value is small ($p = 0.0122$), we conclude that administration of the experimental drug resulted in a significant reduction in the frequency of incontinence episodes. To compare the van Elteren test with the Type II and III analyses in the parametric ANOVA framework, Programs 1.4 and 1.6 were rerun to test the significance of the treatment effect in the urinary incontinence trial. The Type II and III F statistics were equal to 1.4 ($p = 0.2384$) and 2.15 ($p = 0.1446$), respectively. The parametric methods were unable to detect the treatment effect in this data set due to the highly skewed distribution of the primary endpoint.

1.2.4 Summary

This section discussed parametric and nonparametric methods for performing stratified analyses in clinical trials with a continuous endpoint. Parametric analysis methods based on fixed and random effects models are easy to implement using PROC GLM (fixed effects only) or PROC MIXED (both fixed and random effects).

PROC GLM and PROC MIXED support three popular methods of fitting fixed effects models to stratified data. These analysis methods, known as Type I, II and III analyses, are conceptually similar to each other in the sense that they are all based on averaging stratum-specific estimates of the treatment effect. The following is a quick summary of the Type I, II and III methods:

- Each observation receives the same weight when a Type I average of stratum-specific treatment differences is computed. Therefore, the Type I approach ignores the effects of individual strata on the outcome variable.

- The Type II approach is based on a comparison of weighted averages of stratum-specific estimates of the treatment effect, with the weights being inversely proportional to the variances of these estimates. The Type II weighting scheme is optimal when there is no treatment-by-stratum interaction and can also be used when treatment differences vary across strata. It is generally agreed that the Type II method is the preferred way of analyzing continuous outcome variables adjusted for prognostic factors.

- The Type III analysis method relies on a direct comparison of stratum means, which implies that individual observations are weighted according to the size of each stratum. This analysis is typically performed in the presence of a significant treatment-by-stratum interaction. It is important to remember that Type II tests are known to have more power than Type III tests when the treatment difference does not vary much from stratum to stratum.

The information about treatment differences across strata can also be combined using random effects models in which stratum and treatment-by-stratum interaction terms are treated as random variables. Random effects inferences for stratified data can be implemented using PROC MIXED. The advantage of random effects modeling is that it helps the statistician better account for between-stratum variability. However, random effects inferences are generally less powerful than inferences based on fixed effects models. This is one of the reasons why stratified analyses based on random effects models are rarely performed in a clinical trial setting.

A stratified version of the nonparametric Wilcoxon rank-sum test, known as the van Elteren test, can be used to perform inferences in a non-normal setting. It has been shown that the asymptotic distribution of the van Elteren test statistic is not directly affected by the size of individual strata and therefore this testing procedure performs well in the analysis of a large number of small strata.

1.3 Categorical Endpoints

This section covers analysis of stratified categorical data in clinical trials. It discusses both asymptotic and exact approaches, including

- randomization-based Cochran-Mantel-Haenszel approach
- minimum variance methods
- model-based inferences.

Although the examples in this section deal with the case of binary outcomes, the described analysis methods can be easily extended to a more general case of multinomial variables. SAS procedures used below automatically invoke general categorical tests when the analysis variable assumes more than two values.

Also, the section reviews methods that treat stratification factors as fixed variables. It does not cover stratified analyses based on random effects models for categorical data because they are fairly uncommon in clinical applications. For a review of tests for stratified categorical data arising within a random effects modeling framework, see Lachin (2000, Section 4.10) and Agresti and Hartzel (2000).

Measures of Association

There are three common measures of association used with categorical data: risk difference, relative risk and odds ratio. To introduce these measures, consider a clinical trial designed to compare the effects of an experimental drug and a placebo on the incidence of a binary event such as improvement or survival in m strata (see Table 1.2). Let n_{1j1} and n_{2j1} denote the numbers of jth stratum patients in the experimental and placebo groups, respectively, who experienced an event of interest. Similarly, n_{1j2} and n_{2j2} denote the numbers of jth stratum patients in the experimental and placebo groups, respectively, who did not experience an event of interest.

Table 1.2 A two-arm clinical trial with m strata

| Stratum 1 | | | | | Stratum m | | | |
Treatment	Event	No event	Total		Treatment	Event	No event	Total
Drug	n_{111}	n_{112}	n_{11+}		Drug	n_{1m1}	n_{1m2}	n_{1m+}
Placebo	n_{211}	n_{212}	n_{21+}		Placebo	n_{2m1}	n_{2m2}	n_{2m+}
Total	n_{+11}	n_{+12}	n_1		Total	n_{+m1}	n_{+m2}	n_m

The risk difference, relative risk and odds ratio of observing the binary event of interest are defined as follows:

- **Risk difference.** The true event rate in jth stratum is denoted by π_{1j} in the experimental group and π_{2j} in the placebo group and thus the risk difference equals $d_i = \pi_{1j} - \pi_{2j}$. The true event rates are estimated by sample proportions $p_{1j} = n_{1j1}/n_{1j+}$ and $p_{2j} = n_{2j1}/n_{2j+}$, and the risk difference is estimated by $\widehat{d}_j = p_{1j} - p_{2j}$.

- **Relative risk.** The relative risk of observing the event in the experimental group compared to the placebo group is equal to $r_j = \pi_{1j}/\pi_{2j}$ in the jth stratum. This relative risk is estimated by $\widehat{r}_j = p_{1j}/p_{2j}$ (assuming that $p_{2j} > 0$).

- **Odds ratio.** The odds of observing the event of interest in the jth stratum is $\pi_{1j}/(1 - \pi_{1j})$ in the experimental group and $\pi_{2j}/(1 - \pi_{2j})$ in the placebo group. The corresponding odds ratio in the jth stratum equals

$$o_j = \frac{\pi_{1j}}{1 - \pi_{1j}} \bigg/ \frac{\pi_{2j}}{1 - \pi_{2j}}$$

and is estimated by

$$\widehat{o}_j = \frac{p_{1j}}{1 - p_{1j}} \bigg/ \frac{p_{2j}}{1 - p_{2j}}.$$

We assume here that $p_{1j} < 1$ and $p_{2j} > 0$.

Since the results and their interpretation may be affected by the measure of association used in the analysis, it is important to clearly specify whether the inferences are based on risk differences, relative risks or odds ratios.

EXAMPLE: Severe Sepsis Trial

Statistical methods for the analysis of stratified clinical trials with a binary endpoint will be illustrated using the following data. A placebo-controlled clinical trial was conducted on 1690 patients to examine the effect of an experimental drug on 28-day all-cause mortality in patients with severe sepsis. Patients were assigned to one of four strata at randomization, depending on the predicted risk of mortality computed from the APACHE II score (Knaus et al., 1985). The APACHE II score ranges from 0 to 71 and an increased score is correlated with a higher risk of death. The results observed in each of the four strata are summarized in Table 1.3.[3]

Table 1.3 28-day mortality data from a 1690-patient trial in patients with severe sepsis

Stratum	Experimental drug			Placebo		
	Dead	Alive	Total	Dead	Alive	Total
1	33	185	218	26	189	215
2	49	169	218	57	165	222
3	48	156	204	58	104	162
4	80	130	210	118	123	241

Programs 1.11 and 1.12 below summarize the survival and mortality data collected in the sepsis trial. Program 1.11 uses PROC FREQ to compute the risk difference, relative risk and odds ratio of mortality in patients at a high risk of death (Stratum 4).

Program 1.11 Summary of survival and mortality data in the severe sepsis trial example (Stratum 4)

```
data sepsis;
    input stratum therapy $ outcome $ count @@;
    if outcome="Dead" then survival=0; else survival=1;
    datalines;
    1 Placebo Alive 189 1 Placebo Dead 26
    1 Drug    Alive 185 1 Drug    Dead 33
    2 Placebo Alive 165 2 Placebo Dead 57
    2 Drug    Alive 169 2 Drug    Dead 49
    3 Placebo Alive 104 3 Placebo Dead 58
    3 Drug    Alive 156 3 Drug    Dead 48
    4 Placebo Alive 123 4 Placebo Dead 118
    4 Drug    Alive 130 4 Drug    Dead 80
    ;
proc freq data=sepsis;
    where stratum=4;
    table therapy*survival/riskdiff relrisk;
    weight count;
    run;
```

[3]The goal of this example is to introduce statistical tests for binary outcomes stratified by a categorical variable. In general, an analysis of this type does not make the most efficient use of the data and one needs to consider alternative approaches that involve modeling the predicted risk of mortality as a continuous variable.

Output from Program 1.11

```
                      Column 1 Risk Estimates


                                       (Asymptotic) 95%
                    Risk        ASE    Confidence Limits
-----------------------------------------------------------
Row 1              0.3810     0.0335    0.3153      0.4466
Row 2              0.4896     0.0322    0.4265      0.5527
Total              0.4390     0.0234    0.3932      0.4848

Difference        -0.1087     0.0465   -0.1998     -0.0176

                 Difference is (Row 1 - Row 2)


                      (Exact) 95%
                   Confidence Limits
-------------------------------------
Row 1              0.3150     0.4503
Row 2              0.4249     0.5546
Total              0.3926     0.4862

  Difference is (Row 1 - Row 2)

                  Column 2 Risk Estimates


                                       (Asymptotic) 95%
                    Risk        ASE    Confidence Limits
-----------------------------------------------------------
Row 1              0.6190     0.0335    0.5534      0.6847
Row 2              0.5104     0.0322    0.4473      0.5735
Total              0.5610     0.0234    0.5152      0.6068

Difference         0.1087     0.0465    0.0176      0.1998

                 Difference is (Row 1 - Row 2)


                      (Exact) 95%
                   Confidence Limits
-------------------------------------
Row 1              0.5497     0.6850
Row 2              0.4454     0.5751
Total              0.5138     0.6074

  Difference is (Row 1 - Row 2)

          Estimates of the Relative Risk (Row1/Row2)

Type of Study                   Value      95% Confidence Limits
----------------------------------------------------------------
Case-Control (Odds Ratio)       0.6415     0.4404      0.9342
Cohort (Col1 Risk)              0.7780     0.6274      0.9649
Cohort (Col2 Risk)              1.2129     1.0306      1.4276
```

Risk statistics shown under "Column 1 Risk Estimates" in Output 1.11 represent estimated 28-day mortality rates in the experimental (Row 1) and placebo (Row 2) groups. Similarly, risk statistics under "Column 2 Risk Estimates" refer to survival rates in the two treatment groups. PROC FREQ computes both asymptotic and exact confidence intervals for the estimated rates. The estimated risk difference is -0.1087 and thus, among patients with a poor prognosis, patients treated with the experimental drug are 11% more likely to survive (in absolute terms) than those who received the placebo. Note that exact confidence intervals for risk differences are quite difficult to construct (see Coe and Tamhane (1993) for more details) and there is no exact confidence interval associated with the computed risk difference in survival or mortality rates.

Estimates of the ratio of the odds of mortality and relative risks of survival and mortality are given under "Estimates of the Relative Risk (Row1/Row2)." The odds ratio equals 0.6415, which indicates that the odds of mortality are 36% lower in the experimental group compared to the placebo group in the chosen subpopulation of patients. The corresponding relative risks of survival and mortality are 1.2129 and 0.7780, respectively. The displayed 95% confidence limits are based on a normal approximation. An exact confidence interval for the odds ratio can be requested using the EXACT statement with the OR option. PROC FREQ does not currently compute exact confidence limits for relative risks.

Program 1.12 demonstrates how to use the Output Delivery System (ODS) with PROC FREQ to compute risk differences, relative risks and odds ratios of mortality in all four strata.

Program 1.12 Summary of mortality data in the severe sepsis trial example (all strata)

```
proc freq data=sepsis noprint;
    by stratum;
    table therapy*survival/riskdiff relrisk;
    ods output riskdiffcol1=riskdiff relativerisks=relrisk;
    weight count;
* Plot of mortality rates;
data mortrate;
    set riskdiff;
    format risk 3.1;
    if row="Row 1" then therapy="D";
    if row="Row 2" then therapy="P";
    if therapy="" then delete;
axis1 minor=none label=(angle=90 "Mortality rate") order=(0 to 0.6 by 0.2);
axis2 label=none;
pattern1 value=empty color=black;
pattern2 value=r1 color=black;
proc gchart data=mortrate;
    vbar therapy/frame raxis=axis1 maxis=axis2 gaxis=axis2
        sumvar=risk subgroup=therapy group=stratum nolegend;
    run;
* Plot of risk differences;
data mortdiff;
    set riskdiff;
    format risk 4.1;
    if row="Difference";
axis1 minor=none label=(angle=90 "Risk difference")
    order=(-0.2 to 0.1 by 0.1);
axis2 label=("Stratum");
pattern1 value=empty color=black;
proc gchart data=mortdiff;
    vbar stratum/frame raxis=axis1 maxis=axis2 sumvar=risk
    midpoints=1 2 3 4;
    run;
```

```
* Plot of relative risks;
data riskratio;
    set relrisk;
    format value 3.1;
    if studytype="Cohort (Col1 Risk)";
axis1 minor=none label=(angle=90 "Relative risk")
    order=(0.5 to 1.3 by 0.1);
axis2 label=("Stratum");
pattern1 value=empty color=black;
proc gchart data=riskratio;
    vbar stratum/frame raxis=axis1 maxis=axis2 sumvar=value
    midpoints=1 2 3 4;
    run;
* Plot of odds ratios;
data oddsratio;
    set relrisk;
    format value 3.1;
    if studytype="Case-Control (Odds Ratio)";
axis1 label=(angle=90 "Odds ratio") order=(0.4 to 1.4 by 0.2);
axis2 label=("Stratum");
pattern1 value=empty color=black;
proc gchart data=oddsratio;
    vbar stratum/frame raxis=axis1 maxis=axis2 sumvar=value
    midpoints=1 2 3 4;
    run;
```

The output of Program 1.12 is displayed in Figure 1.3. Figure 1.3 shows that there was significant variability among the four strata in terms of 28-day mortality rates. The absolute reduction in mortality in the experimental group compared to the placebo group varied from -3.04% in Stratum 1 to 12.27% in Stratum 3. The treatment effect was most pronounced in patients with a poor prognosis at study entry (i.e., patients in Strata 3 and 4).

1.3.1 Asymptotic Randomization-Based Tests

Fleiss (1981, Chapter 10) described a general method for performing stratified analyses that goes back to Cochran (1954a) and applied it to the case of binary outcomes. Let a_j denote the estimate of a certain measure of association between the treatment and binary outcome in the jth stratum, and let s_j^2 be the sample variance of this estimate. Assume that the measure of association is chosen in such a way that it equals 0 when the treatment difference is 0. Also, w_j will denote the reciprocal of the sample variance, i.e., $w_j = 1/s_j^2$. The total chi-square statistic

$$\chi_T^2 = \sum_{j=1}^{m} w_j a_j^2$$

can be partitioned into a chi-square statistic χ_H^2 for testing the degree of homogeneity among the strata and a chi-square statistic χ_A^2 for testing the significance of overall association across the strata given by

$$\chi_H^2 = \sum_{j=1}^{m} w_j (a_j - \widehat{a})^2, \tag{1.6}$$

$$\chi_A^2 = \left(\sum_{j=1}^{m} w_j \right)^{-1} \left(\sum_{j=1}^{m} w_j a_j \right)^2, \tag{1.7}$$

Figure 1.3 A summary of mortality data in the severe sepsis trial example accompanied by three measures of treatment effect (D = Drug, P = Placebo)

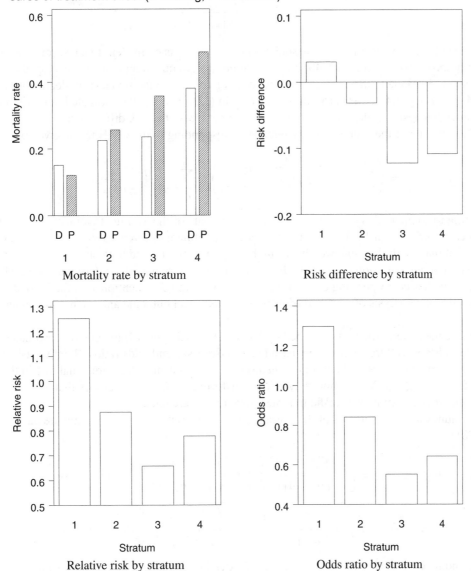

where

$$\widehat{a} = \left(\sum_{j=1}^{m} w_j \right)^{-1} \sum_{j=1}^{m} w_j a_j \tag{1.8}$$

is the associated minimum variance estimate of the degree of association averaged across the m strata. Under the null hypothesis of homogeneous association, χ_H^2 asymptotically follows a chi-square distribution with $m - 1$ degrees of freedom. Similarly, under the null hypothesis that the average association between the treatment and binary outcome is zero, χ_A^2 is asymptotically distributed as chi-square with 1 degree of freedom.

The described method for testing hypotheses of homogeneity and association in a stratified setting can be used to construct a large number of useful tests. For example, if a_j is equal to a standardized treatment difference in the jth stratum,

$$a_j = \frac{\widehat{d}_j}{\overline{p}_j(1 - \overline{p}_j)}, hboxwhere \overline{p}_j = n_{+j1}/n_j \text{ and } \widehat{d}_j = p_{1j} - p_{2j}, \tag{1.9}$$

then

$$w_j = \overline{p}_j(1 - \overline{p}_j)\frac{n_{1j+}n_{2j+}}{n_{1j+} + n_{2j+}}.$$

The associated chi-square test of overall association based on χ_A^2 is equivalent to a test for stratified binary data proposed by Cochran (1954b) and is asymptotically equivalent to a test developed by Mantel and Haenszel (1959). Due to their similarity, it is common to refer to the two tests collectively as the Cochran-Mantel-Haenszel (CMH) procedure. Since a_j in (1.9) involves the estimated risk difference $\widehat{d}_j$, the CMH procedure tests the degree of association with respect to the risk differences $d_1, \ldots, d_m$ in the m strata. The estimate of the average risk difference corresponding to the CMH test is given by

$$\widehat{d} = \left(\sum_{j=1}^{m} \overline{p}_j(1 - \overline{p}_j)\frac{n_{1j+}n_{2j+}}{n_{1j+} + n_{2j+}}\right)^{-1} \sum_{j=1}^{m} \frac{n_{1j+}n_{2j+}}{n_{1j+} + n_{2j+}}\widehat{d}_j. \tag{1.10}$$

It is interesting to compare this estimate to the Type II estimate of the average treatment effect in the continuous case (see Section 1.2.1). The stratum-specific treatment differences $\widehat{d}_1, \ldots, \widehat{d}_m$, are averaged in the CMH estimate with the same weights as in the Type II estimate and thus one can think of the CMH procedure as an extension of the Type II testing method to trials with a binary outcome. Although unweighted estimates corresponding to the Type III method have been mentioned in the literature, they are rarely used in the analysis of stratified trials with a categorical outcome and are not implemented in SAS.

One can use the general method described by Fleiss (1981, Chapter 10) to construct estimates and associated tests for overall treatment effect based on relative risks and odds ratios. Relative risks and odds ratios need to be transformed before the method is applied because they are equal to 1 in the absence of treatment effect. Most commonly, a log transformation is used to ensure that $a_j = 0$, $j = 1, \ldots, m$, when the stratum-specific treatment differences are equal to 0.

The minimum variance estimates of the average log relative risk and log odds ratio are based on the formula (1.8) with

$$a_j = \log\widehat{r}_j, \quad w_j = \left[\left(\frac{1}{n_{1j1}} - \frac{1}{n_{1j+}}\right) + \left(\frac{1}{n_{2j1}} - \frac{1}{n_{2j+}}\right)\right]^{-1} \text{(log relative risk)}, \tag{1.11}$$

$$a_j = \log\widehat{o}_j, \quad w_j = \left(\frac{1}{n_{1j1}} + \frac{1}{n_{1j2}} + \frac{1}{n_{2j1}} + \frac{1}{n_{2j2}}\right)^{-1} \text{(log odds ratio)}. \tag{1.12}$$

The corresponding estimates of the average relative risk and odds ratio, are computed using exponentiation. Adopting the PROC FREQ terminology, we will refer to these estimates as *logit-adjusted* estimates and denote them by $\widehat{r}_L$ and $\widehat{o}_L$.

It is instructive to compare the logit-adjusted estimates $\widehat{r}_L$ and $\widehat{o}_L$ with estimates of the average relative risk and odds ratio proposed by Mantel and Haenszel (1959). The Mantel-Haenszel estimates, denoted by $\widehat{r}_{MH}$ and $\widehat{o}_{MH}$, can also be expressed as weighted averages of stratum-specific relative risks and odds ratios:

$$\widehat{r}_{MH} = \left(\sum_{j=1}^{m} w_j\right)^{-1} \sum_{j=1}^{m} w_j\widehat{r}_j, \text{ where } w_j = \frac{n_{2j1}n_{1j+}}{n_j},$$

$$\widehat{o}_{MH} = \left(\sum_{j=1}^{m} w_j\right)^{-1} \sum_{j=1}^{m} w_j\widehat{o}_j, \text{ where } w_j = \frac{n_{2j1}n_{1j2}}{n_j}.$$

Note that weights in $\widehat{r}_{MH}$ and $\widehat{o}_{MH}$ are not inversely proportional to sample variances of the stratum-specific estimates and thus $\widehat{r}_{MH}$ and $\widehat{o}_{MH}$ do not represent minimum variance estimates. Despite this property, the Mantel-Haenszel estimates are generally comparable to the logit-adjusted estimates $\widehat{r}_L$ and $\widehat{o}_L$ in terms of precision. Also, as shown by Breslow (1981), $\widehat{r}_{MH}$ and $\widehat{o}_{MH}$ are attractive in applications because their mean square error is always less than that of the logit-adjusted estimates $\widehat{r}_L$ and $\widehat{o}_L$. Further, Breslow (1981) and Greenland and Robins (1985) studied the asymptotic behavior of the Mantel-Haenszel estimates and demonstrated that, unlike the logit-adjusted estimates, they perform well in sparse stratifications.

The introduced estimates of the average risk difference, relative risk and odds ratio, as well as associated test statistics, are easy to obtain using PROC FREQ. Program 1.13 carries out the CMH test in the severe sepsis trial controlling for the baseline risk of mortality represented by the STRATUM variable. The program also computes the logit-adjusted and Mantel-Haenszel estimates of the average relative risk and odds ratio. Note that the order of the variables in the TABLE statement is very important; the stratification factor is followed by the other two variables.

Program 1.13 Average association between treatment and survival in the severe sepsis trial example

```
proc freq data=sepsis;
   table stratum*therapy*survival/cmh;
   weight count;
   run;
```

Output from Program 1.13

```
Summary Statistics for therapy by outcome
Controlling for stratum
  Cochran-Mantel-Haenszel Statistics (Based on Table Scores)

Statistic     Alternative Hypothesis     DF      Value      Prob
-----------------------------------------------------------------
    1         Nonzero Correlation         1      6.9677     0.0083
    2         Row Mean Scores Differ      1      6.9677     0.0083
    3         General Association         1      6.9677     0.0083


Estimates of the Common Relative Risk (Row1/Row2)

Type of Study     Method                 Value
-------------------------------------------------
Case-Control      Mantel-Haenszel        0.7438
  (Odds Ratio)    Logit                  0.7426

Cohort            Mantel-Haenszel        0.8173
  (Col1 Risk)     Logit                  0.8049

Cohort            Mantel-Haenszel        1.0804
  (Col2 Risk)     Logit                  1.0397

Type of Study     Method              95% Confidence Limits
-----------------------------------------------------------
Case-Control      Mantel-Haenszel        0.5968      0.9272
  (Odds Ratio)    Logit                  0.5950      0.9267

Cohort            Mantel-Haenszel        0.7030      0.9501
  (Col1 Risk)     Logit                  0.6930      0.9349

Cohort            Mantel-Haenszel        1.0198      1.1447
  (Col2 Risk)     Logit                  0.9863      1.0961
```

```
       Breslow-Day Test for Homogeneity of the Odds Ratios
       ----------------------------------
Chi-Square              6.4950
DF                           3
Pr > ChiSq              0.0899
```

Output 1.13 shows that the CMH statistic for association between treatment and survival adjusted for the baseline risk of death equals 6.9677 and is highly significant ($p = 0.0083$). This means that there is a significant overall increase in survival across the 4 strata in patients treated with the experimental drug.

The central panel of Output 1.13 lists the Mantel-Haenszel and logit-adjusted estimates of the average relative risk and odds ratio as well as the associated asymptotic 95% confidence intervals. The estimates of the odds ratio of mortality, shown under "Case-Control (Odds Ratio)," are 0.7438 (Mantel-Haenszel estimate $\widehat{o}_{MH}$) and 0.7426 (logit-adjusted estimate $\widehat{o}_L$). The estimates indicate that the odds of mortality adjusted for the baseline risk of mortality are about 26% lower in the experimental group compared to the placebo group. The estimates of the average relative risk of mortality, given under "Cohort (Col1 Risk)," are 0.8173 (Mantel-Haenszel estimate $\widehat{r}_{MH}$) and 0.8049 (logit-adjusted estimate $\widehat{r}_L$). Since the Mantel-Haenszel estimate is known to minimize the mean square error, it is generally more reliable than the logit-adjusted estimate. Using the Mantel-Haenszel estimate, the experimental drug reduces the 28-day mortality rate by 18% (in relative terms) compared to the placebo. The figures shown under "Cohort (Col2 Risk)" are the Mantel-Haenszel and logit-adjusted estimates of the average relative risk of survival.

As was mentioned above, confidence intervals for the Mantel-Haenszel estimates $\widehat{r}_{MH}$ and $\widehat{o}_{MH}$ are comparable to those based on the logit-adjusted estimates $\widehat{r}_L$ and $\widehat{o}_L$. The 95% confidence interval associated with $\widehat{o}_L$ is given by (0.5950, 0.9267) and is slightly wider than the 95% confidence interval associated with $\widehat{o}_{MH}$ given by (0.5968, 0.9272). However, the 95% confidence interval associated with $\widehat{r}_L$ (0.6930, 0.9349) is tighter than the 95% confidence interval for $\widehat{r}_{MH}$ (0.7030, 0.9501). Note that the confidence intervals are computed from a very large sample and so it is not surprising that the difference between the two estimation methods is very small.

Finally, the bottom panel of Output 1.13 displays the Breslow-Day chi-square statistic that can be used to examine whether the odds ratio of mortality is homogeneous across the four strata; see Breslow and Day (1980, Section 4.4) for details. The Breslow-Day p-value equals 0.0899 and suggests that the stratum-to-stratum variability in terms of the odds ratio is not very large. It is sometimes stated in the clinical trial literature that the CMH statistic needs to be used with caution when the Breslow-Day test detects significant differences in stratum-specific odds ratios. As pointed out by Agresti (2002, Section 6.3), the CMH procedure is valid and produces a meaningful result even if odds ratios differ from stratum to stratum as long as no pronounced qualitative interaction is present.

It is important to remember that the Breslow-Day test is specifically formulated to compare stratum-specific odds ratios. The homogeneity of relative differences or relative risks can be assessed using other testing procedures, for example, homogeneity tests based on the framework described by Fleiss (1981, Chapter 10) or the simple interaction test proposed by Mehrotra (2001). One can also make use of tests for qualitative interaction proposed by Gail and Simon (1985) and Ciminera et al. (1993, Section 1.5). Note that the tests for qualitative interaction are generally much more conservative than the Breslow-Day test.

1.3.2 Exact Randomization-Based Tests

It is common in the categorical analysis literature to examine the asymptotic behavior of stratified tests under the following two scenarios:

- **Large-strata asymptotics.** The total sample size n is assumed to increase while the number of strata m remains fixed.

- **Sparse-data asymptotics.** The total sample size is assumed to grow with the number of strata.

The majority of estimation and hypothesis testing procedures used in the analysis of stratified categorical data perform well only in a large-strata asymptotic setting. For example, the logit-adjusted estimates of the average relative risk and odds ratio as well as the Breslow-Day test require that all strata contain a sufficiently large number of data points.

It was shown by Birch (1964) that the asymptotic theory for the CMH test is valid under sparse-data asymptotics. In other words, the CMH statistic follows a chi-square distribution even in the presence of a large number of small strata. Mantel and Fleiss (1980) studied the accuracy of the chi-square approximation and devised a simple rule to confirm the adequacy of this approximation in practice. It is appropriate to compute the CMH p-value from a chi-square distribution with 1 degree of freedom if both

$$\sum_{i=1}^{m} \left(\frac{n_{1i+}n_{+i1}}{n_i} - \max(0, n_{+i1} - n_{2i+}) \right) \text{ and } \sum_{i=1}^{m} \left(\min(n_{1i+}, n_{+i1}) - \frac{n_{1i+}n_{+i1}}{n_i} \right)$$

exceed 5. See Breslow and Day (1980, Section 4.4) or Koch and Edwards (1988) for more details.

The Mantel-Fleiss criterion is met with a wide margin in all reasonably large studies and needs to be checked only when most of the strata have low patient counts. As an illustration, consider a subset of the 1690-patient sepsis database, which includes the data collected at three centers (see Table 1.4).

Table 1.4 28-day mortality data from the trial in patients with severe sepsis at three selected centers

Center	Experimental drug			Placebo		
	Alive	Dead	Total	Alive	Dead	Total
1	4	0	4	2	2	4
2	3	1	4	1	2	3
3	3	0	3	3	2	5

It is easy to verify that the Mantel-Fleiss criterion is not met for this subset because

$$\sum_{i=1}^{3} \left(\frac{n_{1i+}n_{+i1}}{n_i} - \max(0, n_{+i1} - n_{2i+}) \right) = 3.464,$$

and

$$\sum_{i=1}^{3} \left(\min(n_{1i+}, n_{+i1}) - \frac{n_{1i+}n_{+i1}}{n_i} \right) = 3.536.$$

When the Mantel-Fleiss criterion is not satisfied, one can resort to exact stratified tests. Although PROC FREQ supports exact inferences in simple binary settings, it does not currently implement exact tests or compute exact confidence intervals for stratified binary data described in the literature (Agresti, 2001). As shown by Westfall et al. (1999, Chapter 12), exact inferences for binary outcomes can be performed by carrying out the Cochran-Armitage permutation test available in PROC MULTTEST. The Cochran-Armitage test is ordinarily used for assessing the strength of a linear relationship between a binary response variable and a continuous covariate. It is known that the Cochran-Armitage permutation test simplifies to the Fisher exact test in the case of two treatment groups and thus we can use a stratified version of the Cochran-Armitage permutation test in PROC MULTTEST to carry out the exact Fisher test for average association between treatment and survival in Table 1.4.

Program 1.14 carries out the CMH test using PROC FREQ and also computes an exact p-value from the Cochran-Armitage permutation test using PROC MULTTEST. The Cochran-Armitage test is requested by the CA option in the TEST statement of PROC MULTTEST. The PERMUTATION option in the TEST statement tells PROC MULTTEST to perform enumeration of all permutations using the multivariate hypergeometric distribution in small strata (stratum size is less than or equal to the specified PERMUTATION parameter) and to use a continuity-corrected normal approximation otherwise.

Program 1.14 Average association between treatment and survival at the three selected centers in the severe sepsis trial

```
data sepsis1;
    input center therapy $ outcome $ count @@;
    if outcome="Dead" then survival=0; else survival=1;
    datalines;
    1 Placebo Alive 2 1 Placebo Dead 2
    1 Drug    Alive 4 1 Drug    Dead 0
    2 Placebo Alive 1 2 Placebo Dead 2
    2 Drug    Alive 3 2 Drug    Dead 1
    3 Placebo Alive 3 3 Placebo Dead 2
    3 Drug    Alive 3 3 Drug    Dead 0
    ;
proc freq data=sepsis1;
    table center*therapy*survival/cmh;
    weight count;
proc multtest data=sepsis1;
    class therapy;
    freq count;
    strata center;
    test ca(survival/permutation=20);
    run;
```

Output from Program 1.14

```
The FREQ Procedure

Summary Statistics for therapy by outcome
Controlling for center

  Cochran-Mantel-Haenszel Statistics (Based on Table Scores)

Statistic    Alternative Hypothesis    DF      Value      Prob
-------------------------------------------------------------
    1        Nonzero Correlation        1      4.6000    0.0320
    2        Row Mean Scores Differ     1      4.6000    0.0320
    3        General Association        1      4.6000    0.0320

Estimates of the Common Relative Risk (Row1/Row2)

Type of Study    Method               Value
---------------------------------------------
Case-Control     Mantel-Haenszel      0.0548
  (Odds Ratio)   Logit **             0.1552

Cohort           Mantel-Haenszel      0.1481
  (Col1 Risk)    Logit **             0.3059

Cohort           Mantel-Haenszel      1.9139
  (Col2 Risk)    Logit                1.8200
```

```
~~~~~~~~~~~~~~~~~~~~~~~~~~~~~~~~~~~~~~~~~~~~~~~~~~~~~~~~~~~~~~~~~~~~
Type of Study     Method              95% Confidence Limits
------------------------------------------------------------------
Case-Control      Mantel-Haenszel         0.0028        1.0801
  (Odds Ratio)    Logit **                0.0223        1.0803

Cohort            Mantel-Haenszel         0.0182        1.2048
  (Col1 Risk)     Logit **                0.0790        1.1848

Cohort            Mantel-Haenszel         1.0436        3.5099
  (Col2 Risk)     Logit                   1.0531        3.1454


** These logit estimators use a correction of 0.5 in every cell
   of those tables that contain a zero.


The Multtest Procedure


                    Model Information


Test for discrete variables:         Cochran-Armitage
Exact permutation distribution used: Everywhere
Tails for discrete tests:            Two-tailed
Strata weights:                      Sample size


              p-Values


Variable    Contrast        Raw


surv        Trend         0.0721
```

Output 1.14 displays the CMH *p*-value as well as the Cochran-Armitage *p*-value for association between treatment and survival in the three selected centers. Since the PERMUTATION parameter specified in PROC MULTTEST is greater than all three stratum totals, the computed Cochran-Armitage *p*-value is exact.

It is important to contrast the *p*-values produced by the CMH and Cochran-Armitage permutation tests. The CMH *p*-value equals 0.0320 and is thus significant at the 5% level. Since the Mantel-Fleiss criterion is not satisfied due to very small cell counts, the validity of the CMH test is questionable. It is prudent to examine the *p*-value associated with the exact Cochran-Armitage test. The exact *p*-value (0.0721) is more than twice as large as the CMH *p*-value and indicates that the adjusted association between treatment and survival is unlikely to be significant.

Since PROC MULTTEST efficiently handles permutation-based inferences in large data sets, the described exact test for stratified binary outcomes can be easily carried out in data sets with thousands of observations. As an illustration, Program 1.15 computes the exact Cochran-Armitage *p*-value for average association between treatment and survival in the severe sepsis trial example.

Program 1.15 Exact test for average association between treatment and survival in the severe sepsis trial example

```
proc multtest data=sepsis;
    class therapy;
    freq count;
    strata stratum;
    test ca(survival/permutation=500);
    run;
```

Output from Program 1.15

	p-Values	
Variable	Contrast	Raw
surv	Trend	0.0097

It is easy to see from Table 1.3 that the PERMUTATION parameter used in Program 1.15 is greater than the size of each individual stratum in the sepsis trial. This means that PROC MULTTEST enumerated all possible permutations in the four strata and the Cochran-Armitage p-value shown in Output 1.15 is exact. Note that the exact p-value equals 0.0097 and is close to the asymptotic CMH p-value from Output 1.13 ($p = 0.0083$). One additional advantage of using the exact Cochran-Armitage test in PROC MULTTEST is that a one-sided p-value can be easily requested by adding the LOWERTAILED option after PERMUTATON=500.

1.3.3   Minimum Risk Tests

Optimal properties of the CMH test have been extensively studied in the literature. Radhakrishna (1965) provided a detailed analysis of stratified tests and demonstrated that the weighting strategy used in the CMH procedure works best (in terms of the power to detect a treatment difference) when odds ratios of an event of interest are constant across strata. This weighting strategy (known as the SSIZE strategy) may not be very effective when this assumption is not met. This happens, for example, when a constant multiplicative or constant additive treatment effect is observed (in other words, strata are homogeneous with respect to the relative risk or risk difference). However, as demonstrated by Radhakrishna (1965), one can easily set up an asymptotically optimal test under these alternative assumptions by utilizing a different set of stratum-specific weights (see also Lachin, 2000, Section 4.7). For example, an optimal test for the case of a constant risk difference (known as the INVAR test) is based on weights that are inversely proportional to the variances of stratum-specific estimates of treatment effect (expressed in terms of risk difference).

Despite the availability of these optimal tests, one can rarely be certain that the pre-specified test is the most efficient one, since it is impossible to tell if the treatment difference is constant on a multiplicative, additive or any other scale until the data have been collected. In order to alleviate the described problem, several authors discussed ways to minimize the power loss that can occur under the worst possible configuration of stratum-specific parameters. Gastwirth (1985) demonstrated how to construct *maximin efficiency robust tests* that maximize the minimum efficiency in a broad class of stratified testing procedures. Mehrotra and Railkar (2000) introduced a family of *minimum risk* tests that minimize the mean square error of the associated estimate of the overall treatment difference. The minimum risk procedures rely on data-driven stratum-specific weights $w_1, \ldots, w_m$ given by

$$
\begin{bmatrix} w_1 \\ w_2 \\ \cdots \\ w_m \end{bmatrix} = \begin{bmatrix} \beta_1 + \alpha_1 \widehat{d_1} & \alpha_1 \widehat{d_2} & \cdots & \alpha_1 \widehat{d_m} \\ \alpha_2 \widehat{d_1} & \beta_2 + \alpha_2 \widehat{d_2} & \cdots & \alpha_2 \widehat{d_m} \\ \vdots & \vdots & \ddots & \vdots \\ \alpha_m \widehat{d_1} & \alpha_m \widehat{d_2} & \cdots & \beta_m + \alpha_m \widehat{d_m} \end{bmatrix}^{-1} \begin{bmatrix} 1 + \alpha_1 \gamma/n \\ 1 + \alpha_2 \gamma/n \\ \cdots \\ 1 + \alpha_m \gamma/n \end{bmatrix},
$$

where

$$
\widehat{d_j} = p_{1j} - p_{2j}, \quad \alpha_i = \widehat{d_i} \sum_{j=1}^{m} V_j^{-1} - \sum_{j=1}^{m} \widehat{d_j} V_j^{-1}, \quad \gamma = \sum_{j=1}^{m} n_j \widehat{d_j},
$$

$$
\beta_i = V_i \sum_{j=1}^{m} V_j^{-1}, \quad V_i = \frac{p_{1j}(1 - p_{1j})}{n_{1j+}} + \frac{p_{2j}(1 - p_{2j})}{n_{2j+}}.
$$

Once the weights have been calculated, the minimum risk estimate of the average treatment difference is computed,

$$\widehat{d}_{MR} = \sum_{j=1}^{m} w_j \widehat{d}_j,$$

and the minimum risk test of association across the m strata is conducted based on the following test statistic:

$$z_{MR} = \left(\sum_{j=1}^{m} w_j^2 V_j^* \right)^{-1/2} \left[|\widehat{d}_{MR}| - \frac{3}{16} \left(\sum_{j=1}^{m} \frac{n_{1j+}n_{2j+}}{n_{1j+} + n_{2j+}} \right)^{-1} \right],$$

where

$$V_j^* = \overline{p}_j(1 - \overline{p}_j)\frac{n_{1j+}n_{2j+}}{n_{1j+} + n_{2j+}}$$

is the sample variance of the estimated treatment difference in the jth stratum under the null hypothesis. Assuming the null hypothesis of no treatment difference, the test statistic z_{MR} is asymptotically normally distributed. Mehrotra and Railkar (2000) showed via simulations that the normal approximation can be used even when the stratum sample sizes are fairly small, i.e., when $n_j \geq 10$.

The principal advantage of the minimum risk test for the strength of average association in a stratified binary setting is that it is more robust than the optimal tests constructed under the assumption of homogeneous odds ratios or risk differences. Unlike the INVAR and SSIZE procedures that are quite vulnerable to deviations from certain optimal configurations of stratum-specific treatment differences, the minimum risk procedure displays much less sensitivity to those configurations. As pointed out by Mehrotra and Railkar (2000), this is a "minimum regret" procedure that minimizes the potential power loss that can occur in the worst-case scenario. To illustrate this fact, Mehrotra and Railkar showed that the minimum risk test is more powerful than the SSIZE test when the latter is not the most efficient test, e.g., when the risk differences (rather than the odds ratios) are constant from stratum to stratum. Likewise, the minimum risk test demonstrates a power advantage over the INVAR test derived under the assumption of homogeneous risk differences when this assumption is not satisfied. This means that the minimum risk strategy serves as a viable alternative to the optimal tests identified by Radhakrishna (1965) when there is little *a priori* information on how the treatment difference varies across the strata.

Program 1.16 uses the minimum risk strategy to test for association between treatment and survival in the severe sepsis trial. The program computes the minimum risk estimate of the average treatment difference and carries out the minimum risk test for association (as well as the INVAR and SSIZE tests) by invoking the %MinRisk macro given in the Appendix. The %MinRisk macro assumes that the input data set includes variables named EVENT1 (number of events of interest in Treatment group 1), EVENT2 (number of events of interest in Treatment group 2) and similarly defined NOEVENT1 and NOEVENT2 with one record per stratum. The EVENT1 and NOEVENT1 variables in the SEPSIS2 data set below capture the number of survivors and nonsurvivors in the experimental group. Likewise, the EVENT2 and NOEVENT2 variables contain the number of survivors and nonsurvivors in the placebo group.

Program 1.16 Minimum risk test for association between treatment and survival in the severe sepsis trial example

```
data sepsis2;
    input event1 noevent1 event2 noevent2 @@;
    datalines;
    185 33 189 26
    169 49 165 57
    156 48 104 58
    130 80 123 118
    ;
%MinRisk(dataset=sepsis2);
```

Output from Program 1.16

```
            MINRISK
Estimate Statistic P-value

   0.0545    2.5838   0.0098

             INVAR
Estimate Statistic P-value

   0.0391    1.9237   0.0544

             SSIZE
Estimate Statistic P-value

   0.0559    2.6428   0.0082
```

Output 1.16 lists the estimates of the average difference in survival between the experimental drug and placebo groups and associated p-values produced by the minimum risk, INVAR and SSIZE procedures. The estimate of the average treatment difference produced by the minimum risk method (0.0545) is very close in magnitude to the SSIZE estimate (0.0559). As a consequence, the minimum risk and SSIZE test statistics and p-values are also very close to each other. Note that, since the SSIZE testing procedure is asymptotically equivalent to the CMH procedure, the p-value generated by the SSIZE method is virtually equal to the CMH p-value shown in Output 1.13 ($p = 0.0083$).

The INVAR estimate of the overall difference is biased downward and the associated test of the hypothesis of no difference in survival yields a p-value that is greater than 0.05. The INVAR testing procedure is less powerful than the SSIZE procedure in this example because the odds ratios are generally more consistent across the strata than the risk differences in survival.

Although the minimum risk test is slightly less efficient than the SSIZE test in this scenario, it is important to keep in mind that the minimum risk approach is more robust than the other two approaches in the sense that it is less dependent on the pattern of treatment effects across strata.

1.3.4 Asymptotic Model-Based Tests

Model-based estimates and tests present an alternative to the randomization-based procedures introduced in the first part of this section. Model-based methods are closely related to the randomization-based procedures and address the same problem of testing for association between treatment and outcome with an adjustment for important covariates. The difference is that this testing problem is now embedded in a modeling framework. The outcome variable is modeled as a function of selected covariates (treatment effect as well as various prognostic and nonprognostic factors) and an inferential method is applied to estimate model parameters and test associated hypotheses. One of the advantages of model-based methods is that one can compute adjusted estimates of the treatment effect in the presence of continuous covariates, whereas randomization-based methods require a contingency table setup: i.e., they can be used only with categorical covariates.

The current section describes asymptotic maximum likelihood inferences based on a logistic regression model, while Section 1.3.5 discusses exact permutation-based inferences. As before, we will concentrate on the case of binary outcome variables. Refer to Stokes, Davis and Koch (2000, Chapters 8 and 9), Lachin (2000, Chapter 7) and Agresti (2002, Chapters 5 and 7) for a detailed overview of maximum likelihood methods in logistic regression models with SAS examples.

Model-based inferences in stratified categorical data can be implemented using several SAS procedures, including PROC LOGISTIC, PROC GENMOD, PROC PROBIT, PROC CATMOD and PROC NLMIXED. Some of these procedures are more general and provide the user with a variety of statistical modeling tools. For example, PROC GENMOD was introduced to support normal, binomial, Poisson and other generalized linear models, and PROC NLMIXED allows the user to fit a large number of nonlinear mixed models. The others, e.g., PROC LOGISTIC and PROC PROBIT, deal with a rather narrow class of models; however, as more specialized procedures often do, they support more useful features. This section will focus mainly on one of these procedures that is widely used to analyze binary data (PROC LOGISTIC) and will briefly describe some of the interesting features of another popular procedure (PROC GENMOD).

Program 1.17 utilizes PROC LOGISTIC to analyze average association between treatment and survival, controlling for the baseline risk of death in the severe sepsis trial example.

Program 1.17 Maximum likelihood analysis of average association between treatment and survival in the severe sepsis trial example using PROC LOGISTIC

```
proc logistic data=sepsis;
    class therapy stratum;
    model survival=therapy stratum/clodds=pl;
    freq count;
    run;
```

Output from Program 1.17

```
         Type III Analysis of Effects

                         Wald
Effect        DF    Chi-Square    Pr > ChiSq

therapy        1       6.9635        0.0083
stratum        3      97.1282        <.0001

         Analysis of Maximum Likelihood Estimates

                         Standard     Wald
Parameter        DF Estimate   Error Chi-Square Pr > ChiSq

Intercept         1  -1.0375  0.0585   314.8468    <.0001
therapy   Drug    1  -0.1489  0.0564     6.9635    0.0083
stratum   1       1  -0.8162  0.1151    50.2692    <.0001
stratum   2       1  -0.1173  0.0982     1.4259    0.2324
stratum   3       1   0.1528  0.1006     2.3064    0.1288

              Odds Ratio Estimates

                         Point        95% Wald
Effect                 Estimate    Confidence Limits

therapy Drug   vs Placebo   0.743     0.595      0.926
stratum 1 vs 4              0.203     0.145      0.282
stratum 2 vs 4              0.407     0.306      0.543
stratum 3 vs 4              0.534     0.398      0.716

Profile Likelihood Confidence Interval for Adjusted Odds Ratios
95% Confidence Limits
    0.595      0.926
    0.144      0.281
    0.305      0.542
    0.397      0.715
```

Output 1.17 lists the Wald chi-square statistics for the THERAPY and STRATUM variables, maximum likelihood estimates of the model parameters, associated odds ratios and confidence intervals. The Wald statistic for the treatment effect equals 6.9635 and is significant at the 5% level ($p = 0.0083$). This statistic is close in magnitude to the CMH statistic in Output 1.13. As shown by Day and Byar (1979), the CMH test is equivalent to the score test in a logistic regression model and is generally in good agreement with the Wald statistic unless the data are sparse and most strata have only a few observations. Further, the maximum likelihood estimate of the overall ratio of the odds of survival is equal to 0.743 and the associated 95% Wald confidence interval is given by (0.595, 0.926). The estimate and confidence limits are consistent with the Mantel-Haenszel and logit-adjusted estimates and their confidence limits displayed in Output 1.13.

The bottom panel of Output 1.17 shows that the 95% profile likelihood confidence interval for the average odds ratio is equal to (0.595, 0.926). This confidence interval is requested by the CLODDS=PL option in the MODEL statement. Note that the profile likelihood confidence limits are identical to the Wald limits in this example. The advantage of using profile likelihood confidence intervals is that they are more stable than Wald confidence intervals in the analysis of very small or very large odds ratios; see Agresti (2002, Section 3.1).

Program 1.18 analyzes the same data set as above using PROC GENMOD. PROC GENMOD is a very flexible procedure for fitting various types of generalized linear models, including the logistic regression. The logistic regression model is requested by the DIST=BIN and LINK=LOGIT options. Alternatively, one can fit a model with a probit link function by setting DIST=BIN and LINK=PROBIT, or one can use any arbitrary link function (defined in the FWDLINK statement) that is consistent with the distribution of the response variable and desired interpretation of parameter estimates.

Program 1.18 Maximum likelihood analysis of average association between treatment and survival in the severe sepsis trial example using PROC GENMOD

```
proc genmod data=sepsis;
   class therapy stratum;
   model survival=therapy stratum/dist=bin link=logit type3;
   freq count;
   run;
```

Output from Program 1.18

```
            Analysis Of Parameter Estimates

                            Standard      Wald 95%
Parameter          DF  Estimate  Error  Confidence Limits

Intercept           1   -0.1079  0.1082  -0.3199   0.1041
therapy   Drug      1   -0.2977  0.1128  -0.5189  -0.0766
therapy   Placebo   0    0.0000  0.0000   0.0000   0.0000
stratum   1         1   -1.5970  0.1695  -1.9292  -1.2648
stratum   2         1   -0.8981  0.1467  -1.1856  -0.6105
stratum   3         1   -0.6280  0.1499  -0.9217  -0.3343
stratum   4         0    0.0000  0.0000   0.0000   0.0000
Scale               0    1.0000  0.0000   1.0000   1.0000


   LR Statistics For Type 3 Analysis

                    Chi-
Source        DF   Square   Pr > ChiSq

therapy        1     6.99      0.0082
stratum        3   105.61     <.0001
```

Output 1.18 displays maximum likelihood estimates of the model parameters and the likelihood ratio test for the THERAPY variable. The computed estimates are different from those shown in Output 1.17 because PROC GENMOD relies on a different parametrization scheme for classification variables. The PROC GENMOD parametrization can be viewed as a more natural one since it is consistent with odds ratio estimates. For example, the maximum likelihood estimate of the overall ratio of the odds of survival (which is equal to 0.743) is easy to obtain by exponentiating the estimate of the treatment effect displayed in Output 1.18 (it equals -0.2977). Further, if one is interested in computing the treatment effect estimate produced by PROC LOGISTIC (-0.1489) and the associated Wald statistic (6.9635), the PROC GENMOD code in Program 1.18 needs to be modified as follows:

```
proc genmod data=sepsis;
   class therapy stratum;
   model survival=therapy stratum/dist=bin link=logit type3;
   freq count;
   estimate "PROC LOGISTIC treatment effect" therapy 1 -1 /divisor=2;
   run;
```

Note that it is also possible to get PROC LOGISTIC to produce the PROC GENMOD estimates of model parameters displayed in Output 1.18. This can be done by adding the PARAM=GLM option to the CLASS statement as shown below:

```
proc logistic data=sepsis;
   class therapy stratum/param=glm;
   model survival=therapy stratum/clodds=pl;
   freq count;
   run;
```

Returning to Output 1.18, the likelihood ratio statistic for the null hypothesis of no treatment effect is requested by adding the TYPE3 option in the MODEL statement of PROC GENMOD. Output 1.18 shows that the statistic equals 6.99 and is thus close to the Wald statistic computed by PROC LOGISTIC. As pointed out by Agresti (2002, Section 5.2), the Wald and likelihood ratio tests produce similar results when the sample size is large; however, the likelihood ratio is generally preferred over the Wald test because of its power and stability.

Comparing the output generated by PROC GENMOD to that produced by PROC LOGISTIC, we can see the latter procedure is more convenient to use as it computes odds ratios for each independent variable and associated confidence limits (both Wald and profile likelihood limits). Although the likelihood-ratio test for assessing the influence of each individual covariate on the outcome is not directly available in PROC LOGISTIC, this test can be carried out, if desired, by fitting two logistic models (with and without the covariate of interest) and then computing the difference in the model likelihood-ratio test statistics. Thus, PROC LOGISTIC matches all features supported by PROC GENMOD. One additional argument in favor of using PROC LOGISTIC in the analysis of stratified categorical data is that this procedure can perform exact inferences (in SAS 8.1 and later versions of SAS) that are supported by neither PROC FREQ or PROC GENMOD. Exact tests available in PROC LOGISTIC are introduced in the next section.

1.3.5   Exact Model-Based Tests

Exact inferences in PROC LOGISTIC are performed by conditioning on appropriate sufficient statistics. The resulting conditional maximum likelihood inference is generally similar to the regular (unconditional) maximum likelihood inference discussed above. The principal difference between the two likelihood frameworks is that the conditional approach enables one to evaluate the exact distribution of parameter estimates and test statistics and therefore construct exact confidence intervals and compute exact p-values. Mehta and Patel (1985), Stokes, Davis and Koch (2000, Chapter 10) and Agresti (2002, Section 6.7) provide a detailed discussion of exact conditional inferences in logistic regression models.

Program 1.19 utilizes PROC LOGISTIC to conduct exact conditional analyses of the data set introduced in Section 1.3.2 (see Table 1.4). This data set contains mortality data collected at three centers in the severe sepsis trial. The EXACTONLY option in PROC LOGISTIC suppresses the regular output (asymptotic estimates and statistics) and the PARAM=REFERENCE option is added to the CLASS statement to allow the computation of exact confidence limits for the overall odds ratio (the limits are computed only if the reference parameterization method is used to code classification variables).

Program 1.19 Exact conditional test of average association between treatment and survival at the three selected centers in the severe sepsis trial example

```
data sepsis1;
    input center therapy $ outcome $ count @@;
    if outcome="Dead" then survival=0; else survival=1;
    datalines;
    1 Placebo Alive 2 1 Placebo Dead 2
    1 Drug    Alive 4 1 Drug    Dead 0
    2 Placebo Alive 1 2 Placebo Dead 2
    2 Drug    Alive 3 2 Drug    Dead 1
    3 Placebo Alive 3 3 Placebo Dead 2
    3 Drug    Alive 3 3 Drug    Dead 0
    ;
proc logistic data=sepsis1 exactonly;
    class therapy center/param=reference;
    model survival(event="0")=therapy center;
    exact therapy/estimate=odds;
    freq count;
    run;
```

Output from Program 1.19

```
Exact Conditional Analysis

            Conditional Exact Tests

                               --- p-Value ---
Effect     Test          Statistic    Exact      Mid

therapy    Score          4.6000     0.0721    0.0544
           Probability    0.0353     0.0721    0.0544

                  Exact Odds Ratios

                             95% Confidence
Parameter       Estimate        Limits          p-Value

therapy  Drug     0.097      0.002    1.168      0.0751
```

Output 1.19 displays the exact *p*-values and confidence limits computed by PROC LOGISTIC. The exact *p*-values associated with the conditional score and probability methods are equal to the *p*-value produced by the Cochran-Armitage permutation test in PROC MULTTEST (see Output 1.14). The estimate of the average odds ratio of mortality in the experimental group compared to the placebo group equals 0.097 and lies in the middle between the Mantel-Haenszel and logit-adjusted estimates shown in Output 1.14 ($\widehat{o}_{MH} = 0.0548$ and $\widehat{o}_L = 0.1552$). The exact 95% confidence interval at the bottom of Output 1.19 is substantially wider than the asymptotic 95% confidence intervals associated with $\widehat{o}_{MH}$ or $\widehat{o}_L$.

It is important to keep in mind that, up to Version 8.2 of the SAS System, the algorithm for exact calculations used in PROC LOGISTIC is rather slow. It may take several minutes to compute exact *p*-values in a data set with a thousand observations. In larger data sets, PROC LOGISTIC often generates the following warning message:

"WARNING: Floating point overflow in the permutation distribution; exact statistics are not computed."

Starting with SAS 9.0, PROC LOGISTIC offers a more efficient algorithm for performing exact inferences and it becomes possible to run exact conditional analyses of binary outcomes even in large clinical trials. For example, it takes seconds to compute exact confidence limits and *p*-values in the 1690-patient sepsis data set (see Program 1.20 below).

Program 1.20 Exact conditional test of average association between treatment and survival in the severe sepsis trial example

```
proc logistic data=sepsis exactonly;
    class therapy stratum/param=reference;
    model survival(event="0")=therapy stratum;
    exact therapy/estimate=odds;
    freq count;
    run;
```

Output from Program 1.20

```
Exact Conditional Analysis

            Conditional Exact Tests

                                --- p-Value ---
Effect     Test           Statistic     Exact      Mid

therapy    Score            6.9677     0.0097    0.0090
           Probability      0.00138    0.0097    0.0090

                 Exact Odds Ratios

                              95% Confidence
Parameter      Estimate         Limits           p-Value

therapy  Drug     0.743      0.592     0.932      0.0097
```

Output 1.20 lists the exact 95% confidence interval for the odds ratio of mortality (0.592, 0.932) and associated exact *p*-value (0.0097). The exact confidence limits are very close to the corresponding Mantel-Haenszel and logit-adjusted confidence limits shown in Output 1.13. Similarly, the exact *p*-value is in good agreement with the CMH *p*-value for average association between treatment and survival ($p = 0.0083$).

Additionally, PROC LOGISTIC in SAS 9.0 supports stratified conditional inferences proposed by Gail, Lubin and Rubinstein (1981). The inferences are based on a logistic regression model with stratum-specific intercepts to better account for between-stratum variability. To request a stratified conditional analysis of the data in PROC LOGISTIC, one needs to add the STRATA statement and specify the name of the stratification variable, e.g.,

```
proc logistic data=sepsis exactonly;
    class therapy/param=reference;
    model survival(event="0")=therapy;
    strata stratum;
    exact therapy/estimate=odds;
    freq count;
    run;
```

An exact stratified conditional analysis of the SEPSIS data set generates confidence limits for the odds ratio of mortality and associated *p*-value that are identical to those displayed in Output 1.20.

1.3.6 Summary

This section reviewed statistical methods for the analysis of stratified categorical outcomes with emphasis on binary data. As was pointed out in the introduction, the analysis methods described in this section (e.g., Cochran-Mantel-Haenszel or model-based methods) are easily extended to a more general case of multinomial responses. PROC FREQ automatically switches to the appropriate extensions of binary estimation and testing procedures when it encounters outcomes variables with three or more levels. Similarly, PROC LOGISTIC can be used to fit proportional-odds models for multinomial variables; see Chapter 3 of this book and Stokes, Davis and Koch (2000, Chapter 9) for details.

The first part of the section dealt with randomization-based estimates of the risk difference, relative risk and odds ratio and associated significance tests. The popular Cochran-Mantel-Haenszel test for overall association as well as the Mantel-Haenszel and logit-adjusted estimates of the average relative risk and odds ratio are easy to compute using PROC FREQ. The %MinRisk macro introduced in Section 1.3.3 implements minimum risk tests for association between treatment and a binary outcome in a stratified setting. The tests are attractive in clinical applications because they minimize the power loss under the worst possible configuration of stratum-specific parameters when patterns of treatment effects across strata are unknown.

Model-based tests for stratified binary data were discussed in the second part of the section. Model-based inferences can be implemented using PROC LOGISTIC and PROC GENMOD. PROC LOGISTIC appears to be more convenient to use in the analysis of stratified binary data because (unlike the more general PROC GENMOD) it generates a complete set of useful summary statistics for each independent variable in the model. For example, one can easily obtain odds ratios and associated Wald and profile likelihood confidence limits for each covariate. PROC LOGISTIC also supports exact inferences for stratified binary data.

When choosing an appropriate inferential method for stratified categorical data, it is important to remember that most of the popular procedures (both randomization- and model-based) need to be used with caution in sparse stratifications. The presence of a large number of under-represented strata either causes these procedures to break down or has a deleterious effect on their statistical power. A commonly used rule of thumb states that one generally needs at least five observations per treatment group per stratum to avoid spurious results. Only a small number of exceptions to this rule occur. Both the Cochran-Mantel-Haenszel test and Mantel-Haenszel estimates of the average relative risk and odds ratio produced by PROC FREQ are known to be fairly robust with respect to stratum-specific sample sizes and perform well as long as the total sample size is large.

1.4   Time-to-Event Endpoints

This section reviews methods for stratified analysis of clinical trials with a time-to-event endpoint. Examples include mortality endpoints and endpoints based on time to the onset of a therapeutic effect or time to worsening/relapse. First, we will discuss randomization-based tests for stratified time-to-event data and review stratified versions of the popular Wilcoxon and log-rank tests implemented in PROC LIFETEST as well as other testing procedures from the broad class of linear rank tests. The second part of this section covers model-based inferences for stratified time-to-event data that can be performed in the framework of the Cox proportional hazards regression. These inferences are implemented using

PROC PHREG. As in Section 1.3, this section deals only with fixed effects models for time-to-event outcomes, and random effects models will not be considered here. The reader interested in random effects models for time-to-event data used in clinical trials is referred to Andersen, Klein and Zhang (1999) and Yamaguchi and Ohashi (1999).

EXAMPLE: Severe Sepsis Trial

In order to illustrate statistical methods for the analysis of stratified time-to-event data, we will consider an artificial data set containing 1600 survival times. The survival times are assumed to follow a Weibull distribution, i.e., the survival function in the ith treatment group and jth stratum is given by

$$S_{ij}(t) = \exp\{-(t/b_{ij})^a\},$$

where the shape parameter a equals 0.5 and the scale parameters represented by b_{ij} in Table 1.5 are chosen in such a way that the generated survival times closely resemble the real survival times observed in the 1690-patient severe sepsis trial described earlier in Section 1.3.

Table 1.5 Scale parameters

Stratum	Experimental group	Placebo group
1	$b_{11} = 13000$	$b_{21} = 25000$
2	$b_{12} = 13000$	$b_{22} = 10000$
3	$b_{13} = 5500$	$b_{23} = 3000$
4	$b_{14} = 2500$	$b_{24} = 1200$

The hazard function that specifies the instantaneous risk of death at time t conditional on survival to t is equal to $h_{ij}(t) = at^{a-1}/b_{ij}^a$. Since a equals 0.5, the hazard function is decreasing in a monotone fashion across all four strata.

Program 1.21 generates the SEPSURV data set with the SURVTIME variable capturing the time from the start of study drug administration to either the patient's death or study completion measured in hours. The SURVTIME values are censored at 672 hours because mortality was monitored only during the first 28 days. The program utilizes PROC LIFETEST to produce the Kaplan-Meier estimates of survival functions across four strata. The strata were formed to account for the variability in the baseline risk of mortality. The TREAT variable in the SEPSURV data set identifies the treatment groups: TREAT=0 for placebo patients and TREAT=1 for patients treated with the experimental drug.

Program 1.21 Kaplan-Meier survival curves adjusted for the baseline risk of mortality

```
data sepsurv;
    call streaminit(9544);
    do stratum=1 to 4;
        do patient=1 to 400;
            if patient<=200 then treat=0; else treat=1;
            if stratum=1 and treat=0 then b=25;
            if stratum=1 and treat=1 then b=13;
            if stratum=2 and treat=0 then b=10;
            if stratum=2 and treat=1 then b=13;
            if stratum=3 and treat=0 then b=3;
            if stratum=3 and treat=1 then b=5.5;
            if stratum=4 and treat=0 then b=1.2;
            if stratum=4 and treat=1 then b=2.5;
            survtime=rand("weibull",0.5,1000*b);
            censor=(survtime<=672);
            survtime=min(survtime,672);
        output;
        end;
    end;
```

```
proc lifetest data=sepsurv notable outsurv=surv;
    by stratum;
    time survtime*censor(0);
    strata treat;

* Plot Kaplan-Meier survival curves in each stratum;
%macro PlotKM(stratum);
    axis1 minor=none label=(angle=90 "Survival") order=(0 to 1 by 0.5);
    axis2 minor=none label=("Time (h)") order=(0 to 700 by 350);
    symbol1 value=none color=black i=j line=1;
    symbol2 value=none color=black i=j line=20;
    data annotate;
        xsys="1"; ysys="1"; hsys="4"; x=50; y=20; position="5";
        size=1; text="Stratum &stratum"; function="label";
    proc gplot data=surv anno=annotate;
        where stratum=&stratum;
        plot survival*survtime=treat/frame haxis=axis2 vaxis=axis1 nolegend;
        run;
        quit;
%mend PlotKM;

%PlotKM(1);
%PlotKM(2);
%PlotKM(3);
%PlotKM(4);
```

The output of Program 1.21 is shown in Figure 1.4. Figure 1.4 displays the Kaplan-Meier survival curves representing increasing levels of mortality risk in the experimental (dashed curve) and placebo (solid curve) groups across the strata. It is clear that survival in the placebo group is significantly reduced in patients in Strata 3 and 4. The beneficial effect of the experimental drug is most pronounced in patients at a high risk of death, and the treatment effect is reversed in Stratum 1.

1.4.1 Randomization-Based Tests

In order to assess the significance of the treatment differences in Output 1.21 and test the null hypothesis of no treatment effect on survival in the four strata, we can make use of three randomization-based methods available in PROC LIFETEST: log-rank, Wilcoxon and likelihood ratio tests.

The log-rank test was developed by Mantel (1966), who adapted the general Mantel-Haenszel approach (Mantel and Haenszel, 1959) to analyze right-censored time-to-event data. Peto and Peto (1972) proposed a more general version of the original Mantel test for a comparison of multiple survival distributions (Peto and Peto also coined the term "log-rank test"). The Wilcoxon test in a two-sample scenario was developed by Gehan (1965). This test was later extended by Breslow (1970) to the case of multiple samples. Both the log-rank and Wilcoxon procedures are based on nonparametric ideas. The likelihood-ratio test is an example a parametric method of comparing survival functions. The test is computed under the assumption that event times follow an exponential distribution. Alternatively, one can compare underlying survival distributions by carrying out generalized versions of *linear rank tests* described by Hájek and Šidák (1967). Examples include testing procedures proposed by Tarone and Ware (1977), Prentice (1978) and Harrington and Fleming (1982). The Tarone-Ware and Harrington-Fleming tests are closely related to the log-rank and Wilcoxon tests. In fact, the four testing procedures perform the same comparison of survival distributions but employ four different weighting strategies; see Collett (1994, Section 2.5) and Lachin (2000, Section 9.3) for more details.

As an illustration, consider a clinical trial with a time-to-event endpoint comparing an experimental therapy to a placebo. Let $t_{(1)} < \ldots < t_{(r)}$ denote r ordered event times in the pooled sample. The

Figure 1.4 Kaplan-Meier survival curves adjusted for the baseline risk of mortality in the experimental (- - -) and placebo (—) groups in the severe sepsis trial example

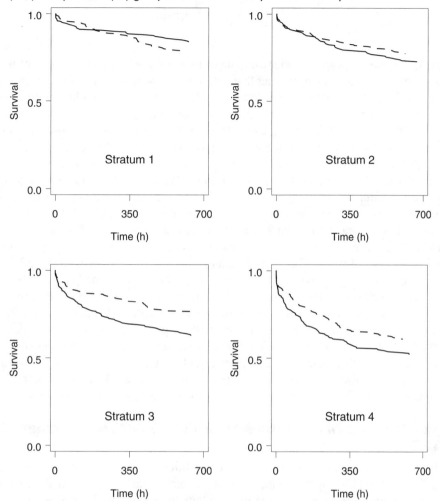

magnitude of the distance between two survival functions is measured in the log-rank test using the statistic

$$d_L = \sum_{k=1}^{r} (d_{1k} - e_{1k}),$$

where d_{1k} is the number of events observed in the experimental group at time $t_{(k)}$, and e_{1k} is the expected number of events at time $t_{(k)}$ under the null hypothesis of no treatment effect on survival. We can see from the definition of d_L that the deviations $d_{1k} - e_{1k}$, $k = 1, \ldots, r$, are equally weighted in the log-rank test.

The Wilcoxon test is based on the idea that early events are more informative than those that occur later when few patients remain alive and survival curves are estimated with low precision. The Wilcoxon distance between two survival functions is given by

$$d_W = \sum_{k=1}^{r} n_k (d_{1k} - e_{1k}),$$

where n_k is the number of patients in the risk set before time $t_{(k)}$ (this includes patients who have not experienced the event of interest or have been censored before $t_{(k)}$).

Similarly, the Tarone-Ware and Harrington-Fleming procedures are based on the distance statistics

$$d_{TW} = \sum_{k=1}^{r} n_k^{1/2} (d_{1k} - e_{1k}), \quad d_{HF} = \sum_{k=1}^{r} S_k^{\rho} (d_{1k} - e_{1k}),$$

respectively. Here S_k denotes the Kaplan-Meier estimate of the combined survival function of the two treatment groups at time $t_{(k)}$, and ρ is a parameter that determines how much weight is assigned to individual event times ($0 \leq \rho \leq 1$). The Tarone-Ware procedure represents the middle point between equally-weighted event times and a Wilcoxon weighting scheme giving considerably more weight to events that occurred early in the trial. To see this, note that the deviation $d_{1k} - e_{1k}$ at time $t_{(k)}$ receives the weight of $n_k^0 = 1$ in the log-rank test and the weight of $n_k^1 = n_k$ in the Wilcoxon test. The Harrington-Fleming procedure provides the statistician with a flexible balance between the log-rank-type and Wilcoxon-type weights. Letting $\rho = 0$ in the Harrington-Fleming procedure yields the log-rank test whereas letting $\rho = 1$ results in a test that assigns greater weights to early events.

An important consideration in selecting a statistical test is its efficiency against a particular alternative. The log-rank test is most powerful when the hazard functions in two treatment groups are proportional to each other, but it can be less efficient than the Wilcoxon test when the proportionality assumption is violated (Peto and Peto, 1972; Lee, Desu and Gehan, 1975; Prentice, 1978). It is generally difficult to characterize the alternative hypotheses that maximize the power of the Wilcoxon test because its efficiency depends on both survival and censoring distributions. It is known that the Wilcoxon test needs to be used with caution when early event times are heavily censored (Prentice and Marek, 1979). The Tarone-Ware procedure serves as a robust alternative to the log-rank and Wilcoxon procedures and maintains power better than these two procedures across a broad range of alternative hypotheses. Tarone and Ware (1977) demonstrated that their test is more powerful than the Wilcoxon test when the hazard functions are proportional and is more powerful than the log-rank test when the assumption of proportional hazards is not met. The same is true for the family of Harrington-Fleming tests.

Comparison of Survival Distributions Using the STRATA Statement in PROC LIFETEST

Randomization-based tests for homogeneity of survival distributions across treatment groups can be carried out using PROC LIFETEST by including the treatment group variable in either the STRATA or TEST statement. For example, Program 1.22 examines stratum-specific survival functions in the severe sepsis trial. In order to request a comparison of the two treatment groups (experimental drug versus placebo) within each stratum, the TREAT variable is included in the STRATA statement.

Program 1.22 Comparison of survival distributions in four strata using the STRATA statement

```
proc lifetest data=sepsurv notable;
    ods select HomTests;
    by stratum;
    time survtime*censor(0);
    strata treat;
    run;
```

Output from Program 1.22

```
stratum=1

The LIFETEST Procedure

        Test of Equality over Strata

                              Pr >
Test        Chi-Square    DF    Chi-Square
Log-Rank      1.4797      1      0.2238
Wilcoxon      1.2748      1      0.2589
-2Log(LR)     1.6271      1      0.2021

stratum=2

The LIFETEST Procedure

        Test of Equality over Strata

                              Pr >
Test        Chi-Square    DF    Chi-Square
Log-Rank      0.9934      1      0.3189
Wilcoxon      0.8690      1      0.3512
-2Log(LR)     1.1345      1      0.2868

stratum=3

The LIFETEST Procedure

        Test of Equality over Strata

                              Pr >
Test        Chi-Square    DF    Chi-Square
Log-Rank      8.8176      1      0.0030
Wilcoxon      8.7611      1      0.0031
-2Log(LR)    10.3130      1      0.0013

stratum=4

The LIFETEST Procedure

        Test of Equality over Strata

                              Pr >
Test        Chi-Square    DF    Chi-Square
Log-Rank      3.5259      1      0.0604
Wilcoxon      3.9377      1      0.0472
-2Log(LR)     4.4858      1      0.0342
```

Including the TREAT variable in the STRATA statement results in a comparison of stratum-specific survival distributions based on the log-rank, Wilcoxon and likelihood ratio tests. Output 1.22 lists the log-rank, Wilcoxon and likelihood ratio statistics accompanied by asymptotic *p*-values. Note that extraneous information has been deleted from the output using the ODS statement (ods select HomTests). We can see from Output 1.22 that the treatment difference is far from being significant in Stratum 1 and Stratum 2, highly significant in Stratum 3 and marginally significant in Stratum 4. The three tests yield similar results within each stratum with the likelihood ratio statistic consistently being larger than the other two. Since the likelihood-ratio test is a parametric procedure that relies heavily on the assumption of an underlying exponential distribution, it needs to be used with caution unless one is certain that the exponential assumption is met.

Comparison of Survival Distributions Using the TEST Statement in PROC LIFETEST

An alternative approach to testing the significance of treatment effect on survival is based on the use of the TEST statement in PROC LIFETEST. If the treatment group variable is included in the TEST statement, PROC LIFETEST carries out only two tests (log-rank and Wilcoxon tests) to compare survival functions across treatment groups. The generated log-rank and Wilcoxon statistics are somewhat different from those shown in Output 1.22.

To illustrate, Program 1.23 computes the stratum-specific log-rank and Wilcoxon statistics and associated *p*-values when the TREAT variable is included in the TEST statement.

Program 1.23 Comparison of survival distributions in four strata using the TEST statement

```
proc lifetest data=sepsurv notable;
    ods select LogUniChisq WilUniChiSq;
    by stratum;
    time survtime*censor(0);
    test treat;
    run;
```

Output from Program 1.23

```
stratum=1

        Univariate Chi-Squares for the Wilcoxon Test

                Test      Standard                  Pr >
Variable      Statistic   Deviation   Chi-Square   Chi-Square
  treat        -4.4090      3.9030      1.2761       0.2586

        Univariate Chi-Squares for the Log-Rank Test

                Test      Standard                  Pr >
Variable      Statistic   Deviation   Chi-Square   Chi-Square
  treat        -5.2282      4.3003      1.4781       0.2241

stratum=2

        Univariate Chi-Squares for the Wilcoxon Test

                Test      Standard                  Pr >
Variable      Statistic   Deviation   Chi-Square   Chi-Square
  treat         4.0723      4.3683      0.8691       0.3512
```

```
            Univariate Chi-Squares for the Log-Rank Test

                    Test        Standard                    Pr >
    Variable     Statistic      Deviation    Chi-Square    Chi-Square
     treat        4.9539         4.9743        0.9918        0.3193

stratum=3

            Univariate Chi-Squares for the Wilcoxon Test

                    Test        Standard                    Pr >
    Variable     Statistic      Deviation    Chi-Square    Chi-Square
     treat       13.8579         4.6821        8.7602        0.0031

            Univariate Chi-Squares for the Log-Rank Test

                    Test        Standard                    Pr >
    Variable     Statistic      Deviation    Chi-Square    Chi-Square
     treat       16.2909         5.4914        8.8007        0.0030

stratum=4

            Univariate Chi-Squares for the Wilcoxon Test

                    Test        Standard                    Pr >
    Variable     Statistic      Deviation    Chi-Square    Chi-Square
     treat       10.3367         5.2107        3.9352        0.0473

            Univariate Chi-Squares for the Log-Rank Test

                    Test        Standard                    Pr >
    Variable     Statistic      Deviation    Chi-Square    Chi-Square
     treat       12.3095         6.5680        3.5125        0.0609
```

Output 1.23 displays the Wilcoxon and log-rank statistics and p-values produced by Program 1.23. Note that the ODS statement (ods select LogUniChisq WilUniChiSq) is used to suppress a redundant set of Wilcoxon and log-rank statistics (under the headings "Forward Stepwise Sequence of Chi-Squares for the Log-Rank Test" and "Forward Stepwise Sequence of Chi-Squares for the Wilcoxon Test") that would otherwise be included in the regular output. These stepwise procedures are identical to the univariate procedures shown above because only one variable was included in the TEST statement in Program 1.23.

It is easy to check that the stratum-specific log-rank and Wilcoxon statistics in Output 1.23 are a bit different from those shown in Output 1.22. The difference is fairly small but tends to increase with the value of a test statistic. To understand the observed discrepancy between the two sets of test statistics, one needs to remember that the TEST statement was added to PROC LIFETEST to enable the user to study effects of continuous covariates on survival distributions. The underlying testing procedures extend the log-rank and Wilcoxon tests for homogeneity of survival functions across treatment groups; see Kalbfleisch and Prentice (1980, Chapter 6). The more general versions of the log-rank and Wilcoxon tests do not always simplify to the ordinary tests when a categorical variable is included in the TEST statement. For example, if there were no identical survival times in the SEPSURV data set, the log-rank statistics in Output 1.23 would match those displayed in Output 1.22. Since this is not the case, the general version of the log-rank test implemented in PROC LIFETEST attempts to adjust for tied observations, which results in a slightly different value of the log-rank statistic. Analysis of time-to-event data with tied event times is discussed in more detail later in this section.

There is another way to look at the difference between inferences performed by PROC LIFETEST when the treatment group variable is included in the STRATA statement as opposed to the TEST statement. Roughly speaking, the tests listed in Output 1.22 (using the STRATA statement) represent a randomization-based testing method whereas the tests in Output 1.23 (using the TEST statement) are fairly closely related to a model-based approach. For example, it will be shown in Section 1.4.2 that the log-rank test in Output 1.23 is equivalent to a test based on the Cox proportional hazards model.

Comparison of Survival Distributions Using Tarone-Ware and Harrington-Fleming Tests

Thus far, we have focused on the log-rank, Wilcoxon and likelihood ratio testing procedures implemented in PROC LIFETEST. It is interesting to compare these procedures to the tests described by Tarone and Ware (1977) and Harrington and Fleming (1982). The latter tests can be implemented using the %LinRank macro written by Cantor (1997, Chapter 3) or, in SAS 9.1, they can be carried out directly in PROC LIFETEST. For example, the following code can be used in SAS 9.1 to compare survival distributions in the SEPSURV data set using the Tarone-Ware and Harrington-Fleming ($\rho = 0.5$) tests.

```
* Tarone-Ware and Harrington-Fleming tests in SAS 9.1;
proc lifetest data=sepsurv notable;
    ods select HomTests;
    by stratum;
    time survtime*censor(0);
    strata treat/test=(tarone fleming(0.5));
    run;
```

The stratum-specific Tarone-Ware and Harrington-Fleming statistics and p-values produced by the %LinRank macro are summarized in Table 1.6. To facilitate the comparison with the log-rank and Wilcoxon tests computed in Program 1.22, the relevant test statistics and p-values from Output 1.22 are displayed at the bottom of the table.

Table 1.6 Comparison of the Tarone-Ware, Harrington-Fleming, log-rank and Wilcoxon tests

Test	Stratum 1	Stratum 2	Stratum 3	Stratum 4
Tarone-Ware test				
Statistic	1.3790	0.9331	8.8171	3.7593
P-value	0.2403	0.3341	0.0030	0.0525
Harrington-Fleming test ($\rho = 0.1$)				
Statistic	1.4599	0.9817	8.8220	3.5766
P-value	0.2269	0.3218	0.0030	0.0586
Harrington-Fleming test ($\rho = 1$)				
Statistic	1.2748	0.8690	8.7611	3.9377
P-value	0.2589	0.3512	0.0031	0.0472
Log-rank test				
Statistic	1.4797	0.9934	8.8176	3.5259
P-value	0.2238	0.3189	0.0030	0.0604
Wilcoxon test				
Statistic	1.2748	0.8690	8.7611	3.9377
P-value	0.2589	0.3512	0.0031	0.0472

Table 1.6 demonstrates that the p-values generated by the Tarone-Ware and Harrington-Fleming tests are comparable to the log-rank and Wilcoxon p-values computed in Program 1.22. By the

definition of the Tarone-Ware procedure, the weights assigned to individual event times are greater than the log-rank weights and less than the Wilcoxon weights. As a consequence, the Tarone-Ware statistics lie between the corresponding log-rank and Wilcoxon statistics, and the Tarone-Ware procedure is always superior to the least powerful of these two procedures. When $\rho = 0.1$, the Harrington-Fleming weights are virtually independent of event times and thus the stratum-specific Harrington-Fleming statistics are generally close in magnitude to the log-rank statistics. On the other hand, the Harrington-Fleming weights approximate the Wilcoxon weights when $\rho = 1$, which causes the two sets of test statistics to be very close to each other.

Stratified Analysis of Time-to-Event Data

In the first part of this section we have concentrated on stratum-specific inferences; however, one is typically more interested in an overall analysis of the treatment effect controlling for important covariates. An adjusted effect of the experimental drug on a time-to-event outcome variable can be assessed by combining the information about the treatment differences across strata. PROC LIFETEST supports stratified versions of the Wilcoxon and log-rank tests. In order to carry out the stratified tests, one needs to include the treatment group variable in the TEST statement and add the stratification variable (e.g., baseline risk of death) to the STRATA statement.

Mathematically, stratified inferences performed by PROC LIFETEST are equivalent to pooling the Wilcoxon and log-rank distance statistics with equal weights across m strata. Specifically, let d_{Lj} denote the value of the log-rank distance between survival functions in the jth stratum and let s_{Lj}^2 be the sample variance of d_{Lj}. The stratified log-rank statistic equals

$$u_L = \left(\sum_{j=1}^{m} d_{Lj} \right)^2 / \sum_{j=1}^{m} s_{Lj}^2.$$

Under the null hypothesis that there is no difference in underlying survival distributions, the stratified statistic asymptotically follows a chi-square distribution with 1 degree of freedom. The stratified Wilcoxon statistic is defined in a similar manner.

Program 1.24 conducts the two stratified tests to evaluate the significance of treatment effect on survival in the severe sepsis trial adjusted for the baseline risk of mortality.

Program 1.24 Stratified comparison of survival distributions in four strata using the Wilcoxon and log-rank tests

```
proc lifetest data=sepsurv notable;
    ods select LogUniChisq WilUniChiSq;
    time survtime*censor(0);
    strata stratum;
    test treat;
    run;
```

Output from Program 1.24

```
        Univariate Chi-Squares for the Wilcoxon Test


              Test        Standard                    Pr >
Variable    Statistic     Deviation    Chi-Square   Chi-Square
  treat      23.8579        9.1317       6.8259       0.0090
```

```
       Univariate Chi-Squares for the Log-Rank Test

                  Test        Standard                     Pr >
  Variable     Statistic     Deviation    Chi-Square    Chi-Square
  treat         28.3261       10.7949       6.8855        0.0087
```

Output 1.24 shows the stratified Wilcoxon and log-rank statistics and *p*-values produced by Program 1.24. As in Program 1.23, the ODS statement is used (ods select LogUniChisq WilUniChiSq) to display the relevant sections of the PROC LIFETEST output. The stratified Wilcoxon and log-rank *p*-values are 0.0090 and 0.0087, respectively. The two *p*-values are almost identical and indicate that the adjusted effect of the experimental drug on survival is very strong. It is worth noting that the stratified Wilcoxon and log-rank statistics are much larger than the corresponding statistics computed in Strata 1, 2 and 4 (see Output 1.23). As expected, stratification increases the power of the testing procedures.

We can also compare the computed stratified Wilcoxon and log-rank *p*-values to those produced by the stratified Tarone-Ware and Harrington-Fleming tests. From the %LinRank macro, the stratified Tarone-Ware statistic is 6.8975 ($p = 0.0086$) and the stratified Harrington-Fleming statistic equals 6.9071 ($p = 0.0086$) if $\rho = 0.1$, and 6.8260 ($p = 0.0090$) if $\rho = 1$. The obtained results are in good agreement with the stratified analysis based on the Wilcoxon and log-rank tests.

1.4.2   Model-Based Tests

As in the case of categorical outcomes considered in Section 1.3, randomization-based tests for time-to-event data generally apply only to rather simple statistical problems, e.g., testing for equality of survival functions. Therefore, if we are interested in investigating effects of mixed (continuous and categorical) covariates on survival distributions or studying the prognostic ability of multiple factors, we need to rely on more flexible methods based on regression models for time-to-event data. Time-to-event outcome variables are analyzed using parametric models that explicitly specify the underlying survival distribution or using semi-parametric models such as proportional hazards models. Parametric regression models are less commonly used in a clinical trial setting and so this section focuses on testing procedures related to proportional hazards regression. See Allison (1995, Chapter 4) and Cantor (1997, Chapter 5) for a review of parametric regression inferences based on PROC LIFEREG.

To define a proportional hazards model introduced in the celebrated paper by Cox (1972), consider a two-arm clinical trial with a time-to-event endpoint. The hazard function $h_{ik}(t)$ for the *k*th patient in the *i*th treatment group is assumed to be

$$h_{ik}(t) = h_0(t) \exp\{X'_{ik}\beta_i\},$$

where $h_0(t)$ denotes the unspecified baseline hazard function, X_{ik} is a covariate vector, and β_i is a vector of unknown regression parameters. The model is called a proportional hazards model because the ratio of the hazard functions in the two treatment groups is constant over time. Cox (1972) proposed to estimate the regression parameters by maximizing the *partial likelihood* that does not involve the unknown baseline hazard function $h_0(t)$. Although the partial likelihood is conceptually different from the ordinary or conditional likelihood (for instance, it lacks a probabilistic interpretation), the resulting estimates of the β_i terms possess the same asymptotic properties as usual maximum likelihood estimates. As shown by Tsiatis (1981), maximum partial likelihood estimates are asymptotically consistent and normally distributed. For an extensive discussion of proportional hazards models, see Kalbfleisch and Prentice (1980, Chapters 4 and 5), Cox and Oakes (1984, Chapters 7 and 8) and Collett (1994, Chapter 3).

Proportional hazards models are implemented in PROC PHREG, which supports a wide range of modeling features, such as stratified models, discrete-time models and models with time-dependent covariates. Here we will focus on proportional hazards models with time-independent covariates because clinical outcome variables are generally adjusted for baseline values of explanatory variables. See Allison (1995, Chapter 5) for examples of fitting proportional hazards models with time-dependent covariates in PROC PHREG.

In order to perform a stratified analysis of time-to-event data in PROC PHREG, the stratification variable needs to be specified in the STRATA statement. The STRATA statement enables one to fit a proportional hazards model when the hazard functions in the two treatment groups are parallel within each stratum but not across the entire sample. Program 1.25 fits a stratified proportional hazards model to the survival data collected in the severe sepsis trial and plots the estimated survival functions. Note that PROC PHREG in SAS 8 does not have a CLASS statement and thus one needs to create dummy indicator variables similar to the TREAT variable in the SEPSURV data set to include categorical covariates and interaction terms in the model. In order to eliminate this tedious preprocessing step, SAS 9 has introduced an experimental version of PROC TPHREG with a CLASS statement.

Program 1.25 Stratified comparison of survival distributions in four strata using the proportional hazards regression

```
data cov;
    treat=0; output;
    treat=1; output;
proc phreg data=sepsurv;
    model survtime*censor(0)=treat/risklimits;
    strata stratum;
    baseline out=curve survival=est covariates=cov/nomean;

%macro PlotPH(stratum);
    axis1 minor=none label=(angle=90 "Survival") order=(0 to 1 by 0.5);
    axis2 minor=none label=("Time (h)") order=(0 to 700 by 350);
    symbol1 value=none color=black i=j line=1;
    symbol2 value=none color=black i=j line=20;
    data annotate;
        xsys="1"; ysys="1"; hsys="4"; x=50; y=20; position="5";
        size=1; text="Stratum &stratum"; function="label";
    proc gplot data=curve anno=annotate;
        where stratum=&stratum;
        plot est*survtime=treat/frame haxis=axis2 vaxis=axis1 nolegend;
        run;
        quit;
%mend PlotPH;

%PlotPH(1);
%PlotPH(2);
%PlotPH(3);
%PlotPH(4);
```

Output from Program 1.25

	Testing Global Null Hypothesis: BETA=0		
Test	Chi-Square	DF	Pr > ChiSq
Likelihood Ratio	6.8861	1	0.0087
Score	6.8855	1	0.0087
Wald	6.8332	1	0.0089

```
          Analysis of Maximum Likelihood Estimates

                    Parameter    Standard
Variable   DF       Estimate      Error    Chi-Square   Pr > ChiSq

treat      1        -0.24308     0.09299     6.8332       0.0089


  Analysis of Maximum Likelihood Estimates

                Hazard      95% Hazard Ratio
Variable        Ratio       Confidence Limits

treat           0.784       0.654        0.941
```

Figure 1.5 Estimated survival curves adjusted for the baseline risk of mortality in the experimental (- - -) and placebo (—) groups in the severe sepsis trial example

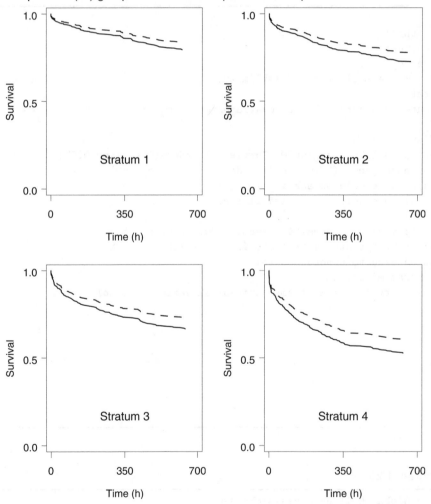

Output 1.25 displays the likelihood ratio, score and Wald statistics for testing the null hypothesis of no treatment effect. The three test statistics are very large in magnitude and indicate that the adjusted effect of the experimental drug on survival is highly significant. The score test is equivalent to the log-rank test for comparing survival distributions described earlier in Section 1.4.1. The two tests produce identical *p*-values when there are no tied event times (i.e., no two survival times are exactly the

same). In the presence of tied observations, the log-rank test is equivalent to the score test in PROC PHREG with a default adjustment for ties (Collett, 1994, Section 3.9). To see this, note that the adjusted log-rank statistic in Output 1.24 is equal to the score statistic in Output 1.25.

While Output 1.25 presents qualitative information similar to that generated by PROC LIFETEST, the lower panel describes the treatment difference in quantitative terms. Specifically, it shows the maximum partial likelihood estimate of the overall hazard ratio adjusted for the baseline risk of mortality and associated 95% confidence limits. The hazard ratio estimate equals 0.784, which means that the experimental drug reduces the hazard of death by 21.6%. The asymptotic 95% confidence interval for the true hazard ratio is equal to (0.654, 0.941). This confidence interval is requested by the RISKLIMITS option in the MODEL statement.

Figure 1.5 displays the estimated survival curves in the four strata from the CURVE data set generated by the BASELINE statement. In order to compute the survival curves in each of the two treatment groups, one needs to create a data set with two records, TREAT=0 and TREAT=1, and pass the name of this data set to the COVARIATES option in the BASELINE statement. Since Program 1.25 performs a stratified analysis of the survival data, the shapes of the estimated survival curves vary from stratum to stratum, but the treatment difference remains constant in the sense that the ratio of the hazard functions is the same in all four strata.

When fitting proportional hazards models in PROC PHREG, it is prudent to check whether the proportional hazards assumption is satisfied, i.e., the hazard ratio in any two treatment groups is approximately constant over time. Lagakos and Schoenfeld (1984) investigated the power of the score test when the assumption of proportional hazards is violated. They demonstrated that the score test is fairly robust with respect to modest deviations from the proportionality assumption but its efficiency decreases dramatically if the hazard functions cross. Allison (1995, Chapter 5) discussed simple graphical checks of the proportional hazards assumption in PROC PHREG.

Analysis of Time-to-Event Data with Ties

In general, analysis of discrete events of any kind becomes quite complicated in the presence of ties, i.e., events that occurred at exactly the same time. A frequency count of the SURVTIME variable shows that there is a fair number of ties in the SEPSURV data set. For example, four patients died 10 hours after the start of study drug administration and five patients died 15 hours after the start of study drug administration. Note that censored observations that occurred at the same time are not counted as ties.

The presence of tied event times considerably complicates the derivation of the partial likelihood function and subsequent inferences. In order to streamline the inferences in data sets with ties, several authors have proposed to ignore the exact partial likelihood function and to construct parameter estimates and significance tests based on an approximate partial likelihood function. Cox (1972) described an approximation to the partial likelihood function that assumes that the underlying time scale is discrete. Breslow (1974) proposed a simple approximation for the continuous-time case. The idea behind the Breslow method is that tied event times are treated as if there is a sequential ordering among them, and the likelihood function is averaged over all possible orderings. The Breslow method was improved by Efron (1977), who developed a more accurate approximation to the exact partial likelihood function. See Collett (1994, Section 3.3.2) for a good discussion of partial likelihood inferences in the presence of tied event times.

It is clear that different approaches to handling tied observations will yield different results and possibly lead to different conclusions. Since the method for handling ties was not explicitly specified in Program 1.25, PROC PHREG invoked the default method for handling ties developed by Breslow (1974). The Breslow method leads to biased parameter estimates in proportional hazards models when the number of ties is large. Since parameter estimates are biased toward 0, one is more likely to miss a significant effect when tied observations are accounted for inappropriately. For this reason, it is generally prudent to rely on more efficient adjustments for tied event times, such as the Efron method or two exact methods available in PROC PHREG (EXACT and DISCRETE methods). The EXACT method utilizes the exact marginal likelihood function considered by Kalbfleisch and Prentice (1973). The DISCRETE method not only changes the method for handling tied observations but also changes the underlying model. Specifically, the TIES=DISCRETE option fits a discrete-time proportional odds model. Note that exact methods requested by the TIES=EXACT and TIES=DISCRETE options are more time consuming than the Breslow or Efron methods; however, the difference is generally very small.

As an illustration, Program 1.26 fits a stratified proportional hazards model to the survival data collected in the severe sepsis trial using the Efron and exact methods for handling ties.

Program 1.26 Stratified comparison of survival distributions in four strata using the proportional hazards regression with the Efron and exact methods for handling ties

```
title "Efron method for handling ties";
proc phreg data=sepsurv;
    model survtime*censor(0)=treat/ties=efron;
    strata stratum;
    run;
title "Exact method for handling ties";
proc phreg data=sepsurv;
    model survtime*censor(0)=treat/ties=exact;
    strata stratum;
    run;
```

Output from Program 1.26

```
Efron method for handling ties

 Testing Global Null Hypothesis: BETA=0

Test                    Chi-Square      DF      Pr > ChiSq

Likelihood Ratio          6.9004         1         0.0086
Score                     6.8998         1         0.0086
Wald                      6.8475         1         0.0089

           Analysis of Maximum Likelihood Estimates

              Parameter     Standard
Variable  DF    Estimate       Error   Chi-Square  Pr > ChiSq

treat      1    -0.24333      0.09299     6.8475       0.0089

 Analysis of Maximum Likelihood Estimates

            Hazard       95% Hazard Ratio
Variable    Ratio       Confidence Limits

treat       0.784         0.653       0.941

Exact method for handling ties

Testing Global Null Hypothesis: BETA=0

Test                    Chi-Square      DF      Pr > ChiSq

Likelihood Ratio          6.9004         1         0.0086
Score                     6.8999         1         0.0086
Wald                      6.8475         1         0.0089
```

```
~~~~~~~~~~~~~~~~~~~~~~~~~~~~~~~~~~~~~~~~~~~~~~~~~~~~~~~~~~~~~~~~~~~~~~~~~
          Analysis of Maximum Likelihood Estimates


                 Parameter    Standard
  Variable  DF    Estimate       Error   Chi-Square   Pr > ChiSq

  treat      1    -0.24333     0.09299      6.8475       0.0089


  Analysis of Maximum Likelihood Estimates


               Hazard     95% Hazard Ratio
  Variable     Ratio     Confidence Limits

  treat        0.784     0.653        0.941
```

Output 1.26 lists the maximum partial likelihood estimates of the adjusted hazard ratio computed using the Efron and exact methods for handling tied survival times. The hazard ratio estimates as well as the 95% confidence limits are identical to those based on the default Breslow method in Output 1.25. Similarly, the likelihood ratio, score and Wald statistics are only slightly different from the corresponding statistics in Output 1.25. Note that the score test in Output 1.26 is no longer equivalent to the stratified log-rank test because Program 1.26 makes use of the Efron and exact methods for handling ties.

1.4.3 Summary

This section reviewed randomization- and model-based testing procedures for stratified time-to-event data implemented in PROC LIFETEST and PROC PHREG. As always, randomization-based procedures can be used only for fairly simple inferences, for example, for comparing survival distributions across treatment groups. Inferences based on regression models such as the Cox proportional hazards regression are more powerful and enable the statistician to examine the effect of both continuous and categorical covariates on survival functions and to study the prognostic ability of multiple factors.

The following properties of randomization-based testing procedures need to be kept in mind when choosing a test for a particular time-to-event endpoint:

- The log-rank test is superior to other tests under the assumption of proportional hazards but is prone to losing power when this assumption is not satisfied.

- The Wilcoxon test is less sensitive to events occurring toward the end of a study when few patients remain alive.

- The Tarone-Ware and Harrington-Fleming procedures serve as a robust alternative to the log-rank and Wilcoxon procedures and maintain power better than these two procedures across a broad range of alternative hypotheses.

In general, given the complex nature of time-to-event data, it may be a good idea to estimate the power of candidate tests against the desirable alternatives via simulations.

Model-based tests for time-to-event data described in this section rely on the Cox proportional hazards regression with partial likelihood inferences. Proportional hazards models implemented in PROC PHREG exhibit several features that are very useful in applications:

- The baseline hazard function is completely removed from the inference and therefore the statistician does not need to specify the underlying survival distribution in order to estimate model parameters.

- Estimation in a proportional hazards model is performed nonparametrically (the inferences are based on ranked event times), which makes the method considerably more robust.

- PROC PHREG supports a wide range of useful features such as stratification, time-dependent covariates and efficient adjustments for tied event times in proportional hazards models.

Inferences in proportional hazards models are generally fairly robust with respect to modest deviations from the proportionality assumption; however, a power loss is likely to occur when underlying hazards functions are not parallel to each other. When this happens, one can use the STRATA statement in PROC PHREG to fit separate proportional hazards models within each stratum.

1.5 Tests for Qualitative Interactions

The importance of an accurate assessment of the heterogeneity of the treatment effect among subgroups of interest has been emphasized in several publications and regulatory guidelines. For example, it is stated in Section 3.2 of the ICH guidance document "Statistical principles for clinical trials" (ICH E9) that

> If positive treatment effects are found in a trial with appreciable numbers of subjects per centre, there should generally be an exploration of the heterogeneity of treatment effects across centres, as this may affect the generalisability of the conclusions. Marked heterogeneity may be identified by graphical display of the results of individual centres or by analytical methods, such as a significance test of the treatment-by-centre interaction.

An appearance of reversed treatment differences in some strata does not always imply a true difference in the outcome variable across the chosen strata and may be due to random variation. In fact, one is virtually certain to encounter various degrees of inconsistency in the treatment effects across the strata. Senn (1997, Chapter 14) demonstrated that the probability of observing at least one effect reversal by chance increases rapidly with the number of strata; this probability exceeds 80% with 10 strata.

The following two definitions help differentiate between the cases of true and possibly random treatment-by-stratum interaction.

- A change in the magnitude of the treatment effect across the strata that does not affect the direction of the treatment difference is called a *quantitative* interaction. Quantitative interactions are very common in clinical trials, and studies in which the treatment difference is constant over all important subsets are rarely seen. Quantitative interactions typically represent natural variability in the outcome variable and need to be contrasted with extreme cases involving qualitative interactions.

- A treatment-by-stratum interaction is termed *qualitative* if the direction of the true treatment difference varies across the strata (it is worth noting that qualitative interactions are sometimes referred to as *crossover* interactions).

Analysis of qualitative interactions have received a considerable amount of attention in the statistical literature (Peto, 1982; Azzalini and Cox, 1984; Gail and Simon, 1985; Ciminera et al., 1993). The presence of qualitative interactions affects the interpretation of the overall trial outcome and influences the analysis of the treatment effect. Some authors, including Ciminera et al. (1993), advised against the use of quantitative interaction tests for judging the heterogeneity of the treatment effect and stressed that the treatment-by-stratum interaction needs to be included in the model only in the rare event of a pronounced qualitative interaction.

In this section we will review two approaches to testing for the presence of qualitative interactions proposed by Gail and Simon (1985) and Ciminera et al. (1993). Although the tests are most frequently applied in the context of multicenter trials, it is clear that they can be used for the analysis of any stratification scheme.

1.5.1 Gail-Simon Test

Gail and Simon (1985) proposed to formulate the problem of testing for qualitative interactions in terms of the following multivariate orthant hypotheses. Let δ_i denote the true treatment difference and let d_i and s_i denote the estimated treatment difference and associated standard error in the ith stratum. No qualitative interactions are present when the vector of the true treatment differences lies either in the positive orthant

$$O^+ = \{\delta_1 \geq 0, \ldots, \delta_m \geq 0\}$$

or in the negative orthant

$$O^- = \{\delta_1 \leq 0, \ldots, \delta_m \leq 0\}$$

of the m-dimensional parameter space. Gail and Simon described a likelihood ratio test for testing the null hypothesis of no qualitative interaction and demonstrated that it can be expressed as

$$Q = \min(Q^+, Q^-) > c,$$

where Q^+ and Q^- are given by

$$Q^+ = \sum_{i=1}^{m} \frac{d_i^2}{s_i^2} I(d_i > 0), \quad Q^- = \sum_{i=1}^{m} \frac{d_i^2}{s_i^2} I(d_i < 0),$$

and c is an appropriate critical value. The Q^+ and Q^- statistics summarize the contribution of the positive and negative treatment differences, respectively. Gail and Simon also showed that the Q statistic follows a fairly complex distribution based on a weighted sum of chi-square distributions. This distribution can be used to derive the following formula for calculating the likelihood ratio p-value:

$$p = \sum_{i=1}^{m-1} (1 - F_i(Q)) \text{Bin}_{i,m-1}(0.5),$$

where $F_i(x)$ is the cumulative distribution function of the chi-square distribution with i degrees of freedom and $\text{Bin}_{i,m-1}(0.5)$ is the binomial probability mass function with success probability 0.5.

The described test is two-sided in the sense that the null hypothesis of no qualitative interaction is rejected when both Q^+ and Q^- are large enough. The Gail-Simon method is easy to extend to one-sided settings to test (i) whether the true treatment differences are all positive or (ii) whether the true treatment differences are all negative. The p-value associated with the likelihood ratio test for (i) is equal to

$$p = \sum_{i=1}^{m} (1 - F_i(Q^-)) \text{Bin}_{i,m}(0.5)$$

and, similarly, the likelihood ratio p-value for testing (ii) is given by

$$p = \sum_{i=1}^{m} (1 - F_i(Q^+)) \text{Bin}_{i,m}(0.5).$$

EXAMPLE: Multicenter Depression Trial

We will first apply the introduced method to test for qualitative interaction in a clinical trial with a continuous endpoint. Program 1.27 carries out the introduced Gail-Simon test to examine the nature of the treatment-by-stratum interaction in the depression trial example of Section 1.2. The program calls the %GailSimon macro provided in the Appendix to compute the one- and two-sided likelihood ratio p-values. The macro has the following parameters:

- DATASET is the data set with test statistics and associated standard errors for each stratum.

- EST specifies the name of the variable containing the test statistics.

- STDERR specifies the name of the variable containing the standard errors.

- TESTTYPE is the type of the test to be carried out, one-sided Gail-Simon test for positive differences ("P"), one-sided Gail-Simon test for negative differences ("N") or two-sided Gail-Simon test ("T"), respectively.

Program 1.27 Analysis of the qualitative interaction in the depression trial example using the Gail-Simon test

```
proc sort data=hamd17;
    by drug center;
proc means data=hamd17 noprint;
    where drug="P";
    by center;
    var change;
    output out=plac mean=mp var=vp n=np;
proc means data=hamd17 noprint;
    where drug="D";
    by center;
    var change;
    output out=drug mean=md var=vd n=nd;
data comb;
    merge plac drug;
    by center;
    d=md-mp;
    n=np+nd;
    stderr=sqrt((1/np+1/nd)*((np-1)*vp+(nd-1)*vd)/(n-2));
%GailSimon(dataset=comb,est=d,stderr=stderr,testtype="P");
%GailSimon(dataset=comb,est=d,stderr=stderr,testtype="N");
%GailSimon(dataset=comb,est=d,stderr=stderr,testtype="T");
```

Output from Program 1.27

```
One-sided Gail-Simon test for positive differences

  Test
statistic    P-value


  7.647      0.0465


One-sided Gail-Simon test for negative differences

  Test
statistic    P-value

 57.750      0.0000


Two-sided Gail-Simon test

  Test
statistic    P-value


  7.647      0.0297
```

We can see from Output 1.27 that all three likelihood ratio p-values are significant at the 5% level. The significance of the one-sided p-value for negative differences ($Q^- = 57.750$, $p < 0.0001$) is hardly surprising because it indicates that the true treatment differences are highly unlikely to be all negative. The other two tests are more informative and convey the same message, namely, the null hypothesis that the positive treatment effect is consistent across the five selected centers can be rejected. This means that the magnitude of the negative treatment difference at Center 101 is too large to be explained by chance and indicates the presence of qualitative interaction. Since Center 101 appears to be an outlier, it is prudent to carefully study the demographic and clinical characteristics of the patients enrolled at that site as well as consistency of the HAMD17 assessments to better understand the observed discrepancy.

EXAMPLE: Severe Sepsis Trial

Program 1.28 illustrates the use of the Gail-Simon test in the analysis of stratified categorical data. Consider the clinical trial in patients with severe sepsis introduced in Section 1.3. As shown in Figure 1.3, the treatment difference varies significantly across the four strata representing different levels of baseline risk of mortality. The survival rates are higher in patients treated with the experimental drug in Strata 2, 3 and 4. However, the treatment difference appears to be reversed in Stratum 1 and thus it is reasonable to ask whether Stratum 1 is qualitatively different from the other strata. The program below utilizes the %GailSimon macro to test the consistency of the treatment differences in 28-day mortality across the 4 strata.

Program 1.28 Analysis of the qualitative interaction in the severe sepsis trial example using the Gail-Simon test

```
proc sort data=sepsis;
    by stratum;
data est;
    set sepsis;
    by stratum;
    retain ad dd ap dp;
    if therapy="Drug" and outcome="Alive" then ad=count;
    if therapy="Drug" and outcome="Dead" then dd=count;
    if therapy="Placebo" and outcome="Alive" then ap=count;
    if therapy="Placebo" and outcome="Dead" then dp=count;
    survd=ad/(ad+dd);
    survp=ap/(ap+dp);
    d=survd-survp;
    stderr=sqrt(survd*(1-survd)/(ad+dd)+survp*(1-survp)/(ap+dp));
    if last.stratum=1;
%GailSimon(dataset=est,est=d,stderr=stderr,testtype="P");
%GailSimon(dataset=est,est=d,stderr=stderr,testtype="N");
%GailSimon(dataset=est,est=d,stderr=stderr,testtype="T");
```

Output from Program 1.28

```
One-sided Gail-Simon test for positive differences

   Test
statistic    P-value

  0.855      0.6005

One-sided Gail-Simon test for negative differences

   Test
statistic    P-value

 12.631      0.0030

Two-sided Gail-Simon test
   Test
statistic    P-value

  0.855      0.4822
```

Both the one-sided statistic for positive differences ($Q^+ = 0.855$) and two-sided statistic ($Q = 0.855$) in Output 1.28 indicate that there is little evidence in the data to reject the null hypothesis of no qualitative interaction. Despite the reversed treatment difference in Stratum 1, the Gail-Simon statistics are not large enough to conclude that this stratum is qualitatively different from the other strata at the 5% significance level. The highly nonsignificant p-values produced by the Gail-Simon test need to be contrasted with the Breslow-Day p-value displayed in Output 1.13. An application of the Breslow-Day test for quantitative homogeneity of odds ratios across the four strata in the same severe sepsis trial yielded a p-value of 0.0899, which is clearly much closer to being significant than the conservative Gail-Simon p-values.

Finally, as in Output 1.27, the significant one-sided Gail-Simon statistic for negative differences ($Q^- = 12.631$) suggests that the stratum-specific treatment differences in survival are very unlikely to be all negative.

1.5.2 Pushback Test

Ciminera et al. (1993) described an alternative test for qualitative interactions based on the following idea. To determine whether or not the observed treatment difference in a particular stratum is consistent with the rest of the data, we can order the standardized treatment differences and then compare them with the expected values computed from the distribution of appropriately defined order statistics. This comparison will show which of the strata, if any, are more extreme than expected under the assumption of homogeneity.

As before, let d_i and s_i denote the estimated treatment difference and the associated standard error in the ith stratum, respectively. Ciminera et al. (1993) proposed the following test for qualitative interactions.

1. Compute the median of $d_1, \ldots, d_m$ and denote it by m. Convert the observed treatment differences into standardized deviations by computing $\tau_i = (d_i - m)/s_i, i = 1, \ldots, m$.

2. Consider the ordered standardized deviations $\tau_{(1)} < \ldots < \tau_{(m)}$ and define the adjusted (or *pushed-back*) standardized deviations $\rho_i = \tau_{(i)} - t_i$, where $t_1, \ldots, t_m$ are pushback adjustments based on the order statistics from a normal or t distribution. Let $\rho_i = 0$ if the sign of $\tau_{(i)} - t_i$ is different from the sign of $\tau_{(i)}$. In other words, only partial adjustment is performed if t_i is more extreme than the standardized deviation $\tau_{(i)}$.

3. Compute the destandardized deviations $d_i^* = s_i \rho_i + m, i = 1, \ldots, m$. The appearance of opposite signs among $d_1^*, \ldots, d_m^*$ is interpreted as evidence of qualitative interaction.

Ciminera et al. (1993) described several methods for calculating the pushback adjustments based on normal and t distributions. The power of the pushback procedure is maximized when $t_1, \ldots, t_m$ are based on medians of normal order statistics, i.e.,

$$t_i = \Phi^{-1}\left(\frac{3i - 1}{3m + 1}\right), \quad i = 1, \ldots, m,$$

where $\Phi(x)$ is the cumulative distribution function of the standard normal distribution. On the other hand, the use of t distribution percentiles leads to the least powerful procedure. In this case,

$$t_i = \begin{cases} T_{v_i}^{-1}(B_{i,m-i+1}^{-1}(\alpha)) & \text{if } d_i \leq m, \\ T_{v_i}^{-1}(B_{i,m-i+1}^{-1}(1-\alpha)) & \text{if } d_i > m, \\ 0 \text{ if } m \text{ is odd and } i = (m+1)/2 & i = 1, \ldots, m, \end{cases}$$

where $T_{v_i}(x)$ is the cumulative distribution function of the t distribution with v_i degrees of freedom, $v_i = n_{1i} + n_{2i} - 2$, $B_{i,m-i+1}(x)$ is the cumulative distribution function of the beta distribution with parameters i and $m - i + 1$, and α is a pre-specified percentile. Ciminera et al. (1993) recommended using $\alpha = 0.1$ and indicated that this value corresponds to the 10% probability of erroneously detecting a qualitative interaction.

%Pushback Macro

We will now demonstrate how to carry out the pushback test in order to evaluate the significance of qualitative treatment-by-center interaction in the depression trial example of Section 1.2. The data from the depression trial are analyzed using the %Pushback macro found in the Appendix. This macro implements the pushback test for qualitative interactions using the weighted median with the normal or *t*-distribution adjustment schemes. The %Pushback macro has the following parameters:

- DATASET is the data set with test statistics, associated standard errors and numbers of patients for each strata.
- EST specifies the name of the variable containing the test statistics.
- STDERR specifies the name of the variable containing the standard errors.
- N specifies the name of the variable containing the numbers of patients.
- TESTTYPE is the type of the test to be carried out, pushback test using the order statistics from a normal distribution ("N") or pushback test using the order statistics from a *t* distribution ("T"), respectively.

Pushback Test Based on Order Statistics from a Normal Distribution

Program 1.29 carries out the pushback test using the medians of normal order statistics. The standardized deviations are computed from the COMB data set created in Program 1.27.

Program 1.29 Analysis of the qualitative interaction in the depression trial example using the pushback test based on the medians of normal order statistics

```
%Pushback(dataset=comb,est=d,stderr=stderr,n=n,
    testtype="N",outdata=pushadj);
axis1 order=(-8 to 12 by 4);
axis2 label=("Ordered strata");
symbol1 value=circle color=black i=none;
proc gplot data=pushadj;
    plot d*ordstr/frame haxis=axis2 vaxis=axis1 vref=0 lvref=34;
    run;
axis1 order=(-8 to 12 by 4);
axis2 label=("Ordered strata");
symbol1 value=circle color=black i=none;
symbol2 value=triangle color=black i=none;
proc gplot data=pushadj;
    plot tau*ordstr t*ordstr/frame overlay haxis=axis2 vaxis=axis1
    vref=0 lvref=34;
    run;
axis1 order=(-8 to 12 by 4);
axis2 label=("Ordered strata");
symbol1 value=circle color=black i=none;
proc gplot data=pushadj;
    plot rho*ordstr/frame haxis=axis2 vaxis=axis1 vref=0 lvref=34;
    run;
axis1 order=(-8 to 12 by 4);
axis2 label=("Ordered strata");
symbol1 value=circle color=black i=none;
proc gplot data=pushadj;
    plot dstar*ordstr/frame haxis=axis2 vaxis=axis1 vref=0 lvref=34;
    run;
```

The output of Program 1.29 is displayed in Figure 1.6. Figure 1.6 illustrates the three data manipulations steps used in the pushback procedure. Note that the centers have been rearranged to

Figure 1.6 Analysis of the qualitative interaction in the depression trial using the pushback test based on the medians of normal order statistics

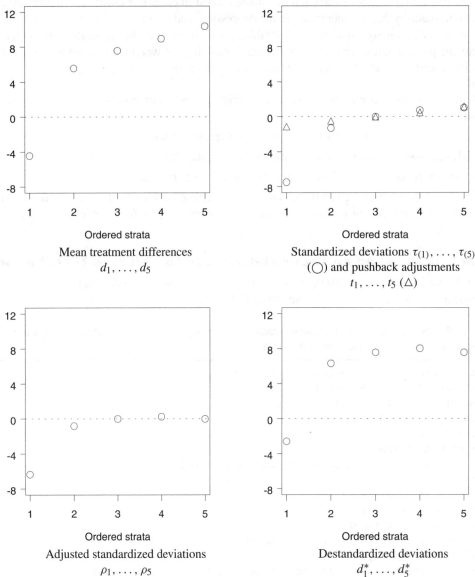

facilitate the interpretation of the findings. The numbers on the horizontal axis represent the ranks chosen in such a way that $\tau_{(1)} < \ldots < \tau_{(5)}$. Table 1.7 shows the ranks assigned to each of the original strata.

Table 1.7 Ordered strata

Ordered strata	1	2	3	4	5
Original strata	2	3	4	1	5
Center	101	102	103	100	104

Comparing the upper-right panel (standardized deviations) and the lower-left panel (adjusted standardized deviations) in Figure 1.6, we can see that the standardized deviations $\tau_{(3)}$ and $\tau_{(5)}$ were set to 0 after the pushback adjustment because they were not extreme enough. Further, the destandardized deviations plotted in the lower-right panel indicate the presence of qualitative treatment-by-center interaction. To see this, note that the four largest destandardized deviations are positive whereas the smallest destandardized deviation has a negative value. This fact indicates that the treatment difference observed at Center 101 is not consistent with the rest of the data.

Pushback Test Based on Order Statistics from a *t* Distribution

To compare the methods for calculating the pushback adjustments proposed by Ciminera et al. (1993), Program 1.30 carries out the pushback test based on the outer 90th percentiles of the *t* distribution.

Program 1.30 Analysis of the qualitative interaction in the depression trial example using the pushback test based on the outer 90th percentiles of the *t* distribution

```
%Pushback(dataset=comb,est=d,stderr=stderr,n=n,
    testtype="T",outdata=pushadj);
axis1 order=(-8 to 12 by 4);
axis2 label=("Ordered strata");
symbol1 value=circle color=black i=none;
proc gplot data=pushadj;
    plot d*ordstr/frame haxis=axis2 vaxis=axis1 vref=0 lvref=34;
    run;
axis1 order=(-8 to 12 by 4);
axis2 label=("Ordered strata");
symbol1 value=circle color=black i=none;
symbol2 value=triangle color=black i=none;
proc gplot data=pushadj;
    plot tau*ordstr t*ordstr/frame overlay haxis=axis2 vaxis=axis1
    vref=0 lvref=34;
    run;
axis1 order=(-8 to 12 by 4);
axis2 label=("Ordered strata");
symbol1 value=circle color=black i=none;
proc gplot data=pushadj;
    plot rho*ordstr/frame haxis=axis2 vaxis=axis1 vref=0 lvref=34;
    run;
axis1 order=(-8 to 12 by 4);
axis2 label=("Ordered strata");
symbol1 value=circle color=black i=none;
proc gplot data=pushadj;
    plot dstar*ordstr/frame haxis=axis2 vaxis=axis1 vref=0 lvref=34;
    run;
```

The output of Program 1.30 is displayed in Figure 1.7. We see from the figure that the smallest destandardized deviation corresponding to Center 101 is closer to 0 and thus there is less evidence of qualitative treatment-by-center interaction when the pushback procedure is based on *t* distribution percentiles. This is explained by the fact that the adjustments computed from a *t* distribution are a bit more extreme than those computed from a normal distribution. Apart from Center 101, the difference between the pushback adjustment schemes based on the normal and *t* distributions is rather small. As demonstrated by Ciminera et al. (1993), this difference becomes more pronounced as the number of strata increases.

Comparison of the Gail-Simon and Pushback Tests

No formal comparison of the Gail-Simon and pushback tests for qualitative interactions has been performed in the literature. Ciminera et al. (1993) briefly compared the performance of the two testing procedures and noted that the pushback procedure had fairly low power but was more sensitive than the Gail-Simon procedure in one example they studied. The following simple exercise indicates that the pushback procedure is also more powerful in the depression trial example. To judge the sensitivity of the

Figure 1.7 Analysis of the qualitative interaction in the depression trial using the pushback test based on the outer 90th percentiles of the *t* distribution

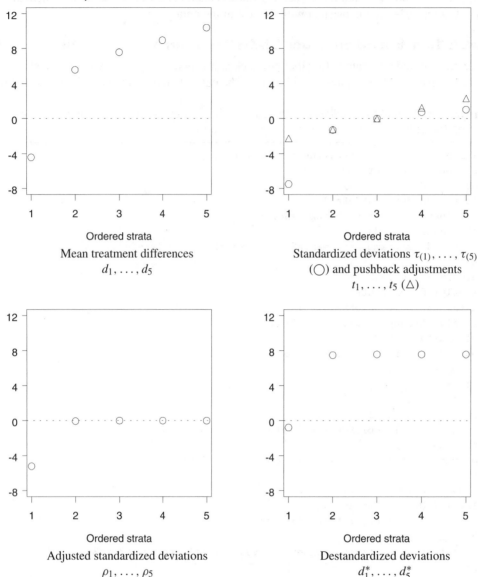

Mean treatment differences
$d_1, \ldots, d_5$

Standardized deviations $\tau_{(1)}, \ldots, \tau_{(5)}$
($\bigcirc$) and pushback adjustments
$t_1, \ldots, t_5$ ($\triangle$)

Adjusted standardized deviations
$\rho_1, \ldots, \rho_5$

Destandardized deviations
$d_1^*, \ldots, d_5^*$

two tests for qualitative interactions, one can consider a range of mean treatment differences at Center 101. By rerunning Program 1.27, one can easily verify that the smallest value of the mean treatment difference at this center that leads to a significant two-sided Gail-Simon statistic is -4.09. Similarly, by rerunning Programs 1.29 and 1.30, one can determine that the corresponding mean treatment differences for the pushback procedures based on the normal and t distributions are equal to -1.85 and -3.7, respectively. We can see that the pushback procedure can show substantial evidence of qualitative interaction when the Gail-Simon statistic is not significant.

1.5.3   Summary

This section discussed the Gail-Simon and pushback tests for qualitative interaction. Both tests rely on stratum-specific summary statistics and therefore they can be carried out in clinical trials with continuous, categorical or time-to-event endpoints. The Gail-Simon procedure can be used in confirmatory analyses and the pushback testing procedure will likely be more useful in exploratory analyses.

As we pointed out in the introduction, tests for qualitative interaction have found many applications in clinical trials. These tests facilitate the analysis of treatment-by-stratum interactions, help identify subgroups of patients who have experienced the most pronounced beneficial effect, and play an important role in sensitivity analyses. For example, one can carry out the tests introduced in this section to find one or several centers in a multicenter trial that are qualitatively different from the rest of the trial population. Although it may be difficult to justify an exclusion of these centers from the final analysis in the present regulatory environment, the obtained knowledge provides a basis for interesting sensitivity analyses and ultimately leads to a better understanding of the trial results.

Multiple Comparisons and Multiple Endpoints

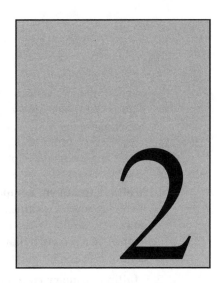

This chapter discusses statistical strategies for handling multiplicity issues arising in clinical trials. It covers basic single-step multiple tests and more advanced closed, fixed-sequence and resampling-based multiple testing procedures. The chapter also reviews methods used in the analysis of multiple endpoints and gatekeeping testing strategies for clinical trials with multiple objectives and for dose-finding studies.

2.1 Introduction

Multiplicity problems arise in virtually every clinical trial. They are caused by multiple analyses performed on the same data. It is well known that performing multiple tests in a univariate manner by using unadjusted p-values increases the overall probability of false-positive outcomes. This problem is recognized by both drug developers and regulators. Regulatory agencies mandate a strict control of the overall Type I error rate in clinical trials because false positive trial findings could lead to approval of inefficacious drugs. The guidance document entitled "Points to consider on multiplicity issues in clinical trials" released by the European Committee for Proprietary Medicinal Products (CPMP) on September 19, 2002, emphasized the importance of addressing multiplicity issues in clinical trials by stating that

> a clinical study that requires no adjustment of the Type I error is one that consists of two treatment groups, that uses a single primary variable, and has a confirmatory statistical strategy that prespecifies just one single null hypothesis relating to the primary variable and no interim analysis.

Along the same line, the ICH E9 guidance document on statistical principles for clinical trials states that

> in confirmatory analyses, any aspects of multiplicity ... should be identified in the protocol; adjustment should always be considered and the details of any adjustment procedure ... should be set out in the analysis plan.

There are several types of multiple testing problems encountered in clinical trials:

1. **Multiple treatment comparisons.** Most commonly, multiple testing is encountered in clinical trials involving several treatment groups. The majority of Phase II trials are designed to assess the efficacy and safety profile of several doses of an experimental drug compared to a placebo or an active control. Performing multiple comparisons of different dose levels of an experimental drug and a control causes multiplicity problems.

2. **Multiple primary endpoints.** Multiplicity is also caused by multiple criteria for assessing the efficacy or safety of an experimental drug. The multiple criteria are required to accurately characterize various aspects of the expected therapeutic benefits. For example, the efficacy profile of cardiovascular drugs is typically evaluated using multiple outcome variables such as all-cause mortality, nonfatal myocardial infarction, or refractory angina/urgent revascularization.

3. **Multiple secondary analyses.** It is commonly accepted that multiplicity issues in the primary analysis must be addressed in all efficacy trials; however, multiplicity adjustments are rarely performed with respect to secondary and subgroup analyses. Recent publications emphasize the need to carefully address these types of multiplicity issues in the trial protocol and to develop a hierarchy of analyses that includes the primary analysis and the most important secondary and subgroup analyses.

Overview

This chapter deals with statistical issues related to multiple comparisons and multiple endpoints in clinical trials. Sections 2.2 and 2.3 discuss single-step tests (e.g., Bonferroni test) and more powerful closed testing procedures such as the Holm and Hommel procedures. Section 2.4 covers fixed-sequence testing methods and Section 2.5 briefly reviews resampling-based methods for multiplicity adjustment with emphasis on clinical trial applications. See Hochberg and Tamhane (1987), Westfall and Young (1993) and Hsu (1996) for a more detailed discussion of issues related to multiple analyses. Westfall et al. (1999) and Westfall and Tobias (2000) provide an excellent overview of multiple comparison procedures with a large number of SAS examples.

Section 2.6 addresses multiplicity problems arising in clinical trials with multiple endpoints. There appears to be no monograph that provides a detailed coverage of statistical issues in the analysis of multiple clinical endpoints. The interested reader is referred to review papers by Pocock, Geller and Tsiatis (1987), Lee (1994) and Wassmer et al. (1999).

Finally, Section 2.7 discusses multiple testing procedures for families of hypotheses with a sequential structure. Sequential families are encountered in clinical trials with multiple objectives (based on primary, secondary and possibly tertiary endpoints) and in dose-finding studies. For a summary of recent research in this area, see Westfall and Krishen (2001) and Dmitrienko, Offen and Westfall (2003).

Weak and Strong Control of Familywise Error Rate

To control the overall error rate in situations involving multiple testing, the statistician needs to answer the billion-dollar question (the billion-dollar part is not an exaggeration in the context of modern drug development!):

> How does one define the family of null hypotheses to be tested and the incorrect decisions whose likelihood needs to be controlled?

In most cases, the family of hypotheses is defined at the trial level. This means that all multiple analyses are to be performed in such a way that the trialwise error rate is maintained at the prespecified level.

Further, there are two definitions of the overall (familywise) error rate. We need to understand what inferences we intend to perform in order to choose the right definition of the overall error rate and an appropriate multiple testing method. To illustrate, consider the following example that will be used throughout Sections 2.2 and 2.3.

EXAMPLE: Dose-Finding Hypertension Trial

Suppose that a dose-finding trial has been conducted to compare low, medium and high doses of a new antihypertensive drug (labeled L, M and H) to a placebo (labeled P). The primary efficacy variable is diastolic blood pressure. Doses that provide a clinically relevant mean reduction in diastolic blood pressure will be declared efficacious.

Let μ_P denote the mean reduction in diastolic blood pressure in the placebo group. Similarly, μ_L, μ_M and μ_H denote the mean reduction in diastolic blood pressure in the low, medium and high dose groups, respectively. The null hypothesis of equality of μ_P, μ_L, μ_M and μ_H (known as the *global null hypothesis*) can be tested in the hypertension trial example using the usual F-test. The F-test is said to preserve the overall Type I error rate in the *weak* sense, which means that it controls the likelihood of rejecting the global null hypothesis when all individual hypotheses are simultaneously true.

The weak control of the familywise error rate is appropriate only if we want to make a statement about the global null hypothesis. In order to test the effects of the individual doses on diastolic blood pressure, we need to control the probability of erroneously rejecting any true null hypothesis regardless of which and how many null hypotheses are true. This is referred to as the *strong control of the familywise error rate*. For example, the procedure proposed by Dunnett (1955) can be used to test the global null hypothesis and, at the same time, to provide information about individual dose-placebo comparisons (e.g., μ_P versus μ_L, μ_P versus μ_M and μ_P versus μ_H). This procedure controls the familywise error rate in the strong sense. Given the importance of the strong control of Type I outcomes in clinical applications, this chapter will focus only on methods that preserve the familywise error rate in the strong sense.

It is worth noting that there are other definitions of the likelihood of an incorrect decision, such as the false discovery rate introduced by Benjamini and Hochberg (1995). Multiple tests controlling the false discovery rate are more powerful (and more liberal) than tests designed to protect the familywise error rate in the strong sense and are useful in multiplicity problems with a large number of null hypotheses. False discovery rate methods are widely used in preclinical research (e.g., genetics) and have recently been applied to the analysis of clinical trial data. Mehrotra and Heyse (2001) used the false discovery rate methodology to develop an efficient strategy for handling multiplicity issues in the evaluation of safety endpoints. Another interesting strategy is to employ Bayesian methods in multiplicity adjustments. Bayesian approaches to multiple testing with clinical trial applications have been investigated in several publications; see, for example, Westfall et al. (1999, Chapter 13) and Gönen, Westfall and Johnson (2003).

Multiple Tests Based on Marginal *p*-Values

Sections 2.2 and 2.3 deal with popular multiple tests based on marginal *p*-values. These tests can be thought of as "distribution-free" tests because they rely on elementary probability inequalities and thus do not depend on the joint distribution of test statistics. Marginal multiple testing procedures are intuitive and easy to apply. These procedures offer a simple way to "fix" Type I error inflation problems in any situation involving multiple testing—e.g., in clinical trials with multiple treatment comparisons, multiple endpoints or interim analyses. Therefore, it should not be surprising that tests based on marginal *p*-values enjoy much popularity in clinical applications (Chi, 1998).

The obvious downside of marginal tests is that they rely on the marginal distribution of individual test statistics and ignore the underlying correlation structure. As a result, multiple tests that make full use of the joint distribution of test statistics outperform marginal tests, especially when the test statistics are highly correlated or the number of multiple analyses is large.

2.2   Single-Step Tests

There are two important classes of multiple testing procedures that will be considered in this and subsequent sections: single-step and stepwise tests. Both single-step and stepwise tests fall in a very broad class of closed testing procedures that will be reviewed in Section 2.3. Single-step methods (e.g., the Bonferroni method) test each null hypothesis of interest independently of the other hypotheses. In other words, the order in which the null hypotheses are examined is not important and the multiple inferences can be thought of as being performed in a single step. In contrast, stepwise testing procedures (e.g., the Holm stepwise procedure) test one hypothesis at a time in a sequential manner. As a result, some of the null hypotheses may not be tested at all. They may be either retained or rejected by implication. Stepwise procedures are superior to simple single-step tests in the sense that they increase the number of rejected null hypotheses without inflating the familywise error rate.

Suppose we plan to carry out m significance tests corresponding to a family of null hypotheses denoted by $H_1, \ldots, H_m$. The global null hypothesis is defined as the intersection of $H_1, \ldots, H_m$, i.e.,

$$\{H_1 \text{ and } H_2 \text{ and } \ldots \text{ and } H_m\}.$$

Let $p_1, \ldots, p_m$ denote the individual p-values generated by the significance tests. The ordered p-values $p_{(1)}, \ldots, p_{(m)}$ are defined in such a way that

$$p_{(1)} \leq p_{(2)} \leq \cdots \leq p_{(m)}.$$

We wish to devise a simultaneous test for the family of null hypotheses. The test will be based on a suitable adjustment for multiplicity to keep the familywise error rate at the prespecified α level. Multiplicity adjustments are performed by modifying the individual decision rules—i.e., by adjusting either the individual p-values or significance levels (p-values are adjusted upward or significance levels are adjusted downward). To define adjusted p-values, we adopt the definition proposed by Westfall and Young (1993). According to this definition, the adjusted p-value equals the smallest significance level for which one would reject the corresponding null hypothesis.

There are three popular multiplicity adjustment methods (the Bonferroni, Šidák and Simes methods) that underlie the majority of multiple testing procedures based on marginal p-values. The methods are briefly discussed below.

Bonferroni and Šidák Methods

The Bonferroni and Šidák methods are perhaps the most widely used multiplicity adjustments. These methods are available in a large number of SAS procedures, such as PROC GLM, PROC MIXED, and PROC MULTTEST. Their implementation is very straightforward. The Bonferroni multiple test rejects H_i if $p_i \leq \alpha/m$, and the Šidák multiple test rejects H_i if $p_i \leq 1 - (1-\alpha)^{1/m}$, where $i = 1, \ldots, m$. The individual adjusted p-values for the two tests are given by

$$\widetilde{p}_i = mp_i \text{ (Bonferroni)}, \quad \widetilde{p}_i = 1 - (1 - p_i)^m \text{ (Šidák)}, \quad i = 1, \ldots, m.$$

Using the Bonferroni inequality, it is easy to show that the Bonferroni multiple test controls the familywise error rate in the strong sense for any joint distribution of the raw p-values. However, the Šidák multiple test does not always preserve the familywise error rate. Šidák (1967) demonstrated that the size of this test does not exceed α when the individual test statistics are either independent or follow a multivariate normal distribution. Holland and Copenhaver (1987) described a broad set of assumptions under which the Šidák test controls the familywise error rate—for example, when the test statistics follow t and some other distributions.

The Bonferroni and Šidák tests can also be used to test the global null hypothesis. The global hypothesis is rejected whenever any of the individual null hypotheses is rejected. This means that the

Bonferroni global test rejects the global hypothesis if $p_i \le \alpha/m$ for at least one $i = 1, \ldots, m$. Likewise, the Šidák global test rejects the global hypothesis if $p_i \le 1 - (1 - \alpha)^{1/m}$ for at least one $i = 1, \ldots, m$.

The adjusted p-values associated with the Bonferroni and Šidák global tests are given by

$$\widetilde{p}_B = m \min(p_1, \ldots, p_m) \text{ (Bonferroni)},$$

$$\widetilde{p}_S = 1 - (1 - \min(p_1, \ldots, p_m))^m \text{ (Šidák)}.$$

In other words, the Bonferroni and Šidák global tests reject the global null hypothesis if $\widetilde{p}_B \le \alpha$ and $\widetilde{p}_S \le \alpha$, respectively. Although it may not be immediately obvious, the Bonferroni and Šidák global tests are more important than the corresponding multiple tests. It will be shown in Section 2.3 that, utilizing these global tests, one can construct closed testing procedures that are uniformly more powerful than the Bonferroni and Šidák multiple tests.

It is easy to show that the Šidák correction is uniformly better than the Bonferroni correction (Hsu, 1996, Section 1.3.5). The difference between these two corrections is rather small when the raw p-values are small. The two tests are known to be very conservative when the individual test statistics are highly correlated. The adjusted p-values generated by the Bonferroni and Šidák procedures are considerably larger than they need to be to maintain the familywise error rate at the desired level.

To illustrate the Bonferroni and Šidák adjustments (as well as other multiple tests that will be discussed later in this section), consider the dose-finding hypertension trial example. Recall that μ_P denotes the mean reduction in diastolic blood pressure in the placebo group and μ_L, μ_M and μ_H denote the mean reduction in diastolic blood pressure in the low, medium and high dose groups, respectively. Negative values of μ_L, μ_M and μ_H indicate an improvement in diastolic blood pressure. The following null hypotheses are tested in the trial:

$$H_L = \{\mu_P - \mu_L \le \delta\}, \quad H_M = \{\mu_P - \mu_M \le \delta\}, \quad H_H = \{\mu_P - \mu_H \le \delta\},$$

where δ represents a clinically significant improvement over placebo. The treatment means are compared using the two-sample t-test. Table 2.1 shows p-values generated by the three dose-placebo comparisons under three scenarios.

Table 2.1 Dose-placebo comparisons in hypertension trial

Comparison	L vs. P	M vs. P	H vs. P
Scenario 1	$p_L = 0.047$	$p_M = 0.0167$	$p_H = 0.015$
Scenario 2	$p_L = 0.047$	$p_M = 0.027$	$p_H = 0.015$
Scenario 3	$p_L = 0.053$	$p_M = 0.026$	$p_H = 0.017$

Program 2.1 computes adjusted p-values produced by the Bonferroni and Šidák tests under Scenario 1. The two tests are requested by the BONFERRONI and SIDAK options in PROC MULTTEST.

Program 2.1 Analysis of the hypertension trial using the Bonferroni and Šidák tests

```
data antihyp1;
    input test $ raw_p @@;
    datalines;
    L 0.047 M 0.0167 H 0.015
    ;

proc multtest pdata=antihyp1 bonferroni sidak out=adjp;
```

```
axis1 minor=none order=(0 to 0.15 by 0.05) label=(angle=90 "P-value");
axis2 minor=none value=("Low" "Medium" "High") label=("Dose")
    order=("L" "M" "H");
symbol1 value=circle color=black i=j;
symbol2 value=diamond color=black i=j;
symbol3 value=triangle color=black i=j;
proc gplot data=adjp;
    plot raw_p*test bon_p*test sid_p*test/frame overlay nolegend
    haxis=axis2 vaxis=axis1 vref=0.05 lvref=34;
    run;
```

Figure 2.1 Analysis of the hypertension trial using the Bonferroni and Šidák tests. Raw *p*-value (◯), Bonferroni-adjusted *p*-value (◇) and Šidák-adjusted *p*-value (△).

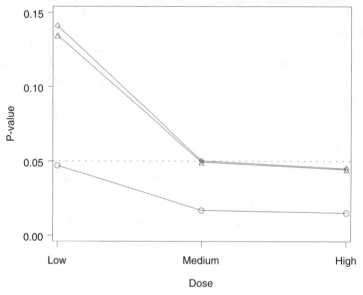

The output of Program 2.1 is shown in Figure 2.1. The figure displays the adjusted *p*-values produced by the Bonferroni and Šidák tests plotted along with the corresponding raw *p*-values. The figure indicates that the raw *p*-values associated with all three dose-placebo comparisons are significant at the 5% level, yet only the high dose is significantly different from placebo after the Bonferroni adjustment for multiplicity ($p = 0.045$). The Šidá k-adjusted *p*-values are consistently less than the Bonferroni-adjusted *p*-values; however, the difference is very small. The Šidák-adjusted *p*-value for the medium dose versus placebo comparison is marginally significant ($p = 0.0493$), whereas the corresponding Bonferroni-adjusted *p*-value is only a notch greater than 0.05 ($p = 0.0501$).

Despite the conservative nature of the Bonferroni adjustment, it has been shown in the literature that the Bonferroni method cannot be improved (Hommel, 1983). One can find fairly exotic *p*-value distributions for which the Bonferroni inequality turns into an equality and therefore it is impossible to construct a single-step test that will be uniformly more powerful than the simple Bonferroni test. The only way to improve the Bonferroni method is by making additional assumptions about the joint distribution of the individual *p*-values. Examples of multiple tests that rely on the assumption of independent *p*-values will be given in the next subsection.

Simes Method

Unlike the Bonferroni and Šidák methods, the Simes method can be used only for testing the global null hypothesis. We will show in Section 2.3 that the Simes global test can be extended to perform inferences on individual null hypotheses, and we will demonstrate how to carry out the extended tests using PROC MULTTEST.

The Simes method is closely related to that proposed by Rüger (1978). Rüger noted that the Bonferroni global test can be written as

Reject the global null hypothesis $\{H_1$ and H_2 and ... and $H_m\}$ if $p_{(1)} \leq \alpha/m$

and uses only a limited amount of information from the sample. It relies on the most significant p-value and ignores the rest of the p-values. Rüger described a family of generalized Bonferroni global tests based on the ordered p-values $p_{(1)}, \ldots, p_{(m)}$. He showed that the global null hypothesis can be tested using any of the following tests:

$$p_{(1)} \leq \alpha/m, \quad p_{(2)} \leq 2\alpha/m, \quad p_{(3)} \leq 3\alpha/m, \quad \ldots, \quad p_{(m)} \leq \alpha.$$

For example, one can test the global null hypothesis by comparing $p_{(2)}$ to $2\alpha/m$ or $p_{(3)}$ to $3\alpha/m$ as long as one prespecifies which one of these tests will be used. Any one of Rüger's global tests controls the Type I error rate in the strong sense for arbitrary dependence structures. However, each test suffers from the same problem as the Bonferroni global test: each individual test is based on only one p-value.

Simes (1986) developed a procedure for combining the information from m individual tests. The Simes global test rejects the global null hypothesis if

$$p_{(i)} \leq i\alpha/m \text{ for at least one } i = 1, \ldots, m.$$

Simes demonstrated that his global test is exact in the sense that its size equals α if $p_1, \ldots, p_m$ are independent. The adjusted p-value for the global hypothesis associated with this test is equal to

$$\widetilde{p}_{SIM} = m \min(p_{(1)}/1, p_{(2)}/2, \ldots, p_{(m)}/m).$$

Since $\widetilde{p}_B = mp_{(1)}$, it is clear that $\widetilde{p}_{SIM} \leq \widetilde{p}_B$ and thus the Simes global test is uniformly more powerful than the Bonferroni global test.

The Simes test achieves higher power by assuming that the individual p-values are independent. Naturally, this assumption is rarely satisfied in clinical applications. What happens if the p-values are correlated? In general, the Simes global test does not preserve the Type I error rate. Hommel (1983) showed that the Type I error rate associated with the Simes test can be considerably higher than α. In fact, it can be as high as

$$\left(1 + \frac{1}{2} + \ldots + \frac{1}{m}\right)\alpha,$$

i.e., 1.5α if $m = 2$ and 2.08α if $m = 4$.

The case of independent p-values often represents the worst-case scenario in terms of the amount of Type I error rate inflation. For example, Simes (1986) showed via simulations that the Type I error rate associated with his test decreases with increasing correlation coefficient when the test statistics follow a multivariate normal distribution. Hochberg and Rom (1995) reported the results of a simulation study based on negatively correlated normal variables in which the size of the Simes test was close to the nominal value. Sarkar and Chang (1997) studied the Simes global test and demonstrated that it preserves the Type I error rate when the joint distribution of the test statistics exhibits a certain type of positive dependence. For example, multiple testing procedures based on the Simes test control the familywise error rate in the problem of performing multiple treatment-control comparisons under normal assumptions.

2.2.1 Summary

This section described simple multiplicity adjustment strategies known as single-step methods. Single-step procedures test each null hypothesis of interest independently of the other hypotheses and therefore the order in which the null hypotheses are examined becomes unimportant. Single-step tests are very easy to implement and have enjoyed much popularity in clinical applications.

The following three single-step tests were discussed in the section:

- The Bonferroni test controls the familywise error rate for any joint distribution of the marginal p-values but is known to be rather conservative. Despite the conservative nature of the Bonferroni method, no single-step test is uniformly more powerful than the Bonferroni test. More powerful tests can be constructed only if one is willing to make additional assumptions about the joint distribution of p-values associated with the null hypotheses of interest.

- The Šidák test is uniformly more powerful than the Bonferroni test; however, its size depends on the joint distribution of the marginal p-values and can exceed the nominal level. The Šidák test controls the familywise error rate when the test statistics are independent or follow a multivariate normal distribution.

- The Simes test can be used only for testing the global null hypothesis. The Simes global test is more powerful than the Bonferroni global test but does not always preserve the Type I error rate. Its size is known to be no greater than the nominal level when the individual test statistics are independent or positively dependent in the sense of Sarkar and Chang (1997).

Multiplicity adjustments based on the Bonferroni and Šidák tests are implemented in PROC MULTTEST and are also available in other SAS procedures, such as PROC GLM and PROC MIXED.

2.3 Closed Testing Methods

The closed testing principle was formulated by Marcus, Peritz and Gabriel (1976) and has since provided mathematical foundation for numerous multiple testing methods. It would not be an exaggeration to say that virtually all multiple testing procedures are either derived using this principle or can be rewritten as closed testing procedures. In fact, Liu (1996) showed that any single-step or stepwise multiple test based on marginal p-values can be formulated as a closed testing procedure. This means that one can always construct a closed testing procedure that is at least as powerful as any single-step or stepwise test.

The principle provides statisticians with a very powerful tool for addressing multiplicity problems in numerous settings. Bauer (1991) described a variety of closed testing procedures with applications to multiple comparisons, multivariate endpoints and repeated significance testing. Rom, Costello and Connell (1994) discussed the problem of testing a dose-response effect in dose-finding trials using a closed testing approach. Koch and Gansky (1996) and Chi (1998) reviewed applications of closed testing procedures in the context of clinical trials including multiple treatment comparisons and multiple subgroup analyses. The only major disadvantage of closed testing procedures is that it is generally difficult, if not impossible, to construct associated simultaneous confidence intervals for parameters of interest.

The closed testing principle is based on a hierarchical representation of a multiplicity problem. As an illustration, consider the three null hypotheses H_L, H_M and H_H tested in the dose-finding hypertension trial introduced earlier in this section. To apply the closed testing principle to this multiple testing problem, we need to construct what is known as the *closed family of hypotheses* associated with the three original hypotheses. This is accomplished by forming all possible intersections of H_L, H_M and H_H. The closed family will contain the following seven intersection hypotheses:

1. Three original hypotheses, H_L, H_M and H_H.

2. Three intersection hypotheses containing two original hypotheses, $\{H_L$ and $H_M\}$, $\{H_L$ and $H_H\}$ and $\{H_M$ and $H_H\}$.

3. One intersection hypothesis containing three original hypotheses, $\{H_L$ and H_M and $H_H\}$.

The next step is to link the intersection hypotheses. The links are referred to as *implication relationships*. A hypothesis that contains another hypothesis is said to imply it. For example,

$$\{H_L \text{ and } H_M \text{ and } H_H\}$$

implies $\{H_L$ and $H_M\}$, which in turn implies H_L. Most commonly, implication relationships are displayed using diagrams similar to that shown in Figure 2.2. Each box in this figure represents a hypothesis in the closed family and is connected to the boxes corresponding to the hypotheses it contains. Note that H_{LMH} denotes the intersection hypothesis $\{H_L$ and H_M and $H_H\}$, H_{LM} denotes the intersection hypothesis $\{H_L$ and $H_M\}$, and so on. The hypothesis at the top is the intersection of the three original hypotheses and therefore it implies H_{LM}, H_{LH} and H_{MH}. Likewise, the three boxes at the second level are connected to the boxes representing the original hypotheses H_L, H_M and H_H. Alternatively, we can put together a list of all intersection hypotheses in the closed family implying the three original hypotheses (Table 2.2).

Figure 2.2 Implication relationships in the closed family of null hypotheses from the hypertension trial. Each box in this diagram represents a hypothesis in the closed family and is connected to the boxes corresponding to the hypotheses it implies.

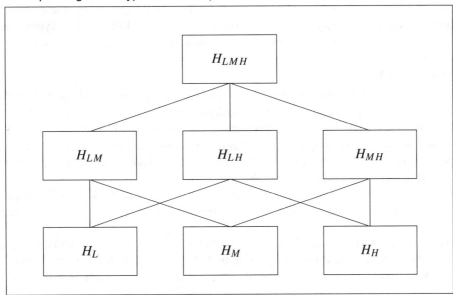

Table 2.2 Intersection hypotheses implying the original hypotheses

Original hypothesis	Intersection hypotheses implying the original hypothesis
H_L	$H_L, H_{LM}, H_{LH}, H_{LMH}$
H_M	$H_M, H_{LM}, H_{MH}, H_{LMH}$
H_H	$H_H, H_{LH}, H_{MH}, H_{LMH}$

Closed Testing Principle

The closed testing principle states that one can control the familywise error rate by using the following multiple testing procedure:

> Test each hypothesis in the closed family using a suitable α-level significance test that controls the error rate at the hypothesis level. A hypothesis is rejected if its associated test and all tests associated with hypotheses implying it are significant.

According to the closed testing principle, to reject any of the original hypotheses in the left column of Table 2.2, we need to test and reject all associated intersection hypotheses shown in the right column.

If any one of the intersection hypotheses is retained then all hypotheses implied by it must also be retained by implication without testing.

Any valid significance test can be used to test intersection hypotheses in the closed family as long as its size does not exceed α at the hypothesis level. One can carry out the global F-test if the individual test statistics are independent or the Bonferroni global test if they are not. Each of these tests will result in a different closed testing procedure. However, as shown by Marcus, Peritz and Gabriel (1976), any multiple test based on the closed testing principle controls the familywise error rate in the strong sense at the prespecified α level.

2.3.1 Stepwise Closed Testing Methods

The reason the closed testing principle has become so popular is that it can be used to construct powerful multiple testing procedures. Consider, for example, the null hypotheses tested in the dose-finding hypertension trial. Choose a single-step test that controls the error rate at the hypothesis level and begin with the global hypothesis H_{LMH}. If the associated test is not significant, we retain the global hypothesis and, according to the closed testing principle, we must retain all other hypotheses in the closed family, including H_L, H_M and H_H. Otherwise, we go on to test the intersection hypotheses H_{LM}, H_{LH} and H_{MH}. If any one of these hypotheses is rejected, we test the hypotheses implied by it and so on. Once we stop, we need to examine the implication relationships to see which of the original hypotheses can be rejected. The obtained closed procedure is more powerful than the single-step test it is based on.

Holm Stepwise Test

In certain cases, the described hierarchical testing algorithm can be significantly simplified. In those cases, the significance testing can be carried out in a straightforward stepwise manner without examining all implication relationships. As an illustration, suppose we wish to enhance the Bonferroni correction by utilizing the closed testing principle. It is a well-known fact that applying the closed testing principle with the Bonferroni global test yields the Bonferroni stepwise procedure introduced by Holm (1979); see Hochberg and Tamhane (1987, Section 2.4).

Choose an arbitrary intersection hypothesis H in the closed family (see Table 2.2). The hypothesis will be tested using the Bonferroni global test; i.e., the following decision rule will be employed:

> Compute the p-value associated with the Bonferroni global test. The p-value is equal to the most significant p-value corresponding to the original hypotheses implied by H times the number of original hypotheses implied by H. Denote the obtained p-value by $\widetilde{p}_B$. Reject H if $\widetilde{p}_B \leq \alpha$.

For example, consider the intersection hypothesis H_{LM}. This intersection hypothesis implies two original hypotheses, namely, H_L and H_M. Therefore, the Bonferroni-adjusted p-value is given by $\widetilde{p}_B = 2\min(p_L, p_M)$. The hypothesis will be rejected if $\widetilde{p}_B \leq \alpha$.

By the Bonferroni inequality, the size of the Bonferroni global test is no greater than α. This means that we have constructed a family of α-level significance tests for each hypothesis in the closed family. Therefore, applying the closed testing principle yields a multiple test for the original hypotheses H_L, H_M and H_H that protects the overall Type I error rate in the strong sense.

The constructed multiple test looks fairly unwieldy at first glance. Despite this first impression, it has a simple stepwise form. Consider a general family of null hypotheses $H_1, \ldots, H_m$. The Holm multiple test is based on a sequentially rejective algorithm that tests the ordered hypotheses $H_{(1)}, \ldots, H_{(m)}$ corresponding to the ordered p-values $p_{(1)}, \ldots, p_{(m)}$. The multiple testing procedure begins with the hypothesis associated with the most significant p-value, i.e., with $H_{(1)}$. This hypothesis is rejected if $p_{(1)} \leq \alpha/m$. Further, $H_{(i)}$ is rejected at the ith step if $p_{(j)} \leq \alpha/(m - j + 1)$ for all $j = 1, \ldots, i$. Otherwise, $H_{(i)}, \ldots, H_{(m)}$ are retained and the algorithm terminates. The details of the Holm test are shown in Table 2.3.

To compare the Holm and Bonferroni testing procedures, note that the Bonferroni procedure tests $H_1, \ldots, H_m$ at the same α/m level. In contrast, the Holm procedure tests $H_{(1)}$ at the α/m level and the other hypotheses are tested at successively higher significance levels. As a result, the Holm stepwise test

Table 2.3 Holm stepwise test

Step	Condition	Condition is met	Condition is not met
1	$p_{(1)} \leq \alpha/m$	Reject $H_{(1)}$ and go to Step 2	Retain $H_{(1)}, \ldots, H_{(m)}$ and stop
...	...	...	...
i	$p_{(i)} \leq \alpha/(m - i + 1)$	Reject $H_{(i)}$ and go to Step $i + 1$	Retain $H_{(i)}, \ldots, H_{(m)}$ and stop
...	...	...	...
m	$p_{(m)} \leq \alpha$	Reject $H_{(m)}$	Retain $H_{(m)}$

rejects at least as many (and possibly more) hypotheses as the Bonferroni test. This means that, by applying the closed testing principle, we have constructed a more powerful test that maintains the familywise error rate at the same level.

To illustrate this important feature of the Holm stepwise procedure, consider Scenario 1 in Table 2.1. Program 2.2 shows how to compute adjusted p-values produced by the Bonferroni and Holm multiple tests using PROC MULTTEST. The Bonferroni and Holm tests are requested by the BONFERRONI and STEPBON options.

Program 2.2 Analysis of the hypertension trial using the Bonferroni and Holm tests

```
proc multtest pdata=antihyp1 bonferroni stepbon out=adjp;

axis1 minor=none order=(0 to 0.15 by 0.05) label=(angle=90 "P-value");
axis2 minor=none value=("Low" "Medium" "High") label=("Dose")
    order=("L" "M" "H");
symbol1 value=circle color=black i=j;
symbol2 value=diamond color=black i=j;
symbol3 value=triangle color=black i=j;
proc gplot data=adjp;
    plot raw_p*test bon_p*test stpbon_p*test/frame overlay nolegend
    haxis=axis2 vaxis=axis1 vref=0.05 lvref=34;
    run;
```

The output of Program 2.2 is displayed in Figure 2.3. Figure 2.3 shows that all three Holm-adjusted p-values are less than 0.05 (note that the adjusted p-value for the low dose versus placebo comparison is equal to the corresponding raw p-value). This means that the Holm stepwise procedure has rejected all three null hypotheses, indicating that all doses of the experimental drug provide a significantly greater reduction in diastolic blood pressure compared to the placebo. In contrast, only the high dose is significantly different from the placebo according to the Bonferroni correction.

2.3.2 Decision Matrix Algorithm

Only a limited number of closed testing procedures have a simple stepwise representation similar to that of the Holm multiple test. Most of the time, the statistician does not have the luxury of being able to set up a stepwise algorithm and needs to carefully review the complex implication relationships to ensure the closed testing principle is applied properly and the familywise error rate is not inflated. Due to the hierarchical nature of closed testing procedures, this can be a challenging task when a large number of hypotheses are being tested.

In this subsection we will introduce the *decision matrix algorithm* for implementing general closed testing procedures. This algorithm streamlines the decision-making process and simplifies the computation of adjusted p-values associated with the intersection and original hypotheses; see Dmitrienko, Offen and Westfall (2003) for details and examples. To illustrate the decision matrix method, we will show how it can be used to carry out the Holm stepwise test. The method will also be

Figure 2.3 Analysis of the hypertension trial using the Bonferroni and Holm tests. Raw p-value ($\bigcirc$), Bonferroni-adjusted p-value ($\diamond$) and Holm-adjusted p-value ($\triangle$).

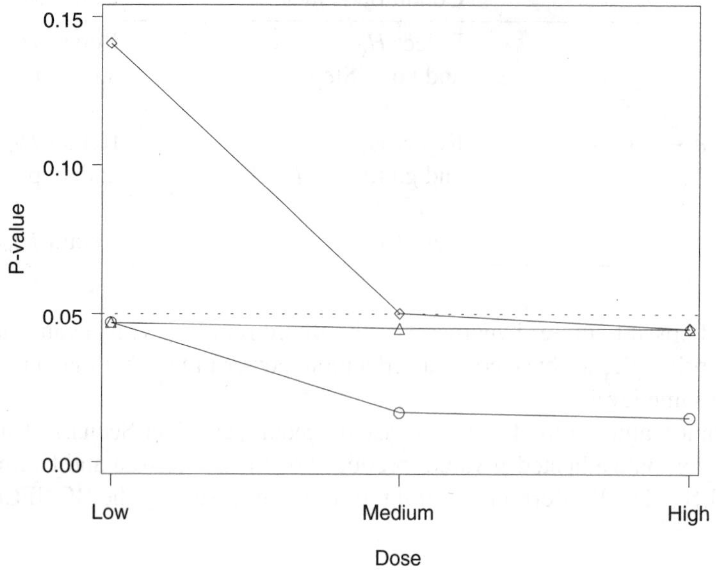

applied to construct closed testing procedures for the identification of individual significant outcomes in clinical trials with multiple endpoints in Section 2.6 and for setting up *gatekeeping procedures* in Section 2.7.

Holm Stepwise Test

Consider the null hypotheses tested in the dose-finding hypertension trial. Table 2.4 presents a decision matrix for the Holm multiple test. It summarizes the algorithm for computing the adjusted p-values that are later used in testing the significance of individual dose-placebo comparisons.

Table 2.4 Decision matrix for the Holm multiple test

Intersection hypothesis	P-value	Implied hypotheses		
		H_L	H_M	H_H
H_{LMH}	$p_{LMH} = 3\min(p_L, p_M, p_H)$	p_{LMH}	p_{LMH}	p_{LMH}
H_{LM}	$p_{LM} = 2\min(p_L, p_M)$	p_{LM}	p_{LM}	0
H_{LH}	$p_{LH} = 2\min(p_L, p_H)$	p_{LH}	0	p_{LH}
H_L	$p_L = p_L$	p_L	0	0
H_{MH}	$p_{MH} = 2\min(p_M, p_H)$	0	p_{MH}	p_{MH}
H_M	$p_M = p_M$	0	p_M	0
H_H	$p_H = p_H$	0	0	p_H

There are seven rows in Table 2.4, each corresponding to a single intersection hypothesis in the closed family. For each of these hypotheses, the three columns on the right side of the table identify the implied hypotheses, while the second column displays the formula for computing the associated p-values denoted by

$$p_{LMH}, p_{LM}, p_{LH}, p_{MH}, p_L, p_M, p_H.$$

In order to make inferences about the three original hypotheses, we first compute these p-values and populate the three columns on the right side of the table. Westfall and Young (1993) stated that the adjusted p-value for each original hypothesis is equal to the largest p-value associated with the intersection hypotheses that imply it. This means that we can obtain the adjusted p-values for H_L, H_M

and H_H by computing the largest p-value in the corresponding column on the right side of the table. For example, the adjusted p-value for the low dose versus placebo comparison is equal to

$$\max(p_L, p_{LM}, p_{LH}, p_{LMH}).$$

Program 2.3 computes the Holm-adjusted p-values using the decision matrix algorithm.

Program 2.3 Analysis of the hypertension trial using the Holm multiple test (decision matrix approach)

```
proc iml;
    use antihyp1;
    read all var {raw_p} into p;
    h=j(7,3,0);
    decision_matrix=j(7,3,0);
    adjusted_p=j(1,3,0);
    do i=1 to 3;
        do j=0 to 6;
            k=floor(j/2**(3-i));
            if k/2=floor(k/2) then h[j+1,i]=1;
        end;
    end;
    do i=1 to 7;
        decision_matrix[i,]=h[i,]*sum(h[i,])*min(p[loc(h[i,])]);
    end;
    do i=1 to 3;
        adjusted_p[i]=max(decision_matrix[,i]);
    end;
    title={"L vs P", "M vs P", "H vs P"};
    print decision_matrix[colname=title];
    print adjusted_p[colname=title];
    quit;
```

Output from Program 2.3

```
        DECISION_MATRIX
   L vs P     M vs P     H vs P


   0.045      0.045      0.045
   0.0334     0.0334     0
   0.03       0          0.03
   0.047      0          0
   0          0.03       0.03
   0          0.0167     0
   0          0          0.015


         ADJUSTED_P
   L vs P     M vs P     H vs P


   0.047      0.045      0.045
```

The DECISION_MATRIX table in Output 2.3 represents the three columns on the right of Table 2.4 and serves as a helpful tool for visualizing the decision-making process behind the closed testing procedure. As was noted earlier, the adjusted p-values for H_L, H_M and H_H can be obtained by computing the maximum over all p-values in the corresponding column. The computed p-values are shown at the bottom of Output 2.3. Note that these adjusted p-values are identical to those produced by PROC MULTTEST in Program 2.2.

2.3.3 Popular Closed Testing Procedures

It was shown in the previous subsection that one can significantly improve the performance of the Bonferroni correction by constructing a closed testing procedure based on the Bonferroni global test (i.e., the Holm procedure). The same idea can be used to enhance any single-step test for the global null hypothesis described in Section 2.2, such as the Šidák or Simes global test. While no one appears to have taken credit for developing a closed testing procedure based on the Šidák global test, several authors have proposed closed testing procedures derived from the Bonferroni and Simes global tests. We will briefly review multiple tests developed by Shaffer (1986), Hommel (1988) and Hochberg (1988).

All of the multiple tests discussed in this subsection are superior to the Holm procedure in terms of power. However, it is important to remember that the Holm procedure is based on the Bonferroni global test, which cannot be sharpened unless additional assumptions about the joint distributions of p-values are made. This means that one needs to pay a price to improve the Holm test. Some of the multiple tests described below are efficient only for certain types of multiple testing problems and some of them lose the strict control of the overall Type I error rate.

Shaffer Multiple Test

Shaffer (1986) proposed an enhanced version of the stepwise Bonferroni procedure by assuming that the hypotheses of interest are linked to each other; i.e., a rejection of one hypothesis immediately implies that another one is rejected. The Shaffer method is highly efficient in multiple testing problems involving a large number of pairwise comparisons, such as dose-finding studies. When the hypotheses being tested are not logically interrelated (e.g., when multiple comparisons with a control are performed), the Shaffer procedure reduces to the Holm procedure.

Hommel Multiple Test

A closed testing procedure based on the Simes test was proposed by Hommel (1986, 1988). Unlike the Simes test, which can be used only for testing the global null hypothesis, the Hommel testing procedure starts with the global hypothesis and then "steps down" to examine the individual hypotheses. Since the Simes global test is more powerful than the Bonferroni global test, the Hommel procedure rejects all hypotheses rejected by the Holm closed procedure based on the Bonferroni procedure, and possibly more. However, the improvement comes with a price. The Hommel test no longer guarantees that the probability of an overall Type I error is at most α. The Hommel procedure protects the familywise error rate only when the Simes global test does—e.g., when the individual test statistics are independent or positively dependent (Sarkar and Chang, 1997).

Unlike the Holm multiple test, the Hommel test cannot be carried out in a simple sequentially rejective manner. The test can be implemented using the decision matrix algorithm and one can write a SAS program similar to Program 2.3 to compute the Hommel-adjusted p-values for H_L, H_M and H_H. Here, we will present an efficient solution that utilizes PROC MULTTEST. The Hommel multiple test is available in PROC MULTTEST in SAS 8.1 and later versions of the SAS System. It can be requested using the HOMMEL option. PROC MULTTEST produces the same adjusted p-values as the decision matrix approach.

Program 2.4 computes the Holm- and Hommel-adjusted p-values for the individual dose-placebo comparisons in the hypertension trial under Scenario 2 shown in Table 2.1.

Program 2.4 Analysis of the hypertension trial using the Holm and Hommel tests

```
data antihyp2;
    input test $ raw_p @@;
    datalines;
    L 0.047 M 0.027 H 0.015
    ;
proc multtest pdata=antihyp2 stepbon hommel out=adjp;
```

```
axis1 minor=none order=(0 to 0.06 by 0.02) label=(angle=90 "P-value");
axis2 minor=none value=("Low" "Medium" "High") label=("Dose")
    order=("L" "M" "H");
symbol1 value=circle color=black i=j;
symbol2 value=diamond color=black i=j;
symbol3 value=triangle color=black i=j;
proc gplot data=adjp;
    plot raw_p*test stpbon_p*test hom_p*test/frame overlay nolegend
    haxis=axis2 vaxis=axis1 vref=0.05 lvref=34;
    run;
```

Figure 2.4 Analysis of the hypertension trial using the Holm and Hommel tests. Raw p-value ($\bigcirc$), Holm-adjusted p-value ($\diamond$) and Hommel-adjusted p-value ($\triangle$).

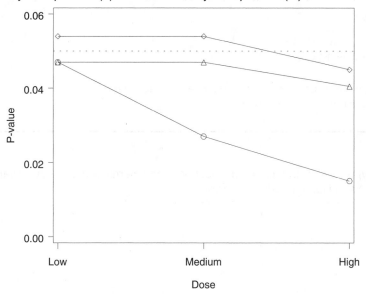

The output of Program 2.4 is displayed in Figure 2.4. The figure demonstrates that the Hommel testing procedure has rejected all three null hypotheses and thus it is clearly more powerful than the Holm procedure, which rejected only one hypothesis (note that the Hommel-adjusted p-value for the low dose versus placebo comparison is equal to the corresponding raw p-value). The figure also illustrates an interesting property of the Hommel procedure. Since the Hommel procedure is based on the Simes test, it rejects all null hypotheses whenever all raw p-values are significant.

Hochberg Multiple Test

Another popular stepwise test supported by PROC MULTTEST is the Hochberg test (Hochberg, 1988). This test is virtually identical to the Holm test except for the order in which the null hypotheses are tested. As was explained earlier, the Holm multiple test examines the most significant p-value first and then works downward. For this reason, it is commonly referred to as a *step-down test*. In contrast, the Hochberg procedure examines the ordered p-values $p_{(1)}, \ldots, p_{(m)}$ starting with the largest one and thus falls into the class of *step-up tests*.

The Hochberg multiple test rejects all hypotheses rejected by the Holm test but is uniformly less powerful than the Hommel procedure (Hommel, 1989). Also, like the Hommel test, the Hochberg test does not always preserve the familywise error rate. Its size can potentially exceed α but it is no greater than α when the individual p-values are independent. This means that in all situations when both of these tests can be carried out, the Hommel multiple test should be given a preference.

The Hochberg procedure is available in MULTTEST and can be requested using the HOCHBERG option. Program 2.5 computes the Hochberg- and Hommel-adjusted *p*-values for the three null hypotheses tested in the dose-finding hypertension trial under Scenario 3 shown in Table 2.1.

Program 2.5 Analysis of the hypertension trial using the Hochberg and Hommel tests

```
data antihyp3;
    input test $ raw_p @@;
    datalines;
    L 0.053 M 0.026 H 0.017
    ;
proc multtest pdata=antihyp2 hochberg hommel out=adjp;

axis1 minor=none order=(0 to 0.06 by 0.02) label=(angle=90 "P-value");
axis2 minor=none value=("Low" "Medium" "High") label=("Dose")
    order=("L" "M" "H");
symbol1 value=circle color=black i=j;
symbol2 value=diamond color=black i=j;
symbol3 value=triangle color=black i=j;
proc gplot data=adjp;
    plot raw_p*test hoc_p*test hom_p*test/frame overlay nolegend
    haxis=axis2 vaxis=axis1 vref=0.05 lvref=34;
    run;
```

Figure 2.5 Analysis of the hypertension trial using the Hochberg and Hommel tests. Raw *p*-value (○), Hochberg-adjusted *p*-value (◇) and Hommel-adjusted *p*-value (△).

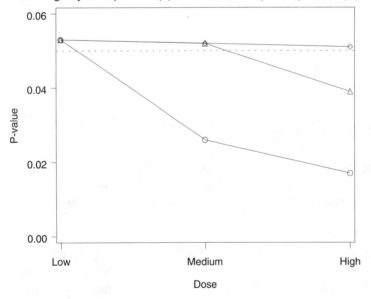

The output of Program 2.5 is shown in Figure 2.5. We can see from Figure 2.5 that the Hommel multiple test has rejected more null hypotheses than the Hochberg test. Note that both the Hochberg- and Hommel-adjusted *p*-values for the low dose versus placebo comparison are equal to the corresponding raw *p*-value.

Power Comparisons

Figure 2.6 displays the relationship among the two single-step and three stepwise multiple tests discussed in this and previous sections. The multiple tests shown in Figure 2.6 are arranged in the order of increasing power. The tests on the right-hand side are uniformly more powerful than the tests on the

Figure 2.6 A comparison of five popular multiple tests. Tests displayed on the right-hand side are uniformly more powerful than tests on the left-hand side. An asterisk indicates that the test does not always control the familywise error rate.

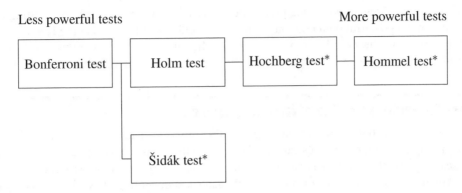

left-hand side. Although the testing procedures derived from the Simes and related multiple tests (i.e., Hochberg and Hommel procedures) are more powerful than the Holm and Bonferroni tests, one needs to remember that these procedures do not always control the familywise error rate. The familywise error rate is protected if the individual test statistics are independent or positively dependent (Sarkar and Chang, 1997).

A number of authors investigated the Type I and Type II error rates associated with popular multiple tests. Dunnett and Tamhane (1992) performed a simulation study to compare several stepwise procedures in the context of multiple treatment-control tests under normal theory. Dunnett and Tamhane observed marginal increases in power when they compared the Hommel procedure with the Holm procedure.

Brown and Russell (1997) reported the results of an extensive simulation study of 17 multiple testing procedures based on marginal p-values. The simulation study involved multiple comparisons of equally correlated normal means. Although the authors did not find the uniformly best multiple testing procedure, they generally recommended the empirical modification of the Hochberg test proposed by Hochberg and Benjamini (1990) because it had the smallest Type II error rate and its overall Type I error rate was close to the nominal value. It is worth noting that the performance of the modified Hochberg test was generally comparable to that of the Holm, Hochberg and Hommel procedures.

Sankoh, Huque and Dubey (1997) studied the performance of the Hochberg and Hommel tests. They ran a simulation study to examine familywise error rates associated with the two testing procedures using a multivariate normal model with equally correlated components. The Hochberg and Hommel methods had comparable overall Type I error rates that decreased as the number of endpoints and correlation coefficient increased. For example, the overall Type I error rate associated with the Hommel method was below 0.04 in the three-dimensional case and below 0.03 in the ten-dimensional case when the correlation coefficient was 0.9.

2.3.4   Summary

The closed testing principle provides clinical statisticians with a very powerful tool for addressing multiplicity problems and has found numerous applications in a clinical trial setting. This section discussed three popular closed testing procedures implemented in PROC MULTTEST:

- The Holm test is derived from the Bonferroni test and therefore it controls the familywise error rate for arbitrarily dependent marginal p-values. The Holm testing procedure is based on a sequentially rejective algorithm that tests the hypothesis associated with the most significant p-value at the same level as the Bonferroni test, but tests the other hypotheses at successively higher significance levels. As a consequence, the stepwise Holm test is uniformly more powerful than the single-step Bonferroni test

- The Hochberg test is set up as a step-up test that examines the least significant *p*-value first and then works upward. This test is superior to the Holm test but its size can potentially exceed the nominal level. The Hochberg test controls the familywise error rate in all situations that the Simes test does.

- The Hommel test is a closed testing procedure derived from the Simes test. This testing procedure is uniformly more powerful than both the Holm and Hochberg tests and, like the Hochberg test, is known to preserve the Type I error rate only when the Simes test does. For this reason, the Hommel multiple test should be given a preference in all situations when one can carry out the Hochberg test.

2.4 Fixed-Sequence Testing Methods

So far we have talked about stepwise multiple tests that rely on a data-driven ordering of *p*-values. Stepwise multiple testing procedures can also be constructed using any prespecified sequence of hypotheses. Suppose that there is a natural ordering among the null hypotheses $H_1, \ldots, H_m$ and the order in which the testing is performed is fixed. If each subsequent hypothesis is tested only if all previously tested hypotheses have been rejected, the principle of closed testing implies that we don't need to make any adjustments to control the familywise error rate.

There is a very important distinction between the described fixed-sequence testing approach and the closed testing procedures discussed in Section 2.3. Both methodologies can be used to set up hierarchical multiple testing procedures. However, the manner in which the stepwise testing is carried out is completely different. Closed testing procedures are adaptive in the sense that the order in which the null hypotheses of interest are tested is driven by the data. The hypotheses that are likely to be false are tested first and testing ceases when none of the untested hypotheses appears to be false. For example, the Holm multiple test examines the individual *p*-values from the most significant ones to the least significant ones. The tests stops when all remaining *p*-values are too large to be significant. In contrast, fixed-sequence testing procedures rely on the assumption that the order in which the null hypotheses are tested is predetermined. As a result, one runs a risk of retaining false hypotheses because they happened to be placed late in the sequence.

2.4.1 Testing *a priori* Ordered Hypotheses

Fixed-sequence testing procedures can be used in a wide variety of multiplicity problems with *a priori* ordered hypotheses. Problems of this kind arise in clinical trials when longitudinal measurements are analyzed in a sequential manner to identify the onset of therapeutic effect or to study its duration.

EXAMPLE: Allergen-Induced Asthma Trial

Consider a trial designed to assess the efficacy profile of a bronchodilator. Twenty patients with mild asthma were enrolled in this trial and were randomly assigned to receive either an experimental drug or a placebo (10 patients in each treatment group). The efficacy of the experimental drug was studied using an allergen-induced asthma model; see Taylor et al. (1991) for a detailed description of an allergen-induced asthma trial. Patients were given a dose of the drug and then asked to inhale allergen to induce bronchoconstriction. Spirometry measurements were taken every 15 minutes for the first hour and every hour up to 3 hours to measure the forced expiratory volume in one second (FEV1). To assess how the drug attenuated the allergen-induced bronchoconstriction, the FEV1 curves were constructed by averaging the FEV1 values at each time point in the placebo and treated groups. The collected FEV1 data are summarized in Table 2.5.

A very important indicator of therapeutic effect is the time to the onset of action—that is, the first time point at which a clinically and statistically significant separation between the FEV1 curves is observed. Since the time points at which spirometry measurements are taken are naturally ordered, the onset of action analyses can be performed using fixed-sequence testing methods. The inferences are performed without an adjustment for multiplicity and without modeling the longitudinal correlation. Thus, the resulting tests are more powerful than the multiple tests introduced in Sections 2.2 and 2.3.

Table 2.5 Reduction in FEV1 measurements from baseline by time after the allergen challenge (L)

Time (hours)	Experimental drug			Placebo		
	n	Mean	SD	n	Mean	SD
0.25	10	0.58	0.29	10	0.71	0.35
0.5	10	0.62	0.31	10	0.88	0.33
0.75	10	0.51	0.33	10	0.73	0.36
1	10	0.34	0.27	10	0.68	0.29
2	10	−0.06	0.22	10	0.37	0.25
3	10	0.05	0.23	10	0.43	0.28

Program 2.6 computes and plots the mean treatment differences in FEV1 changes, the associated lower 95% confidence limits, and one-sided p-values for the treatment effect from two-sample t-tests at each of the six time points when the spirometry measurements were taken.

Program 2.6 Treatment comparisons in the allergen-induced asthma trial

```
data fev1;
    input time n1 mean1 sd1 n2 mean2 sd2;
    datalines;
    0.25 10 0.58  0.29 10 0.71 0.35
    0.5  10 0.62  0.31 10 0.88 0.33
    0.75 10 0.51  0.33 10 0.73 0.36
    1    10 0.34  0.27 10 0.68 0.29
    2    10 -0.06 0.22 10 0.37 0.25
    3    10 0.05  0.23 10 0.43 0.28
    ;
data summary;
    set fev1;
    meandif=mean2-mean1;
    se=sqrt((1/n1+1/n2)*(sd1*sd1+sd2*sd2)/2);
    t=meandif/se;
    p=1-probt(t,n1+n2-2);
    lower=meandif-tinv(0.95,n1+n2-2)*se;
axis1 minor=none label=(angle=90 "Treatment difference (L)")
    order=(-0.2 to 0.5 by 0.1);
axis2 minor=none label=("Time (hours)") order=(0 to 3 by 1);
symbol1 value=none i=j color=black line=1;
symbol2 value=none i=j color=black line=20;
proc gplot data=summary;
    plot meandif*time lower*time/overlay frame vaxis=axis1 haxis=axis2
    vref=0 lvref=34;
    run;
axis1 minor=none label=(angle=90 "Raw p-value") order=(0 to 0.2 by 0.05);
axis2 minor=none label=("Time (hours)") order=(0 to 3 by 1);
symbol1 value=dot i=j color=black line=1;
proc gplot data=summary;
    plot p*time/frame vaxis=axis1 haxis=axis2 vref=0.05 lvref=34;
    run;
```

The output of Program 2.6 is shown in Figure 2.7. When reviewing the one-sided confidence limits and raw p-values in Figure 2.7, it is tempting to examine the results in a "step-up" manner—i.e., to start with the first spirometry measurement and stop testing as soon as a statistically significant mean difference is observed (30 minutes after the allergen challenge). However, this approach does not control

Figure 2.7 Treatment comparisons in the allergen-induced asthma trial. Left-hand panel: Mean treatment difference (—) and lower confidence limit (- - -) by time. Right-hand panel: Raw *p*-values by time.

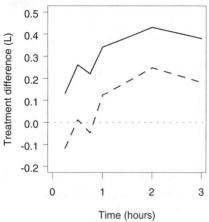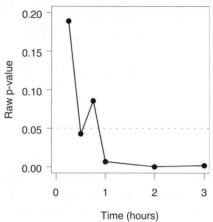

the familywise error rate. To protect the Type I error rate, fixed-sequence testing should be performed in a sequentially *rejective* fashion. This means that each subsequent hypothesis is tested only if all previously tested hypotheses have been *rejected*. This can be achieved if we examine the treatment differences in a "step-down" fashion—i.e., by starting with the last spirometry measurement and working backwards. With the step-down approach, the lower 95% confidence limit includes zero (or, equivalently, a non-significant *p*-value is observed) for the first time 45 minutes after the allergen inhalation. This means that a statistically significant separation between the mean FEV1 values in the two groups occurs 1 hour after the allergen challenge.

This example illustrates the importance of "monotonicity" assumptions in fixed-sequence testing. Fixed-sequence testing methods perform best when the magnitude of the treatment effect can be assumed to change monotonically with respect to time or dose. When the assumption is not met, fixed-sequence tests are prone to producing spurious results. Coming back to the data summarized in Table 2.5, suppose that the mean difference in FEV1 changes between the experimental drug and the placebo is very small at the last spirometry measurement. If the associated *p*-value is not significant, one cannot determine the onset of therapeutic effect despite the fact that the experimental drug separated from the placebo at several time points.

Similarly, Hsu and Berger (1999) proposed to use intersection-union testing methods to help identify the minimum effective dose (MED) in dose-finding trials. One starts with comparing the highest dose to the placebo and then steps down to the next dose if the comparison is significant. Testing continues in this manner until an ineffective dose is reached. Hsu and Berger argued that the described algorithm guarantees a contiguous set of efficacious doses. This contiguous set of doses is helpful for establishing a therapeutic window for drug regimens. Note that the outlined testing procedure can be used only if the response increases monotonically with dose. It is clear that one runs a risk of missing the MED if the true dose-response curve is umbrella-shaped.

As a side note, one can also perform multiple inferences in studies with serial measurements per subject by taking into account the longitudinal correlation. See Littell et al. (1996) for a review of repeated-measures models for continuous endpoints and associated multiple testing procedures with a large number of SAS examples.

2.4.2 Hsu-Berger Method for Constructing Simultaneous Confidence Intervals

In the previous subsection, we described the use of fixed-sequence testing in applications with *a priori* ordered hypotheses and demonstrated how to interpret unadjusted confidence intervals and *p*-values in order to identify the onset of therapeutic effect in an allergen-induced asthma trial. An interesting feature of fixed-sequence tests is that, unlike closed tests, they are easily inverted to set up simultaneous confidence intervals for the parameters of interest. In this subsection we will briefly outline a stepwise method proposed by Hsu and Berger (1999) for constructing simultaneous confidence sets.

Consider a clinical trial with two treatment groups (experimental drug and placebo) in which a continuous endpoint is measured at m consecutive time points. The numbers of patients in the two groups are denoted by n_1 and n_2. Let Y_{ijk} denote the measurement collected from the jth patient in the ith treatment group at the kth time point. Assume that Y_{ijk} is normally distributed with mean μ_{ik} and variance σ_k^2. Assuming that higher values of the endpoint indicate improvement, let $H_1, \ldots, H_m$ denote the null hypotheses stating that the mean response in the experimental group is not meaningfully higher than that in the placebo group, i.e.,

$$H_k = \{\mu_{1k} - \mu_{2k} \leq \delta\}, \quad k = 1, \ldots, m,$$

where δ denotes the clinically relevant difference. The hypotheses are logically ordered and thus they can be tested in a step-down manner using a fixed-sequence procedure. Let l equal the index of the first retained hypothesis if at least one hypothesis has been retained. If all hypotheses have been rejected, let $l = 0$.

Hsu and Berger (1999) proposed the following algorithm for setting up lower confidence limits for the true treatment difference at the kth time point, i.e., $\mu_{1k} - \mu_{2k}, k = 1, \ldots, m$. First, construct one-sided confidence intervals for the treatment differences at each time point (as was done in Program 2.6). The confidence interval for $\mu_{1k} - \mu_{2k}$ is given by

$$I_k = \{\mu_{1k} - \mu_{2k} \geq \widehat{\mu}_{1k} - \widehat{\mu}_{2k} - t_{\alpha,\nu} s_k\},$$

where

$$\widehat{\mu}_{ik} = \sum_{j=1}^{n_i} Y_{ijk}/n_i, \quad s_k = \widehat{\sigma}_k \sqrt{1/n_1 + 1/n_2}$$

and $\widehat{\sigma}_k$ is the pooled sample standard deviation at the kth time point, $\nu = n_1 + n_2 - 2$, and $t_{\alpha,\nu}$ denotes the upper 100α percentile of the t distribution with ν degrees of freedom. If the fixed-sequence test has rejected all hypotheses, i.e.,

$$\widehat{\mu}_{1k} - \widehat{\mu}_{2k} - t_{\alpha,\nu} s_k \geq \delta, \quad k = 1, \ldots, m,$$

set the lower limit of the adjusted confidence intervals to the same value, namely,

$$\min_{k=1,\ldots,m} (\widehat{\mu}_{1k} - \widehat{\mu}_{2k} - t_{\alpha,\nu} s_k).$$

Otherwise, the adjusted confidence interval $\widetilde{I}_k$ is defined as

$$\widetilde{I}_k = \{\mu_{1k} - \mu_{2k} \geq \min(\delta, \widehat{\mu}_{1k} - \widehat{\mu}_{2k} - t_{\alpha,\nu} s_k)\}$$

for $k = l, \ldots, m$ and $\widetilde{I}_k$ is empty for $k = 1, \ldots, l - 1$.

We can see from the outlined algorithm that the adjusted confidence intervals for the treatment difference are constructed in a step-down manner. Beginning with the last time point, the one-sided confidence interval for $\mu_{1k} - \mu_{2k}$ is given by

$$\{\mu_{1k} - \mu_{2k} \geq \delta\}$$

if the fixed-sequence test has rejected the null hypotheses $H_k, \ldots, H_m$, and the unadjusted one-sided $100(1 - \alpha)\%$ confidence interval is used otherwise. Hsu and Berger (1999) proved that the coverage probability of the constructed set is no less than $100(1 - \alpha)\%$.

To illustrate the Hsu-Berger method, consider the data collected in the allergen-induced asthma trial (see Table 2.5) and assume that δ is equal to zero; that is, the trial is declared successful if any statistically significant treatment is observed. Program 2.7 employs the Hsu-Berger procedure to construct the adjusted lower 95% confidence limits for the mean difference in FEV1 changes between the two treatment groups (experimental group minus placebo).

Program 2.7 Hsu-Berger simultaneous confidence intervals

```
proc sort data=summary;
    by descending time;
data rejcount;
    set summary nobs=m;
    retain index 1 minlower 100;
    if lower>0 and index=_n_ then index=_n_+1;
    if lower<minlower then minlower=lower;
    keep index minlower;
    if _n_=m;
data adjci;
    set summary nobs=m;
    if _n_=1 then set rejcount;
    if index=m+1 then adjlower=minlower;
    if index<=m and _n_<=index then adjlower=min(lower,0);
axis1 minor=none label=(angle=90 "Treatment difference (L)")
    order=(-0.2 to 0.5 by 0.1);
axis2 minor=none label=("Time (hours)") order=(0 to 3 by 1);
symbol1 value=none i=j color=black line=1;
symbol2 value=none i=j color=black line=20;
proc gplot data=adjci;
    plot meandif*time lower*time/overlay frame vaxis=axis1 haxis=axis2
    vref=0 lvref=34;
    run;
axis1 minor=none label=(angle=90 "Treatment difference (L)")
    order=(-0.2 to 0.5 by 0.1);
axis2 minor=none label=("Time (hours)") order=(0 to 3 by 1);
symbol1 value=none i=j color=black line=1;
symbol2 value=none i=j color=black line=20;
proc gplot data=adjci;
    plot meandif*time adjlower*time/overlay frame vaxis=axis1 haxis=axis2
    vref=0 lvref=34;
    run;
```

The output of Program 2.7 is shown in Figure 2.8. The left-hand panel of the figure displays the unadjusted lower 95% confidence limits for the treatment difference in FEV1 changes and is identical to the left-hand panel of Figure 2.6. It is reproduced here to facilitate the comparison with the right-hand panel, which presents the simultaneous 95% confidence limits computed using the Hsu-Berger algorithm. The unadjusted confidence intervals exclude zero at 3 hours, 2 hours and 1 hour after the allergen challenge and thus, according to the Hsu-Berger algorithm, the adjusted lower limits are set to zero at these time points. The hypothesis of no treatment difference is retained for the first time 45 minutes after the allergen inhalation, which implies that the adjusted confidence interval is equal to the unadjusted one at 45 minutes and is undefined at the first two spirometry measurements.

2.4.3 Summary

Fixed-sequence tests introduced in this section provide an attractive alternative to closed tests when the null hypotheses of interest are naturally ordered. In the presence of an *a priori* ordering, one can test the individual hypotheses in a sequentially rejective fashion without any adjustment for multiplicity. Each subsequent hypothesis is tested only if all previously tested hypotheses have been rejected.

Figure 2.8 Hsu-Berger simultaneous confidence intervals in the allergen-induced asthma trial. Left-hand panel: Mean treatment difference (—) and unadjusted lower confidence limit (- - -) by time. Right-hand panel: Mean treatment difference (—) and Hsu-Berger adjusted lower confidence limit (- - -) by time.

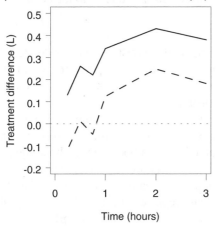
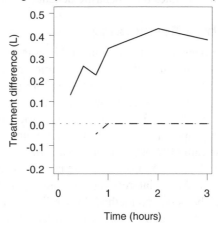

In clinical trials, it is natural to carry out fixed-sequence tests when the endpoint is measured under several different conditions—for instance, when testing is performed over time and thus the order of null hypotheses is predetermined. As an example, it was demonstrated in this section how to perform fixed-sequence inferences to identify the onset of therapeutic effect in an asthma study. Fixed-sequence testing methods are known to perform best when the magnitude of treatment effect can be assumed to change monotonically with respect to time or dose. When the assumption is not met, fixed-sequence tests are likely to produce spurious results.

Unlike closed testing procedures described in Section 2.3, fixed-sequence procedures are easily inverted to construct simultaneous confidence intervals for the parameters of interest. To illustrate this interesting feature of fixed-sequence tests, this section briefly outlined a stepwise method proposed by Hsu and Berger (1999) for constructing simultaneous confidence sets.

2.5 Resampling-Based Testing Methods

This section provides a brief overview of the method of resampling-based multiplicity adjustment introduced in Westfall and Young (1989) and further developed in Westfall and Young (1993) and Westfall et al. (1999).

Consider the problem of simultaneously testing m null hypotheses $H_1, \ldots, H_m$ and let $p_1, \ldots, p_m$ denote the p-values generated by the associated significance tests. Assume for a moment that we know the exact distribution of the individual p-values. Westfall and Young (1989) proposed to define adjusted p-values $\widetilde{p}_1, \ldots, \widetilde{p}_m$ as

$$\widetilde{p}_i = P\{\min(P_1, \ldots, P_m) \leq p_i\}, \quad i = 1, \ldots, m,$$

where $P_1, \ldots, P_m$ are random variables that follow the same distribution as $p_1, \ldots, p_m$ assuming that the m null hypotheses are simultaneously true. Once the adjusted p-values have been computed, the null hypotheses can be tested in a straightforward manner. Specifically, the null hypothesis H_i is rejected if $\widetilde{p}_i \leq \alpha$ and retained otherwise. Under some natural assumptions, the strong sense familywise error rate associated with this single-step multiple testing procedure equals α (the assumptions are related to the so-called *subset pivotality condition* discussed later in this section). The described testing method is more powerful than the Bonferroni and Šidák methods because it takes into account the empirical correlation structure of the individual p-values.

Westfall and Young (1993, Section 2.6) also derived adjusted p-values associated with a step-down procedure similar to that proposed by Holm (1979). The adjusted p-values are given by

$$\widetilde{p}_{(1)} = P\{\min(P_1, \ldots, P_m) \leq p_1\},$$

$$\widetilde{p}_{(i)} = \max[\widetilde{p}_{(i-1)}, P\{\min(P_{(i)}, \ldots, P_{(m)}) \leq p_{(i)}\}], \quad i = 2, \ldots, m.$$

Again, the computations are done under the assumption that $H_1, \ldots, H_m$ are simultaneously true. This testing procedure will dominate the Holm, Hommel or any other step-down procedure in terms of power since it incorporates the stochastic dependence among the individual p-values into the decision rule.

Bootstrap Resampling

A natural question that comes up at this point is how to compute the adjusted p-values defined above when we do not know the exact distribution of the p-values observed in an experiment. Westfall and Young (1989, 1993) described a resampling-based solution to this problem. The unknown joint distribution of the p-values can be estimated using the bootstrap.

The bootstrap methods have found a variety of applications since they were introduced in the pioneering paper of Efron (1979). A large number of references on the bootstrap can be found in Efron and Tibshirani (1993). To briefly review the rationale behind the Efron bootstrap methodology, consider a sample $(X_1, \ldots, X_n)$ of independent, identically distributed observations from an unknown distribution. We are interested in computing multiplicity-adjusted p-values using the Westfall-Young formula. The bootstrap methodology relies on resampling with replacement. Let $(X_1^*, \ldots, X_n^*)$ denote a *bootstrap sample* of size n drawn with replacement from $(X_1, \ldots, X_n)$. Further, let $p_1^*, \ldots, p_m^*$ denote the raw p-values computed from the bootstrap sample. These bootstrap p-values are derived in exactly the same way as the original p-values $p_1, \ldots, p_m$ with the only exception that $H_1, \ldots, H_m$ are assumed to be simultaneously true.

Suppose we have generated all possible bootstrap samples and computed raw bootstrap p-values from each of them. For each p_i, calculate the proportion of bootstrap samples in which $\min(p_1^*, \ldots, p_m^*)$ is less than or equal to p_i. This quantity is a bootstrap estimate of the true adjusted p-value (it is often called the *ideal bootstrap estimate*). The total number of all possible bootstrap samples generated from a given sample of observations is extremely large. It grows exponentially with increasing n and thus ideal bootstrap estimates are rarely available. In all practical applications ideal bootstrap estimates are approximated using Monte Carlo methods.

EXAMPLE: Ulcerative Colitis Trial

The Westfall-Young resampling-based multiplicity adjustment method is implemented in PROC MULTTEST (in fact, PROC MULTTEST was created to support this methodology). To show how to perform a resampling-based multiplicity adjustment in PROC MULTTEST, consider a data set from a dose-finding ulcerative colitis trial in which a placebo (Dose 0) is compared to three doses of an experimental drug (with 12 patients in each treatment group). The primary trial endpoint is the reduction in a 15-point endoscopy score in the four treatment groups. The endoscopy scores are not normally distributed; however, they are likely to follow a location shift model which is effectively handled by PROC MULTTEST.

Let y_{0j} and y_{ij}, $i = 1, 2, 3$, denote the changes in the endoscopy score in the jth patient in the placebo and ith dose group, respectively. Since there are 12 patients in each treatment group, the within-group residuals ε_{ij} are defined as

$$\varepsilon_{ij} = y_{ij} - \frac{1}{12} \sum_{j=1}^{12} y_{ij}, \quad i = 0, 1, 2, 3, \quad j = 1, \ldots, 12.$$

Let p_1, p_2 and p_3 be the raw p-values produced by the three two-sample t-tests comparing the individual doses of the experimental drug to the placebo.

The following is an algorithm for computing Monte Carlo approximations to the multiplicity-adjusted p-values in the ulcerative colitis trial example:

* Select a bootstrap sample ε_{ij}^*, $i = 0, 1, 2, 3$, $j = 1, \ldots, 12$, by sampling with replacement from the pooled sample of 48 within-group residuals. The obtained residuals can be assigned to any treatment group because the sampling process is performed under the assumption that the three doses of the drug are no different from the placebo.

- Let p_1^*, p_2^* and p_3^* denote the p-values computed from each bootstrap sample using the two-sample t-tests for the three dose-placebo comparisons.

- Repeat this process a large number of times.

- Lastly, consider each one of the raw p-values (for example, p_1) and compute the proportion of bootstrap samples in which $\min(p_1^*, p_2^*, p_3^*)$ was less than or equal to p_1. This is a Monte Carlo approximation to the true adjusted p_1. Monte Carlo approximations for the multiplicity-adjusted p_2 and p_3 are computed in a similar manner.

Program 2.8 estimates the adjusted p-values for the three dose-placebo comparisons using single-step and stepwise algorithms (BOOTSTRAP and STEPBOOT options) that are conceptually similar to single-step and stepwise marginal tests discussed earlier in Sections 2.2 and 2.3. The adjusted p-values are computed based on the two-sample t-test using 10,000 bootstrap samples.

Program 2.8 Resampling-based multiplicity adjustment in the dose-finding ulcerative colitis trial

```
data colitis;
    do dose="Dose 0", "Dose 1", "Dose 2", "Dose 3";
        do patient=1 to 12;
            input reduct @@; output;
        end;
    end;
    datalines;
    -2 -1 -1 -1 0 0 0 0 0 2 4  5
    -1  0  1  1 1 2 3 3 3 4 7  9
     1  2  2  3 3 3 3 4 6 8 8  8
     1  4  5  5 6 7 7 8 8 11 12
     ;
proc multtest data=colitis bootstrap stepboot seed=47292 n=10000;
    class dose;
    test mean(reduct);
    contrast "Dose 0 vs Dose 1" 1 -1 0 0;
    contrast "Dose 0 vs Dose 2" 1 0 -1 0;
    contrast "Dose 0 vs Dose 3" 1 0 0 -1;
    run;
```

Output from Program 2.8

		p-Values		Stepdown
Variable	Contrast	Raw	Bootstrap	Bootstrap
reduct	Dose 0 vs Dose 1	0.0384	0.0973	0.0397
reduct	Dose 0 vs Dose 2	0.0028	0.0090	0.0067
reduct	Dose 0 vs Dose 3	<.0001	<.0001	<.0001

Output 2.8 displays the raw and bootstrap-adjusted p-values for each of the three dose-placebo comparisons computed by PROC MULTTEST. The single-step resampling-based procedure has rejected two null hypotheses. The two highest doses of the experimental drug demonstrated a significantly larger mean reduction in the endoscopy score compared to the placebo. The stepwise procedure has produced a smaller adjusted p-value for the placebo versus lowest dose comparison and therefore rejected all three null hypotheses. As in the case of multiple tests based on marginal p-values, the stepwise resampling-based test is more powerful than the single-step resampling-based test. Note that, even though the bootstrap resampling is performed under the assumption that all three null hypotheses are true, the resulting testing procedure controls the familywise error rate in the strong sense.

The resampling-based methodology is sometimes criticized because it relies heavily on Monte Carlo approximations. Westfall and Young (1993) also introduced permutation versions of their bootstrap tests and showed that permutation testing methods often deliver exact solutions. Westfall and Young demonstrated via simulations that permutation multiple testing procedures are generally more conservative than bootstrap procedures. The difference between the two methods is rather small in the continuous case and becomes more pronounced in the binary case. Permutation-based multiplicity adjustments are available in PROC MULTTEST and can be requested using the PERMUTATION and STEPPERM options.

Subset Pivotality Condition

The concept of *subset pivotality* is one of the key concepts of resampling-based inference. It was introduced by Westfall and Young (1993) to describe conditions under which resampling-based multiple tests control the familywise error rate in the strong sense. To define the subset pivotality condition, consider again the null hypotheses $H_1, \ldots, H_m$. Partition the hypotheses into two subsets. The subset pivotality condition holds if the joint distribution of the p-values corresponding to the hypotheses in the first subset does not depend on the hypotheses in the second subset for any partitioning scheme. In other words, the hypotheses in the second subset may be true or false but this will not affect our inferences with respect to the hypotheses in the first subset. See Westfall and Young (1993, Section 2.2) for details and examples.

The subset pivotality condition is met in a large number of practical situations. There are, however, some exceptions, the most important of which is the case of binary outcomes. The subset pivotality condition does not hold in problems involving multiple pairwise or treatment-control comparisons of proportions. In simple terms, this is caused by the heteroscedastic nature of binary data. Under normal theory, different populations can have a common variance even if their means are dramatically different. In contrast, the variances of sample proportions are constant across several populations only if the underlying true proportions are all the same. Westfall et al. (1999, Section 12.3) gave an example of a study with a binary endpoint in which a permutation multiple testing procedure based on the Fisher exact test produced a clearly incorrect result.

To alleviate this problem, Westfall and Young (1993) recommended to apply a variance-stabilizing transformation (e.g., the well-known arcsine transformation) before performing a resampling-based multiplicity adjustment. The Freeman-Tukey test in PROC MULTTEST is based on the arcsine transformation and generally does a better job in terms of controlling the overall Type I error rate than the Fisher exact test.

Program 2.9 compares the performance of the one-sided Fisher exact and Freeman-Tukey tests on a data set similar to the one used by Westfall et al. (1999, Program 12.5). The Fisher and Freeman-Tukey tests are requested in the program by using the FISHER and FT options in the TEST statement of PROC MULTTEST.

Program 2.9 Multiple testing procedures based on Fisher exact and Freeman-Tukey tests

```
data trouble;
    input group outcome count @@;
    datalines;
    1 0 4   1 1 0   2 0 1   2 1 3   3 0 3   3 1 1
    ;
proc multtest data=trouble stepboot seed=443 n=20000;
    title "Adjustment based on the Fisher exact test";
    class group;
    freq count;
    test fisher(outcome/lower);
    contrast "1 vs 2" 1 -1 0;
    contrast "1 vs 3" 1  0 -1;
    contrast "2 vs 3" 0  1 -1;
```

```
proc multtest data=trouble stepboot seed=443 n=20000;
    title "Adjustment based on the Freeman-Tukey test";
    class group;
    freq count;
    test ft(outcome/lower);
    contrast "1 vs 2" 1 -1 0;
    contrast "1 vs 3" 1  0 -1;
    contrast "2 vs 3" 0  1 -1;
    run;
```

Output from Program 2.9

Adjustment based on the Fisher exact test
                    p-Values

Variable	Contrast	Raw	Stepdown Bootstrap
outcome	1 vs 2	0.0714	0.0698
outcome	1 vs 3	0.5000	0.4956
outcome	2 vs 3	0.9857	0.7972

Adjustment based on the Freeman-Tukey test
                    p-Values

Variable	Contrast	Raw	Stepdown Bootstrap
outcome	1 vs 2	0.0109	0.0698
outcome	1 vs 3	0.1522	0.3361
outcome	2 vs 3	0.8975	0.9162

Output 2.9 shows that all three adjusted *p*-values produced by the Fisher exact test are less than the corresponding raw *p*-values. This is obviously a serious error. In repeated sampling, this procedure will demonstrate excessive Type I error rates. In contrast, the adjusted *p*-values associated with the Freeman-Tukey test are greater than the raw *p*-values. Generally, multiple testing procedures based on the Freeman-Tukey test have a more reasonable Type I error rate. See Westfall and Wolfinger (2000) for more details about subset pivotality and PROC MULTTEST documentation, and Westfall et al. (1999, Section 12.3) for other approaches to resampling-based multiple inference in binary applications.

2.5.1 Summary

This section briefly described the method of resampling-based multiplicity adjustment introduced by Westfall and Young (1989). The resampling-based methodology is very appealing in clinical applications because it combines the simplicity of marginal tests and the power of tests that make distributional assumptions. Resampling-based multiple tests are easy to implement and yet they can be applied to a wide variety of settings including univariate and multivariate models. PROC MULTTEST has extensive capabilities for carrying out bootstrap- and permutation-based multiple tests. For a further discussion of resampling-based multiplicity adjustments, their applications and PROC MULTTEST examples, see Westfall et al. (1999).

2.6 Testing Procedures for Multiple Endpoints

A large number of clinical trials employ multiple co-primary endpoints to study the efficacy or safety of new therapies. Multiple endpoints are popular in a clinical trial setting for several reasons. In their review of clinical trials with multiple outcome measures, Huque and Sankoh (1997) pointed out that it is often difficult to fully characterize the efficacy profile of an experimental therapy using a single endpoint when the disease of interest has a complex etiology. They illustrated their point using ulcerative colitis trials, which commonly include a variety of patient and physician assessments. Drug developers encounter similar problems in many other areas. For example, it is known that no single outcome variable defines a clinically relevant therapeutic benefit for patients with lupus (Siegel, 1999). This section describes several approaches to the simultaneous analysis of multiple endpoints in a clinical trial setting. We will discuss parametric and resampling-based testing procedures for multiple endpoints.

2.6.1 Global Tests for Multiple Endpoints

Consider a clinical trial in which g therapies are compared to each other and the therapeutic effect of each of them is assessed using m continuous endpoints. There are n_i patients in the ith treatment group and $n = \sum_{i=1}^{g} n_i$. Let X_{ijk} denote a normally distributed measurement taken from the jth patient in the ith treatment group with respect to the kth endpoint. Let μ_{ik} and σ_k denote the mean and standard deviation of X_{ijk}, respectively. Further, assume a common correlation matrix in the g treatment groups and denote it by R. We are interested in constructing a test that combines the evidence from the individual endpoints, i.e., a test that evaluates the drug effect in a global fashion.

In a clinical trial setting, there is an important distinction between favorable and unfavorable treatment differences. A good global test needs to be able to detect the direction of treatment differences with respect to the individual endpoints. Assume that larger values of X_{ijk} reflect a clinical improvement. In mathematical terms, we wish to test the global null hypothesis H of no treatment effect,

$$H = \{\mu_{1k} = \mu_{2k} = \ldots = \mu_{gk}, \quad k = 1, \ldots, m\},$$

against a "one-sided" alternative hypothesis H^* that represents an improvement with respect to some or all of the m endpoints,

$$H^* = \{\mu_{tk} \leq \mu_{uk} \text{ with at least one strict inequality}$$
$$\text{for some } t \text{ and } u, \quad k = 1, \ldots, m\}.$$

Note that *directionless* tests such as the Hotelling T^2 test will not work in clinical applications because they test the global null hypothesis H against a "two-sided" alternative representing any departure from H. Clinical statisticians are interested in methods for directing Hotelling-type tests toward narrow, clinically important alternatives.

Tests Based on Marginal *p*-Values

As we stressed in Sections 2.2 and 2.3, multiple tests based on marginal p-values are widely used in the analysis of multiple endpoints. Single-step and stepwise marginal tests such as the Bonferroni or Holm tests are easy to implement in SAS using PROC MULTTEST. It is important to remember that marginal tests for multiple endpoints ignore the stochastic dependence among the individual endpoints. As a result, these tests are often very conservative in a clinical setting because multiple endpoints are typically biologically related and thus likely to exhibit a significant amount of correlation. Several authors presented the results of Monte Carlo simulations conducted to assess the performance of marginal tests such as the Bonferroni test and to compare it to the performance of tests that account for the correlation among the endpoints. Pocock, Geller and Tsiatis (1987) indicated that the Bonferroni test is most powerful when a significant improvement is observed only with respect to one of the endpoints, which is rarely the case in clinical applications. On the other hand, the Bonferroni test seriously lacks power in more realistic scenarios involving favorable changes in all of the endpoints.

EXAMPLE: Rheumatoid Arthritis Trial

We will illustrate the limitations of marginal tests for multiple endpoints using a small "proof-of-concept" trial in patients with rheumatoid arthritis. The efficacy of rheumatoid arthritis therapies is typically assessed using the American College of Rheumatology (ACR) definition of improvement (Felson et al., 1995). This definition was derived from seven measures of disease activity, including joint counts, patient and physician assessments, and an inflammation biomarker. The ACR response criterion is typically defined based on a 20% improvement in some or all of the listed measures. The use of this response criterion is required in registration trials for therapies aimed at improving the signs and symptoms of rheumatoid arthritis.

Note that the ACR response criterion is constructed by dichotomizing continuous outcome variables. It is well known that one should generally expect a loss of power in the statistical analysis when a continuous endpoint is converted into a categorical one. For this reason, the ACR response criterion is less frequently used as the primary endpoint in early proof-of-concept trials in patients with rheumatoid arthritis. Global tests based on some of the continuous endpoints comprising the ACR definition of improvement are generally more powerful than ACR response analyses in this setting.

Consider a clinical trial conducted to compare a new rheumatoid arthritis therapy to a placebo. Twenty-four rheumatoid arthritis patients were enrolled in the trial. The primary analysis in this trial was based on the number of swollen joints (SJC), number of tender joints (TJC), physician global assessment (PHA) and patient global assessment (PTA). The number of swollen and tender joints was computed using a 28-joint count, and the physician and patient global assessments were performed on a 100-mm visual analog scale. The changes from baseline in the four efficacy measures are summarized in Program 2.10.

Program 2.10 Rheumatoid arthritis data

```
data ra;
    input group $ sjc tjc pta pha @@;
    datalines;
    Placebo    -5  -9  -14  -21 Placebo    -3  -7   -5  -25
    Placebo    -7  -4  -28  -15 Placebo    -3   0  -17   -6
    Placebo    -4  -1   -5    5 Placebo     0   5   -8  -11
    Placebo    -3   1   15    0 Placebo     2   6   15   27
    Placebo    -1  -4  -11   -8 Placebo     0   1    8   12
    Placebo     2  -2    6   -9 Placebo     8   2   11   33
    Therapy    -7  -1  -21   -9 Therapy    -6 -11  -36  -12
    Therapy    -3  -7  -14  -21 Therapy    -4   2   10  -10
    Therapy   -11  -4  -28  -45 Therapy    -4  -1  -11  -23
    Therapy    -3  -1   -7  -15 Therapy    -5  -9  -36  -15
    Therapy    -4  -9  -35  -32 Therapy   -11 -10  -47  -31
    Therapy     3  -1    6   17 Therapy    -1  -9   -5  -27
    ;
```

The four selected outcome measures represent closely related aspects of patient outcome and it should not be surprising that they are highly correlated. The sample correlation matrix is equal to

$$\widehat{R} = \begin{bmatrix} 1 & 0.51 & 0.75 & 0.76 \\ 0.51 & 1 & 0.72 & 0.65 \\ 0.75 & 0.72 & 1 & 0.67 \\ 0.76 & 0.65 & 0.67 & 1 \end{bmatrix}.$$

Program 2.11 performs simple univariate analyses of the four efficacy endpoints using the two-sample t-tests under the assumption of equal variances (we used `ods listing close` to suppress the regular PROC TTEST output and `ods listing` to enable printing in PROC PRINT).

Program 2.11 Analysis of the rheumatoid arthritis data using univariate two-sample *t*-tests

```
ods listing close;
proc ttest data=ra;
    class group;
    var sjc tjc pta pha;
    ods output ttests=ttest(where=(method="Pooled"));
proc print data=ttest noobs label;
    ods listing;
    run;
```

Output from Program 2.11

Variable	Method	Variances	t Value	DF	Pr >|t|
sjc	Pooled	Equal	2.18	22	0.0403
tjc	Pooled	Equal	2.21	22	0.0375
pta	Pooled	Equal	2.43	22	0.0239
pha	Pooled	Equal	2.50	22	0.0205

Note that all four raw *p*-values in Output 2.11 are significant at the usual 5% level. However, if we employ a crude Bonferroni correction for multiplicity, our conclusions about the overall effect of the experimental therapy will change. The Bonferroni global test produces a non-significant *p*-value of 0.082 (this *p*-value equals 4 times the smallest raw *p*-value in Output 2.11).

Likelihood-Based Tests

Under normal theory, a natural choice for a hypothesis-testing problem with multiple endpoints is a likelihood ratio test. As pointed out in Wassmer, Reitmeir, Kieser and Lehmacher (1999), several authors (including Perlman (1969)) considered likelihood ratio tests for the one-sided problem outlined above. However, the likelihood-based solutions turned out to be very complex, especially in the case when the correlation matrix R is unknown. Since the likelihood ratio test for the multiple endpoint problem is computationally intractable, alternative solutions based on approximations were proposed in the literature. For instance, Tang, Gnecco and Geller (1989a) derived an approximation to the likelihood ratio test by suitably transforming the original data. Although the proposed approximate likelihood ratio test is more attractive than the full-blown likelihood ratio test, it still presents considerable computational problems. The null distribution of the test statistic developed by Tang, Gnecco and Geller belongs to the class of *chi-bar-squared distributions* and numerical integration is required to compute the associated critical points and *p*-values.

Ordinary Least Squares Test

A different and more flexible approach was proposed by O'Brien (1984). O'Brien developed a general method for testing for the global null hypothesis of no treatment effect based on a weighted sum of the individual test statistics. Suppose that the effect sizes associated with the individual endpoints are equal within each treatment group, i.e.,

$$\frac{\mu_{i1}}{\sigma_1} = \frac{\mu_{i2}}{\sigma_2} = \ldots = \frac{\mu_{im}}{\sigma_m}, \quad i = 1, \ldots, g.$$

Let λ_i denote the common effect size in the ith treatment group.

When the assumption of equal effect sizes is met, the complex multivariate problem of analyzing the m endpoints reduces to a simpler univariate problem of comparing the common effect sizes across the treatment groups. O'Brien (1984) proposed to estimate $\lambda_1, \ldots, \lambda_g$ using the method of ordinary least squares (OLS) and then perform across-group comparisons with the help of standard ANOVA techniques.

First, individual observations need to be standardized to ensure that the m endpoints are expressed in common units. Let

$$Y_{ijk} = (X_{ijk} - m_k)/s_k,$$

where m_k is the overall mean and s_k is the usual pooled sample standard deviation for the kth endpoint. To carry out the O'Brien OLS test, combine the standardized observations across the m endpoints by defining

$$Y_{ij}^* = \sum_{k=1}^{m} Y_{ijk}$$

and perform a one-way analysis of variance on these composite scores. The resulting F-test statistic follows the F distribution with $g - 1$ and $n - mg$ degrees of freedom (it is worth noting that the F-test in a one-way ANOVA setting has more degrees of freedom in the denominator).

In two-arm studies, the two-sample t-test can be employed. It is interesting to note that the OLS t-test statistics can be expressed as

$$t_{OLS} = \frac{1}{\sqrt{J'\widehat{R}J}} \sum_{k=1}^{m} t_k,$$

where t_k is the usual t-test statistic for the kth endpoint, i.e.,

$$t_k = \frac{\bar{X}_{1 \cdot k} - \bar{X}_{2 \cdot k}}{s_k\sqrt{1/n_1 + 1/n_2}},$$

$\widehat{R}$ is the sample correlation matrix of the original observations, and $J' = [1\ 1\ \ldots\ 1]$. (In other words, $J'\widehat{R}J$ is the sum of all entries in the sample correlation matrix.) This representation of t_{OLS} highlights the fact that the O'Brien OLS method simply combines the individual t-test statistics for each of the m endpoints with equal weights.

Let us now analyze the rheumatoid arthritis data introduced earlier in this section using the O'Brien OLS test. Figure 2.9 presents a simple plot of the data that indicates that the effect sizes associated with

Figure 2.9 Plot of the effect sizes associated with the physician global assessment (PHA), patient global assessment (PTA), number of swollen joints (SJC) and number of tender joints (TJC) in the placebo (△) and experimental (○) groups in the rheumatoid arthritis trial

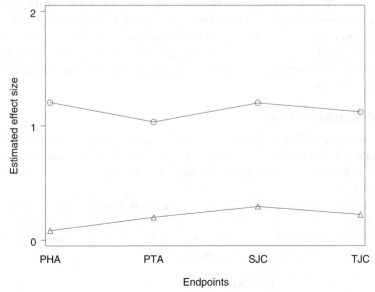

the four efficacy measures are fairly consistent within the experimental and placebo groups. It is safe to conclude that the assumption of equal effect sizes is met.

Program 2.12 assesses the overall effect of the experimental therapy on the selected efficacy measures of disease activity using the O'Brien OLS test. The program is based on the %GlobTest macro given in the Appendix. This powerful macro implements the O'Brien OLS test as well as three other global tests that will be introduced later in this section.

Program 2.12 Analysis of the rheumatoid arthritis data using the O'Brien OLS test

```
%GlobTest(dataset=ra,group=group,ngroups=2,varlist=sjc tjc pta pha,
    test="OLS");
```

The %GlobTest macro has five arguments described below:

- DATASET is the data set to be analyzed.
- GROUP is the name of the group variable in the data set.
- NGROUPS is the number of groups in the data set.
- VARLIST is the list of variable names corresponding to the multiple endpoints of interest.
- TEST is the name of the test to be used, OLS test ("OLS"), GLS test ("GLS"), modified GLS test ("MGLS") or rank-sum test ("RS"), respectively.

Output from Program 2.12

F-value	ndf	ddf	Global p-value
7.73	1	16	0.0134

Output 2.12 shows that the *p*-value associated with the O'Brien OLS test equals 0.0134. Comparing this finding with the Bonferroni-adjusted *p*-value of 0.082 displayed in Output 2.11, we see that incorporating the correlation structure into the decision rule has resulted in a substantial increase in power. Moreover, due to strong positive dependence among the four variables, the O'Brien OLS *p*-value is more significant than any of the raw *p*-values from the univariate *t*-tests. Based on the OLS test, we conclude that the experimental therapy is statistically superior to the placebo when the four efficacy measures are treated as one instrument.

We have considered a multiple endpoint scenario in which the effect sizes were fairly similar within the treatment groups. The O'Brien OLS test also performs well when the effect sizes associated with the multiple endpoints vary within treatment groups. However, it loses power as the spread in the effect sizes increases. One needs to carefully examine both the univariate *p*-values and the global OLS *p*-value when no treatment effect is observed with respect to some of the endpoints, because the OLS test may break down in this situation.

Generalized Least Squares Test

Along with the OLS test, O'Brien (1984) proposed a global test based on a generalized least squares (GLS) estimate of the treatment effect under the assumption of equal effect sizes. The GLS test is more efficient than the OLS test in the presence of heteroscedasticity because it better accounts for the underlying correlation structure.

The important difference between the OLS and GLS approaches is that the GLS test statistic is based on a *weighted* sum of individual test statistics with the weights reflecting the correlation among multiple endpoints. To define the test statistic, consider again normally distributed observations X_{ijk}. As with the OLS test, we first standardize the individual observations and let

$$Y_{ijk} = (X_{ijk} - m_k)/s_k.$$

Now, to combine the standardized observations across the m endpoints, we will take into account the correlation structure. Let r^{tu} denote the (t, u) entry in the inverse of the sample correlation matrix $\widehat{R}$, i.e.,

$$\widehat{R}^{-1} = \begin{bmatrix} r^{11} & \cdots & r^{1m} \\ \vdots & \ddots & \vdots \\ r^{m1} & \cdots & r^{mm} \end{bmatrix}.$$

The composite scores Y_{ij}^* are defined as

$$Y_{ij}^* = \sum_{t=1}^{m} \sum_{u=1}^{m} r^{tu} Y_{iju}$$

and thus endpoints receive greater weights when they are less correlated with the other endpoints. The computed composite scores are analyzed using a one-way analysis of variance. The GLS F-test statistic follows the F distribution with $g - 1$ and $n - mg$ degrees of freedom.

Although the GLS test is generally more powerful than the OLS test, it may be less attractive in clinical applications because it is prone to producing uninterpretable results. As shown above, the weighting scheme in the GLS test is based on the inverse of the sample correlation matrix and it is theoretically possible that some of the endpoints can receive negative weights. Clinically, this means that the GLS test can reject the global null hypothesis of no treatment effect even if the new therapy is inferior to the control on all of the endpoints. See Pocock, Geller and Tsiatis (1987) and Follmann (1995) for a detailed discussion of this phenomenon and examples.

To fix the outlined problem, Tang, Geller and Pocock (1993) proposed to modify the O'Brien GLS test in such a way that individual endpoints always receive non-negative weights. The modified GLS test is based on the composite scores given by

$$Y_{ij}^* = \sum_{t=1}^{m} \sqrt{r^{tt}} Y_{ijt}.$$

As explained in Tang, Geller and Pocock (1993), this choice of weights often possesses an important maximin property. The modified GLS test maximizes the minimum power over all treatment differences in the favorable direction.

Program 2.13 analyzes the rheumatoid arthritis data using both the GLS test and its modification proposed by Tang, Geller and Pocock (1993). The program utilizes the %GlobTest macro.

Program 2.13 Analysis of the rheumatoid arthritis data using the O'Brien GLS test and modified GLS test proposed by Tang, Geller and Pocock (1993)

```
%GlobTest(dataset=ra,group=group,ngroups=2,varlist=sjc tjc pta pha,
    test="GLS");
%GlobTest(dataset=ra,group=group,ngroups=2,varlist=sjc tjc pta pha,
    test="MGLS");
```

Output from Program 2.13

```
          O'Brien GLS test
                        Global
  F-value    ndf    ddf    p-value

    7.41      1     16     0.0151
```

```
           Modified O'Brien GLS test
                             Global
   F-value    ndf    ddf    p-value

    7.71       1      16     0.0135
```

Output 2.13 lists the *p*-values produced by the regular and modified GLS tests. The modified GLS *p*-value equals 0.0135 and is virtually identical to that produced by the OLS test (see Output 2.12). The *p*-value associated with the GLS test is slightly less significant.

It is important to check whether the GLS test assigned non-negative weights to the four individual endpoints. The inverse of the sample correlation matrix $\widehat{R}$ is given by

$$\widehat{R}^{-1} = \begin{bmatrix} 3.45 & 0.87 & -1.95 & -1.88 \\ 0.87 & 2.56 & -1.7 & -1.19 \\ -1.95 & -1.7 & 3.56 & 0.18 \\ -1.88 & -1.19 & 0.18 & 3.08 \end{bmatrix}$$

and it is easy to verify that the column sums in this matrix are positive. This implies that all four endpoints received positive weights and the GLS test is a valid test for comparing the experimental drug to the placebo with respect to the four selected endpoints.

The introduced O'Brien OLS and GLS methods can be extended to a variety of multiple endpoint problems involving normally distributed test statistics. For example, the next subsection introduces a nonparametric version of the O'Brien methods. Further, Pocock, Geller and Tsiatis (1987) demonstrated how the O'Brien GLS test can be applied to the analysis of binary and survival data. Other interesting extensions of this methodology are found in Follmann (1996) and Läuter (1996).

Rank-Sum Test

When clinical measurements are not normally distributed, one can perform an analysis of multiple endpoints using a nonparametric test proposed by O'Brien (1984). This rank-sum test is similar to the OLS and GLS testing procedures introduced earlier in the sense that it reduces the dimensionality of the multiple endpoint problem by combining data across the endpoints in a straightforward manner.

Consider the kth endpoint, and let R_{ijk} denote the rank of X_{ijk} in the pooled sample of g treatment groups with respect to the kth endpoint. The composite score Y_{ij}^* is defined for the jth patient in the ith treatment group as the sum of the obtained ranks, i.e.,

$$Y_{ij}^* = \sum_{t=1}^{m} R_{ijt}.$$

O'Brien proposed to analyze the composite scores by a one-way analysis of variance. The constructed test is conceptually similar to the Kruskal-Wallis test for a nonparametric comparison of multiple samples.

Program 2.14 carries out the O'Brien rank-sum test to compare the experimental drug to the placebo in the rheumatoid arthritis trial example. The rank-sum test statistic is computed by calling the %GlobTest macro.

Output 2.14 shows that the nonparametric *p*-value equals 0.0087 and is highly significant, which indicates that the experimental drug is clearly superior to the placebo when the four selected endpoints are examined simultaneously.

Program 2.14 Analysis of the rheumatoid arthritis data using the O'Brien rank-sum test

```
%GlobTest(dataset=ra,group=group,ngroups=2,varlist=sjc tjc pta pha,
    test="RS");
```

Output from Program 2.14

F-value	ndf	ddf	Global p-value
8.28	1	22	0.0087

Resampling-Based Tests

Section 2.5 outlined applications of the Westfall-Young resampling-based methodology to multiplicity problems arising in the context of multiple comparisons. It is easy to extend this powerful methodology to the analysis of multiple endpoints. Westfall et al. (1999, Section 11.3) discussed the use of bootstrap and permutation tests in clinical trials with multiple outcome measures and showed how to carry out these tests using PROC MULTTEST.

Following Westfall et al. (1999), we will utilize resampling-based multiplicity adjustment techniques in the analysis of the rheumatoid arthritis data. As we have shown earlier in this section, a univariate approach to the analysis of the four outcome measures in the rheumatoid arthritis trial lacks power because it ignores the multivariate nature of the problem. To simultaneously test the four null hypotheses associated with the outcome measures of interest, we need to account for the stochastic dependence among the individual t-test statistics. The resampling-based methodology provides a way to estimate the underlying correlation structure and to compute adjusted p-values for each of the endpoints.

Program 2.15 computes adjusted p-values for the four endpoints in the rheumatoid arthritis trial example using the stepwise bootstrap algorithm.

Program 2.15 Analysis of the rheumatoid arthritis data using the resampling-based test

```
proc multtest data=ra stepboot n=10000 seed=57283;
    class group;
    test mean(sjc tjc pta pha);
    contrast "Treatment effect" 1 -1;
    run;
```

Output from Program 2.15

Variable	Contrast	p-Values Raw	Stepdown Bootstrap
sjc	Treatment effect	0.0403	0.0702
tjc	Treatment effect	0.0375	0.0702
pta	Treatment effect	0.0239	0.0646
pha	Treatment effect	0.0205	0.0646

Output 2.15 demonstrates that the bootstrap-based multiplicity adjustment is not very efficient in this example. The global p-value associated with the bootstrap algorithm equals 0.0646 and is much larger than the O'Brien p-values in Output 2.12 and Output 2.13. It is important to point out that the disproportionately large adjusted p-values produced by the resampling-based procedure in this example do not imply that resampling-based inferences always lack power in statistical problems involving multiple endpoints. The observed difference between the resampling-based and O'Brien tests may simply reflect the fact that the latter testing procedures are very powerful under the assumption of equal effect sizes.

2.6.2 Individual Tests for Multiple Endpoints

The goal of global tests is to examine a significant overall difference across treatment groups with respect to the endpoints of interest. Global tests provide no information about the significance of treatment differences for individual endpoints. However, if the overall analysis yields a significant result, both the trial sponsor and regulatory reviewers are naturally interested in determining which of the individual treatment differences are significant after a proper adjustment for multiplicity.

Statistical inferences about individual endpoints are also very important in clinical trials designed to pursue multiple regulatory claims. It may not be appropriate to combine endpoints if they describe unrelated aspects of the patient response, in which case a global test of the endpoints needs to be replaced with suitably adjusted individual tests.

The easiest way to identify individual significant outcome variables is to analyze the data using a multiple rather than a global test. For example, Troendle and Legler (1998) discussed the application of marginal tests in a multiple endpoint setting. All of the marginal tests described earlier in Sections 2.2 and 2.3 allow the clinical statistician to test the null hypotheses associated with each of the endpoints. Resampling-based tests for multiple endpoints also support inferences for individual outcome measures.

Alternatively, one can start with a global test (e.g., O'Brien and related tests) and utilize the closed testing principle introduced in Section 2.3 to step down to the individual hypotheses; see Lehmacher, Wassmer and Reitmeir (1991) and Westfall and Tobias (2000, Chapter 8) for more details. As we pointed out in Section 2.3, the closed testing principle provides clinical statisticians with a powerful tool for extending global tests to the level of individual hypotheses.

As an illustration, we will apply the method based on the closed testing principle to analyze the data from the rheumatoid arthritis trial example. The primary analysis in this trial was based on four efficacy measures, the swollen joint count, tender joint count, physician global assessment and patient global assessment. Let H_1, H_2, H_3, and H_4 denote the null hypotheses of no treatment effect for the four endpoints. Consider a closed family of hypotheses associated with the four null hypotheses. The closed family contains 15 hypotheses representing all possible intersections of H_1, H_2, H_3 and H_4 (see Section 2.3 for a more detailed description of closed families of hypotheses). Each member of the closed family can be viewed as a global hypothesis and, therefore, can be tested using a global test, e.g., the O'Brien OLS test. To test the individual null hypotheses, we will need to combine the results and compute the adjusted p-values associated with H_1, H_2, H_3 and H_4. The adjusted p-value for each individual null hypothesis is defined as the largest p-value for the intersection hypotheses that imply it.

In practice, adjusted p-values for H_1, H_2, H_3 and H_4 can be computed using the decision matrix algorithm introduced in Section 2.3.2. Program 2.16 utilizes the decision matrix approach to compute the adjusted p-values for the four efficacy variables in the rheumatoid arthritis trial. The %GlobTest macro is invoked in Program 2.16 to carry out the O'Brien OLS test for each member of the closed family of hypotheses associated with H_1, H_2, H_3 and H_4.

Program 2.16 Analysis of the rheumatoid arthritis data using the closed version of the O'Brien OLS test

```
%let varname=sjc tjc pta pha;
data hyp;
    length varlist $50;
    array h{*} h1-h4;
    do i=15 to 1 by -1;
        string=put(i,binary4.);
        hypnum=16-i;
        do j=1 to 4;
            h{j}=substr(string,j,1);
        end;
        varlist=" ";
        do j=1 to 4;
            if h{j}=1 then varlist=
            trim(varlist) || " " || scan("&varname",j);
```

```
            end;
        output;
        end;
        keep hypnum h1-h4 varlist;
data pvalcomb;
%macro pval;
    %do j=1 %to 15;
    data _null_;
        set hyp;
        if hypnum=&j then call symput("varlist",trim(varlist));
        run;
        %GlobTest(ra,group,2,&varlist,"OLS");
    data pvalcomb;
        set pvalcomb pval;
        keep adjp;
        run;
    %end;
%mend pval;

%pval;

data decrule;
    merge hyp pvalcomb(where=(adjp^=.));
    array h{*} h1-h4;
    array hyp{*} hyp1-hyp4;
    do i=1 to 4;
        hyp{i}=adjp*h{i};
    end;
    keep hyp1-hyp4;
proc means data=decrule noprint;
    var hyp1-hyp4;
    output out=indadjp(keep=adjp1-adjp4)
    max(hyp1-hyp4)=adjp1-adjp4;
data indadjp;
    set indadjp;
    format adjp1-adjp4 6.4;
proc print data=indadjp noobs;
    title "Adjusted p-values for individual hypotheses";
    run;
```

Output from Program 2.16

```
Adjusted p-values for individual hypotheses

  adjp1     adjp2     adjp3     adjp4

 0.0403    0.0375    0.0239    0.0205
```

Output 2.16 lists the adjusted p-values for the individual null hypotheses in the rheumatoid trial example. The p-values correspond to the swollen joint count, tender joint count, physician global assessment and patient global assessment, respectively. It is instructive to compare these adjusted p-values to the raw p-values displayed in Output 2.11. Output 2.16 indicates that here we are dealing with a unique situation in which the adjusted p-values generated by the O'Brien OLS test are equal to the raw p-values produced by the univariate t-tests. Due to a common treatment effect across the variables considered, not only has the global OLS test yielded a significant result, but also the treatment differences with respect to all four endpoints are significant.

Needless to say, scenarios in which adjusted p-values are equal to raw p-values are very uncommon in clinical applications. Adjusted p-values for the individual endpoints are typically larger than the corresponding raw univariate p-values. In fact, one is likely to see non-significant adjusted p-values in univariate analyses following a significant global test. This happens because global tests are generally substantially more powerful than univariate inferences with respect to each individual endpoint. Theoretically, one may run into situations when the global test yields a significant result yet none of the adjusted univariate analyses is even remotely significant.

2.6.3 Summary

In this section we discussed statistical methods for the analysis of clinical trials with multiple endpoints and described the following testing procedures used in a clinical trial setting:

- Tests based on marginal p-values (e.g., the Bonferroni test) are often very conservative in clinical applications because they ignore the correlation among multiple endpoints.

- The ordinary least squares (OLS) test is an example of a global test for a simultaneous analysis of multiple endpoints. The OLS method combines equally weighted test statistics for the individual endpoints. The OLS test is most powerful under the assumption of equal effect sizes.

- The generalized least squares (GLS) test is a global test based on a weighted sum of individual test statistics. The test statistics are weighted to account for heteroscedasticity. The GLS test is generally more efficient than the OLS test but can sometimes produce uninterpretable results when it assigns negative weights to some of the endpoints.

- The modified generalized least squares test is similar to the GLS test. This test is set up in such a way that individual endpoints always receive non-negative weights.

- The rank-sum test is a natural extension of the OLS test to a nonparametric setting.

- Resampling-based testing procedures account for the stochastic dependence among multiple endpoints via bootstrap or permutation methods. These procedures can be used both for testing the global hypothesis and for testing the effects of individual endpoints.

The listed testing procedures for the analysis of clinical trials with multiple endpoints are easy to implement in SAS using PROC MULTTEST or the %GlobTest macro introduced in this section.

The section also addressed the issue of making inferences with respect to the individual endpoints after a global test has been carried out. Univariate analyses of this type are based on the closed testing principle and can be performed using the decision matrix algorithm.

2.7 Gatekeeping Strategies

This section describes testing procedures for families of hypotheses encountered in clinical trials with hierarchically ordered endpoints and in dose-finding studies. The families are tested in a sequential manner in the sense that the acceptance or rejection of hypotheses in a particular family depends on the outcome of the significance tests carried out in the preceding families. In other words, the families of hypotheses examined earlier serve as *gatekeepers*, and one can test hypotheses in a particular family only if the preceding gatekeepers have been successfully passed.

Several types of gatekeeping testing procedures for sequential families of hypotheses have been proposed in the literature.

- Bauer et al. (1998) and Westfall and Krishen (2001) considered multiple testing procedures that are closely related to fixed-sequence procedures discussed in Section 2.4. The proposed procedures pass a gatekeeper family only if all hypotheses in the family have been rejected. To make an analogy with reliability theory, this approach can be called a *serial* gatekeeping approach because serial gatekeepers correspond to systems in which basic elements are connected in series. With this type of connection, each element plays a very important role in defining the strength of the overall system.

Similarly, a serial gatekeeping procedure terminates as soon as it fails to reject any of the individual hypotheses.

- An alternative type of gatekeeping inferences (known as *parallel* inferences) was discussed by Dmitrienko, Offen and Westfall (2003). Within the parallel gatekeeping framework, only one hypothesis needs to be rejected to pass a gatekeeper and thus one has more power to evaluate inferences in the subsequent families.

This section discusses procedures for hypothesis-testing problems with serial or parallel families of hypotheses as well as problems involving a mixture of serial and parallel families. The outlined framework of gatekeeping inferences is very flexible and can be used to effectively manage multiple analyses in a variety of clinical applications.

It is important to note that the hypothesis-testing problems considered within the gatekeeping framework are different from those discussed earlier in Section 2.6. The focus of Section 2.6 was on the analysis of clinical trials with multiple outcome variables that carry the same weight in terms of determining the overall outcome of the trial. Within the gatekeeping framework, the trial endpoints are classified in a hierarchical manner, e.g., primary, secondary and possibly tertiary endpoints. Gatekeeping testing procedures are set up to account for this hierarchy of endpoints when making multiple inferences.

2.7.1 Examples of Sequential Families of Hypotheses in Clinical Trials

Trials with Hierarchically Ordered Endpoints

Hypotheses tested in clinical trials are commonly divided into primary and secondary categories. The primary hypothesis is formulated in terms of the primary trial endpoint, which describes the most important features of an experimental drug. In most registration trials, the primary analysis determines the overall outcome of the trial and provides the basis for the regulatory claim. Secondary hypotheses may also play an important role in determining the overall outcome, and it is often desirable to present secondary findings in the product label. However, a significant improvement in a secondary endpoint is not generally considered as substantial evidence of therapeutic benefit (O'Neill, 1997).

Relative merits of various methods for performing flexible data-driven analyses of secondary endpoints in clinical trials have been debated in the drug development literature over the past several years. The interpretation of a positive finding with respect to a secondary outcome variable depends heavily on its clinical importance. The guideline entitled "Points to consider on multiplicity issues in clinical trials" published by the CPMP on September 19, 2002, classified secondary variables as

- variables that may potentially provide the basis for a new regulatory claim
- variables that may become the basis for additional claims
- variables yielding supportive evidence.

The following two examples present two scenarios in which the secondary analyses can potentially lead to additional regulatory claims.

EXAMPLE: Depression Trial

Consider a clinical trial in patients with clinical depression. The primary endpoint is the mean improvement from baseline in the 17-item Hamilton Depression Scale (HAMD17 score) and the important secondary endpoints include the response and remission rates based on the HAMD17 score. (See Hamilton (1967) and Faries et al. (2000) for a detailed discussion of depression rating scales.) The primary regulatory claim will be based on the primary outcome variable, and the secondary variables will be analyzed to evaluate the evidence for additional regulatory claims. The primary hypothesis serves as a gatekeeper in the sense that the secondary hypotheses will be tested only after the primary analysis has yielded a statistically significant result. We wish to develop a gatekeeping strategy for testing the primary and two secondary hypotheses in a manner that preserves the familywise error rate in the strong sense.

EXAMPLE: Acute Respiratory Distress Syndrome Trial

Next, we will consider a clinical trial in patients with acute respiratory distress syndrome (ARDS). The trial is conducted to compare one dose of an investigational drug to a placebo. The therapeutic benefits of experimental treatments in ARDS trials are commonly measured using the number of days alive and off mechanical ventilation during a 28-day study period and 28-day all-cause mortality. Either of these two endpoints can be used to make regulatory claims. Additional regulatory claims can be made with respect to secondary outcome variables such as the number of ICU-free days (the number of days the patient was out of the intensive care unit) and general quality of life. Our interest lies in developing a multiple testing procedure that will allow us to test the statistical significance of the secondary endpoints after at least one primary outcome variable has been found significant. Note that the mathematics underlying gatekeeping inferences in this example is more sophisticated than in the previous example due to the presence of multiple hypotheses in the primary gatekeeper family.

Multiple Comparisons in Dose-Finding Trials

One can also encounter hierarchically ordered hypotheses in clinical trials designed to test several doses of an experimental drug versus a placebo or an active control. Westfall and Krishen (2001) described serial gatekeeping procedures and Denne and Koch (2002) discussed sequential families of hypotheses with parallel gatekeepers in dose-response studies. The following example deals with a trial in patients with hypertension in which four doses of an experimental drug are compared to placebo.

EXAMPLE: Dose-Finding Hypertension Trial

Suppose that four doses of a new antihypertensive drug (labeled D1, D2, D3 and D4) are tested against a placebo. If the highest two doses D3 and D4 are considered to be most efficacious, it is prudent to compare them to the placebo at the first stage of the procedure. If at least one of the two dose-placebo comparisons is significant, one can proceed to testing D1 and D2 versus the placebo. Again, if at least one of the two tests produces a significant result, various pairwise comparisons (e.g., D4 versus D1, D4 versus D2, D3 versus D1, D3 versus D2) can be performed to study the shape of the dose-response relationship. We are interested in setting up a gatekeeping procedure for testing the three families of hypotheses in a sequential manner without inflating the overall Type I error rate. The gatekeeping procedure needs to properly account for the fact that the hypotheses in the first two families are tested in a parallel manner.

2.7.2 General Principles of Gatekeeping Inferences

In order to explain how to set up gatekeeping testing procedures in the examples presented above, we will describe the general framework for performing gatekeeping inferences. Consider a family of n null hypotheses grouped into m families denoted by $F_1, \ldots, F_m$. The ith family contains n_i hypotheses $H_{i1}, \ldots, H_{in_i}, i = 1, \ldots, m$, and $n_1 + \ldots + n_m = n$. Let $p_{i1}, \ldots, p_{in_i}$ denote the raw p-values for the hypotheses in the ith family and $\widetilde{p}_{i1}, \ldots, \widetilde{p}_{in_i}$ denote the corresponding multiplicity adjusted p-values, $i = 1, \ldots, m$. Additionally, as will be explained later in this section, we can assign weights both within each family and across families. Within-family weights may reflect the clinical importance of individual hypotheses/endpoints. A more important hypothesis with a larger weight is more likely to be rejected than a hypothesis with a lower weight. Similarly, one can assign greater importance to a certain family and, by doing so, increase the likelihood of rejecting all hypotheses in that family.

The individual families $F_1, \ldots, F_m$ are referred to as *gatekeepers* and are tested in the following sequential manner. The null hypotheses in F_1 are examined first and tested at the prespecified α level with a suitable adjustment for multiplicity. Next, the hypotheses in F_2 are tested with an appropriate adjustment for multiplicity provided the gatekeeper F_1 has been successfully passed. Further, if the gatekeeper F_2 has also been successfully passed, we examine the hypotheses in F_3 and so on. As was noted earlier, a serial gatekeeper F_i is passed if one rejects all hypotheses in F_i, i.e., if

$$\max(\widetilde{p}_{i1}, \ldots, \widetilde{p}_{in_i}) \leq \alpha.$$

In contrast, in order to pass a parallel gatekeeper F_i, it is sufficient to reject only one hypothesis, which occurs when

$$\min(\widetilde{p}_{i1}, \ldots, \widetilde{p}_{in_i}) \leq \alpha.$$

The three clinical examples in Section 2.7.1 represent special cases of this general formulation of the problem of sequential hypothesis-testing. As shown in Figures 2.10 and 2.11, the depression and ARDS trial examples involve two families of hypotheses with one and two hypotheses in the gatekeeper family, respectively. The two primary hypotheses H_{11} and H_{12} in the ARDS trial example are represented by two vertically stacked boxes to emphasize that the hypotheses are tested in a parallel fashion; i.e., only one of them needs to be rejected to proceed to the secondary hypotheses H_{21} and H_{22}.

Figure 2.10 Two families of null hypotheses in the depression trial example. The primary hypothesis based on the mean improvement in the HAMD17 score serves as a gatekeeper. The secondary hypotheses will be tested only after the primary hypothesis has been rejected.

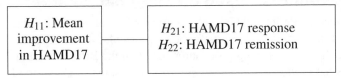

Figure 2.11 Two families of null hypotheses in the ARDS trial example. The co-primary endpoints (number of ventilator-free days and 28-day all-cause mortality) form a gatekeeper. The secondary endpoints will be analyzed provided at least one primary outcome variable has been found significant.

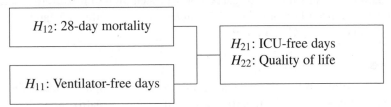

Figure 2.12 shows that the dose-finding hypertension trial involves three sequential families of hypotheses. The first two families in this example are tested in a parallel manner and thus there are four decision-making paths leading to the hypotheses in the third family of hypotheses. For instance, pairwise comparisons in the third family can be performed after rejecting H_{11} and H_{21}, or H_{12} and H_{21}, etc.

Figure 2.12 Three families of null hypotheses in the dose-finding hypertension trial example. The first family includes the null hypotheses corresponding to the D4 vs. placebo and D3 vs. placebo comparisons. If at least one of these comparisons is significant, proceed to testing the null hypotheses in the second family (D2 vs. placebo and D1 vs. placebo). Now if at least one of the two tests in the second family produces a significant outcome, test the null hypotheses in the third family (pairwise comparisons).

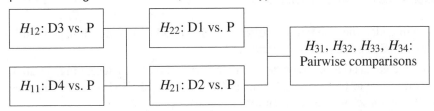

In general, gatekeeping procedures are required to satisfy either one of the following two conditions:

Condition A. Inferences for the null hypotheses in F_i may depend on inferences in the subsequent families $F_{i+1}, \ldots, F_m$. It is possible to reject any null hypothesis in F_i regardless of how many hypotheses have been rejected in $F_{i+1}, \ldots, F_m$; however, a rejection of a hypothesis in F_i may be due to certain significant outcomes in $F_{i+1}, \ldots, F_m$.

Condition B. Inferences for the null hypotheses in F_i do not depend on inferences for the hypotheses in $F_{i+1}, \ldots, F_m$. In other words, the adjusted p-values associated with the hypotheses in F_i do not depend on the raw p-values for the hypotheses in $F_{i+1}, \ldots, F_m$ and, therefore, a decision to reject a hypothesis in F_i is completely independent of decisions made in $F_{i+1}, \ldots, F_m$.

Note that Condition B is stronger and generally more desirable than Condition A in clinical trial applications because it implies that inferences with respect to more important hypotheses are unaffected by which and how many secondary hypotheses have been rejected. On the other hand, gatekeeping procedures that satisfy the more desirable Condition B are typically less powerful than those satisfying Condition A only.

2.7.3   Gatekeeping Procedures Based on Marginal *p*-Values

The principle of closed testing of Marcus, Peritz and Gabriel (1976) provides clinical statisticians with a powerful tool for setting up gatekeeping strategies that satisfy the two formulated conditions.

In this section we will introduce three gatekeeping procedures based on the Bonferroni and Simes tests. The first procedure, known as the *Bonferroni gatekeeping procedure*, satisfies Condition B. The second procedure, known as the *modified Bonferroni gatekeeping procedure*, is uniformly more powerful than the first procedure; however, it does not always satisfy Condition B. In general, it can be shown that the modified Bonferroni gatekeeping procedure satisfies Condition A only, which means that inferences for any particular family of hypotheses may depend on whether or not some hypotheses are rejected in the subsequent families. Lastly, the Simes gatekeeping procedure is similar to the modified Bonferroni procedure in that it is uniformly more powerful than the regular Bonferroni gatekeeping procedure and, in general, does not satisfy Condition B.

%GateKeeper Macro

The Bonferroni, modified Bonferroni and Simes gatekeeping procedures are implemented in the %GateKeeper macro given in the Appendix. The macro relies on the decision matrix algorithm introduced in Section 2.3.2 to perform the gatekeeping inferences (see Section 2.7.5 for more details).

The %GateKeeper macro has the following three parameters:

- DATASET is the name of the input data set with information about sequential families of hypotheses (testing type, weights, relative importance of gatekeeper hypotheses and raw p-values).

- TEST is the name of the test to be used: "B," MB," or "S" for Bonferroni, modified Bonferroni or Simes gatekeeping procedure, respectively.

- OUTDATA is the name of the output data set with adjusted p-values.

The %GateKeeper macro assumes that the input data set contains one record per individual hypothesis and includes the following variables:

- The FAMILY variable identifies the family index for each individual hypothesis. The families of hypotheses are assumed to be sequentially numbered.

- The SERIAL variable equals 0 if the hypotheses in the current family are tested in a parallel manner and 1 if the hypotheses are tested in a serial manner. Note that the SERIAL variable must have the same value for all hypotheses within each family.

- The WEIGHT variable specifies the relative importance of hypotheses within each family. The values of the WEIGHT variable must be between 0 and 1 and must add up to 1 within each family.

- The RELIMP variable specifies the importance of each family of hypotheses relative to hypotheses in subsequent families (and thus the RELIMP variable must have the same value for all hypotheses within each family). The RELIMP variable equals 0 if the family is tested in a serial manner and is equal to a number between 0 and 1 (0 is included but 1 is excluded) in the case of parallel testing. Larger values of this variable increase the importance of the current family of hypotheses. Mathematically, increasing the RELIMP variable results in a higher probability of rejecting hypotheses in the current family at the price of reducing the likelihood of rejecting hypotheses in the subsequent families.

- Finally, the RAW_P variable contains the raw p-values for the individual hypotheses.

The output data set includes the same five variables plus the ADJP variable containing the adjusted p-values for the hypotheses in the input data set.

Bonferroni Gatekeeping Procedure in the Depression Trial Example

Here we will demonstrate how to test two families of hypotheses in the depression trial using a simple gatekeeping strategy based on the Bonferroni test. To describe the theory behind the Bonferroni gatekeeping procedure, we will show how to set up a closed test that accounts for the hierarchical structure of this hypothesis-testing problem. We will then construct the corresponding decision matrix. See Section 2.7.5 for a description of multiple testing algorithms implemented in the %GateKeeper macro.

The three null hypotheses tested in the depression trial are defined as

H_{11} (no treatment effect with respect to mean HAMD17 improvement)

H_{21} (no treatment effect with respect to HAMD17 response rate)

H_{22} (no treatment effect with respect to HAMD17 remission rate).

The associated raw p-values will be denoted by p_{11}, p_{21} and p_{22}.

The gatekeeper family, denoted by F_1, comprises the primary hypothesis H_{11}, and the other family, denoted by F_2, comprises the secondary hypotheses H_{21} and H_{22}. As with any closed test, we need to define a closed family of hypotheses associated with the three original hypotheses. The closed family includes seven possible intersections of H_{11}, H_{21} and H_{22} known as intersection hypotheses. It is convenient to adopt the following binary representation of the intersection hypotheses. The original hypotheses H_{11}, H_{21} and H_{22} are denoted by H^*_{100}, H^*_{010} and H^*_{001}, respectively. Similarly,

$$H^*_{110} = H_{11} \cap H_{21}, \quad H^*_{101} = H_{11} \cap H_{22}, \quad H^*_{011} = H_{21} \cap H_{22}, \text{ etc.}$$

Now, to define a gatekeeping procedure based on the principle of closed testing, choose an intersection hypothesis H^* in the closed family. Suppose first that H^* is equal to H^*_{100}, H^*_{110}, H^*_{101} or H^*_{111}, and thus it implies the primary hypothesis H_{11}. In this case, H^* will be tested by comparing p_{11} to α, which means that the adjusted p-value associated with H^* is simply p_{11}. Note that the described decision rule ignores the p-values for the secondary hypotheses. This is done to ensure that the tests of the secondary hypotheses will not affect the inferences with respect to the primary hypothesis. Further, if H^* equals H^*_{011}, it will be tested using the Bonferroni procedure and thus the adjusted p-value for H^* is given by $2\min(p_{21}, p_{22})$. Finally, if H^* is equal to H^*_{010} or H^*_{001}, it will be tested by comparing p_{21} or p_{22} to α, respectively. This implies that the adjusted p-value associated with H^* is p_{21} or p_{22}.

Once all hypotheses in the closed family have been examined, one can compute the adjusted p-values associated with the original hypotheses H_{11}, H_{21} and H_{22}. The adjusted p-value $\widetilde{p}_{11}$ for H_{11} is defined as the largest p-value associated with the closed family hypotheses that imply H_{11}—i.e., H^*_{100}, H^*_{110}, H^*_{101} and H^*_{111}. The adjusted p-values $\widetilde{p}_{21}$ and $\widetilde{p}_{22}$ are defined in a similar manner. The original hypotheses H_{11}, H_{21} and H_{22} are tested by comparing $\widetilde{p}_{11}$, $\widetilde{p}_{21}$ and $\widetilde{p}_{22}$ to α.

Table 2.6 Decision matrix for the Bonferroni gatekeeping procedure in the depression trial

Intersection hypothesis	P-value	Implied hypotheses		
		H_{11}	H_{21}	H_{22}
H_{111}^*	$p_{111}^* = p_{11}$	p_{111}^*	p_{111}^*	p_{111}^*
H_{110}^*	$p_{110}^* = p_{11}$	p_{110}^*	p_{110}^*	0
H_{101}^*	$p_{101}^* = p_{11}$	p_{101}^*	0	p_{101}^*
H_{100}^*	$p_{100}^* = p_{11}$	p_{100}^*	0	0
H_{011}^*	$p_{011}^* = 2\min(p_{21}, p_{22})$	0	p_{011}^*	p_{011}^*
H_{010}^*	$p_{010}^* = p_{21}$	0	p_{010}^*	0
H_{001}^*	$p_{001}^* = p_{22}$	0	0	p_{001}^*

Table 2.6 displays the decision matrix for the constructed closed testing procedure. Each of the seven rows in the table corresponds to an intersection hypothesis in the closed family. As in Section 2.3.2, the adjusted p-values for the original hypotheses H_{11}, H_{21} and H_{22} equal the largest p-value in the corresponding column on the right side of the table. For example, the adjusted p-value for the primary hypothesis H_{11} is defined as

$$\widetilde{p}_{11} = \max(p_{111}^*, p_{110}^*, p_{101}^*, p_{100}^*) = p_{11}.$$

This adjusted p-value does not depend on p_{21} or p_{22}, which means that the primary hypothesis is tested independently of the secondary hypotheses, and thus the constructed closed test appropriately accounts for the hierarchical structure of the multiple testing problem.

The outlined decision matrix algorithm for setting up gatekeeping tests is implemented in the %GateKeeper macro. Program 2.17 demonstrates how to use this macro in the depression trial example. The EXAMPLE1 data set contains three records, one for each of the three null hypotheses. The gatekeeper family F_1 includes one hypothesis and F_2 includes two hypotheses, so FAMILY=1 in the first record and FAMILY=2 in the second and third records. The SERIAL variable is set to 1 to indicate that multiple inferences in the two families are performed in a serial fashion (note that hypotheses in the last family are always tested in a serial manner). The secondary hypotheses are assumed to be equally weighted and therefore WEIGHT=0.5 when FAMILY=2.[1] The RELIMP variable is 0 because SERIAL=1. The p-value for the primary analysis equals 0.046 and the p-values associated with the HAMD17 response and remission rates are 0.048 and 0.021, respectively. Lastly, the HYP variable is optional and is used here to help identify the individual hypotheses.

Program 2.17 Bonferroni gatekeeping procedure in the depression trial example

```
data example1;
    input hyp $ family serial weight relimp raw_p;
    datalines;
    H11 1 1 1   0 0.046
    H21 2 1 0.5 0 0.048
    H22 2 1 0.5 0 0.021
    ;

%GateKeeper(dataset=example1,test="B",outdata=out1);

axis1 minor=none order=(0 to 0.06 by 0.02) label=(angle=90 "P-value");
axis2 minor=none label=("Hypothesis") order=("H11" "H21" "H22");
symbol1 value=circle color=black i=j;
symbol2 value=triangle color=black i=j;
proc gplot data=out1;
```

---

[1]Note that, in general, the weights assigned to individual null hypotheses can affect the significance of various trial outcomes and thus they need to be discussed with an appropriate regulatory agency and included in the study protocol.

```
plot raw_p*hyp adjp*hyp/frame overlay nolegend haxis=axis2 vaxis=axis1
    vref=0.05 lvref=34;
run;
```

Figure 2.13 Bonferroni gatekeeping procedure in the depression trial example. Raw *p*-value (◯) and adjusted *p*-value (△).

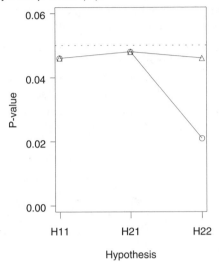

The output of Program 2.17 is shown in Figure 2.13. The figure displays the adjusted *p*-values produced by the Bonferroni gatekeeping procedure plotted along with the corresponding raw *p*-values (note that the adjusted *p*-values for H_{11} and H_{21} are equal to the corresponding raw *p*-values). We can see from the figure that the three adjusted *p*-values are significant at the 5% level and therefore the Bonferroni gatekeeping procedure rejects the primary (gatekeeper) hypothesis as well as all secondary hypotheses.

It is interesting to note that in the case of serial gatekeepers the Bonferroni gatekeeping procedure has a simple stepwise version. In this scenario, the primary hypothesis is examined first using a test based on the raw *p*-value. The hypothesis is retained and testing ceases if the raw *p*-value is greater than 0.05. Otherwise, the secondary hypotheses are tested simultaneously using the Holm test discussed in Section 2.3.1. Using PROC MULTTEST with the STEPBON option, it is easy to verify that the Holm-adjusted *p*-values associated with the secondary hypotheses equal 0.048 and 0.042, respectively. These *p*-values need to be further adjusted for the fact that the testing of the secondary hypotheses is contingent upon the outcome of the gatekeeper test. The final adjusted *p*-value for each of the secondary hypotheses equals the maximum of the raw primary *p*-value and the associated Holm-adjusted *p*-value. Specifically, the adjusted *p*-values for H_{21} and H_{22} are equal to 0.048 and 0.046, respectively. Therefore, the two secondary hypotheses are rejected.

The example from the depression trial illustrates the difference between closed gatekeeping procedures, such as the outlined Bonferroni procedure, and fixed-sequence gatekeeping procedures. As was noted in Section 2.4, one can test the secondary hypotheses without any adjustment for multiplicity provided the primary analysis is significant and the order in which the secondary hypotheses are tested is predetermined. This fixed-sequence testing approach is similar to the hierarchical testing strategy described in the guidance document entitled "Points to consider on multiplicity issues in clinical trials" published by the CPMP on September 19, 2002. It is prudent to employ the fixed-sequence approach if there are sufficient historical data to prioritize the secondary endpoints. Otherwise, drug developers run a serious risk of erroneously retaining false secondary hypotheses that happened to be placed at the end of the sequence. Along the same line, Moyé (2000) argued that determining the significance of endpoints based on the order in which they are examined may not always be acceptable from a broad scientific prospective.

Bonferroni Gatekeeping Procedure in the ARDS Trial Example

The next step is to utilize the constructed Bonferroni procedure in the ARDS trial example to set up gatekeeping strategies involving two families of hypotheses with a parallel gatekeeper. Let H_{11} and H_{12} denote the null hypotheses of no treatment effect with respect to the number of ventilator-free days (VFD) and 28-day all-cause mortality. Also, denote the hypotheses associated with the secondary endpoints by H_{21} and H_{22}. The weights representing the importance of the VFD and mortality endpoints are equal to 0.9 and 0.1, respectively, and the secondary hypotheses are assumed to be equally weighted. Lastly, the associated raw p-values will be denoted by p_{11}, p_{12}, p_{21} and p_{22}.

The gatekeeper family F_1 in the ARDS trial comprises H_{11} and H_{12}, and the family of secondary hypotheses, denoted by F_2, includes H_{21} and H_{22}. Table 2.7 shows the decision matrix for the Bonferroni gatekeeping procedure. The decision matrix was generated using Algorithm 1 of Dmitrienko, Offen and Westfall (2003). Here we adopted a binary representation of the intersection hypotheses similar to the one used in the previous subsection. For example, the original hypotheses H_{11}, H_{12}, H_{21} and H_{22} are denoted by H^*_{1000}, H^*_{0100}, H^*_{0010} and H^*_{0001}, respectively.

Table 2.7 Decision matrix for the Bonferroni gatekeeping procedure in the ARDS trial

Intersection hypothesis	P-value	Implied hypotheses			
		H_{11}	H_{12}	H_{21}	H_{22}
H^*_{1111}	$p^*_{1111} = \min(p_{11}/0.9,\, p_{12}/0.1)$	p^*_{1111}	p^*_{1111}	p^*_{1111}	p^*_{1111}
H^*_{1110}	$p^*_{1110} = \min(p_{11}/0.9,\, p_{12}/0.1)$	p^*_{1110}	p^*_{1110}	p^*_{1110}	0
H^*_{1101}	$p^*_{1101} = \min(p_{11}/0.9,\, p_{12}/0.1)$	p^*_{1101}	p^*_{1101}	0	p^*_{1101}
H^*_{1100}	$p^*_{1100} = \min(p_{11}/0.9,\, p_{12}/0.1)$	p^*_{1100}	p^*_{1100}	0	0
H^*_{1011}	$p^*_{1011} = \min(p_{11}/0.9,\, p_{21}/0.05,\, p_{22}/0.05)$	p^*_{1011}	0	p^*_{1011}	p^*_{1011}
H^*_{1010}	$p^*_{1010} = \min(p_{11}/0.9,\, p_{21}/0.1)$	p^*_{1010}	0	p^*_{1010}	0
H^*_{1001}	$p^*_{1001} = \min(p_{11}/0.9,\, p_{22}/0.1)$	p^*_{1001}	0	0	p^*_{1001}
H^*_{1000}	$p^*_{1000} = p_{11}/0.9$	p^*_{1000}	0	0	0
H^*_{0111}	$p^*_{0111} = \min(p_{12}/0.1,\, p_{21}/0.45,\, p_{22}/0.45)$	0	p^*_{0111}	p^*_{0111}	p^*_{0111}
H^*_{0110}	$p^*_{0110} = \min(p_{12}/0.1,\, p_{21}/0.9)$	0	p^*_{0110}	p^*_{0110}	0
H^*_{0101}	$p^*_{0101} = \min(p_{12}/0.1,\, p_{22}/0.9)$	0	p^*_{0101}	0	p^*_{0101}
H^*_{0100}	$p^*_{0100} = p_{12}/0.1$	0	p^*_{0100}	0	0
H^*_{0011}	$p^*_{0011} = \min(p_{21}/0.5,\, p_{22}/0.5)$	0	0	p^*_{0011}	p^*_{0011}
H^*_{0010}	$p^*_{0010} = p_{21}$	0	0	p^*_{0010}	0
H^*_{0001}	$p^*_{0001} = p_{22}$	0	0	0	p^*_{0001}

The decision rule presented in Table 2.7 incorporates the weights assigned to the primary hypotheses and accounts for the fact that the first family of hypotheses is a parallel gatekeeper. In fact, a careful examination of the adjusted p-values for the four null hypotheses in the ARDS trial example reveals that the closed test corresponding to the decision matrix in Table 2.7 meets the following criteria that define a parallel gatekeeping strategy:

- The adjusted p-values for the primary hypotheses H_{11} and H_{12} are no greater than α if $p_{11} \leq \alpha/0.9$ and $p_{12} \leq \alpha/0.1$, respectively. This implies that the gatekeeper hypotheses will be rejected whenever their Bonferroni-adjusted p-values are significant, regardless of the outcome of the secondary analyses. The analyses in the gatekeeper family do not depend on the significance of the secondary p-values.

- The adjusted p-values associated with the secondary hypotheses H_{21} and H_{22} are greater than the minimum of the adjusted primary p-values $\tilde{p}_{11}$ and $\tilde{p}_{12}$. In other words, none of the secondary hypotheses can be rejected if all of the gatekeeper analyses failed to reach significance.

Program 2.18 uses the %GateKeeper macro to perform the outlined gatekeeping inferences under two scenarios:

- Scenario 1 (EXAMPLE2a data set) assumes that the experimental therapy provides a statistically significant improvement with respect to both the number of ventilator-free days and 28-day all-cause mortality compared to the placebo.
- Under Scenario 2 (EXAMPLE2b data set), the VFD analysis yields a significant result but the treatment difference with respect to 28-day all-cause mortality is only marginally significant.

The secondary analyses are assumed to produce highly significant results under both scenarios.

Program 2.18 Bonferroni gatekeeping procedure in the ARDS trial example

```
data example2a;
    input hyp $ family serial weight relimp raw_p @@;
    datalines;
    H11 1 0 0.9 0 0.024   H12 1 0 0.1 0 0.002
    H21 2 1 0.5 0 0.010   H22 2 1 0.5 0 0.005
    ;
data example2b;
    input hyp $ family serial weight relimp raw_p @@;
    datalines;
    H11 1 0 0.9 0 0.024   H12 1 0 0.1 0 0.006
    H21 2 1 0.5 0 0.010   H22 2 1 0.5 0 0.005
    ;

%GateKeeper(dataset=example2a,test="B",outdata=out2a);
%GateKeeper(dataset=example2b,test="B",outdata=out2b);

axis1 minor=none order=(0 to 0.06 by 0.02) label=(angle=90 "P-value");
axis2 minor=none label=("Hypothesis") order=("H11" "H12" "H21" "H22");
symbol1 value=circle color=black i=j;
symbol2 value=triangle color=black i=j;
proc gplot data=out2a;
    plot raw_p*hyp adjp*hyp/frame overlay nolegend haxis=axis2 vaxis=axis1
        vref=0.05 lvref=34;
    run;
proc gplot data=out2b;
    plot raw_p*hyp adjp*hyp/frame overlay nolegend haxis=axis2 vaxis=axis1
        vref=0.05 lvref=34;
    run;
```

The output of Program 2.18 is displayed in Figure 2.14. We see from the left-hand panel of Figure 2.14 that the adjusted p-values for the primary hypotheses are both significant at the 5% level in Scenario 1. Since the primary hypotheses have been rejected, the Bonferroni gatekeeping procedure proceeded to testing the secondary hypotheses, both of which were also rejected. The right-hand panel of Figure 2.14 presents a more interesting scenario. The adjusted p-value associated with H_{11} is less than 0.05 whereas the adjusted p-value for H_{12} is greater than 0.05. This means that only one of the primary comparisons is significant at the 5% level after a multiplicity adjustment (it is the comparison with respect to the VFD endpoint). Since the primary hypotheses are tested in a parallel manner, the Bonferroni gatekeeping procedure needs only one significant primary comparison to continue to the second stage and test the secondary hypotheses. The raw p-values associated with the secondary hypotheses are highly significant and, as a consequence, the Bonferroni procedure successfully rejected both H_{21} and H_{22}.

Figure 2.14 Bonferroni gatekeeping procedure in the ARDS trial example under Scenario 1 (left-hand panel) and Scenario 2 (right-hand panel). Raw *p*-value (○) and adjusted *p*-value (△).

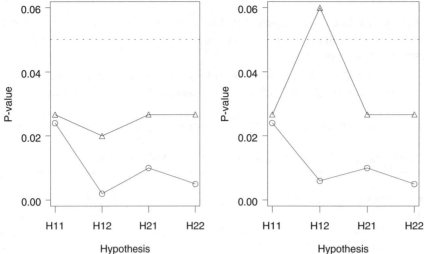

Modified Bonferroni Gatekeeping Procedure in the ARDS Trial Example

A notable feature of the decision matrix displayed in Table 2.7 is the definition of the *p*-values associated with the primary and secondary hypotheses. Consider the intersection hypotheses H^*_{1000}, H^*_{0100}, H^*_{0010} and H^*_{0001}. These hypotheses are the same as the original hypotheses H_{11}, H_{12}, H_{21} and H_{22} and thus it is natural to expect that the *p*-values corresponding to the four intersection hypotheses will be equal to the raw *p*-values. This is, however, not the case. It can be seen from Table 2.7 that

$$p^*_{0010} = p_{21} \text{ and } p^*_{0001} = p_{22},$$

which means that our conjecture is true for the secondary hypotheses. Examining the *p*-values associated with H^*_{1000} and H^*_{0100}, we see that they are greater than the corresponding raw *p*-values:

$$p^*_{1000} = p_{11}/0.9 > p_{11} \text{ and } p^*_{0100} = p_{12}/0.1 > p_{12}.$$

Although it might seem counterintuitive at first, this definition of p^*_{1000} and p^*_{0100} is driven by the requirement that the primary analyses be independent of the secondary ones (it is known as Condition B).

In cases when Condition B can be relaxed and replaced by Condition A, one can improve the power of the Bonferroni gatekeeping procedure by modifying the definition of the *p*-values associated with the intersection hypotheses H^*_{1000} and H^*_{0100} (the rest of the *p*-values remain unchanged). Specifically,

$$p^*_{1000} = p_{11} \text{ and } p^*_{0100} = p_{12}.$$

The resulting gatekeeping procedure will be referred to as the *modified Bonferroni gatekeeping procedure*.

Program 2.19 illustrates the power advantage of the modified Bonferroni gatekeeping procedure. By its definition, the modified Bonferroni procedure rejects all hypotheses rejected by the regular Bonferroni procedure and possibly more. To facilitate the comparison, Program 2.19 utilizes the %GateKeeper macro to apply the modified Bonferroni gatekeeping procedure to the two data sets analyzed in Program 2.18.

Program 2.19 Modified Bonferroni gatekeeping procedure in the ARDS trial example

```
%GateKeeper(dataset=example2a,test="MB",outdata=out2a);
%GateKeeper(dataset=example2b,test="MB",outdata=out2b);
```

```
axis1 minor=none order=(0 to 0.06 by 0.02) label=(angle=90 "P-value");
axis2 minor=none label=("Hypothesis") order=("H11" "H12" "H21" "H22");
symbol1 value=circle color=black i=j;
symbol2 value=triangle color=black i=j;
proc gplot data=out2a;
    plot raw_p*hyp adjp*hyp/frame overlay nolegend haxis=axis2 vaxis=axis1
        vref=0.05 lvref=34;
    run;
proc gplot data=out2b;
    plot raw_p*hyp adjp*hyp/frame overlay nolegend haxis=axis2 vaxis=axis1
        vref=0.05 lvref=34;
    run;
```

Figure 2.15 Modified Bonferroni gatekeeping procedure in the ARDS trial example under Scenario 1 (left-hand panel) and Scenario 2 (right-hand panel). Raw *p*-value (○) and adjusted *p*-value (△).

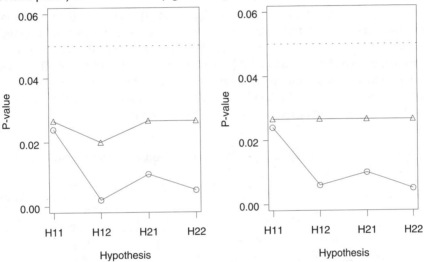

The output of Program 2.19 is shown in Figure 2.15. We can see from the left-hand panel of the figure that the adjusted *p*-values generated by the modified Bonferroni gatekeeping procedure are identical to those produced by the regular Bonferroni procedure in Scenario 1. However, there is a notable difference between the two testing procedures under the assumptions of Scenario 2. The right-hand panel of Figure 2.15 demonstrates that the adjusted *p*-values for H_{11} and H_{12} are less than 0.05. Therefore, unlike the regular procedure, the modified procedure has been able to reject both the mortality and VFD hypotheses in the gatekeeper family.

It is important to keep in mind that the modified procedure does not satisfy Condition B and therefore inferences with respect to the primary endpoints can be influenced by the secondary analyses. Roughly speaking, the modified procedure borrows strength from the secondary analyses and yields more significant results in the gatekeeper family only if the *p*-values associated with the secondary hypotheses H_{21} and H_{22} are highly significant. It is easy to check that the modified Bonferroni gatekeeping procedure can no longer find a significant difference with respect to 28-day mortality if at least one of the raw *p*-values for the secondary hypotheses is sufficiently large.

Bonferroni Gatekeeping Procedure with a Large RELIMP Variable in the ARDS Trial Example

As we explained in the previous subsection, the modified Bonferroni gatekeeping procedure is introduced to improve the power of the primary inferences by dropping the requirement that the primary analyses be independent of the secondary ones. Alternatively, the power of the regular Bonferroni gatekeeping procedure can be increased by shifting the power balance between the primary and secondary analyses. This is achieved by choosing a positive value of the RELIMP parameter in the %GateKeeper macro. Recall that the RELIMP parameter quantifies the relative importance of each family of hypotheses and thus, in the ARDS trial example, larger values of RELIMP will improve the power of the primary tests by decreasing the power of the secondary tests.

Table 2.8 displays the structure of the decision matrix underlying a general version of the Bonferroni gatekeeping procedure with a positive RELIMP value. A careful review of the matrix entries shows that the adjusted p-values for the primary hypotheses are monotonically decreasing functions of the r parameter representing the RELIMP variable. Setting r to 0 causes the decision matrix in Table 2.8 to be identical to that displayed in Table 2.7 and thus we end up with the regular Bonferroni gatekeeping procedure. On the other hand, the adjusted p-value for a primary hypothesis is "shrunk" toward the corresponding raw p-value and thus becomes more significant when r approaches 1. Note that we buy more power for the primary endpoints by reducing the probability of observing a significant secondary outcome. The adjusted p-values associated with the secondary hypotheses become less significant with increasing r.

Program 2.20 implements the outlined method for improving the power of the Bonferroni gatekeeping procedure in the ARDS trial example. Recall that multiple analyses in Program 2.18 were performed with the relative importance of the primary family set to 0 (i.e., the RELIMP variable is 0 when FAMILY=1 in the EXAMPLE2a and EXAMPLE2b data sets). In order to shift the power balance between the primary and secondary tests, we need to use a larger value of the RELIMP variable. For instance, if one is interested mainly in finding significant results with respect to the primary analyses, it is prudent to set RELIMP to a value close to 1, such as 0.8 or even 0.9.

Table 2.8 Decision matrix for the Bonferroni gatekeeping procedure with a positive RELIMP value in the ARDS trial (RELIMP is denoted by r)

Intersection hypothesis	P-value	Implied hypotheses			
		H_{11}	H_{12}	H_{21}	H_{22}
H_{1111}^*	$p_{1111}^* = \min(p_{11}/0.9, p_{12}/0.1)$	p_{1111}^*	p_{1111}^*	p_{1111}^*	p_{1111}^*
H_{1110}^*	$p_{1110}^* = \min(p_{11}/0.9, p_{12}/0.1)$	p_{1110}^*	p_{1110}^*	p_{1110}^*	0
H_{1101}^*	$p_{1101}^* = \min(p_{11}/0.9, p_{12}/0.1)$	p_{1101}^*	p_{1101}^*	0	p_{1101}^*
H_{1100}^*	$p_{1100}^* = \min(p_{11}/0.9, p_{12}/0.1)$	p_{1100}^*	p_{1100}^*	0	0
H_{1011}^*	$p_{1011}^* = \min(p_{11}/[(1-r)0.9+r],$ $p_{21}/[(1-r)0.05], p_{22}/[(1-r)0.05])$	p_{1011}^*	0	p_{1011}^*	p_{1011}^*
H_{1010}^*	$p_{1010}^* = \min(p_{11}/[(1-r)0.9+r],$ $p_{21}/[(1-r)0.1])$	p_{1010}^*	0	p_{1010}^*	0
H_{1001}^*	$p_{1001}^* = \min(p_{11}/[(1-r)0.9+r],$ $p_{22}/[(1-r)0.1])$	p_{1001}^*	0	0	p_{1001}^*
H_{1000}^*	$p_{1000}^* = p_{11}/[(1-r)0.9+r]$	p_{1000}^*	0	0	0
H_{0111}^*	$p_{0111}^* = \min(p_{12}/[(1-r)0.1+r],$ $p_{21}/[(1-r)0.45], p_{22}/[(1-r)0.45])$	0	p_{0111}^*	p_{0111}^*	p_{0111}^*
H_{0110}^*	$p_{0110}^* = \min(p_{12}/[(1-r)0.1+r],$ $p_{21}/[(1-r)0.9])$	0	p_{0110}^*	p_{0110}^*	0
H_{0101}^*	$p_{0101}^* = \min(p_{12}/[(1-r)0.1+r],$ $p_{22}/[(1-r)0.9])$	0	p_{0101}^*	0	p_{0101}^*
H_{0100}^*	$p_{0100}^* = p_{12}/[(1-r)0.1+r]$	0	p_{0100}^*	0	0
H_{0011}^*	$p_{0011}^* = \min(p_{21}/0.5, p_{22}/0.5)$	0	0	p_{0011}^*	p_{0011}^*
H_{0010}^*	$p_{0010}^* = p_{21}$	0	0	p_{0010}^*	0
H_{0001}^*	$p_{0001}^* = p_{22}$	0	0	0	p_{0001}^*

The output of Program 2.20 is shown in Figure 2.16. One can see from Figure 2.16 that the Bonferroni gatekeeping procedure with RELIMP=0.9 in the primary family is clearly more powerful than the Bonferroni procedure with RELIMP=0. Further, the Bonferroni procedure in Program 2.20 rejected all hypotheses rejected by the modified Bonferroni procedure. An important difference between the regular Bonferroni procedure with a large RELIMP value and the modified Bonferroni procedure is that the former satisfies Condition B, and thus the inferences in the primary family are unaffected by the outcome of the secondary analyses.

Program 2.20 Bonferroni gatekeeping procedure with a large RELIMP variable in the ARDS trial example

```
data example2c;
    set example2a;
    if family=1 then relimp=0.9;
data example2d;
    set example2b;
    if family=1 then relimp=0.9;

%GateKeeper(dataset=example2c,test="B",outdata=out2c);
%GateKeeper(dataset=example2d,test="B",outdata=out2d);

axis1 minor=none order=(0 to 0.06 by 0.02) label=(angle=90 "P-value");
axis2 minor=none label=("Hypothesis") order=("H11" "H12" "H21" "H22");
symbol1 value=circle color=black i=j;
symbol2 value=triangle color=black i=j;
proc gplot data=out2c;
    plot raw_p*hyp adjp*hyp/frame overlay nolegend haxis=axis2 vaxis=axis1
        vref=0.05 lvref=34;
    run;
proc gplot data=out2d;
    plot raw_p*hyp adjp*hyp/frame overlay nolegend haxis=axis2 vaxis=axis1
        vref=0.05 lvref=34;
    run;
```

Figure 2.16 Bonferroni gatekeeping procedure with a large RELIMP variable in the ARDS trial example under Scenario 1 (left-hand panel) and Scenario 2 (right-hand panel). Raw *p*-value (○) and adjusted *p*-value (△).

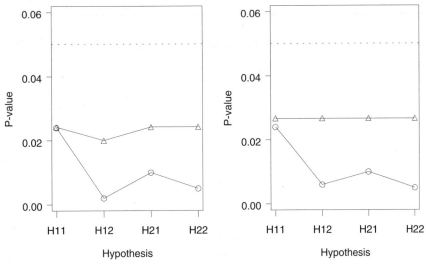

Bonferroni Gatekeeping Procedure in the Hypertension Trial Example

In this subsection we will construct a gatekeeping procedure for the dose-finding hypertension trial. Program 2.21 computes and plots the mean reduction in diastolic blood pressure (expressed in mmHg) in the placebo group and in four dose groups. The output of Program 2.21 is displayed in Figure 2.17.

Program 2.21 The dose-finding hypertension trial

```
data dftrial(drop=dose0-dose4);
    array dose{*} dose0-dose4;
    input dose0-dose4 @@;
    do group=0 to 4;
        change=dose{group+1};
        if change^=. then output;
    end;
    datalines;
    -7.5 -4.8  0.9  1.9 19.3 -6.2  -0.9 -3.2 13.7 -5.9
    17.5 10.6 18.6  4.4  7.9  8.7 -10.2  5.6  5.8 -1.2
     5.6 -3.2  6.6  8.1 -0.3  1.3  -5.1  4.6  2.2 10.3
    -6.1  3.6  7.6  8.2  3.3 -2.0   3.5  6.0 -3.2 14.0
    -6.8 13.3 12.2 19.4 15.0  4.0   9.5  9.8  0.5  5.3
    -1.5 -2.9  5.9 -7.6 11.6 -2.9 -13.3 -7.7 12.1  0.1
     0.0  2.0 -3.0  0.0  3.9  0.6   2.1 15.6  9.8 11.2
     3.5  7.3  3.9 -6.6 11.1 -6.3  -5.5 13.8 23.1  4.0
    10.7  0.3 12.0 11.8  4.8  0.5   3.6  2.8  2.3 16.1
    -1.1 13.2  5.3  0.7  7.6  2.1   0.3  5.0 12.1  3.3
    12.5  2.6 -3.0  1.4  9.5 -5.2  -8.7  2.4 14.5 -0.5
    -9.8 -7.4 -2.6  0.1 12.8  4.8    .   7.9   .   9.9
     1.2 -9.7  4.0  0.4 13.7   .     .   5.6   .   3.8
    ;
proc multtest data=dftrial;
    class group;
    test mean(change);
    ods output continuous=doseresp;
axis1 minor=none order=(0 to 10 by 5) label=(angle=90 "Mean reduction (mmHg)");
axis2 minor=none value=("P" "D1" "D2" "D3" "D4") label=("Treatment group");
symbol1 value=dot color=black i=j;
proc gplot data=doseresp;
    plot mean*group/frame haxis=axis2 vaxis=axis1;
    run;
```

Figure 2.17 Mean reduction in diastolic blood pressure (mmHg) by treatment group in the hypertension trial example

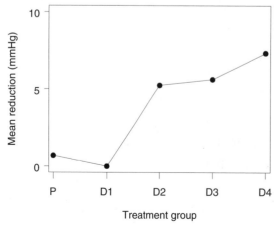

As was pointed out earlier, an efficient way of analyzing the dose-response relationship in the hypertension trial is based on a gatekeeping strategy that first compares doses D3 and D4 to the placebo and then tests doses D1 and D2 versus the placebo if either dose D3 or dose D4 separated from the placebo. Additional pairwise comparisons are performed if at least one significant comparison was found at the second stage.

Specifically, assume that

- F_1 comprises the null hypotheses H_{11} and H_{12} related to the D4 vs. P and D3 vs. P comparisons
- F_2 comprises the null hypotheses H_{21} and H_{22} related to the D2 vs. P and D1 vs. P comparisons
- F_3 comprises the null hypotheses H_{31}, H_{32}, H_{33} and H_{34} related to the D4 vs. D1, D4 vs. D2, D3 vs. D1, D3 vs. D2 comparisons, respectively.

The hypotheses are assumed equally weighted within each family, reflecting equal importance of the four doses.

As in the previous subsections, we can construct a decision matrix for the outlined hypothesis-testing problem. Since the problem involves eight null hypotheses, the decision matrix will have $2^8 - 1 = 255$ rows, and a manual calculation of the adjusted p-values can easily take a couple of hours. Program 2.22 automates this process by utilizing the %GateKeeper macro to test the null hypotheses in the three sequential families using a gatekeeping strategy based on the Bonferroni test. In order to compare the gatekeeping strategy with a stepwise testing approach, the program also tests the eight null hypotheses using the Hommel procedure (the Hommel procedure is described in Section 2.3.3).

Program 2.22 Bonferroni gatekeeping procedure versus Hommel procedure in the hypertension trial example

```
proc multtest data=dftrial;
    class group;
    test mean(change);
    contrast "H11" -1 0 0 0 1;
    contrast "H12" -1 0 0 1 0;
    contrast "H21" -1 0 1 0 0;
    contrast "H22" -1 1 0 0 0;
    contrast "H31" 0 -1 0 0 1;
    contrast "H32" 0 0 -1 0 1;
    contrast "H33" 0 -1 0 1 0;
    contrast "H34" 0 0 -1 1 0;
    ods output pvalues=pval;
data seqfam;
    set pval;
    relimp=0; raw_p=raw;
    if contrast in ("H11","H12") then
        do; family=1; serial=0; weight=0.5; end;
    if contrast in ("H21","H22") then
        do; family=2; serial=0; weight=0.5; end;
    if contrast in ("H31","H32","H33","H34") then
        do; family=3; serial=1; weight=0.25; end;
    keep contrast family serial weight relimp raw_p;

%GateKeeper(dataset=seqfam,test="B",outdata=out);

proc multtest pdata=seqfam noprint hommel out=hommel;

symbol1 value=circle color=black i=none;
symbol2 value=triangle color=black i=none;
axis1 minor=none order=(0 to 0.1 by 0.05) label=(angle=90 "P-value");
```

```
axis2 label=("Hypothesis")
    order=("H11" "H12" "H21" "H22" "H31" "H32" "H33" "H34");
proc gplot data=out;
    plot raw_p*contrast adjp*contrast/frame overlay
    haxis=axis2 vaxis=axis1 vref=0.05 lvref=34;
    run;
proc gplot data=hommel;
    plot raw_p*contrast hom_p*contrast/frame overlay
    haxis=axis2 vaxis=axis1 vref=0.05 lvref=34;
    run;
```

Figure 2.18 Bonferroni gatekeeping procedure (left-hand panel) versus Hommel procedure (right-hand panel) in the hypertension trial example. Raw *p*-value (○) and adjusted *p*-value (△).

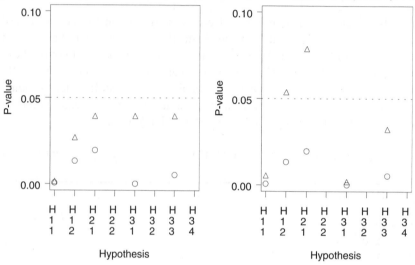

The output of Program 2.22 is shown in Figure 2.18 (note that the raw and adjusted *p*-values greater than 0.1 are not included in the figure). We can see from the left-hand panel of Figure 2.18 that the adjusted *p*-values associated with H_{11} and H_{12} are less than 0.05 and thus the Bonferroni gatekeeping procedure found doses D3 and D4 significantly different from the placebo in terms of the mean reduction in diastolic blood pressure. Since the first gatekeeper was passed, the Bonferroni procedure proceeded to testing doses D1 and D2 versus the placebo. Since the adjusted *p*-value for H_{21} was significant at a 5% level, testing continued to family F_3 comprising the null hypotheses related to the four pairwise dose comparisons. The analysis of the four comparisons revealed that the adjusted *p*-values associated with H_{31} and H_{33} were less than 0.05. This means that the reduction in diastolic blood pressure associated with doses D3 and D4 is significantly higher than that in dose group D1. Further, comparing the left- and right-hand panels of Figure 2.18, it is clear that the Bonferroni gatekeeping procedure is more powerful than the Hommel procedure in this example. Although the gatekeeping procedure is based on the Bonferroni test and the Hommel procedure is derived from the more powerful Simes test, the gatekeeping method gains efficiency by accounting for the hierarchical structure of the three sequential families.

Simes Gatekeeping Procedure in the Hypertension Trial Example

This subsection introduces a gatekeeping procedure based on the Simes test discussed in Section 2.2. The Simes test is uniformly more powerful than the Bonferroni global test and thus the Simes gatekeeping procedure rejects as many null hypotheses as the Bonferroni gatekeeping procedure and possibly more. One of the disadvantages of using the Simes gatekeeping procedure is that it satisfies Condition A but not the more desirable Condition B. This means that the Simes procedure can sometimes reject null hypotheses in a family even though it failed to reject any hypotheses in all preceding families.

Program 2.23 utilizes the %GateKeeper macro to test the three sequential families of hypotheses in the dose-finding hypertension trial using the Simes gatekeeping procedure.

Program 2.23 Simes gatekeeping procedure in the hypertension trial example

```
%GateKeeper(dataset=seqfam,test="S",outdata=out);

symbol1 value=circle color=black i=none;
symbol2 value=triangle color=black i=none;
axis1 minor=none order=(0 to 0.1 by 0.05) label=(angle=90 "P-value");
axis2 label=("Hypothesis")
    order=("H11" "H12" "H21" "H22" "H31" "H32" "H33" "H34");
proc gplot data=out;
    plot raw_p*contrast adjp*contrast/frame overlay
    haxis=axis2 vaxis=axis1 vref=0.05 lvref=34;
    run;
```

Figure 2.19 Simes gatekeeping procedure in the hypertension trial example. Raw *p*-value (◯) and adjusted *p*-value (△).

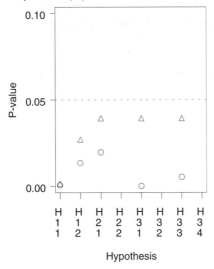

The output of Program 2.23 is shown in Figure 2.19. A quick comparison of the left-hand panel of Figure 2.18 and Figure 2.19 reveals that the Simes gatekeeping procedure has rejected the same number of null hypotheses as the Bonferroni gatekeeping procedure, and the adjusted *p*-values produced by the two testing procedure are either identical or very close to each other. Although the Simes procedure is uniformly more powerful than the Bonferroni procedure, the power advantage generally decreases with the increasing number of families. The two procedures are known to yield different results when all of the raw *p*-values are significant, in which case the Simes procedure rejects all of the null hypotheses whereas the Bonferroni procedure tends to reject only the hypotheses with highly significant raw *p*-values.

2.7.4   Resampling-Based Gatekeeping Procedures

In the previous subsections we have discussed gatekeeping strategies based on the Bonferroni and Simes tests. Both of these tests rely on marginal *p*-values and do not efficiently account for the correlation among the test statistics. Test statistics arising in multiple endpoint or dose-finding settings are often highly correlated and therefore it seems natural to incorporate the underlying correlation structure into the decision rule in order to increase the efficiency of gatekeeping inferences.

In this subsection we will utilize the Westfall-Young resampling-based methodology introduced in Section 2.5 to construct gatekeeping dose-finding strategies that account for the joint distribution of individual p-values. Consider the problem of testing the three sequential families of hypotheses related to the individual dose-placebo and pairwise comparisons in the hypertension trial example. A resampling-based algorithm for testing the sequential families can be carried out using the %ResamGate macro given in the Appendix. This macro is similar to the %GateKeeper macro in that it utilizes the decision matrix algorithm of Section 2.3.2 to implement the Bonferroni, modified Bonferroni and Simes gatekeeping procedures; however, unlike the %GateKeeper macro, the macro used in this subsection produces resampling-based versions of the three procedures.

The %ResamGate macro has four arguments. The DATASET, TEST and OUTDATA arguments are the same as in the %GateKeeper macro. The additional RESP argument specifies the name of the data set containing the raw bootstrap p-values. The macro assumes that the ith variable in RESP corresponds to the bootstrap p-values for the null hypothesis in the ith row of DATASET.

Program 2.24 uses the %ResamGate macro to test the three families of hypotheses in the dose-finding hypertension trial using the resampling gatekeeping procedures based on the Bonferroni and Simes tests. The program relies on the short %Resam macro to generate a set of bootstrap p-values that are later passed to the %ResamGate macro to perform the resampling-based gatekeeping inferences. In order to efficiently produce bootstrap p-values, the %Resam macro takes advantage of the built-in resampling generator in PROC MULTTEST. In the first run of PROC MULTTEST, it generates a bootstrap sample from the pooled sample of within-group residuals. The second run of PROC MULTTEST is used to compute the raw p-values for each of the eight null hypotheses. This process is repeated 20,000 times. Lastly, note that the program uses the PVAL and SEQFAM data sets created in Program 2.22.

Program 2.24 Resampling-based gatekeeping procedures in the hypertension trial example

```
%let contrasts=%str(
    contrast "H11" -1 0 0 0 1;
    contrast "H12" -1 0 0 1 0;
    contrast "H21" -1 0 1 0 0;
    contrast "H22" -1 1 0 0 0;
    contrast "H31" 0 -1 0 0 1;
    contrast "H32" 0 0 -1 0 1;
    contrast "H33" 0 -1 0 1 0;
    contrast "H34" 0 0 -1 1 0;
    );

%macro resam(n);
    data resam;
    proc transpose data=pval out=raw_p prefix=p;
        var raw;
    %do i=1 %to &n;
    proc multtest data=dftrial noprint bootstrap n=1 seed=388&i
        outsamp=resdata;
        class group;
        test mean(change);
        &contrasts;
    proc multtest data=resdata noprint out=p;
        class _class_;
        test mean(change);
        &contrasts;
    proc transpose data=p out=boot_p prefix=p;
        var raw_p;
    data resam;
```

```
          set resam boot_p;
          run;
      %end;
      data resam;
          set resam; if p1^=.;
%mend resam;


%resam(20000);


%ResamGate(dataset=seqfam,resp=resam,test="B",outdata=out1);
%ResamGate(dataset=seqfam,resp=resam,test="S",outdata=out2);


symbol1 value=circle color=black i=none;
symbol2 value=triangle color=black i=none;
axis1 minor=none order=(0 to 0.1 by 0.05) label=(angle=90 "P-value");
axis2 label=("Hypothesis")
      order=("H11" "H12" "H21" "H22" "H31" "H32" "H33" "H34");
proc gplot data=out1;
      plot raw_p*contrast adjp*contrast/frame overlay
      haxis=axis2 vaxis=axis1 vref=0.05 lvref=34;
      run;
proc gplot data=out2;
      plot raw_p*contrast adjp*contrast/frame overlay
      haxis=axis2 vaxis=axis1 vref=0.05 lvref=34;
      run;
```

Figure 2.20 Resampling-based Bonferroni procedure (left-hand panel) and Simes procedure (right-hand panel) in the hypertension trial example. Raw p-value ($\bigcirc$) and adjusted p-value ($\triangle$).

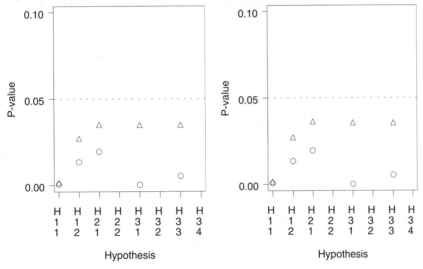

The output of Program 2.24 is displayed in Figure 2.20. The figure indicates that both resampling-based gatekeeping procedures have rejected the null hypotheses H_{11}, H_{12} and H_{21} and proceeded to test the hypotheses related to the four pairwise comparisons in the third family. The resampling-based gatekeeping procedures generated adjusted p-values that are very close to the adjusted p-values produced by the Bonferroni and Simes procedures without the resampling modification (see Figures 2.18 and 2.19). As pointed out by Dmitrienko, Offen and Westfall (2003), the resampling methodology generally improves the performance of gatekeeping procedures based on marginal p-values; however, with the exception of borderline cases, the magnitude of this improvement is small.

2.7.5   Computational Algorithms

Here we will provide a detailed description of computational algorithms underlying the gatekeeping testing procedures introduced earlier in this section. First, consider n null hypotheses tested in a clinical trial and assume that they are grouped into m families denoted by $F_1, \ldots, F_m$. As indicated in Table 2.9, F_i contains the null hypotheses $H_{i1}, \ldots, H_{in_i}$ ($n_1 + \ldots + n_m = n$). Let $p_{i1}, \ldots, p_{in_i}$ denote the raw p-values for the null hypotheses in F_i, and let $w_{i1}, \ldots, w_{in_i}$ be the weights representing the importance of the null hypotheses ($w_{i1} + \ldots + w_{in_i} = 1$). The individual families $F_1, \ldots, F_m$ are classified as parallel or serial gatekeepers (note that F_m is always tested in a serial manner). If F_i is a parallel gatekeeper, let r_i denote its relative importance ($0 \leq r_i < 1$).

Table 2.9 Families of null hypotheses

Family	Relative importance	Null hypotheses	Hypothesis weights	Unadjusted p-values
F_1	r_1	$H_{11}, \ldots, H_{1n_1}$	$w_{11}, \ldots, w_{1n_1}$	$p_{11}, \ldots, p_{1n_1}$
$\ldots$	$\ldots$	$\ldots$	$\ldots$	$\ldots$
F_i	r_i	$H_{i1}, \ldots, H_{in_i}$	$w_{i1}, \ldots, w_{in_i}$	$p_{i1}, \ldots, p_{in_i}$
$\ldots$	$\ldots$	$\ldots$	$\ldots$	$\ldots$
F_m	r_m	$H_{m1}, \ldots, H_{mn_m}$	$w_{m1}, \ldots, w_{mn_m}$	$p_{m1}, \ldots, p_{mn_m}$

Note: The relative importance is defined for parallel gatekeepers only.

In order to define a gatekeeping procedure for testing the null hypotheses in $F_1, \ldots, F_m$, we will need the following notation. Let K_i be the set of two-dimensional indices corresponding to F_i, i.e., $K_i = \{(i, 1), \ldots, (i, n_i)\}$. Let A be the union of $K_1, \ldots, K_m$, i.e.,

$$A = \cup_{i=1}^m K_i.$$

This union helps define the closed family of hypotheses associated with $F_1, \ldots, F_m$. For any $S \subseteq A$,

$$H_S = \cap_{(i,j) \in S} H_{ij}$$

represents an intersection hypothesis in the closed family. Let $\mathcal{S}_{ij}$ denote the set of all S such that $(i, j) \in S$. The intersection hypotheses H_S, $S \in \mathcal{S}_{ij}$, are said to imply H_{ij}. Let $\delta_{ij}(S)$ denote an indicator variable that identifies the original hypotheses implied by H_S, i.e., let $\delta_{ij}(S) = 1$ if $S \in \mathcal{S}_{ij}$, and 0 otherwise.

The closed testing principle requires that any original hypothesis H_{ij} should be rejected only when all intersection hypotheses implying it, i.e., H_S with $S \in \mathcal{S}_{ij}$, are rejected. To control the familywise error rate at the α level for all null hypotheses in $F_1, \ldots, F_m$, each intersection hypothesis H_S needs to be tested at the α level.

Lastly, to define the adjusted p-value for an original hypothesis H_{ij} (denoted by $\tilde{p}_{ij}$), let p_S denote an unadjusted p-value for testing the intersection hypothesis H_S. Note that when $S = \{(i, j)\}$, we have $p_S = p_{ij}$, the unadjusted p-value for testing H_{ij}. The adjusted p-value for H_{ij} is the smallest significance level for which one would reject H_{ij} using the given multiple testing procedure (Westfall and Young, 1993). Therefore, the adjusted p-value is given by

$$\tilde{p}_{ij} = \max_{S \in \mathcal{S}_{ij}} p_S.$$

Bonferroni Gatekeeping Procedures

The outlined general framework can be applied to set up the Bonferroni gatekeeping procedures considered in Section 2.7.3. Toward this end, assume that each intersection hypothesis H_S is tested using the weighted Bonferroni test. The weights $v_{ij}(S)$ are chosen to satisfy

$$0 \leq v_{ij}(S) \leq 1, \quad v_{ij}(S) = 0 \text{ if } \delta_{ij}(S) = 0, \quad \sum_{i=1}^m \sum_{j=1}^{n_i} v_{ij}(S) \leq 1.$$

The Bonferroni p-value for H_S is

$$p_S = \min_{1 \le i \le m} \min_{1 \le j \le n_i} \delta_{ij}(S) p_{ij} / v_{ij}(S),$$

where $\delta_{ij}(S)/v_{ij}(S) = 0$ if $v_{ij}(S) = 0$, and H_S is rejected if $p_S \le \alpha$.

The weights $v_{ij}(S)$ play a very important role in this definition and determine main characteristics of the resulting gatekeeping procedure. In what follows, we will show how to define the weights corresponding to the original and modified Bonferroni gatekeeping procedures.

Original Bonferroni Gatekeeping Procedure

Choose an intersection hypothesis H_S from the closed family corresponding to $F_1, \ldots, F_m$ and define the weights $v_{ij}(S)$ using the following procedure (we will assume below that $0/0=0$).

Step 1. Consider F_1 and let

$$v_{1l}(S) = \delta_{1l}(S) w_{1l} \left\{ (1 - r_1) + r_1 / \sum_{k=1}^{n_1} \delta_{1k}(S) w_{1k} \right\}, \quad 0 \le r_1 < 1,$$

if F_1 is a parallel gatekeeper, and

$$v_{1l}(S) = \delta_{1l}(S) w_{1l} / \sum_{k=1}^{n_1} \delta_{1k}(S) w_{1k}$$

if F_1 is a serial gatekeeper, $l = 1, \ldots, n_1$. Further, let

$$v_2^* = 1 - \sum_{l=1}^{n_1} v_{1l}(S).$$

Go to Step 2 if $v_2^* > 0$, and let $v_{ij}(S) = 0$, $i = 2, \ldots, m$, $j = 1, \ldots, n_i$, otherwise.

Step 2. Consider F_2. Let

$$v_{2l}(S) = v_1^* \delta_{2l}(S) w_{2l} \left\{ (1 - r_2) + r_2 / \sum_{k=1}^{n_2} \delta_{2k}(S) w_{2k} \right\}, \quad 0 \le r_2 < 1,$$

if F_2 is a parallel gatekeeper, and

$$v_{2l}(S) = v_1^* \delta_{2l}(S) w_{2l} / \sum_{k=1}^{n_2} \delta_{2k}(S) w_{2k}$$

if F_2 is a serial gatekeeper, $l = 1, \ldots, n_2$. Let

$$v_3^* = v_2^* - \sum_{l=1}^{n_2} v_{2l}(S).$$

Go to Step 3 if $v_3^* > 0$, and let $v_{ij}(S) = 0$, $i = 3, \ldots, m$, $j = 1, \ldots, n_i$, otherwise.

$\ldots$

Step m. Consider F_m. Let

$$v_{ml}(S) = v_m^* \delta_{ml}(S) w_{ml} / \sum_{k=1}^{n_m} \delta_{mk}(S) w_{mk},$$

$l = 1, \ldots, n_m$, and stop.

Modified Bonferroni Gatekeeping Procedure

The modified Bonferroni gatekeeping procedure relies on a similar algorithm for defining the weights associated with intersection hypotheses. The only difference is that the modified weights are forced to add up to 1, i.e.,

$$\sum_{i=1}^{m} \sum_{j=1}^{n_i} v_{ij}(S) = 1,$$

for any intersection hypothesis H_S.

Simes Gatekeeping Procedure

To define the Simes gatekeeping procedure, we will use the weighted Simes test introduced by Benjamini and Hochberg (1997). For any intersection hypothesis H_S in the closed family of hypotheses associated with $F_1, \ldots, F_m$, let

$$p_{(1)S} \leq p_{(2)S} \leq \cdots \leq p_{(t)S}$$

denote the ordered p-values for the original hypotheses contained in H_S (here t is the number of original hypotheses contained in H_S). Let $v_{(1)S}, \ldots, v_{(t)S}$ denote the modified Bonferroni weights corresponding to the ordered p-values. The weighted Simes p-value for the intersection hypothesis H_S is given by

$$p_S = \min_{1 \leq l \leq t} p_{(l)S} / \sum_{k=1}^{l} v_{(k)S}.$$

After we have computed weighted Simes p-values for each intersection hypothesis in the closed family, a closed testing procedure for the null hypotheses in $F_1, \ldots, F_m$ can be constructed using the principles outlined above. The resulting testing procedure is known as the Simes gatekeeping procedure.

Resampling-Based Bonferroni and Simes Gatekeeping Procedure

Resampling-based gatekeeping procedures extend the Bonferroni and Simes gatekeeping procedures defined above by incorporating the estimated correlation structure into the decision rules for the individual null hypotheses in $F_1, \ldots, F_m$. Resampling-based multiplicity adjustments are defined as follows:

- Consider the original data sample and generate N bootstrap or permutation samples from it.
- Using the original Bonferroni, modified Bonferroni or Simes gatekeeping procedure, compute the adjusted p-values for the null hypotheses in $F_1, \ldots, F_m$ from the original sample and denote them by $\widetilde{p}_{i1}, \ldots, \widetilde{p}_{in_i}$, $i = 1, \ldots, m$.
- Similarly, compute the adjusted p-values from each one of the N bootstrap or permutation samples. Denote the adjusted p-values for the null hypotheses in $F_1, \ldots, F_m$ from the kth bootstrap or permutation sample by $\widetilde{p}_{i1}(k), \ldots, \widetilde{p}_{in_i}(k)$, $i = 1, \ldots, m, k = 1, \ldots, N$.
- The final adjusted p-value for H_{ij} is given by

$$\frac{1}{N} \sum_{k=1}^{N} I\{\widetilde{p}_{ij}(k) < \widetilde{p}_{ij}\},$$

where $I\{\}$ is an indicator function.

2.7.6 Summary

In this section we described methods for addressing multiplicity issues arising in clinical trials with multiple objectives. Efficient solutions for multiplicity problems of this kind can be obtained using gatekeeping strategies in which the primary analyses are treated as gatekeepers and the secondary analyses are performed only if one or more primary hypotheses have been rejected. This section discussed multiple testing procedures for serial and parallel families of hypotheses defined as follows:

- A serial gatekeeping procedure passes a gatekeeper only after it has rejected all of the individual hypotheses. It is worth noting that fixed-sequence tests described in Section 2.4 serve as an example of serial gatekeeping procedures. Specifically, a serial gatekeeping procedure simplifies to a fixed-sequence test when each gatekeeper contains only one hypothesis.

- A parallel gatekeeping procedure passes a gatekeeper every time it has rejected at least one of the hypotheses.

We first reviewed the general framework for performing gatekeeping inferences and then illustrated it using examples from clinical trials with hierarchically ordered endpoints and from dose-finding studies. The following gatekeeping procedures were introduced in this section:

- The ordinary and modified Bonferroni gatekeeping procedures can be implemented using the %GateKeeper macro. The modified procedure is uniformly more powerful than the ordinary procedure with respect to the primary analyses. However, it is important to remember that the modified Bonferroni gatekeeping procedure gains power for more important analyses by borrowing strength from less important analyses. As a consequence, inferences with respect to primary analyses can potentially be influenced by secondary analyses. This can be a concern in situations when the hierarchy among the primary and secondary endpoints needs to be strictly observed. Alternatively, we can improve the power of the ordinary Bonferroni gatekeeping procedure by increasing the relative importance of primary analyses (i.e., by using larger values of the RELIMP variable in the %GateKeeper macro). An advantage of this approach is that primary analyses are not longer affected by the outcome of secondary analyses.

- The Simes gatekeeping procedure is superior to both the ordinary and modified Bonferroni gatekeeping procedures. It is similar to the modified Bonferroni procedure in that it also borrows strength from less important analyses.

- Gatekeeping procedures based on the Westfall-Young resampling methodology are performed using the %ResamGate macro. The resampling-based gatekeeping procedures are generally more powerful than the Bonferroni and Simes gatekeeping procedures because they incorporate the underlying correlation structure into the decision rule.

Analysis of Safety and Diagnostic Data

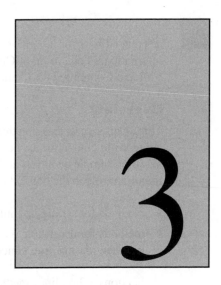

This chapter describes methods for constructing reference intervals for safety and diagnostic measures in clinical trials. It discusses the computation of reference limits based on sample quantiles and tolerance limits, and it focuses on several issues that play an important role in drug development, such as methods for adjusting reference intervals for important prognostic factors. The second part of the chapter reviews statistical methods for the analysis of shift tables produced after reference intervals have been applied to safety and diagnostic data.

3.1 Introduction

Quantitative diagnostic and safety data, such as laboratory measurements, vital signs or electrocardiographic parameters, are typically analyzed in clinical trials by computing measures of center and dispersion and by examining extreme observations. It is commonly agreed that the analysis of extreme observations often plays a more important role than the analysis of mean trends because it allows a more accurate evaluation of the safety profile of an experimental therapy. For example, the draft guidance document "Assessment of the QT Prolongation Potential of Non-Antiarrhythmic Drugs" released by Health Canada on March 15, 2001, emphasized that

> Electrocardiogram data should always be presented both as group means for the test drug and placebo/active comparator treatments and the proportion of individual subjects in each treatment group experiencing abnormal values. An increase in the proportion of patients experiencing abnormal values should be considered a cause for concern, regardless of whether statistically significant differences are present between group mean values.

The analysis of extreme safety and diagnostic measures in clinical trials relies on reference intervals that help drug developers quickly determine whether a particular value is typical or atypical. A large number of publications deal with the problem of constructing reference intervals for quantitative safety and diagnostic measurements. For example, Wilson (2000) presented reference intervals for routine clinical laboratory analyses computed from a sample of more than 20,000 patients. Dmitrienko et al. (2004) derived a set of reference intervals for electrocardiographic parameters from a database of 13,000 patients. A number of guidelines have been published recently that outline the principles for developing reference limits for laboratory and other data. Solberg (1987) summarized the standards proposed by the International Federation of Clinical Chemistry. A similar set of guidelines was published by the National Committee for Clinical Laboratory Standards (1995).

Overview

This chapter describes practical methods for constructing reference intervals for diagnostic and safety variables in clinical trials. Section 3.2 discusses the computation of nonparametric reference limits based on sample quantiles and tolerance limits. The section also focuses on several issues that play an important role in the context of pharmaceutical drug development:

- methods for setting up multivariate reference intervals adjusted for important prognostic factors
- methods for describing a relationship among multiple numerical endpoints (e.g., the relationship between plasma drug concentration and safety markers).

Sections 3.3 outlines methods for the analysis of shift tables produced after reference intervals have been applied to safety and diagnostic data. Although the section focuses on categorical outcomes that are produced after reference intervals have been applied to diagnostic data, the methods discussed are useful in a variety of situations, for instance, in the analysis of repeated efficacy measurements.

3.2 Reference Intervals for Safety and Diagnostic Measures

As was emphasized in the introduction, reference intervals play an important role in the analysis of safety and diagnostic measures. In the first part of this section we will review statistical methods for setting up univariate reference intervals based on sample quantiles (Section 3.2.1) and an alternative definition that relies on the method of tolerance limits (Section 3.2.2).

The second part of the section deals with multivariate quantile functions that are used in the construction of covariate-adjusted reference limits. Covariate-adjusted reference intervals allow more accurate assessment of safety and diagnostic data in clinical trials than univariate reference intervals because they match a patient's result with the results collected from other patients with similar demographic characteristics. Sections 3.2.3 and 3.2.4 discuss reference limits based on the method of global smoothing, and Sections 3.2.5 and 3.2.6 review local smoothing techniques for setting up reference intervals. Finally, Section 3.2.7 introduces other interesting applications of multivariate quantile functions in clinical trials.

This section focuses on a cross-sectional setting in which only one measurement per patient is used for establishing reference limits. This is the most common scenario in clinical applications. With multiple observations per patient, one needs to properly account for serial correlation in the process of setting up reference intervals. Methods for constructing reference limits based on serial measurements within individuals have recently been discussed in the literature; see, for example, Berkey et al. (1993) and Wade and Ades (1998).

EXAMPLE: Analysis of QTc Interval

The methods for defining reference intervals presented in this section will be illustrated using an artificial data set of QTc interval measurements in males aged 10 to 60 years of age (QTc is the QT interval corrected for heart rate). Clinical researchers use the QTc interval as a surrogate endpoint for cardiac repolarization abnormalities. It is stated in the concept paper "The clinical evaluation of QT/QTc interval prolongation and proarrhythmic potential for non-antiarrhythmic drugs" released by the FDA on November 15, 2002, that

> Certain drugs have the ability to delay cardiac repolarization, an effect that is manifested on surface electrocardiogram as prolongation of the QT interval.... QT interval prolongation creates

an electrophysiological environment that favours development of cardiac arrhythmias, most clearly torsade de pointes (TdP), but possibly other arrhythmias as well. . . . A feature of TdP is pronounced prolongation of the QT interval in the beats preceding the arrhythmia. TdP can degenerate into life-threatening cardiac rhythms, such ventricular fibrillation, which can result in sudden death.

For this reason, analysis of the QTc interval plays a very important role in evaluating cardiac liability of new therapies. See Dmitrienko and Smith (2002) for further details and references.

Program 3.1 creates the QTC data set with two variables representing the length of the QTc interval in milliseconds (Y variable) and patient's age in years (X variable). Patient's age is included in this data set to illustrate methods for constructing age-adjusted reference limits for the QTc interval.

Program 3.1 QTC data set

```
data qtc;
    length x 6.4;
    do id=1 to 3000;
        x=input(10+50*ranuni(343+23*id),6.4);
        if x<=20 then mean=-0.5*(x-10)+415; else mean=x+390;
        sigma=mean/20;
        upper=mean+probit(0.9)*sigma;
        y=mean+sigma*normal(623+84*id);
        output;
    end;
    run;
```

The distribution of randomly generated QTc values in the QTC data set was chosen to mimic the distribution of real QTc measurements collected in clinical trials. Several authors, including Rautaharju et al. (1992) and Dmitrienko et al. (2004), pointed out that the duration of the QTc interval in males exhibits an interesting pattern. The QTc interval generally increases with age but there is a notable shortening in young males that is attributed to the onset of puberty. In order to reproduce this complex relationship between the duration of the QTc interval and patient's age, the Y variable in the QTC data set was assumed to be normally distributed with

$$\text{Mean}(Y|X = x) = \begin{cases} -0.5(x - 10) + 415, & \text{if } 0 \leq x \leq 20, \\ x + 390, & \text{if } 20 < x \leq 60. \end{cases}$$

Since the coefficient of variation estimated from real QTc data is close to 5%, the standard deviation of the Y variable was set to

$$\text{Standard deviation}(Y|X = x) = \text{Mean}(Y|X = x)/20.$$

Figure 3.1 displays the generated QTc values plotted versus age with the two curves representing the mean (solid curve) and 90th quantile (dashed curve) of the QTc interval as a function of age.

3.2.1 Reference Intervals Based on Sample Quantiles

The simplest and most popular way for setting up univariate reference limits for safety and diagnostic variables is based on excluding a certain proportion of extreme data points in the lower and upper tails of the distribution. In other words, reference intervals are defined by the range between two sample quantiles centered around the median. For example, the 1st and 99th quantiles define a reference interval capturing 98% of the measurements.

Sample quantiles are easy to compute using PROC UNIVARIATE. For example, Program 3.2 calculates the 10th and 90th quantiles based on the sample distribution of the QTc interval in the QTC data set.

Figure 3.1 The mean (—) and 90th quantile (- - -) of the QTc interval in 3,000 male patients

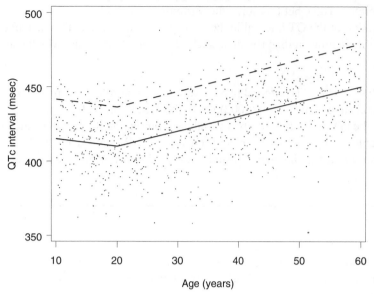

Program 3.2 The 10th and 90th quantiles of the sample distribution of the QTc interval

```
proc univariate data=qtc noprint;
    var y;
    output out=quantile pctlpts=10, 90 pctlpre=quantile;
proc print data=quantile noobs label;
    run;
```

Output from Program 3.2

```
    the            the
  10.0000        90.0000
percentile,    percentile,
    y              y


  394.292        458.076
```

Output 3.2 shows that the estimated 10th and 90th quantiles of the QTc interval are equal to 394.292 and 458.076, respectively. The two quantiles have been computed using the default definition of the sample quantile based on the empirical distribution function with averaging. PROC UNIVARIATE supports four more algorithms for computing sample quantiles that can be requested using the PCTLDEF option in PROC UNIVARIATE. The differences among the five algorithms may become important when the number of observations is small or the data around the estimated quantile are sparse (for example, when you are trying to estimate the 99.9th quantile). However, these differences are rarely of any practical significance in large data sets from which reference limits are typically computed. For example, it is easy to check by modifying Program 3.2 that the smallest 90th quantile produced by the five algorithms is 457.989 and the largest 90th quantile is 458.146.

It is important to point out that, despite being mathematically correct, the computed 10% and 90% reference limits for the QTc interval need to be used with caution because their use will bias the analysis of extreme QTc values. The bias is caused by the fact that the univariate reference limits ignore the patient's age, which is directly related to the duration of the QTc interval. In order to illustrate this fact, Program 3.3 uses PROC UNIVARIATE to plot the distribution of QTc values as a function of the patient's age.

Program 3.3 Distribution of the QTc interval in four age groups

```
data age1 age2 age3 age4;
    set qtc;
    if x<22.5 then output age1;
    if 22.5<=x<35 then output age2;
    if 35<=x<47.5 then output age3;
    if 47.5<=x then output age4;

%macro DistPlot(dataset);
    proc univariate data=&dataset noprint;
        histogram y/outhist=hist;
    axis1 minor=none major=none value=none label=none
        order=(0 to 25 by 5);
    axis2 minor=none label=("QTc interval (msec)")
        order=(350 to 510 by 40);
    symbol1 value=none i=j;
    data annotate;
        xsys="1"; ysys="1"; hsys="4"; x=50; y=90; position="5";
        size=1; text="&label"; function="label";
    proc gplot data=hist anno=annotate;
        plot _obspct_*_midpt_/haxis=axis2 vaxis=axis1
            href=394.292, 458.076 lhref=34;
        run;
        quit;
%mend DistPlot;

%DistPlot(age1,Age<22.5);
%DistPlot(age2,22.5<=Age<35);
%DistPlot(age3,35<=Age<47.5);
%DistPlot(age4,47.5<=Age);
```

The output of Program 3.3 is displayed in Figure 3.2. The figure depicts the distribution of the QTc interval in four age groups of approximately the same size. The dotted lines are drawn at the univariate 10% and 90% reference limits produced by Program 3.2. It is clear from Figure 3.2 that the proportion of younger patients whose QTc interval is above the 90% reference limit is less than 10%. On the other hand, the likelihood that a patient 47.5 years of age or older will be classified as having an abnormally long QTc interval is substantially greater than 10%; in fact, it is close to 40%. Figure 3.2 demonstrates that univariate reference limits that ignore important covariates are quite unreliable. It will be shown in Sections 3.2.3 through 3.2.6 that more accurate limits for the QTc interval and other safety or diagnostic parameters can be constructed using multivariate quantile functions adjusted for important covariates such as the patient's age.

3.2.2   Tolerance Limits

Section 3.2.1 discussed methods for setting up univariate reference intervals based on sample quantiles. This section provides a brief review of an alternative approach that is becoming increasingly popular in clinical applications. This alternative approach is based on univariate tolerance limits. Several authors have recently advocated the use of tolerance intervals for defining extreme measurements in clinical research. Nickens (1998) and Chuang-Stein (1998) argued that reference limits derived from sample quantiles operate at the sample level and cannot be used to make inferences about the underlying population of patients. Specifically, the methods described in Section 3.2.1 do not address the likelihood that a specified proportion of the patients in the underlying population will have their diagnostic or safety measurements between the lower and upper limits of the reference interval. In order to set up reference intervals that will be valid at the population level, one needs to employ the methodology of tolerance limits developed by Wilks (1941), Tukey (1947) and others.

Figure 3.2 Distribution of the QTc interval in four age groups

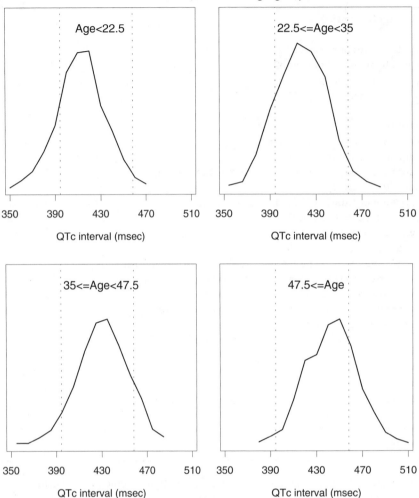

To introduce this methodology, consider n observations $y_1, \ldots, y_n$ that represent independent realizations of a random variable Y with a continuous distribution function. We are interested in constructing a tolerance interval (L, U) that covers at least 100γ percent of the population with the confidence of at least 100β percent ($0 < \beta < 1$ and $0 < \gamma < 1$). In other words, the interval (L, U) is chosen to satisfy the following condition:

$$P\left(\int_L^U f(y)dy \geq \gamma \right) \geq \beta,$$

where $f(y)$ is the unknown probability density function of the random variable Y. In a clinical trial setting, tolerance intervals can serve as prediction tools because they define the probability with which a future measurement will fall between the lower and upper limits.

Univariate tolerance limits can be set up using a parametric or a nonparametric approach. To be consistent with earlier sections covering nonparametric reference intervals based on sample quantiles, this section will focus on nonparametric tolerance limits. Let $y_{(1)}, \ldots, y_{(n)}$ denote a sample of ordered observations and let

$$T(r, s) = \int_{y_{(r)}}^{y_{(s)}} f(y)dy.$$

The derivation of nonparametric tolerance limits is based on the fundamental fact that the distribution of $T(r, s)$ does not depend on the form of the probability density function $f(y)$. Tukey (1947) proved that $T(r, s)$ follows the beta distribution with the parameters $s - r$ and $n - s + r + 1$. Using this fact, it is easy to show that equitailed two-sided tolerance limits can be set equal to $L = y_{(r)}$ and $U = y_{(n-r+1)}$, where r is the largest integer with

$$B_{n-2r+1,2r}(\gamma) \leq 1 - \beta,$$

and $B_{n-2r+1,2r}(\gamma)$ denotes the cumulative distribution function of the beta distribution with the parameters $n - 2r + 1$ and $2r$. Similarly, a one-sided upper tolerance limit is given by $U = y_{(n-r+1)}$, where r is the largest integer such that

$$B_{n-r+1,r}(\gamma) \leq 1 - \beta.$$

The defined tolerance limits are easy to implement in SAS using the PROBBETA function. Program 3.4 computes two-sided and one-sided 90% tolerance limits for the QTc interval in the QTC data set with a 95% confidence level: i.e., $\gamma = 0.9$ and $\beta = 0.95$. This program is based on a simple call of the %TolLimit macro given in the Appendix. The macro has the following arguments:

- DATASET is the data set to be analyzed.
- VAR is the name of the variable for which tolerance limits will be computed.
- GAMMA is the content of the tolerance interval.
- BETA is the confidence of the tolerance interval.
- OUTDATA is the output data set with one-sided and two-sided tolerance limits.

The %TolLimit macro first determines the ranks of the measurements constituting the upper and lower tolerance limits and then computes the actual values of the limits using PROC RANK.

Program 3.4 Computation of the 90% tolerance limits for the QTc interval in the QTC data set with a 95% confidence level

```
%TolLimit(dataset=qtc,var=y,gamma=0.9,beta=0.95,outdata=tollimit);
proc print data=tollimit noobs label;
    run;
```

Output from Program 3.4

Upper one-sided tolerance limit	Lower two-sided tolerance limit	Upper two-sided tolerance limit
459.307	384.471	468.109

Output 3.4 lists the reference limits computed by the %TolLimit macro. The upper one-sided 90% tolerance limit at the 95% confidence level is 459.307. Note that the upper reference limit based on the 90th quantile produced by PROC UNIVARIATE in Program 3.2 varied between 457.989 and 458.146. Thus, the tolerance-based upper reference limit for the QTc interval is numerically close to the upper limit computed in Section 3.2.1 using sample quantiles.

Due to the conceptual difference between the two outlined approaches to defining reference limits in clinical trials, one should generally avoid a direct comparison of the two sets of limits. As we stressed in the beginning of this subsection, quantile-based limits operate at fsample level whereas tolerance limits are aimed at population/predictive inferences. If one is interested in studying how the use of the tolerance limit methodology influences the width of the reference interval, one needs to remember that tolerance-based reference intervals are wider than quantile-based reference intervals when the confidence level β is greater than 0.5 and narrower otherwise. Confidence levels used in practice are larger than 0.8 and thus the use of the tolerance limit methodology always results in wider reference intervals.

3.2.3 Multivariate Reference Intervals Based on Global Smoothing

In the previous sections we discussed the computation of upper reference limits for the QTc interval based on univariate sample quantiles and tolerance limits. Univariate reference limits are unlikely to be useful in practice because they ignore an important covariate that affects the length of the QTc interval. As shown in Figures 3.1 and 3.2, QTc values tend to be shorter in younger patients and longer in older patients. Therefore, to produce accurate and scientifically sound reference limits for the QTc interval, we need to account for the effect of the patient's age on the upper tail of the QTc interval distribution. Similar problems arise when one is interested in analyzing multiple correlated variables—for instance, in estimating the average value and variability of a safety marker as a function of plasma drug concentration (see Section 3.2.7 for details and examples).

This section describes a simple approach based on global smoothing to establish covariate-adjusted reference limits for safety and diagnostic variables. Unlike statistical methods for local smoothing that will be described later in Section 3.2.5, global smoothing methods yield a single model that approximates the unknown quantile function over the entire covariate space.

Koenker-Bassett Method for Constructing Univariate Reference Limits

In Section 3.2.1 we talked about univariate reference intervals based on sample quantiles. Koenker and Bassett (1978) introduced an alternative computational algorithm for estimating population quantiles that will be used extensively in this section. Consider n observations, denoted by $y_1, \ldots, y_n$, from an unknown distribution $F(y)$, and suppose we are interested in estimating the 100γth quantile of this distribution ($0 < \gamma < 1$). Koenker and Bassett noted that the 100γth quantile of the unknown distribution minimizes

$$S(a) = \sum_{i=1}^{n} \rho_\gamma(y_i - a)$$

with respect to a, where $\rho_\gamma(u)$ is the so-called *check function* given by

$$\rho_\gamma(u) = (|u| + (2\gamma - 1)u)/2.$$

The check functions for the sample median $\rho_{0.5}(u)$ and 90th quantile $\rho_{0.9}(u)$ are plotted in Figure 3.3.

Figure 3.3 Koenker-Bassett check function for the sample median (left-hand panel) and 90th quantile (right-hand panel)

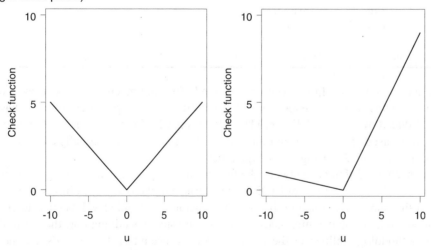

We see from Figure 3.3 that the two check functions assign different sets of weights to the residuals

$$y_1 - a, \ldots, y_n - a.$$

The check function for the median places equal weights on positive and negative residuals and, as a consequence, the sum of weighted residuals $S(a)$ is minimized when a lies exactly in the middle of the sample. In contrast, the check function for the 90th quantile assigns much more weight to positive residuals and this shifts the optimal value a toward the higher values. In general, the larger the value of γ, the more the optimal value a is pushed toward the extreme values in the sample.

The problem of minimizing the sum of weighted residuals $S(a)$ with respect to a can be solved using the iteratively reweighted least squares (IRLS) algorithm widely used in the world of robust regression. For a detailed description of the IRLS methodology, see Holland and Welsch (1977).

IRLS Algorithm for Computing the 100γth Quantile

Step 1. Start with some initial estimate $\widehat{a}(0)$, e.g., the sample mean or 75th quantile.

Step 2. Compute the residuals $r_i = y_i - \widehat{a}(0)$, $i = 1, \ldots, n$, and then the weights $w_i = \tau_\gamma(r_i)/r_i$, $i = 1, \ldots, n$, where

$$\tau_\gamma(u) = \begin{cases} \gamma - 1, & \text{if } u < 0, \\ 0, & \text{if } u = 0, \\ \gamma, & \text{if } u > 0. \end{cases}$$

Note that $\tau_\gamma(u)$ is equal to the derivative of the check function $\rho_\gamma(u)$ when $u \neq 0$.

Step 3. The new estimate $\widehat{a}(1)$ is obtained by minimizing

$$\sum_{i=1}^{n} w_i (y_i - a)^2$$

with respect to a, i.e.,

$$\widehat{a}(1) = \left(\sum_{i=1}^{n} w_i \right)^{-1} \sum_{i=1}^{n} w_i y_i.$$

Step 4. Repeat Steps 2 and 3 until convergence.

Note that if the weights $w_1, \ldots, w_n$ were fixed, the IRLS algorithm would converge in just one step because the problem of minimizing

$$\sum_{i=1}^{n} w_i (y_i - a)^2$$

with respect to a has a simple closed-form solution. However, the weights change from iteration to iteration to selectively discount the observations with large residuals and force the sequence

$$\{\widehat{a}(1), \widehat{a}(2), \widehat{a}(3), \ldots\}$$

to converge to the 100γth sample quantile.

The outlined IRLS algorithm has a simple structure and can be implemented in PROC IML using the NLP routines. However, PROC NLIN provides a much more elegant solution. PROC NLIN is a powerful procedure for the analysis of nonlinear regression models based on the method of weighted least squares. One interesting feature of the weighted least squares algorithm implemented in PROC NLIN is that it gives the user an option to update the weights at each step of the algorithm. Thanks to this option, the algorithm becomes a highly versatile tool for solving a variety of optimization problems, including the one stated above.

Program 3.5 utilizes PROC NLIN to approximate the 90th quantile of the QTc interval in the QTC data set. The sample mean of the QTc values serves as an initial estimate of the 90th quantile and is passed to PROC NLIN using the INITIAL macro variable. As shown in Program 3.5, the weights

$w_1, \ldots, w_n$ are re-computed at each step of the IRLS algorithm using the special variable named _WEIGHT_. The CONVERGE parameter in PROC NLIN controls the convergence of the IRLS algorithm.

Program 3.5 An IRLS approximation to the 90th quantile of the QTc interval in the QTC data set

```
proc means data=qtc noprint;
    var y;
    output out=initial mean=mean;
data _null_;
    set initial;
    call symput("initial",mean);
proc nlin data=qtc nohalve converge=0.001;
    ods select EstSummary ParameterEstimates;
    parms quantile=&initial;
    model y=quantile;
    der.quantile=1; resid=y-model.y;
    if resid>0 then _weight_=0.9/resid;
    if resid<0 then _weight_=-0.1/resid;
    if resid=0 then _weight_=0;
    run;
```

Output from Program 3.5

```
          Estimation Summary

Method                   Gauss-Newton
Iterations                         51
R                            0.000844
PPC(quantile)                 0.00001
RPC(quantile)                0.000028
Object                        2.938E-6
Objective                    13126.41
Observations Read                3000
Observations Used                3000
Observations Missing                0



                          Approx
Parameter     Estimate  Std Error    Approximate 95% Confidence Limits

quantile         457.9     0.1011      457.7       458.1
```

Output 3.5 lists the estimation summary and IRLS estimate of the 90th quantile (note that the iteration history was suppressed using the ODS statement ods select EstSummary ParameterEstimates). Output 3.5 shows that, starting with the sample mean, it took PROC NLIN 51 iterations to estimate the 90th quantile of the QTc interval when the CONVERGE parameter was set to 0.001. The estimate of the 90th quantile produced by the Koenker-Bassett algorithm in Program 3.5 equals 457.9 and is very close to the estimates produced by PROC UNIVARIATE in Program 3.2. As was indicated earlier, the smallest 90th quantile generated by the five algorithms in PROC UNIVARIATE was 457.989 and the largest 90th quantile was 458.146.

Koenker-Bassett Method for Constructing Multivariate Reference Limits

The global smoothing approach to setting up multivariate reference limits relies on an extension of the univariate Koenker-Bassett method. As an illustration, consider a sample of independent bivariate observations (x_i, y_i), $i = 1, \ldots, n$, that follow an unknown distribution $F(x, y)$. Here x_i and y_i represent the values of the continuous covariate and the response variable for the ith patient, respectively. Let $q_\gamma(x)$ denote the 100γth quantile of the conditional distribution of Y given $X = x$ ($0 < \gamma < 1$). We are interested in estimating the quantile function $q_\gamma(x)$ from this sample and using it to construct a one-sided reference limit for the response variable Y adjusted for the covariate X.

Since the 100γth quantile of the marginal distribution of Y equals the value a that minimizes

$$\sum_{i=1}^{n} \rho_\gamma(y_i - a),$$

Koenker and Bassett proposed to define the linear quantile regression as the function $a + bx$ that minimizes

$$\sum_{i=1}^{n} \rho_\gamma(y_i - a - bx_i).$$

The obtained linear approximation to $q_\gamma(x)$ will likely be overly simplistic in most clinical applications. Instead of this linear quantile model, we can utilize more general polynomial models considered by Dmitrienko (2003a). It is natural to define a quantile polynomial of the pth degree by minimizing

$$S(a_0, \ldots, a_p) = \sum_{i=1}^{n} \rho_\gamma(y_i - a_0 - a_1 x_i - \ldots - a_p x_i^p)$$

with respect to the model parameters $a_0, \ldots, a_p$.

As in the case of univariate quantiles considered earlier in this section, this optimization problem can be solved using an IRLS algorithm.

IRLS Algorithm for Computing a pth Degree Polynomial Approximation to the Quantile Function $q_\gamma(x)$

Step 1. Start with some initial estimates $\widehat{a}_0(0), \ldots, \widehat{a}_p(0)$ of the model coefficients. The initial estimates can be obtained by fitting a pth degree polynomial to the conditional mean of the response variable Y given the covariate X based on the method of least squares.

Step 2. Compute the residuals

$$r_i = y_i - \widehat{a}_0(0) - \widehat{a}_1(0)x_i - \ldots - \widehat{a}_p(0)x_i^p, \quad i = 1, \ldots, n,$$

and the weights $w_i = \tau_\gamma(r_i)/r_i$, $i = 1, \ldots, n$. Here

$$\tau_\gamma(u) = \begin{cases} \gamma - 1, & \text{if } u < 0, \\ 0, & \text{if } u = 0, \\ \gamma, & \text{if } u > 0. \end{cases}$$

Step 3. The new set of model coefficients $\widehat{a}_0(1), \ldots, \widehat{a}_p(1)$ is computed by fitting a pth degree polynomial to the original observations based on the method of weighted least squares, i.e., by minimizing

$$\sum_{i=1}^{n} w_i(y_i - a_0 - a_1 x_i - \ldots - a_p x_i^p)^2.$$

with respect to $a_0, \ldots, a_p$.

Step 4. Repeat Steps 2 and 3 until convergence.

Program 3.6 fits second- and tenth-degree polynomials to estimate the age-adjusted one-sided upper 90% reference limit of the QTc interval based on the outlined IRLS algorithm and compares the obtained polynomials with the true age-adjusted 90% limit. The program utilizes the %GlobalQSmooth macro provided in the Appendix. The macro has the following five arguments:

- DATASET is the data set to be analyzed.
- GRID is the name of the input data set with the grid points at which the computed polynomial will be evaluated (X variable).
- P is the degree of the polynomial approximation.
- GAMMA is the quantile of the conditional distribution function of the response variable Y given the covariate $X = x$ that needs to be estimated.
- OUTDATA is the name of the output data set containing the fitted polynomial (POLY variable), its first derivative (FIRSTDER variable) and second derivative (SECDER variable) evaluated at the grid points.

Program 3.6 Age-adjusted one-sided upper 90% reference limit for the QTc interval based on second- and tenth-degree polynomials

```
ods listing close;
data grid100;
    do i=0 to 100;
        x=10+50*i/100;
        output;
    end;

%GlobalQSmooth(dataset=qtc,grid=grid100,gamma=0.9,p=2,
    outdata=poly2);
%GlobalQSmooth(dataset=qtc,grid=grid100,gamma=0.9,p=10,
    outdata=poly10);

data comb;
    set qtc(in=in1) poly2(in=in2) poly10(in=in3);
    group=in1+2*in2+3*in3;
    if (in1) then y=upper; else y=poly;
    keep y x group;
axis1 minor=none label=(angle=90 "QTc interval (msec)")
    order=(420 to 480 by 20);
axis2 minor=none label=("Age (years)") order=(10 to 60 by 10);
symbol1 value=none color=black i=join line=1;
symbol2 value=none color=black i=join line=20;
symbol3 value=none color=black i=join line=34;
ods listing;
proc gplot data=comb;
    plot y*x=group/frame nolegend haxis=axis2 vaxis=axis1;
    run;
```

The output of Program 3.6 is shown in Figure 3.4 (the PROC NLIN output was suppressed using the ODS statement ods listing close). The figure displays the age-adjusted 90% reference limit for the QTc interval based on the second- and tenth-degree polynomial approximations. The polynomials are evaluated at 100 equally spaced points on the age axis specified in the GRID100 data set. Since the second-degree polynomial has fewer degrees of freedom, it produces an oversmoothed approximation to the true age-adjusted 90% limit in Figure 3.4. By contrast, the tenth-degree polynomial has too many fluctuations and masks the important fact that the QTc interval shortens with increasing age in males younger than 20 years old.

Figure 3.4 Reference limits for the QTc interval. Age-adjusted upper 90% reference limit based on a second-degree polynomial (- - -), age-adjusted upper 90% reference limit based on a tenth-degree polynomial (···) and true age-adjusted 90% reference limit (—).

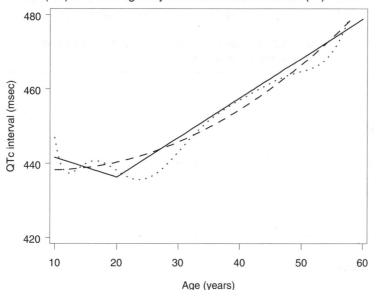

3.2.4 Selecting a Quantile Polynomial in Global Smoothing

It is clear from Figure 3.4 that the degree of a quantile polynomial greatly affects the accuracy of the estimated age-adjusted reference limit for the QTc interval. In what follows we will describe a simple criterion that can be used for choosing the degree of a quantile polynomial model in clinical applications. The first step in this process is determining the degree of a polynomial approximation that results in overfitting. This degree is denoted by p^*. The value of p^* is determined empirically depending on the shape of the quantile function. For example, based on the analysis of the age-adjusted reference limit for the QTc interval, it seems reasonable to let $p^* = 10$ since going beyond the tenth degree will likely result in overfitting. Once p^* has been fixed, the optimal degree is defined as the value p between 1 and p^* minimizing a suitably chosen criterion that balances the model fit and the number of parameters. In a linear regression setting, variable selection is commonly performed using the C_p criterion introduced by Mallows (1973). This criterion is based on comparing the residual sum of squares for all possible submodels of the full model and penalizing submodels with a large number of variables. This basic idea can be applied to the comparison of quantile polynomials. Since a quantile polynomial of the pth degree is computed by minimizing the sum of the weighted residuals

$$S(a_0, \ldots, a_p) = \sum_{i=1}^{n} \rho_\gamma (y_i - a_0 - a_1 x_i - \ldots - a_p x_i^p),$$

Dmitrienko (2003a) proposed to modify the Mallows criterion by replacing the residual sum of squares with the minimum value of $S(a_0, \ldots, a_p)$. Let $S(p)$ denote the minimum value of $S(a_0, \ldots, a_p)$ with respect to the model parameters $a_0, \ldots, a_p$. The modified Mallows criterion C_p^* for a quantile polynomial of the pth degree is defined as

$$C_p^* = \frac{S(p)}{S(p^*)/(n - p^* - 1)} - n + 2(p + 1).$$

Although the obtained C_p^* has a different interpretation from that of the classical Mallows C_p in a least squares setting, it can serve as a simple "rule of thumb" for selecting the degree of a polynomial approximation to quantile functions. Specifically, one needs to choose the value p between 1 and p^* that minimizes C_p^*.

To illustrate the process of selecting the degree of a quantile polynomial, Program 3.7 computes the value of $S(p)$ as well as C_p^* for 10 quantile polynomials ($p = 1, \ldots, 10$) approximating the age-adjusted one-sided upper 90% reference limit for the QTc interval. The program is based on the %Cp macro that calls the %GlobalQSmooth macro to fit each of the 10 quantile polynomials and then

Program 3.7 The sum of weighted residuals and modified Mallows criterion for polynomial approximations to the age-adjusted 90% reference limit for the QTc interval

```
ods listing close;
%macro cp(dataset,gamma,pmax);
    data comb;
    %do j=&pmax %to 1 %by -1;

        %GlobalQSmooth(dataset=&dataset,grid=&dataset,gamma=&gamma,p=&j,
        outdata=poly);

        data res;
            set poly;
            res=0.5*(abs(y-poly)+2*(&gamma-1)*(y-poly));
            keep res;
        proc means data=res noprint;
            var res;
            output out=cp sum(res)=s;
        data _null_;
            set cp;
            if &j=&pmax then call symput("smax",s);
        data _null_;
            set &dataset nobs=m;
            call symput("n",m);
            run;
        data cp;
            set cp;
            degree=&j;
            smax=&smax/(&n-&pmax-1);
            cp=s/smax-&n+2*(&j+1);
            keep s cp degree;
        data comb;
            set comb cp;
            run;
    %end;
%mend cp;

%cp(dataset=qtc,gamma=0.9,pmax=10);

axis1 minor=none label=(angle=90 "S(p)") order=(50000 to 52000 by 1000);
axis2 minor=none label=("Degree (p)") order=(1 to 10 by 1);
symbol1 value=dot color=black i=none;
proc gplot data=comb;
    plot s*degree/frame nolegend haxis=axis2 vaxis=axis1;
    run;
axis1 minor=none label=(angle=90 "Cp") order=(0 to 100 by 50);
axis2 minor=none label=("Degree (p)") order=(1 to 10 by 1);
symbol1 value=dot color=black i=none;
ods listing;
proc gplot data=comb;
    plot cp*degree/frame nolegend haxis=axis2 vaxis=axis1;
    run;
```

computes the $S(p)$ and C_p^* statistics. Note that, in order to compute these statistics, the 10 polynomials are evaluated at each X value in the QTC data set.

The output of Program 3.7 is shown in Figure 3.5. The left-hand and right-hand panels in Figure 3.5 convey a similar message about the fit of the 10 quantile polynomials because the number of observations in the QTC data set is very large and thus the value of the modified Mallows criterion C_p^* is driven primarily by the sum of weighted residuals $S(p)$. Examining the modified Mallows criterion C_p^* as a function of p, it is clear that the first- to fourth-degree quantile polynomials provide roughly the same fit to the 90% reference limit. There is, however, a notable improvement between the fourth- and fifth-degree polynomials ($C_4^* = 77.7$ and $C_5^* = 13.2$). Any further increase in the degree of a polynomial approximation does not affect its accuracy and $C_6^* = 12.8$ is the local minimum. Although C_{10}^* is slightly smaller than C_6^*, the principle of parsimony suggests selecting the sixth-degree polynomial as an optimal approximation to the age-adjusted 90% reference limit for the QTc interval. Further, it is easy to verify that the modified Mallows achieves a local minimum at $p = 6$ over a range p^* values—for example, when $p^* = 8$, $p^* = 12$ or $p^* = 15$—which confirms our conclusion that the sixth-degree polynomial provides an optimal approximation to the QTc reference curve.

Figure 3.5 Selecting the degree of a quantile polynomial. The sum of weighted residuals (left-hand panel) and modified Mallows criterion (right-hand panel) for polynomial approximations to the age-adjusted 90% reference limit for the QTc interval.

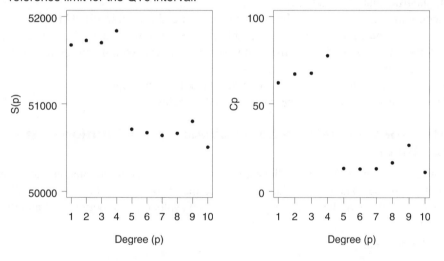

3.2.5   Multivariate Reference Intervals Based on Local Smoothing

We pointed out in the beginning of Section 3.2.3 that the idea behind global smoothing is to derive a single model to approximate a multivariate quantile function over the entire covariate space. For example, Program 3.6 computes polynomials that approximate the age-adjusted 90% reference limit for the QTc interval over a 50-year range of age values. The global approach provides the clinical statistician with a simple means for setting up covariate-adjusted reference limits for safety and diagnostic parameters. However, the effectiveness of global methods may be limited when the underlying quantile function is irregularly shaped. It is often difficult, if not impossible, to capture complex relationships between a response variable and quantitative covariates using global optimization criteria.

This section discusses quantile estimators based on local optimization criteria. As their name suggests, local smoothing methods rely on approximating the unknown quantile function independently in each of multiple partitions of the covariate space. This allows local quantile estimators to be more flexible than the global quantile estimators introduced in the previous subsection.

An important example of local quantile estimators is a kernel-based estimator. Kernel smoothing methods are easy to implement in practice and their properties have been studied in a large number of publications. For example, Fan, Hu and Truong (1994) and Yu and Jones (1998) described a kernel quantile estimation method based on local linear fitting. To define the local linear quantile estimator, consider again a sample of independent bivariate observations (x_i, y_i), $i = 1, \ldots, n$, representing the values of the continuous covariate and the response variable. According to the local linear method, the 100γth quantile of the conditional distribution of Y given $X = x_0$, denoted by $q_\gamma(x_0)$, is estimated by fitting a linear model in a suitably chosen neighborhood of x_0. Specifically, the local linear estimator $\widehat{q}_\gamma(x_0)$ is defined as the value a that minimizes

$$\sum_{i=1}^{n} \rho_\gamma(y_i - a - b(x_i - x_0)) \frac{1}{h} K\left(\frac{x_i - x_0}{h}\right),$$

where $\rho_\gamma(u)$ is the check function defined in Section 3.2.3, $K(u)$ is a kernel function, i.e.,

$$K(u) \geq 0 \text{ and } \int K(u)du = 1,$$

and h is the bandwidth parameter that determines the smoothness of the resulting quantile estimator and hence the smoothness of the resulting reference curves. When h is large, the local linear estimation method combines a larger number of data points to approximate $q_\gamma(x)$ and this has an effect of averaging out fluctuations. On the other hand, using small values of h results in a fairly wiggly approximation to the true quantile function.

It is worth mentioning that similar kernel-based estimators are also used in PROC LOESS for estimating the conditional mean of the response variable Y given the covariate X. While PROC LOESS focuses on the estimation of the conditional mean, this subsection deals with the problem of estimating quantiles of the conditional distribution of Y given X.

Since the local linear estimator $\widehat{q}_\gamma(x)$ is based on the check function approach, it can be computed using the IRLS algorithm for fitting local linear models shown below.

IRLS Algorithm for Computing a Local Linear Approximation to the Quantile Function $q_\gamma(x)$

Step 1. Fix a point x_0 and start with some initial estimates $\widehat{a}(0)$ and $\widehat{b}(0)$ of the intercept and slope of the local linear model. The initial values can be obtained by fitting a global polynomial approximation to the quantile function $q_\gamma(x)$ and then evaluating the polynomial and its first derivative at x_0.

Step 2. Compute the residuals

$$r_i = y_i - \widehat{a}(0) - \widehat{b}(0)(x_i - x_0), \quad i = 1, \ldots, n,$$

and the weights

$$w_i = \frac{1}{h} K\left(\frac{x_i - x_0}{h}\right) \frac{\tau_\gamma(r_i)}{r_i}, \quad i = 1, \ldots, n.$$

Here

$$\tau_\gamma(u) = \begin{cases} \gamma - 1, & \text{if } u < 0, \\ 0, & \text{if } u = 0, \\ \gamma, & \text{if } u > 0. \end{cases}$$

Step 3. Compute the new values of the intercept and slope $\widehat{a}(1)$ and $\widehat{b}(1)$ by fitting a local linear model using the method of weighted least squares, i.e., by minimizing

$$\sum_{i=1}^{n} w_i(y_i - a - b(x_i - x_0))^2 \frac{1}{h} K\left(\frac{x_i - x_0}{h}\right)$$

with respect to a and b.

Step 4. Repeat Steps 2 and 3 until convergence.

Step 5. Once the approximation at x_0 has been computed, repeat the same process over the entire range of X values.

The introduced IRLS algorithm can be implemented using the NLP optimization routines in PROC IML or, alternatively, one can rely on the built-in optimization algorithms in PROC NLIN. The PROC NLIN solution with a normal kernel

$$K(u) = \frac{1}{\sqrt{2\pi}} e^{-u^2/2}$$

is implemented in the %LocalQSmooth macro found in the Appendix. The macro has the following parameters:

- DATASET is the data set to be analyzed.
- GRID is the name of the input data set with the grid points at which the computed polynomial will be evaluated (X variable).
- P is the degree of the polynomial approximation.
- GAMMA is the quantile of the conditional distribution function of the response variable Y given the covariate $X = x$ that needs to be estimated.
- INITIAL is the name of the input data set with the grid points (X variable), initial values of the intercept and slope of the local linear model (POLY and FIRSTDER variables), and the bandwidth parameter (H variable).
- OUTDATA is the name of the output data set containing the local linear estimates of the quantile function evaluated at the grid points (ESTIMATE variable).

Program 3.8, based on the %LocalQSmooth macro, estimates the age-adjusted upper 90% reference limit for the QTc interval for the bandwidth parameters of 2 and 4. To compute the initial values of the intercept and slope of the local linear model, a sixth-degree polynomial was fitted to the QTC data set. The polynomial was evaluated along with its first derivative at 50 and 500 equally spaced age points (GRID50 and GRID500 data sets). The obtained initial values and the pre-specified bandwidth parameter ($h = 2$ or $h = 4$) were then passed to the %LocalQSmooth macro in the INITIAL data set. Note that computing the local linear estimate $\widehat{q}_\gamma(x)$ for each X value in the QTC data set is fairly time-consuming and may take up to an hour.

Program 3.8 Age-adjusted upper 90% reference limit for the QTc interval based on local smoothing

```
ods listing close;
data grid50;
    do i=0 to 50;
        x=10+50*i/50;
        output;
    end;
data grid500;
    do i=0 to 500;
        x=10+50*i/500;
        output;
    end;

%GlobalQSmooth(dataset=qtc,grid=grid50,gamma=0.9,p=6,outdata=poly6a);
%GlobalQSmooth(dataset=qtc,grid=grid500,gamma=0.9,p=6,outdata=poly6b);
```

```
* Bandwidth=2;
data initial1;
    set poly6a;
    h=2;

%LocalQSmooth(dataset=qtc,gamma=0.9,initial=initial1,outdata=loc1);

* Bandwidth=2;
data initial2;
    set poly6b;
    h=2;

%LocalQSmooth(dataset=qtc,gamma=0.9,initial=initial2,outdata=loc2);

* Bandwidth=4;
data initial3;
    set poly6a;
    h=4;

%LocalQSmooth(dataset=qtc,gamma=0.9,initial=initial3,outdata=loc3);

* Bandwidth=4;
data initial4;
    set poly6b;
    h=4;

%LocalQSmooth(dataset=qtc,gamma=0.9,initial=initial4,outdata=loc4);

ods listing;

* Plot the reference limits;
%macro QPlot(dataset,label1,label2);
axis1 minor=none label=(angle=90 "QTc interval (msec)")
    order=(420 to 480 by 20);
axis2 minor=none label=("Age (years)") order=(10 to 60 by 10);
symbol1 value=none color=black i=join line=1;
data temp;
    set &dataset;
    format estimate 3.0 x 3.0;
proc sort data=temp;
    by x;
data annotate;
    length text $50;
    xsys="1"; ysys="1"; hsys="4"; x=50; y=16; position="5";
    size=0.8; text="&label1"; function="label"; output;
    xsys="1"; ysys="1"; hsys="4"; x=50; y=8; position="5";
    size=0.8; text="&label2"; function="label"; output;
proc gplot data=temp anno=annotate;
    plot estimate*x/frame haxis=axis2 vaxis=axis1;
    run;
    quit;
%mend QPlot;

ods listing;
```

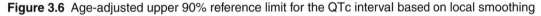

```
%QPlot(dataset=loc1,label1=Bandwidth=2,label2=50 grid points);
%QPlot(dataset=loc2,label1=Bandwidth=2,label2=500 grid points);
%QPlot(dataset=loc3,label1=Bandwidth=4,label2=50 grid points);
%QPlot(dataset=loc4,label1=Bandwidth=4,label2=500 grid points);
```

The output of Program 3.8 is displayed in Figure 3.6. As expected, a larger value of the bandwidth parameter H yields a smoother approximation to the age-adjusted 90% reference limit for the QTc interval. We can also see from Figure 3.6 that the number of points at which the local linear quantile estimator is computed does not affect the accuracy of the approximation. Reducing the number of grid points by a factor of 10 (from 500 to 50 points) eliminates some of the occasional spikes but hardly changes the shape of the age-adjusted reference limit.

Figure 3.6 Age-adjusted upper 90% reference limit for the QTc interval based on local smoothing

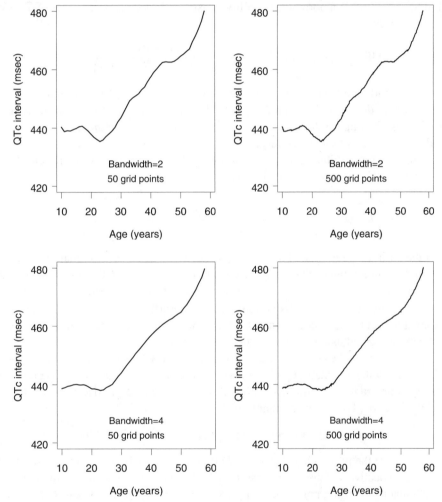

On a practical note, when running the %LocalQSmooth macro, you may encounter warning messages indicating that PROC NLIN failed to converge. Most of the time, this is caused by the fact that the IRLS algorithm quickly reaches the point of convergence and therefore additional iterations produce no further improvement in the PROC NLIN criteria. Despite the theoretical possibility that the IRLS algorithm can sometimes fail to converge, convergence problems are very rare in practice.

3.2.6 Bandwidth Selection in Local Smoothing

Figure 3.6 demonstrates that the magnitude of the bandwidth parameter H affects the shape of the estimated quantile function and thus the shape of the resulting covariate-adjusted reference limits. The bandwidth plays a role similar to that of the degree of a polynomial approximation in global smoothing in that it determines the smoothness and accuracy of quantile estimators. In an exploratory setting, one can often select the bandwidth by visual examination and comparison of several sets of reference curves. However, the choice of the optimal bandwidth parameter becomes a much more important issue when one intends to establish covariate-adjusted reference limits for safety and diagnostic variables that will be used across multiple drug development projects or for regulatory submission purposes. This section reviews an algorithm for computing an optimal bandwidth parameter based on the work of Fan, Hu and Truong (1994).

Consider a local linear estimator for the 100γth quantile of the conditional distribution of the response variable Y given the covariate $X = x_0$ introduced in the previous subsection. The estimator, denoted by $\widehat{q}_\gamma(x_0)$, is computed from a sample of n independent bivariate observations. When the kernel function used in the estimator is a normal probability density, the mean squared error of $\widehat{q}_\gamma(x_0)$ has the following asymptotic representation:

$$\text{MSE} \sim \frac{1}{4}h^4\{q_\gamma''(x_0)\}^2 + \frac{\gamma(1-\gamma)}{2\sqrt{\pi}nhg(x_0)\{f(q_\gamma(x_0)|x_0)\}^2},$$

where $q_\gamma''(x)$ is the second derivative of the true quantile function, $g(x)$ is the marginal density of X and $f(y|x)$ is the conditional density of Y given $X = x$. This representation of the mean squared error was derived by Fan, Hu and Truong (1994) under the assumption that x_0 lies in the interior of the covariate space, h is small, n is large, and nh is also large.

Given the asymptotic representation, the optimal bandwidth can be chosen by minimizing the mean squared error of $\widehat{q}_\gamma(x_0)$. The resulting optimal value is given by

$$h_\gamma^*(x_0) = \left[\frac{\gamma(1-\gamma)}{2\sqrt{\pi}ng(x_0)\{q_\gamma''(x_0)f(q_\gamma(x_0)|x_0)\}^2}\right]^{1/5}.$$

The formula for the optimal value of the bandwidth parameter involves several quantities that need to be estimated from the bivariate sample. The marginal density function $g(x)$ and the second derivative of the true conditional quantile function $q_\gamma''(x)$ are relatively easy to estimate. To compute an estimate of $g(x_0)$, we can employ any popular kernel-smoothing method. Further, to estimate $q_\gamma''(x)$, we can fit a quantile polynomial model to the bivariate sample and compute its second derivative. This estimation procedure can be implemented using the %GlobalQSmooth macro.

Estimating $f(q_\gamma(x_0)|x_0)$—the conditional density of Y given $X = x$ evaluated at $q_\gamma(x_0)$—is a more difficult task. To simplify this estimation problem, it is reasonable to assume that $f(y|x)$ is a member of a parametric family. For example, Dmitrienko (2003a) proposed to assume that $f(y|x)$ is a normal probability density function. Under this assumption,

$$f(q_\gamma(x)|x) = \phi(\Phi^{-1}(\gamma))/(q_{\Phi(1)}(x) - q_{1/2}(x)),$$

where $\phi(x)$ and $\Phi(x)$ are the probability density and cumulative distribution functions of the standard normal distribution, respectively. This means that $f(q_\gamma(x_0)|x_0)$ can be estimated using the %GlobalQSmooth macro by fitting polynomial approximations to $q_{\Phi(1)}(x)$ and $q_{1/2}(x)$ and then evaluating the obtained functions at x_0. It is important to point out that the normality assumption is used here only to simplify the process of computing the optimal bandwidth. The assumption does not affect the performance of the nonparametric estimator $\widehat{q}_\gamma(x)$.

Program 3.9 demonstrates how to implement the described algorithm for computing the optimal bandwidth function $h_\gamma^*(x)$ in the problem of estimating the age-adjusted 90% reference limit of the QTc interval. The program is based on the %Bandwidth macro that calls the %LocalQSmooth macro to obtain sixth-degree and tenth-degree polynomial approximations to $q_\gamma(x)$, $q_{\Phi(1)}(x)$ and $q_{1/2}(x)$. The marginal density function $g(x)$ is estimated using the weighted kernel method implemented in PROC

KDE. The estimated functions are then utilized to compute the optimal bandwidth function $h_\gamma^*(x)$ at 100 equally spaced points on the age axis.

Program 3.9 The optimal bandwidth function for the computation of the age-adjusted upper 90% reference limit for the QTc interval based on local smoothing

```
ods listing close;
%macro bandwidth(dataset,gamma,p,outdata);
    data _null_;
        set &dataset nobs=m;
        call symput("n",m);
        run;

    %GlobalQSmooth(dataset=&dataset,grid=grid100,gamma=&gamma,
    p=&p,outdata=q1);
    %GlobalQSmooth(dataset=&dataset,grid=grid100,gamma=probnorm(1),
    p=&p,outdata=q2);
    %GlobalQSmooth(dataset=&dataset,grid=grid100,gamma=0.5,
    p=&p,outdata=q3);

    data q1;
        set q1;
        keep x secder;
    data q2;
        set q2;
        qprob1=poly;
        keep x qprob1;
    data q3;
        set q3;
        median=poly;
        keep x median;
    proc kde data=&dataset ngrid=101 gridl=10 gridu=60 out=margdens;
        var x;
    proc sort data=margdens;
        by x;
    data comb;
        merge q1 q2 q3 margdens;
        by x;
    data &outdata;
        set comb;
        dens=pdf("normal",probit(&gamma))/(qprob1-median);
        denom=3.546*&n*density*secder*secder*dens*dens;
        h=(&gamma*(1-&gamma)/denom)**0.2;
%mend bandwidth;

data grid100;
    do i=0 to 100;
        x=10+50*i/100;
        output;
    end;

%bandwidth(dataset=qtc,gamma=0.9,p=6,outdata=h6);
%bandwidth(dataset=qtc,gamma=0.9,p=10,outdata=h10);
axis1 minor=none label=(angle=90 "Bandwidth") order=(0 to 20 by 5);
axis2 minor=none label=("Age (years)") order=(10 to 60 by 10);
symbol1 value=none color=black i=join line=1;
ods listing close;
```

```
proc gplot data=h6;
    plot h*x;
    run;
proc gplot data=h10;
    plot h*x;
    run;
```

The output of Program 3.9 is shown in Figure 3.7. The left-hand panel of the figure displays the optimal bandwidth function derived from a sixth-degree polynomial and the right-hand panel displays the optimal bandwidth function based on a tenth-degree polynomial approximation. Although the degree of the polynomial approximation can potentially influence the final estimate of the optimal bandwidth function $h_\gamma^*(x)$, Figure 3.7 indicates that this effect is not very pronounced. Due to their peculiar shapes the two bandwidth functions in the figure appear to be dissimilar at first glance; however, it is easy to check that their median values are fairly close to each other. The median values of the bandwidth functions are equal to 2.84 (sixth-degree polynomial approximation) and 2.95 (tenth-degree polynomial approximation). The peaks in Figure 3.7 correspond to the inflection points of the polynomials approximating the true quantile curves. By its definition, the optimal bandwidth function $h_\gamma^*(x)$ is inversely proportional to the second derivative of the true quantile function $q_\gamma''(x)$. The optimal bandwidth function assumes very large values when $q_\gamma''(x)$ is close to zero, which occurs at the inflection points of the true quantile function $q_\gamma(x)$. Similarly, the estimated bandwidth function spikes at the inflection points of the polynomial approximating the true quantile curve.

Figure 3.7 Reference limits for the QTc interval. The optimal bandwidth function for the computation of the age-adjusted upper 90% reference limit for the QTc interval based on local smoothing. Left-hand panel: optimal bandwidth function based on a sixth-degree polynomial. Right-hand panel: optimal bandwidth function based on a tenth-degree polynomial.

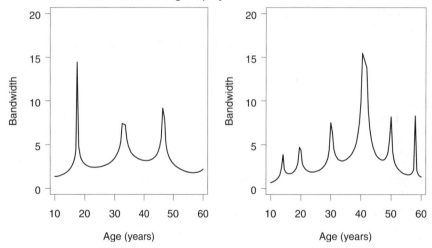

3.2.7 Other Applications of Quantile Estimation Methods

It is important to emphasize that the SAS macros for global and local quantile smoothing %GlobalQSmooth and %LocalQSmooth can be successfully utilized in the analysis of various types of clinical data. This section introduces two clinical applications in which quantile functions enhance the analysis of multiple correlated variables.

Effect of Plasma Drug Concentration on Changes in the QTc Interval

As was stated in the beginning of this section, analysis of the QTc interval prolongation plays a key role in the assessment of cardiac liability of experimental therapies. To help characterize the effect of a new drug on the duration of the QTc interval, it is common to pool QTc data collected in multiple trials and examine QTc changes matched with plasma concentrations of the parent drug and its major metabolites. The concept paper "The clinical evaluation of QT/QTc interval prolongation and proarrhythmic potential for non-antiarrhythmic drugs" released by the FDA on November 15, 2002, recommended that drug developers perform the following analyses of the concentration-response relationship:

> ... collection of plasma samples near the time of the ECG measurement is encouraged to permit exploration of the relationship between parent drug and active metabolite concentrations and resulting ECG changes. Important considerations in characterizing the dose- or concentration-response relationship include the following: ... the steepness of the relationship between the dose/concentration of the drug QT/QTc interval prolongation, the linearity or nonlinearity of the dose/concentration-effect dependency...

The following example will be used to illustrate analysis of concentration-dependent changes in the QTc interval.

EXAMPLE: Meta-analysis of QTc Interval Data

A set of 267 paired ECG recordings (representing baseline and follow-up recordings for the same person) with blood samples collected at the time of the second ECG recording was pooled from early studies in healthy subjects and patients with the disease of interest. A change in the QTc interval from baseline to the follow-up assessment was computed for each individual and was matched with the plasma drug concentration at the follow-up time point. The obtained data are included in the QTCCONC data set shown in the Appendix. The QTCCHANGE variable in this data set represents the change in the QTc interval duration and the CONC variable is the logarithm of the drug concentration measured in ng/mL.

In what follows, we will examine the QTc and drug concentration data in the QTCCONC data set to see whether or not higher levels of drug concentration are associated with larger positive changes in the QTc interval. As pointed out in the FDA concept paper, concentration-response relationships are commonly analyzed by testing the steepness of the regression line fitted to the QTc-drug concentration data. To illustrate this process, Program 3.10 plots the changes in the QTc interval versus plasma drug concentration from the QTCCONC data set and fits a linear regression model to the bivariate measurements.

Program 3.10 Scatter plot of QTc changes and plasma drug concentrations with a linear regression model

```
data qtcconc1;
    set qtcconc;
    y=qtcchange;
    x=conc;
    keep x y;
axis1 minor=none order=(-40 to 40 by 20) label=(angle=90 "Change in QTc (msec)");
axis2 minor=none order=(0 to 6 by 1) label=("Log plasma drug concentration");
symbol1 value=dot color=black i=rlcli90;
proc gplot data=qtcconc1;
    plot y*x/frame overlay haxis=axis2 vaxis=axis1;
    run;
```

The output of Program 3.10 is shown in Figure 3.8. The regression line and 90% confidence limits are requested by using the i=rlcli90 option in the SYMBOL statement. The fitted linear regression model is given by $y = -1.755 + 0.737x$. The slope of the regression model is positive and thus higher concentrations of the experimental drug are associated with larger positive changes in the QTc interval. The mean change in the QTc interval estimated from the model equals -1.755 msec when no drug is

Figure 3.8 Meta-analysis of QTc interval data. Scatter plot of plasma drug concentrations versus QTc changes with a linear regression model (—) and 90% confidence limits (- - -).

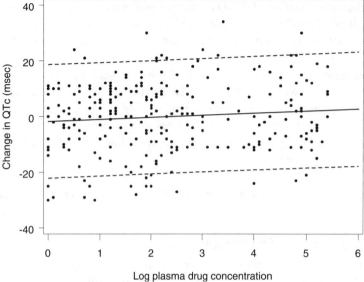

Log plasma drug concentration

detected in the blood and increases to 2.667 msec when the log concentration is equal to 6. This observation may raise safety concerns because it suggests that the experimental drug will likely cause QTc interval prolongation at very high systemic exposures.

To confirm the findings based on a linear regression analysis of QTc interval changes, Program 3.11 uses PROC LOESS (available in SAS 8.0 and later versions of SAS) to fit a local regression model for the mean change in the QTc interval as a function of plasma drug concentration.

Program 3.11 Scatter plot of QTc changes and plasma drug concentrations with a local linear regression model

```
proc loess data=qtcconc1;
    model y=x;
    ods output outputstatistics=smooth;
data smooth;
    set smooth;
    format x 3.0 depvar pred 5.1;
axis1 minor=none order=(-40 to 40 by 20) label=(angle=90 "Change in QTc (msec)");
axis2 minor=none order=(0 to 6 by 1) label=("Log plasma drug concentration");
symbol1 value=dot color=black i=rl line=1;
symbol2 value=none i=j line=20;
proc gplot data=smooth;
    plot depvar*x pred*x/frame haxis = axis2 vaxis = axis1 overlay;
    run;
```

The output of Program 3.11 is displayed in Figure 3.9. The figure shows that the mean change in the QTc interval predicted by the local linear model is smaller in individuals with a low concentration of the experimental drug and gradually increases with increasing exposure. A close examination of Figure 3.9 reveals that the QTc interval is prolonged by 5 msec at higher concentrations compared to lower concentrations, and therefore higher doses of the experimental drug may be associated with abnormal electrophysiological effects.

The methods for estimating multivariate quantile functions introduced earlier in this chapter provide an alternative set of tools for exploring relationships among multiple continuous variables. Recall that the two outlined approaches to examining concentration-response relationships relied on models for the mean change in the QTc interval. The quantile function approach allows one to perform a nonparametric analysis of QTc interval changes and, for this reason, will lead to more robust inferences.

Figure 3.9 Meta-analysis of QTc interval data. Scatter plot of plasma drug concentrations versus QTc changes with a linear regression model (—) and local linear regression model (- - -) generated by PROC LOESS.

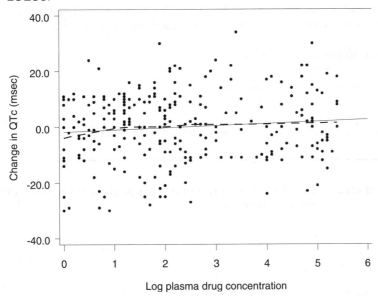

In order to perform a nonparametric analysis of the relationship between systemic exposure and changes in the QTc interval, we will employ the %VarPlot macro given in the Appendix. The macro was developed to facilitate the analysis of trends and variability in data sets with bivariate measurements.

The %VarPlot macro has the following seven parameters:

- DATASET is the name of the input data set to be analyzed.
- GRID specifies the name of the input data set with the grid points (X variable).
- Q1, Q2 and Q3 specify the three quantiles to be estimated, e.g, the lower, middle and upper quantiles.
- H is the value of the bandwidth parameter used in local smoothing.
- OUTDATA is the name of the output data set containing the three quantile functions estimated using the method of local smoothing along with the raw data points. The quantile functions are evaluated at the grid points (ESTIMATE variable).

Program 3.12 utilizes the %VarPlot macro to compute the 10th, 50th and 90th quantiles of the QTc interval change adjusted for plasma concentration of the experimental drug. The quantile functions are computed using the bandwidth parameter of 1 and then evaluated at 20 equally spaced points on the horizontal axis.

Program 3.12 Scatter plot of QTc changes and plasma drug concentrations with three quantile curves

```
ods listing close;
data grid20;
    do i=0 to 20;
        x=6*i/20;
        output;
    end;

%VarPlot(dataset=qtcconc1,grid=grid20,q1=0.1,q2=0.5,q3=0.9,
    h=1,outdata=qtcsmooth);
```

```
data temp;
    set qtcsmooth;
    format estimate 3.0 x 3.0;
axis1 minor=none order=(-40 to 40 by 20) label=(angle=90 "Change in QTc (msec)");
axis2 minor=none order=(0 to 6 by 1) label=("Log plasma drug concentration");
symbol1 value=dot color=black i=none;
symbol2 value=none color=black i=join line=20;
symbol3 value=none color=black i=join line=1;
symbol4 value=none color=black i=join line=20;
ods listing;
proc gplot data=temp;
    plot estimate*x=quantile/nolegend frame haxis=axis2 vaxis=axis1;
    run;
```

Figure 3.10 Meta-analysis of QTc interval data. Scatter plot of plasma drug concentrations versus QTc changes with 50th (—), 10th and 90th quantile curves (- - -).

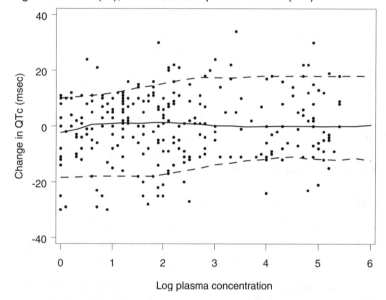

The output of Program 3.12 is displayed in Figure 3.10 (as before, the regular PROC NLIN output was suppressed using the ODS statement `ods listing close`). Figure 3.10 demonstrates the advantages of a nonparametric analysis of multivariate relationships. Both Figure 3.8 and Figure 3.9 showed that higher concentrations of the experimental drug are associated with greater mean changes in the QTc interval. By contrast, the median of the QTc changes is virtually independent of plasma drug concentration in Figure 3.10. The median appears to provide a more reliable estimate of central tendency than the mean because the drug concentration affects primarily the tails of the QTc distribution. Indeed, comparing the estimated 10th and 90th quantiles to the median, we can see that a small number of outliers causes the distribution of QTc changes to be skewed downward at low concentrations and skewed upward at high concentrations. Given the skewness of the distribution and results of the nonparametric analysis of the concentration-response relationship, we conclude that the experimental drug is unlikely to cause QTc prolongation and associated electrophysiological abnormalities.

EXAMPLE: Physician and Patient Assessments in a Rheumatoid Arthritis Trial

This subsection provides another example of a nonparametric analysis of correlated variables. The RACOUNT data set in the Appendix contains a subset of data collected in a Phase II clinical trial in 251 patients with rheumatoid arthritis. The PTPAIN variable is the baseline patient pain assessment measured on a 100-millimeter visual analog scale, and the TJCOUNT and SJCOUNT variables represent the number of tender and swollen joints computed using a 28-joint count. The joint assessments were performed by a physician and the study sponsor was interested in determining which one of the two joint counts is more correlated with the subjective level of pain reported by patients.

In order to answer this question, Program 3.13 utilizes the %VarPlot macro to compute the 10th, 50th and 90th quantiles of the patient pain assessment as a function of both tender and swollen joint counts. The quantile functions are estimated using the method of local smoothing with the bandwidth parameter of 4 and are evaluated at 20 equally spaced points on the horizontal axis.

Program 3.13 Scatter plots of patient pain assessment versus tender and swollen joint counts with three quantile curves

```
ods listing close;
data tender;
    set racount;
    y=ptpain;
    x=tjcount;
    keep x y;
data swollen;
    set racount;
    y=ptpain;
    x=sjcount;
    keep x y;
data grid20;
    do i=0 to 20;
        x=30*i/20;
    output;
    end;

%VarPlot(dataset=tender,grid=grid20,q1=0.1,q2=0.5,q3=0.9,
    h=4,outdata=tsmooth);

data temp;
    set tsmooth;
    format estimate 3.0 x 3.0;
axis1 minor=none order=(0 to 100 by 20)
    label=(angle=90 "Pain assessment (mm)");
axis2 minor=none order=(3 to 28 by 5) label=("Tender joint count");
symbol1 value=dot color=black i=none;
symbol2 value=none color=black i=join line=20;
symbol3 value=none color=black i=join line=1;
symbol4 value=none color=black i=join line=20;
proc gplot data=temp;
    plot estimate*x=quantile/nolegend frame haxis=axis2 vaxis=axis1;
    run;

%VarPlot(dataset=swollen,grid=grid20,q1=0.1,q2=0.5,q3=0.9,
    h=4,outdata=ssmooth);

data temp;
    set ssmooth;
    format estimate 3.0 x 3.0;
axis1 minor=none order=(0 to 100 by 20)
    label=(angle=90 "Pain assessment (mm)");
axis2 minor=none order=(3 to 28 by 5) label=("Swollen joint count");
symbol1 value=dot color=black i=none;
```

```
symbol2 value=none color=black i=join line=20;
symbol3 value=none color=black i=join line=1;
symbol4 value=none color=black i=join line=20;
ods listing;
proc gplot data=temp;
    plot estimate*x=quantile/nolegend frame haxis=axis2 vaxis=axis1;
    run;
```

Figure 3.11 displays the 10th, 50th and 90th quantiles of the patient pain assessment adjusted for the number of tender and swollen joints. We can see from the left-hand panel of the figure that the distribution of the patient pain assessment shifts upward with the increasing number of tender joints in a fairly regular fashion. A quick examination of the quantile curves in the right-hand panel reveals that the 50th and 90th quantiles of the patient pain assessment also increase with increasing swollen joint count. However, the 10th quantile exhibits a great deal of variability and assumes virtually the same value at 3 and 28 swollen joints. This simple analysis of quantile curves indicates that the tender and swollen joint counts demonstrate similar predictive ability in patients with mild disease (i.e., patients with a small number of tender and swollen joints) and the tender joint count better predicts the level of pain compared to the swollen joint count in patients with moderate to severe rheumatoid arthritis.

Figure 3.11 Scatter plots of patient pain assessment versus tender joint count (left-hand panel) and patient pain assessment versus swollen joint count (right-hand panel) in the rheumatoid arthritis trial, with 50th (—), 10th and 90th quantile curves (- - -)

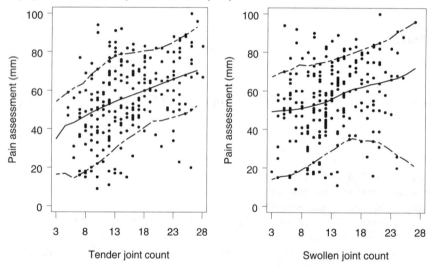

It is worth noting that similar conclusions can theoretically be drawn from scatter plots of pain scores versus tender and swollen joint counts. However scatter plots often suffer from overplotting that limits one's ability to accurately assess changes in conditional distributions.

3.2.8 Summary

This section reviewed methods for constructing reference intervals to facilitate the detection of extreme safety and diagnostic measurements in clinical trials. Sections 3.2.1 and 3.2.2 showed how to set up univariate reference limits based on sample quantiles and tolerance intervals using PROC UNIVARIATE and the %TolLimit macro. Reference limits derived from sample quantiles describe a sample of patients, whereas tolerance intervals can be used to make inferences about the entire underlying population of patients. Due to the conceptual difference between the two approaches to defining reference limits, one should generally avoid a direct comparison of the two sets of limits. As demonstrated in this section, the numerical difference between reference limits based on the two approaches is relatively small.

Section 3.2.3 through 3.2.6 covered two methods for estimating multivariate quantile functions (global and local smoothing). It was shown how the two methods can be used for setting up reference intervals adjusted for important covariates such as the patient's age or baseline disease severity. The global and local quantile smoothing methods are easy to implement in SAS using the %GlobalQSmooth and %LocalQSmooth macros. This section also outlined simple rules for determining optimal parameters of quantile estimation procedures. This includes selecting the degree of a polynomial approximation in global smoothing and the bandwidth parameter in local smoothing. Although the section focused on reference limits adjusted for a single quantitative covariate, the proposed methodology and its implementation in PROC NLIN is easy to extend to the important case of multiple covariates.

Section 3.2.7 demonstrated that applications of multivariate quantile functions are not limited to reference intervals for safety and diagnostic parameters but also include other important problems such as a nonparametric analysis of correlated continuous variables. For example, it was shown that bivariate quantile functions help reveal important trends in the relationship between systemic exposure and changes in the QTc interval. The same methodology can be applied to analyze relationships among multiple continuous variables.

3.3 Analysis of Shift Tables

The previous section discussed statistical methods for constructing reference limits for quantitative diagnostic and safety data. Once the limits have been established, quantitative results are converted into categorical outcomes. For example, laboratory test results are commonly labeled as "low", "high" or "normal" depending on whether the observed value is below the lower reference limit, above the upper reference limit or between the limits. This section reviews methods for handling the obtained categorical outcomes that are commonly summarized using *shift tables* (square contingency tables). To simplify the discussion, we will focus on the case of paired categorical variables. Safety and diagnostic assessments are typically performed only a few times in the course of a clinical trial, most commonly at baseline (prior to the start of study drug administration) and at endpoint (the end of the study period). The general case involving multiple repeated measurements on the same subject is reviewed in Section 5.10.

We begin with a brief description of the method of generalized estimating equations (GEE) in Section 3.3.1. The GEE methodology was introduced by Liang and Zeger (1986) and has since become one of the most important tools in the arsenal of applied statisticians. Several recently published books provide an extensive review of GEE methods; see, for example, Diggle, Liang and Zeger (1994, Chapter 8) and Agresti (2002, Chapter 11). A detailed discussion of this methodology with a large number of SAS examples can be found in Stokes, Davis and Koch (2000, Chapter 15). Section 3.3.2 discusses random effects models for correlated categorical outcomes implemented in a new powerful SAS procedure (PROC NLMIXED) introduced in SAS 8.0. Finally, Section 3.3.3 outlines a multinomial likelihood approach to modeling the joint distribution of paired categorical measurements that complements the GEE and random effects models.

It is important to note that statistical methods reviewed in this section are not limited to the analysis of safety and diagnostic variables and can be applied to a wide variety of repeated categorical measurements, including efficacy data.

The following example from a clinical trial in patients with ulcerative colitis will be used in this section to illustrate methods for the analysis of paired categorical measurements.

EXAMPLE: Analysis of Safety Data in an Ulcerative Colitis Trial

A trial in patients with ulcerative colitis was conducted to compare several doses of an experimental drug to a placebo. This example focuses on the safety profile of the highest dose of the drug. The safety analyses in this trial were based on several laboratory assessments, including tests for aspartate transaminase (AST). High AST levels represent a serious safety concern because they may indicate that the drug impairs the liver function. Table 3.1 presents a summary of AST findings in the trial after the AST results have been converted into two binary outcomes (normal value and elevated value). These binary outcomes are summarized in two shift tables with the rows and columns corresponding to the baseline and endpoint assessments.

In order to test whether or not the high dose of the experimental drug is likely to cause liver damage, we need to compare the patterns of AST changes from baseline to endpoint between the two treatment groups in Table 3.1.

Table 3.1 The distribution of AST results at baseline and endpoint in the placebo and high dose groups

Placebo group			High dose group		
	Endpoint			Endpoint	
Baseline	Normal	Elevated	Baseline	Normal	Elevated
Normal	34	1	Normal	30	7
Elevated	2	3	Elevated	1	1

3.3.1   Generalized Estimating Equations

The GEE methodology was developed by Liang and Zeger (1986) as a way of extending generalized linear models and associated estimation methods to a longitudinal setting. Generalized linear models, introduced by Nelder and Wedderburn (1972), represent a broad class of statistical models based on exponential family distributions. This class includes various linear and nonlinear models such as ordinary normal regression, logistic regression, log-linear models, etc. Refer to McCullagh and Nelder (1989) for a detailed discussion of generalized linear models and related topics.

GEE Methods for Binary Responses

We will first discuss the use of GEE methods in the analysis of paired binary responses and then show how to extend this approach to ordinal measurements. Consider a sample of independent multivariate observations (y_{ij}, X_{ij}), $i = 1, \ldots, n$, $j = 1, 2$. Here y_{i1} and y_{i2} are the values of a binary response variable for the ith subject measured at two time points in a clinical trial, e.g., baseline and endpoint. Further, X_{i1} and X_{i2} are r-dimensional vectors of covariates for the ith subject collected at the same two time points. The covariates may include treatment effect as well as important prognostic factors that need to be adjusted for in the analysis of the response variable. The binary outcomes are coded as 0 and 1, and p_{ij} is the probability that $y_{ij} = 1$. Since y_{ij} is binary, this probability defines the marginal distribution of the response variable at the jth time point. At each of the two time points, the marginal distribution of the response variable is related to the covariates via the *link function* $g(p)$ using the following model:

$$g(p_{ij}) = X'_{ij}\beta, \quad j = 1, 2, \tag{3.1}$$

where β is an r-dimensional vector of regression parameters, $\beta = (\beta_1, \ldots, \beta_r)'$. The most frequently used link function $g(p)$ is a logit function given by $g(p) = \ln(p/(1 - p))$. With a logit link function, the analysis of the binary responses is performed based on a logistic regression model:

$$p_{ij} = \frac{\exp(X'_{ij}\beta)}{1 + \exp(X'_{ij}\beta)}, \quad j = 1, 2.$$

Note that the joint distribution of the binary measurements is completely specified at each of the two time points and therefore it is easy to estimate the baseline and endpoint parameters—say, $(\beta_{1B}, \ldots, \beta_{rB})$ and $(\beta_{1E}, \ldots, \beta_{rE})$—using the method of maximum likelihood. Because we are interested in obtaining one set of estimates, we have to find a way of combining the baseline and endpoint binary outcomes. Specifically, we need to develop a model that accounts for the correlation between the repeated measurements on the same subject, such as a model for the joint distribution of y_{i1} and y_{i2}, $i = 1, \ldots, n$, as a function of covariates that incorporates an estimated covariance matrix into the equation for $\beta_1, \ldots, \beta_r$. The problem with this approach is that modeling the joint distribution of non-Gaussian repeated measurements and estimating the longitudinal correlation matrix is generally a very complex process. Unlike a multivariate normal distribution, this joint distribution is not fully specified by the first and second moments.

To alleviate the problem, Liang and Zeger (1986) decided to bypass the challenging task of estimating the true covariance matrix and proposed to estimate an approximation to the true covariance matrix instead. This approximated covariance matrix is termed a *working covariance matrix*. The working covariance matrix is chosen by the statistician based on objective or subjective criteria. In the case of paired binary outcomes the working covariance matrix for the ith subject is defined as

$$V_i(\alpha) = \begin{bmatrix} v_{i1} & \alpha\sqrt{v_{i1}v_{i2}} \\ \alpha\sqrt{v_{i1}v_{i2}} & v_{i2} \end{bmatrix},$$

where α is a parameter that determines the correlation between y_{i1} and y_{i2}. Liang and Zeger (1986) proposed the following modified score equations for the parameter vector β that incorporate the working covariance matrix:

$$\sum_{i=1}^{n} \left(\frac{\partial P_i}{\partial \beta}\right)' V_i^{-1}(\alpha)(Y_i - P_i) = 0,$$

where $\partial P_i/\partial \beta$ is a $2 \times r$ matrix of partial derivatives, $Y_i = (y_{i1}, y_{i2})'$ and $P_i = (p_{i1}, p_{i2})'$. The α parameter is estimated from the data using an iterative algorithm.

It is important to emphasize that the equations proposed by Liang and Zeger are no longer based on a likelihood analysis of the joint distribution of the paired binary responses. They represent a multivariate generalization of a quasi-likelihood approach known as *estimating equations* and, for this reason, they are termed *generalized estimating equations*. The GEE approach extends ordinary estimating equations (to non-Gaussian responses) and quasi-likelihood theory (to incorporate multivariate distributions). The generalized estimating equations simplify to the regular likelihood-based score equations when the paired binary outcomes are assumed independent, i.e., $\alpha = 0$.

The outlined GEE approach possesses a very interesting property that plays an important role in applications. It was pointed out by Zeger and Liang (1986) that GEE methods consistently estimate the regression parameters $(\beta_1, \ldots, \beta_r)$ even if one misspecifies the correlation structure, as long as one correctly selects the link function $g(p)$. The same is true for the covariance matrix of the regression coefficients. One can construct an estimate of the covariance matrix that will be asymptotically consistent despite the wrong choice of the working correlation structure.

The GEE methodology is implemented in PROC GENMOD. Program 3.14 illustrates the capabilities of this procedure using the AST data from the ulcerative colitis trial example. Specifically, the program uses PROC GENMOD to fit a logistic model to the dichotomized AST values and assess the significance of the treatment effect. The dichotomized AST data from Table 3.1 are included in the AST data set (the BASELINE and ENDPOINT variables are recorded as 0 for normal and 1 for elevated AST results). Note that the AST results are summarized in the AST data set using frequency counts and need to be converted into one record per patient and time point in order to allow the assessment of group and time effects and their interaction in PROC GENMOD.

Program 3.14 Analysis of AST changes in an ulcerative colitis trial using generalized estimating equations

```
data ast;
    input therapy $ baseline endpoint count @@;
    datalines;
    Placebo 0 0 34 Placebo 1 0 2 Placebo 0 1 1 Placebo 1 1 3
    Drug    0 0 30 Drug    1 0 1 Drug    0 1 7 Drug    1 1 1
    ;
```

```
data ast1;
    set ast;
    do i=1 to count;
        if therapy="Placebo" then group=1; else group=0;
        subject=10000*group+1000*baseline+100*endpoint+i;
        outcome=baseline; time=0; output;
        outcome=endpoint; time=1; output;
    end;
proc genmod data=ast1 descending;
    ods select GEEEmpPEst Type3;
    class subject group time;
    model outcome=group|time/link=logit dist=bin type3;
    repeated subject=subject/type=unstr;
    run;
```

Output from Program 3.14

```
                  Analysis Of GEE Parameter Estimates
                  Empirical Standard Error Estimates


                          Standard   95% Confidence
Parameter        Estimate   Error        Limits            Z  Pr > |Z|

Intercept         -2.1972   0.5270  -3.2302  -1.1642   -4.17   <.0001
group       0      0.8427   0.6596  -0.4501   2.1354    1.28   0.2014
group       1      0.0000   0.0000   0.0000   0.0000      .       .
time        0      0.2513   0.4346  -0.6005   1.1031    0.58   0.5631
time        1      0.0000   0.0000   0.0000   0.0000      .       .
group*time 0 0    -1.8145   0.8806  -3.5404  -0.0886   -2.06   0.0393
group*time 0 1     0.0000   0.0000   0.0000   0.0000      .       .
group*time 1 0     0.0000   0.0000   0.0000   0.0000      .       .
group*time 1 1     0.0000   0.0000   0.0000   0.0000      .       .


   Score Statistics For Type 3 GEE Analysis


                          Chi-
Source           DF      Square   Pr > ChiSq

group             1       0.01      0.9188
time              1       2.38      0.1231
group*time        1       4.58      0.0323
```

The DESCENDING option in PROC GENMOD causes Program 3.14 to model the probability of an abnormal AST result. Note, however, that inferences with respect to the significance of the drug effect will not change if we request an analysis of normal AST results because the logit link function is symmetric. Further, to properly analyze repeated measurements in the AST data set, one needs to use the SUBJECT option in the REPEATED statement to identify the cluster variable, i.e., the variable that defines groups of related observations made on the same person. In this case, it is the SUBJECT variable. Lastly, the ODS statement `ods select GEEEmpPEst Type3` selects the output related to the GEE parameter estimates and Type 3 statistics.

Output 3.14 displays the point estimates and confidence intervals for the individual levels of the GROUP, TIME and GROUP*TIME variables. Note that most of the parameters of the fitted GEE model are not estimable in the binary case and therefore the output contains quite a few zeroes. Our main focus in Output 3.14 is the GROUP*TIME variable that captures the difference in AST changes from baseline to endpoint between the two treatment groups. The GROUP variable represents a time-independent component of the treatment effect.

Since the binary data are analyzed based on a logistic model, the obtained parameter estimates can be interpreted in terms of odds ratios of observing abnormal AST values. To compute the odds of observing elevated AST levels, we begin by computing the log-odds from the fitted GEE model (see Output 3.14):

$$\text{Placebo group at baseline:} \ -1.9459 = -2.1972 + 0.2513$$

$$\text{Placebo group at endpoint:} \ -2.1972 = -2.1972$$

$$\text{Experimental group at baseline:} \ -2.9177 = -2.1972 + 0.8427 + 0.2513 - 1.8145$$

$$\text{Experimental group at endpoint:} \ -1.3545 = -2.1972 + 0.8427.$$

Exponentiating the obtained log-odds, we conclude that the odds of elevated AST levels decreased in the placebo group from $e^{-1.95} = 0.1429$ at baseline to $e^{-2.2} = 0.1111$ at endpoint. In contrast, the odds of elevated AST levels increased in the high dose group from $e^{-2.92} = 0.0541$ to $e^{-1.35} = 0.2581$.

Note that the odds of elevated AST levels can be computed using the LSMEANS statement in PROC GENMOD as shown below.

```
proc genmod data=temp descending;
    class subject group time;
    model outcome=group time group*time/link=logit dist=bin type3;
    repeated subject=subject/type=unstr;
    lsmeans time*group;
    ods output LSMeans=LogOdds;

data odds;
    set LogOdds;
    LogOdds=estimate;
    Odds=exp(estimate);
    keep group time Odds LogOdds;
proc print data=odds noobs;
    run;
```

This program produces the following output:

group	time	LogOdds	Odds
0	0	-2.91777	0.05405
0	1	-1.35455	0.25806
1	0	-1.94591	0.14286
1	1	-2.19722	0.11111

Since `group=0` corresponds to the high dose group and `time=0` corresponds to the baseline, it is easy to verify that the odds of observing elevated AST levels in this output are identical to the odds computed above.

The magnitude of the group and time effects and the group-by-time interaction are assessed in Output 3.14 using the Wald test (upper panel) and the Type 3 likelihood score test (lower panel). As pointed out by Stokes, Davis and Koch (2000, Chapter 15), the Type 3 statistics are generally more conservative than the Wald test when the number of patients is small. Therefore, it is generally prudent to focus on p-values computed from the Type 3 statistics. The score statistics for the group and time effects are not significant at the 5% level but the interaction term is significant ($p = 0.0323$). This finding suggests that the patterns of change in AST levels from baseline to endpoint are not the same in the two treatment groups. The patients who received the high dose of the experimental drug were significantly more likely to develop abnormal AST levels during the course of the study than those in the placebo group.

Although this section focuses on the case of paired measurements, it is worth noting that the PROC GENMOD code shown in Program 3.14 can handle more general scenarios with multiple repeated measurements on the same subject. Since TIME is defined as a classification variable, Type 3 analyses can be used to assess the overall pattern of change over time with any number of time points. See Section 5.10 for a detailed review of GEE methods for multiple repeated measurements.

The TYPE option in the REPEATED statement of PROC GENMOD allows the user to specify the working covariance matrix. The choice of the working covariance matrix becomes unimportant in the case of paired observations. With two measurements per subject, the exchangeable, unstructured and more complicated correlation structures are identical to each other. When a data set contains multiple measurements per subject, one needs to make a decision with respect to which correlation structure to use in modeling the association of binary outcomes over time. This decision is driven primarily by prior information. As was noted before, an incorrect specification of the working covariance matrix does not affect the asymptotic consistency of GEE parameter estimates. However, it can have an impact on small sample properties of the estimates. Several authors, including Zeger and Liang (1986) and Zeger, Liang and Albert (1988), examined the sensitivity of GEE parameter estimates to the choice of the working covariance matrix using real and simulated data. The general conclusion is that the effect of the working covariance matrix on parameter estimates is small for time-independent parameters and is more pronounced for time-varying parameters. Although these findings might imply that one can safely run GEE analyses with the independent working structure, it is important to keep in mind that the wrong choice of the correlation structure lowers the efficiency of GEE estimates. Based on the analysis of a generalized linear model with 10 measurements per subject, Liang and Zeger (1986) concluded that a correct specification of the correlation matrix substantially reduces the standard errors of GEE parameter estimates when the repeated measurements are highly correlated.

The last remark is concerned with the use of GEE methods in the analysis of shift tables with empty cells. Shift tables summarizing safety and diagnostic data in clinical trials often contain a large number of cells with zero counts. Just like the majority of categorical analysis methods, GEE methods will likely fail when the data are very sparse. As an illustration, consider a modified version of the AST data set shown in Table 3.2. Note that two off-diagonal cells in the placebo group and one off-diagonal cell in the high dose group have zero counts.

Table 3.2 Modified AST data at baseline and endpoint in the placebo and high dose groups

	Placebo group			High dose group	
	Endpoint			Endpoint	
Baseline	Normal	Elevated	Baseline	Normal	Elevated
Normal	34	0	Normal	30	7
Elevated	0	3	Elevated	0	1

The paired binary outcomes shown Table 3.2 are analyzed in Program 3.15.

Program 3.15 Analysis of the modified AST data set

```
data modast;
    input therapy $ baseline endpoint count @@;
    datalines;
    Placebo 0 0 34 Placebo 1 0 0 Placebo 0 1 0 Placebo 1 1 3
    Drug    0 0 30 Drug    1 0 0 Drug    0 1 7 Drug    1 1 1
    ;
data modast1;
    set modast;
```

```
    do i=1 to count;
        if therapy="Placebo" then group=1; else group=0;
        subject=10000*group+1000*baseline+100*endpoint+i;
        outcome=baseline; time=0; output;
        outcome=endpoint; time=1; output;
    end;
proc genmod data=modast1 descending;
    ods select GEEEmpPEst Type3;
    class subject group time;
    model outcome=group time group*time/link=logit dist=bin type3;
    repeated subject=subject/type=unstr;
    run;
```

Output from Program 3.15

```
                    Analysis Of GEE Parameter Estimates
                    Empirical Standard Error Estimates


                            Standard   95% Confidence
Parameter          Estimate   Error       Limits           Z  Pr > |Z|

Intercept          -2.4277   0.6023  -3.6082  -1.2473   -4.03   <.0001
group        0      1.1060   0.7219  -0.3088   2.5208    1.53   0.1255
group        1      0.0000   0.0000   0.0000   0.0000      .       .
time         0      0.0000   0.0000  -0.0000   0.0000    0.00   1.0000
time         1      0.0000   0.0000   0.0000   0.0000      .       .
group*time 0 0     -2.2892   0.9636  -4.1779  -0.4005   -2.38   0.0175
group*time 0 1      0.0000   0.0000   0.0000   0.0000      .       .
group*time 1 0      0.0000   0.0000   0.0000   0.0000      .       .
group*time 1 1      0.0000   0.0000   0.0000   0.0000      .       .
WARNING: The generalized Hessian matrix is not positive definite.
Iteration will be terminated.
```

Output 3.15 lists parameter estimates produced by Program 3.15. Since the GEE method relies on the off-diagonal cells in Table 3.2 to estimate the time effect and these cells are mostly empty, PROC GENMOD produced a warning message that the GEE score statistic algorithm failed to converge for the TIME and GROUP*TIME variables. As a result, PROC GENMOD cannot perform the Type 3 analyses for these variables and cannot assess the significance of the treatment effect on AST levels.

GEE Methods for Ordinal Responses

More general variables measured on an ordinal scale can be analyzed in PROC GENMOD using an extended version of the simple logistic model. Consider a sample of paired independent observations (y_{ij}, X_{ij}), $i = 1, \ldots, n$, $j = 1, 2$, where y_{ij} is the value of an ordinal response variable with m ordered categories recorded for the ith subject at the jth time point. Let p_{ijk} denote the probability that y_{ij} falls in the lower k categories, $k = 1, \ldots, m - 1$. The marginal distribution of the response variable is uniquely defined by a set of $m - 1$ cumulative probabilities $p_{ij1}, \ldots, p_{ij,m-1}$. Therefore, in order to relate the marginal distribution to the covariates, one needs to define a system of $m - 1$ equations. For example, consider the following model for the marginal distribution of the response variable at the jth time point:

$$g(p_{ij1}) = \mu_1 + X'_{ij}\beta, \tag{3.2}$$

$$\cdots$$

$$g(p_{ij,m-1}) = \mu_{m-1} + X'_{ij}\beta.$$

Here μ_k is the intercept associated with the kth cumulative probability and β is an r-dimensional vector of regression parameters.

When the analysis of ordinal responses is based on the cumulative logit link function, i.e., $g(p) = \ln(p/(1-p))$, the parameters of the model are easy to express in terms of odds ratios, which facilitates the interpretation of the findings. For example, we can see from model (3.2) that the odds of observing a response in the lowest category are $\exp(\mu_1 + X'_{ij}\beta)$ and the odds of observing a response in the two lowest categories are $\exp(\mu_2 + X'_{ij}\beta)$. The odds ratio equals $\exp(\mu_1 - \mu_2)$ and is independent of X_{ij}. This means that adding a category proportionately increases the odds of the corresponding outcome by the same amount regardless of the covariate values. Due to this interesting property, model (3.2) is commonly referred to as the *proportional odds model*.

The GEE methodology outlined in the previous section can be extended to the more general case of repeated measurements on an ordinal scale. See Liang, Zeger and Qaqish (1992) and Lipsitz, Kim and Zhao (1994) for a description of GEE methods for ordinal responses.

The GEE methods for proportional odds models will be illustrated using the following example.

EXAMPLE: Analysis of QTc Interval Prolongation

Table 3.3 summarizes QTc interval data collected in a Phase II study comparing the effects of one dose of an experimental drug to a placebo. As was indicated earlier in this chapter, the QTc interval is analyzed in clinical trials to assess the potential for inducing cardiac repolarization abnormalities linked to sudden death. The analysis of QTc values was performed based on the set of reference intervals published in the document "Points to consider: The assessment of the potential for QT interval prolongation by non-cardiovascular medicinal products" released by the Committee for Proprietary Medicinal Products Points to Consider on December 17, 1997. According to this guidance document, the length of QTc interval is classified as normal ($\leq$ 430 msec in adult males and $\leq$ 450 msec in adult females), borderline (431-450 msec in adult males and 451-470 msec in adult females) or prolonged (> 450 msec in adult males and > 470 msec in adult females).

Table 3.3 The distribution of QTc interval values at baseline and endpoint in the placebo and experimental groups (N, B and P stand for normal, borderline and prolonged QTc intervals)

Placebo group				Experimental group			
	Endpoint				Endpoint		
Baseline	N	B	P	Baseline	N	B	P
N	50	3	0	N	42	11	0
B	1	7	1	B	1	5	0
P	0	1	0	P	0	1	0

Program 3.16 shows how to modify the PROC GENMOD code in Program 3.14 to examine the treatment effect on the QTc interval based on the analysis of change patterns in the two 3×3 shift tables.

The categorized QTc values from Table 3.3 are included in the QTCPROL data set. The normal, borderline and prolonged QTc values are coded as 0, 1 and 2, respectively. The trinomial responses are analyzed using the cumulative logit link function in PROC GENMOD (LINK=CUMLOGIT). The DESCENDING option in PROC GENMOD specifies that the model for the trinomial responses is based on the ratio of the probability of higher levels of the response variable to the probability of lower levels. In other words, Program 3.16 fits two separate logistic models, one for the likelihood of observing a prolonged QTc interval and the other one for the likelihood of observing a prolonged or borderline QTc interval. As in the binary case, dropping the DESCENDING option changes the signs of the parameter estimates but does not have any impact on the associated p-values. The TYPE option in the REPEATED statement is set to IND, which means that the data are modeled using the independent working covariance matrix. PROC GENMOD does not currently support any other correlation structures for ordinal response variables.

Program 3.16 Analysis of QTc interval changes

```
data qtcprol;
    input therapy $ baseline endpoint count @@;
    datalines;
    Placebo 0 0 50 Placebo 1 0  1 Placebo 2 0  0
    Placebo 0 1  3 Placebo 1 1  7 Placebo 2 1  1
    Placebo 0 2  0 Placebo 1 2  1 Placebo 2 2  0
    Drug    0 0 42 Drug    1 0  1 Drug    2 0  0
    Drug    0 1 11 Drug    1 1  5 Drug    2 1  1
    Drug    0 2  0 Drug    1 2  0 Drug    2 2  0
    ;
data qtcprol1;
    set qtcprol;
    do i=1 to count;
        if therapy="Placebo" then group=1; else group=0;
        subject=10000*group+1000*baseline+100*endpoint+i;
        outcome=baseline; time=0; output;
        outcome=endpoint; time=1; output;
    end;
proc genmod data=qtcprol1 descending;
    ods select GEEEmpPEst Type3;
    class subject group time;
    model outcome=group time group*time/link=cumlogit dist=multinomial
    type3;
    repeated subject=subject/type=ind;
    run;
```

Output from Program 3.16

```
             Analysis Of GEE Parameter Estimates
             Empirical Standard Error Estimates


                  Standard  95% Confidence
Parameter         Estimate    Error       Limits          Z  Pr > |Z|


Intercept1         -4.3936   0.6516  -5.6707  -3.1165  -6.74   <.0001
Intercept2         -1.4423   0.3201  -2.0697  -0.8149  -4.51   <.0001
group        0      0.4867   0.4284  -0.3530   1.3263   1.14   0.2559
group        1      0.0000   0.0000   0.0000   0.0000     .       .
time         0     -0.2181   0.2176  -0.6445   0.2083  -1.00   0.3161
time         1      0.0000   0.0000   0.0000   0.0000     .       .
group*time 0 0     -0.8395   0.4293  -1.6809   0.0020  -1.96   0.0505
group*time 0 1      0.0000   0.0000   0.0000   0.0000     .       .
group*time 1 0      0.0000   0.0000   0.0000   0.0000     .       .
group*time 1 1      0.0000   0.0000   0.0000   0.0000     .       .


   Score Statistics For Type 3 GEE Analysis


                        Chi-
Source           DF    Square    Pr > ChiSq


group            1      0.02       0.8769
time             1      8.78       0.0031
group*time       1      3.88       0.0489
```

Output 3.16 contains the GEE parameter estimates as well as the Type 3 analysis results for the group and time effects and their interaction. Since Program 3.16 fitted two logistic models, the output lists estimates of two intercept terms. INTERCEPT1 represents the estimated intercept in the model for prolonged QTc intervals and INTERCEPT2 is the estimated intercept in the model for borderline and prolonged QTc intervals. INTERCEPT1 is substantially less than INTERCEPT2 because the probability of observing a prolonged QTc interval is very small.

The time effect in Output 3.16 is very pronounced ($p = 0.0031$), which reflects the fact that the marginal distribution of the categorized QTc values changed from baseline to endpoint. Table 3.3 shows that the odds of having a borderline or prolonged QTc interval increased from baseline to endpoint in both treatment groups. The p-value for the treatment effect, represented here by the GROUP*TIME interaction, is marginally significant ($p = 0.0489$), suggesting that the change patterns in Table 3.3 are driven more by an overall shift toward higher QT values than by the effect of the experimental drug.

3.3.2 Random Effects Models

An important feature of the GEE approach is that it concentrates on modeling the marginal distribution of the response variable at each of the time points of interest and avoids a complete specification of the joint distribution of the multivariate responses. It was noted in the previous section that the primary interest in the GEE approach centers on the analysis of expected values of a subject's categorical responses in a longitudinal setting. The within-subject correlation structure is treated as a nuisance parameter and is not directly modeled within the GEE framework. In other words, the GEE inferences are performed at the population level and, using the terminology introduced in Zeger, Liang and Albert (1988), the GEE approach can be referred to as a *population-averaged* approach. As pointed out by Liang and Zeger (1986), treating the longitudinal correlation matrix as a nuisance parameter may not always be appropriate, and alternative modeling approaches need to be used when one is interested in studying the time course of the outcome for each subject. Lindsey and Lambert (1998) concurred with this point by emphasizing that the population-averaged approach assumes that subjects' responses are homogeneous and should be used with caution when this assumption is not met.

An alternative approach to the analysis of repeated categorical responses relies on modeling the conditional probability of the responses given subject-specific random effects and, for this reason, is termed a *subject-specific* approach. This section reviews categorical analysis methods developed within the subject-specific framework and demonstrates how they can be implemented in PROC NLMIXED.

To introduce random effects models for repeated categorical outcomes, consider a sample of n subjects and assume that binary observations have been made on each of the subjects at two different occasions. Denote the paired binary responses by (y_{i1}, y_{i2}), $i = 1, \ldots, n$ and let p_{ij} be the probability that $y_{ij} = 1$. The distribution of the ith pair of observations depends on covariate vectors (X_{i1}, X_{i2}), $i = 1, \ldots, n$.

The relationship between (y_{i1}, y_{i2}) and (X_{i1}, X_{i2}) is described by the following random effects model, which represents an extension of Model (3.1):

$$g(p_{ij}) = \theta_i + X'_{ij}\beta, \quad j = 1, 2, \tag{3.3}$$

where $g(p)$ is a link function (e.g., the logit link function), θ_i is a random variable representing an unobservable subject effect, and β is an r-dimensional vector of regression parameters. Models of this type were discussed by Cox (1958) and Rasch (1961) in the context of case-control studies and educational testing, respectively. For this reason, model (3.3) will be referred to as the Cox-Rasch model.

It is important to note that, unlike model (3.1) underlying the GEE methodology, the Cox-Rasch model contains a random term for each subject. This term helps account for between-subject heterogeneity and allows the explicit modeling of the correlation among the repeated observations made on the same subject. In this respect, the Cox-Rasch model is analogous to random effects models (e.g., models with random subject-specific terms) in a linear regression setting.

Since the Cox-Rasch model explicitly specifies the joint distribution of the responses, one can employ likelihood-based methods for estimating the vector of regression parameters β. To eliminate the dependence of the obtained parameter estimates on unobservable subject effects, it is common to work with the marginal likelihood function. Let Y_i denote the vector of repeated observations made on the ith subject. Denote the probability density of the observations given the subject effect θ_i and the probability density of θ_i by $f(Y_i|\theta_i)$ and $h(\theta_i)$, respectively. The marginal likelihood function for the response variables integrated over the subject effects is given by

$$L(\beta) = \prod_{i=1}^{n} \int f(Y_i|\theta_i)h(\theta_i)d\theta_i$$

and the vector of regression parameters β is estimated by maximizing $L(\beta)$. The specific details of this procedure depend on the assumptions about $h(\theta_i)$ and may involve an empirical Bayes approach, the EM algorithm and other methods. The general theory of random effects models for repeated categorical data is outlined in Stiratelli, Laird and Ware (1984), Diggle, Liang and Zeger (1994, Chapter 9) and Agresti (2002, Chapter 12).

The integral in the definition of $L(\beta)$ does not, in general, have a closed form. The process of fitting nonlinear random effects models requires a substantial amount of numerical integration and is very computationally intensive even in small studies. The NLMIXED procedure, introduced in SAS 8.0, implements the described marginal likelihood approach and considerably simplifies inferences in random effects models for repeated categorical measurements. To estimate the vector of regression parameters, PROC NLMIXED uses a numerical integration routine to approximate the marginal likelihood function $L(\beta)$ and then maximizes the obtained approximation with respect to β.

Random Effects Models for Binary Responses

The following example demonstrates how to fit random effects models for repeated binary measurements in PROC NLMIXED. Consider the ulcerative colitis trial example introduced earlier in this section. Program 3.17 fits a random effects model to the dichotomized AST data collected at baseline and endpoint in the two treatment groups. The PROC NLMIXED code in the program shows that the probability of an abnormal AST result (P variable) is linked to four fixed effects (intercept, group, time and group-by-time interaction) as well as a random subject effect using the logit link function. The random subject effects are assumed to follow a normal distribution with mean 0 and unknown variance SIGMASQ that will be estimated from the data.

Program 3.17 Analysis of AST changes in the ulcerative colitis trial using a logistic random effects model

```
data ast2;
    set ast;
    do i=1 to count;
        if therapy="Placebo" then gr=1; else gr=0;
        subject=10000*gr+1000*baseline+100*endpoint+i;
        outcome=baseline; tm=0; int=tm*gr; output;
        outcome=endpoint; tm=1; int=tm*gr; output;
    end;
proc nlmixed data=ast2 qpoints=50;
    ods select ParameterEstimates;
    parms intercept=-2.2 group=0.8 time=0.3 interaction=-1.8 sigmasq=1;
    logit=intercept+group*gr+time*tm+interaction*int+se;
    p=exp(logit)/(1+exp(logit));
    model outcome~binary(p);
    random se~normal(0,sigmasq) subject=subject;
    run;
```

Output from Program 3.17

```
                        Parameter Estimates


                     Standard
Parameter    Estimate   Error    DF  t Value  Pr > |t|  Alpha    Lower

intercept     -5.4303   1.8028   78   -3.01    0.0035    0.05   -9.0193
group          1.4347   1.4529   78    0.99    0.3265    0.05   -1.4579
time           2.6406   1.2456   78    2.12    0.0372    0.05    0.1608
interaction   -3.1207   1.6412   78   -1.90    0.0609    0.05   -6.3880
sigmasq        8.4967   6.8737   78    1.24    0.2201    0.05   -5.1878


            Parameter Estimates


Parameter      Upper    Gradient

intercept     -1.8412   -0.00003
group          4.3273   -7.12E-6
time           5.1204   -0.00006
interaction    0.1466   -7.25E-6
sigmasq       22.1813    4.024E-6
```

As in Program 3.14, the paired binary responses in the AST data set are first transformed to construct a data set with one record per patient and time point. One needs to manually create the INT variable representing the group-by-time interaction because PROC NLMIXED, unlike PROC GENMOD, has no mechanism for creating this variable. As in PROC GENMOD, the SUBJECT parameter in the RANDOM statement identifies the cluster variable. The parameter tells PROC NLMIXED how to define groups of related observations made on the same individual. It is important to keep in mind that PROC NLMIXED assumes that a new realization of the random effects occurs whenever the cluster variable changes from the previous observation. Thus, to avoid spurious results, one needs to make sure the analysis data is sorted by the cluster variable. The starting values used in Program 3.17 are derived from the estimates produced by the GEE method (see Output 3.14).

Output 3.17 lists parameter estimates produced by PROC NLMIXED. Comparing Output 3.17 to the corresponding GEE model in Output 3.14, we see that the estimates from the Cox-Rasch model have the same signs as the GEE estimates but they are uniformly larger in the absolute value (McCulloch and Searle (2001, Chapter 8) showed this is true in the general case). Note that parameter estimates obtained from random effects models have a different interpretation and should not be directly compared to GEE estimates.

Output 3.17 indicates that the addition of subject-specific random terms in the model affects the inferences with respect to the time and group-by-time interaction effects in the AST data set. Comparing Output 3.17 to Output 3.14, we see that the group-by-time interaction in the logistic random effects model is no longer significant at the 5% level ($p = 0.0609$), whereas the time effect is fairly influential with $p = 0.0372$.

It was pointed out earlier that GEE methods often fail to converge in the analysis of sparse data sets. Experience shows that numerical algorithms underlying random effects models tend to be less sensitive to empty cells. Using the MODAST data set, we demonstrated that the GEE approach cannot assess the significance of the treatment effect on AST levels when both of the off-diagonal cells in the placebo shift table and one off-diagonal cell in the high dose shift table are set to zero. Running Program 3.17 against the MODAST data set with the initial values obtained from Output 3.15 produces the following output.

Output from Program 3.17 with the MODAST data set

```
                        Parameter Estimates

                         Standard
Parameter    Estimate      Error      DF    t Value    Pr > |t|
intercept    -36.7368    15.3590      74     -2.39      0.0193
group         10.0661     8.9702      74      1.12      0.2654
time          21.0261    10.6290      74      1.98      0.0516
interaction  -20.8554    11.1549      74     -1.87      0.0655
sigmasq       422.85     333.91       74      1.27      0.2094
```

We can see from this output that PROC NLMIXED converged and produced meaningful inferences in the MODAST data set with three empty cells. Estimation methods in random effects models are generally more stable and perform better than GEE methods in the analysis of shift tables with empty cells.

Numerical Integration Algorithm

The PROC NLMIXED code in Program 3.17 uses the default numerical integration algorithm to approximate the marginal likelihood function of the binary responses (see Section 5.10 for a detailed discussion of numerical integration algorithms implemented in PROC NLMIXED). This is a very popular algorithm known as Gauss-Hermite quadrature (Liu and Pierce, 1994). The performance of the Gauss-Hermite quadrature approximation depends on the number of quadrature points specified by the QPOINTS parameter in PROC NLMIXED (Agresti and Hartzel, 2000). Choosing a large value of QPOINTS increases the accuracy of the numerical integration algorithm. Figure 3.12 demonstrates the relationship between the four parameter estimates in the logistic random effects model for AST levels and the value of the QPOINTS parameter. Figure 3.12 reveals that the parameter estimates do not stabilize until QPOINTS=30. Using the Gauss-Hermite quadrature algorithm with the default value of QPOINTS (5 points) will likely result in biased parameter estimates. It is prudent to routinely choose large values of the QPOINTS parameter (e.g., 50) in PROC NLMIXED when fitting nonlinear random effects models.

Random Effects Models for Ordinal Responses

The logistic random effects model for paired binary responses introduced in the previous subsection is easy to extend to the general case of ordinal variables. In order to show how to fit logistic random effects models for ordinal outcomes in PROC NLMIXED, it is convenient to adopt a slightly different specification of the likelihood function. As was mentioned above, the PROC NLMIXED code in Program 3.17 is fairly transparent and easy to follow. For example, it is clear from Program 3.17 that the P variable (probability of an abnormal AST result) is modeled as a function of four fixed effects and one normally distributed random effect with the logit link.

A less transparent but more flexible approach to modeling correlated categorical responses in PROC NLMIXED involves a direct specification of the conditional likelihood of responses given random subject effects. To illustrate, consider again the ulcerative colitis trial example with paired binary outcomes. Program 3.18 uses PROC NLMIXED to fit a logistic model with random subject effects to the data by maximizing the marginal likelihood function. However, unlike Program 3.17, this program does not explicitly indicate that the OUTCOME variable follows a binary distribution with the success probability P but rather tells SAS to work with the user-specified log-likelihood function. Since the specified log-likelihood function is a log-likelihood function for binary observations, the resulting PROC NLMIXED code is equivalent to the PROC NLMIXED code shown in Program 3.17 and produces identical output.

The advantage of the outlined alternative specification of the likelihood function is that it can be used to pass any likelihood function to PROC NLMIXED, including a likelihood function of observations on an ordinal scale. Consider the QTc interval prolongation example involving a comparison of QTc values

Figure 3.12 Effect of quadrature approximation on parameter estimates in a logistic random effects model

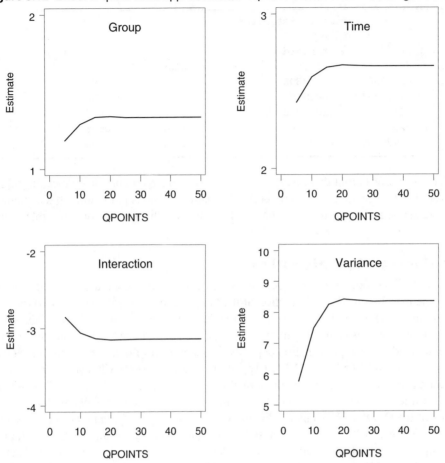

Program 3.18 Analysis of AST changes in the ulcerative colitis trial using a logistic random effects model

```
proc nlmixed data=ast2 qpoints=50;
    parms intercept=-2.2 group=0.8 time=0.3 interaction=-1.8 sigmasq=1;
    logit=intercept+group*gr+time*tm+interaction*int+se;
    p0=1/(1+exp(logit));
    p1=exp(logit)/(1+exp(logit));
    if outcome=0 then logp=log(p0);
    if outcome=1 then logp=log(p1);
    model outcome~general(logp);
    random se~normal(0,sigmasq) subject=subject;
    run;
```

classified as normal, borderline and prolonged between two treatment groups (see Table 3.3). Program 3.19 fits a proportional odds model with random subject effects to the 3×3 shift tables in the placebo and experimental drug groups (with the initial values of the six parameters taken from Output 3.16). This model is similar to the GEE proportional odds model introduced in Section 3.3.1 (see Program 3.16) in that they both have two components (one for assessing the treatment effect on prolonged QTc intervals and the other for examining the treatment effect on both borderline and prolonged QTc intervals). However, the GEE and random effects models differ in the way they

Program 3.19 Analysis of QTc interval changes using a logistic random effects model

```
data qtcprol1;
    set qtcprol;
    do i=1 to count;
        if therapy="Placebo" then gr=1; else gr=0;
        subject=10000*gr+1000*baseline+100*endpoint+i;
        outcome=baseline; tm=0; int=tm*gr; output;
        outcome=endpoint; tm=1; int=tm*gr; output;
    end;
proc nlmixed data=qtcprol1 qpoints=50;
    ods select ParameterEstimates;
    parms intercept1=-4.4 intercept2=-1.4 group=0.5 time=-0.2
        interaction=-0.8 sigmasq=1;
    logit1=intercept1+group*gr+time*tm+interaction*int+se;
    logit2=intercept2+group*gr+time*tm+interaction*int+se;
    p0=1/(1+exp(logit2));
    p1=exp(logit2)/(1+exp(logit2))-exp(logit1)/(1+exp(logit1));
    p2=exp(logit1)/(1+exp(logit1));
    if outcome=0 then logp=log(p0);
    if outcome=1 then logp=log(p1);
    if outcome=2 then logp=log(p2);
    model outcome~general(logp);
    random se~normal(0,sigmasq) subject=subject;
    run;
```

Output from Program 3.19

```
                           Parameter Estimates

                      Standard
Parameter    Estimate    Error    DF   t Value  Pr > |t|  Alpha    Lower

intercept1   -11.1595    2.4940   122   -4.47   <.0001    0.05   -16.0966
intercept2    -5.0064    1.3380   122   -3.74    0.0003   0.05    -7.6552
group          0.3814    1.2437   122    0.31    0.7596   0.05    -2.0806
time           2.1535    0.8254   122    2.61    0.0102   0.05     0.5196
interaction   -1.6065    1.0830   122   -1.48    0.1406   0.05    -3.7505
sigmasq       17.4644    9.3402   122    1.87    0.0639   0.05    -1.0255


          Parameter Estimates

Parameter     Upper    Gradient

intercept1   -6.2223   0.000107
intercept2   -2.3576  -0.00004
group         2.8434   0.000198
time          3.7874  -0.00012
interaction   0.5375  -0.00019
sigmasq      35.9543   0.000033
```

incorporate correlation between repeated measurements on the same subject. Since PROC GENMOD currently supports only the independent working covariance matrix for ordinal variables, Program 3.16 accounts for the correlations in repeated observations implicitly (through the empirical covariance matrix estimate). By contrast, the logistic model in Program 3.19 includes subject-specific random terms and thus explicitly accounts for the correlation between paired outcomes.

Output 3.19 displays estimates of the six model parameters produced by PROC NLMIXED. Note that the two logistic regression models fitted to the paired trinomial outcomes in the QTc prolongation example share all parameters with the exception of the intercept that becomes model-specific. INTERCEPT1 is the estimated intercept in the logistic model for prolonged QTc intervals and INTERCEPT2 is equal to the estimated intercept in the logistic model for borderline and prolonged QTc intervals.

We can see from Output 3.19 that the computed *p*-value for the TIME term is consistent in magnitude with the *p*-value produced by the GEE method (see Output 3.16). However, the *p*-value for the treatment effect, represented here by the INTERACTION term, is larger than that produced by the GEE method and is clearly non-significant. There is clearly not enough evidence to conclude that the two shift tables in the QTc interval prolongation example exhibit different change patterns.

3.3.3 Multinomial Likelihood Methods

This section reviews analysis methods for paired categorical variables based on direct models for cell probabilities in shift tables. The outlined modeling approach complements the methods described earlier in this chapter.

As was pointed out above, it is helpful to summarize paired categorical outcomes computed from quantitative diagnostic and safety measurements using shift tables. Once the shift tables have been constructed, the analysis of the categorical outcomes can be performed by comparing the patterns of change across the shift tables representing different treatment groups. Popular methods for the analysis of changes in shift tables described in Sections 3.3.1 and 3.3.2 rely primarily on comparing marginal distributions over time. For instance, the GEE approach focuses on regression parameters that characterize the marginal distribution of responses at each time point, whereas parameters describing the association across time points are treated as nuisance parameters. Although methods for performing simultaneous analyses of the regression and correlation parameters have been discussed in the literature (see, for example, Zhao and Prentice (1990)), they are rarely used in practice, partly due to their complexity.

By concentrating on the analysis of regression parameters, one essentially assumes that the marginal distribution of the endpoint measurements is a location shift of the baseline marginal distribution. This assumption may be fairly restrictive in a clinical trial setting. Tests of marginal homogeneity fail to capture clinically important trends when the location shift assumption is not met. To illustrate this fact, Dmitrienko (2003b) used an example from a two-arm Phase II clinical trial in which 205 patients underwent electrocardiographic (ECG) evaluations at baseline and endpoint. The ECG evaluations were all performed by the same cardiologist, who classified each ECG recording as normal or abnormal. Two 2×2 shift tables summarizing the results of these evaluations are presented in Table 3.4.

Table 3.4 The distribution of the overall ECG evaluations at baseline and endpoint in the two treatment groups

| | Treatment group 1 | | | Treatment group 2 | |
| | Endpoint | | | Endpoint | |
Baseline	Normal	Abnormal	Baseline	Normal	Abnormal
Normal	83	1	Normal	80	7
Abnormal	1	18	Abnormal	8	7

It is easy to verify from Table 3.4 that the difference between the baseline and endpoint distributions of the overall ECG evaluations is very small. The likelihood of observing a normal overall ECG evaluation in Treatment group 1 is equal to 84/103=0.816 at baseline and 84/103=0.816 at endpoint. In Treatment group 2, this likelihood is equal to 87/102=0.853 at baseline and 88/102=0.863 at endpoint. As a result, using tests for homogeneity of marginal changes, one will likely conclude that the patterns of change are identical in the two treatment groups. For example, the following output was generated when the ECG data in Table 3.4 were analyzed using GEE and random effects models.

Analysis of changes in the overall ECG evaluations using a GEE model

```
 Score Statistics For Type 3 GEE Analysis


                           Chi-
 Source           DF     Square    Pr > ChiSq

 group             1       0.80        0.3724
 time              1       0.06        0.8042
 group*time        1       0.06        0.8042
```

Analysis of changes in the overall ECG evaluations using a random effects model

```
                    Parameter Estimates


                       Standard
 Parameter   Estimate    Error     DF   t Value   Pr > |t|
 intercept    -3.8464    0.7262    204    -5.30    <.0001
 group         0.3767    0.8407    204     0.45     0.6546
 time         -0.1673    0.5790    204    -0.29     0.7729
 interaction   0.1673    0.8303    204     0.20     0.8405
 sigmasq      10.1600    2.9416    204     3.45     0.0007
```

The output shown above lists the parameter estimates and associated test statistics produced by Programs 3.14 and 3.17. The treatment effect is represented here by the GROUP*TIME variable in the upper panel and the INTERACTION variable in the lower panel. The test statistics corresponding to these variables are very small, which means that the GEE and random effects models failed to detect the difference between the two shift tables. However, even a quick look at the data summarized in Table 3.4 reveals that the change patterns in the two shift tables are quite different. We can see from Table 3.4 that only one patient experienced worsening and only one patient experienced spontaneous improvement in Treatment group 1. In contrast, seven patients experienced worsening and eight patients experienced improvement in Treatment group 2. This finding may translate into a safety concern because the identified groups of improved and worsened patients most likely represent two different patient populations and do not cancel each other out. The observed difference in change patterns warrants additional analyses because it may imply that the drug administered to patients in Treatment group 2 causes harmful side effects. Similar examples can be found in Lindsey and Lambert (1998).

Inferences based on the regression parameters in GEE and random effects models fail to detect the treatment difference in Table 3.4 because the analysis of marginal changes is equivalent to the analysis of the off-diagonal cells and ignores the information in the main-diagonal cells. To improve the power of inferences based on marginal shifts, one needs to account for treatment-induced changes in both diagonal and off-diagonal cells. This can be accomplished by joint modeling of all cell probabilities in shift tables, rather than modeling the margins. A simple joint modeling method is based on grouping response vectors in 2×2 and more general shift tables into clinically meaningful categories and specifying a multinomial probability model for the defined response profiles. This approach was discussed by Dmitrienko (2003b) and is conceptually related to the modeling framework proposed by McCullagh (1978) and transition models described by Bonney (1987) and others.

To introduce the multinomial likelihood approach, suppose that a binary variable is measured at baseline and endpoint in a clinical trial with m treatment groups. The binary outcomes are coded as 0 and 1 and are summarized in m shift tables. Let X_i and Y_i be selected at random from the marginal distribution of the rows and columns of the ith shift table. Since the response variable is binary and is measured at two time points, the response vector (X_i, Y_i) assumes four values: (0,0), (0,1), (1,0) and

(1,1). The paired observations with $X_i = Y_i$ and $X_i \neq Y_i$ are commonly termed *concordant* and *discordant* pairs, respectively.

The response vectors can be grouped in a variety of ways depending on the objective of the analysis. For example, one can consider the following partitioning scheme based on three categories in the ith treatment group:

$$\text{Category } C_i^- : \quad (1, 0), \tag{3.4}$$

$$\text{Category } C_i^0 : \quad (0, 0) \text{ and } (1, 1),$$

$$\text{Category } C_i^+ : \quad (0, 1).$$

Note that the concordant pairs are pooled together in this partitioning scheme to produce the C_i^0 category in the ith group because these cells do not contain information about treatment-induced changes. Next, consider the following model for this partitioning scheme:

$$P(C_i^-) = \alpha_i(1 - \beta_i), \quad P(C_i^0) = 1 - \alpha_i, \quad P(C_i^+) = \alpha_i \beta_i, \tag{3.5}$$

where α_i and β_i are model parameters. It is instructive to compare this trinomial model to model (3.1) with a logit link function. Assuming two treatment groups, the group-by-time interaction in model (3.1) on the logit scale equals the difference in the β parameters in model (3.5). This means that by comparing the β parameters across the shift tables, one can draw conclusions about the homogeneity of marginal changes. Unlike model (3.1), the trinomial model includes the α parameters that summarize the relative weight of discordant pairs compared to concordant pairs (known as the *discordance rate*) in each shift table. A comparison of the α parameters helps detect treatment-induced changes in the diagonal cells.

The introduced model for paired binary data can be extended to more general scenarios involving ordinal responses (Dmitrienko, 2003b). This section will concentrate on the analysis of the simple binary case. Let n_i be the number of subjects in ith group and denote the numbers of subjects in Categories C_i^-, C_i^0 and C_i^+ by n_i^-, n_i^0 and n_i^+, respectively. Change patterns can be compared across the m treatment groups by testing the homogeneity of marginal changes ($\beta_1 = \ldots = \beta_m$) and the equality of discordance rates ($\alpha_1 = \ldots = \alpha_m$). Dmitrienko (2003b) showed that the likelihood-ratio test of this hypothesis is equivalent to the likelihood-ratio test for association in the $m \times 3$ contingency table shown in Table 3.5.

Table 3.5 Contingency table used in comparing change patterns across m treatment groups

Treatment group	Number of subjects		
	Category C_i^-	Category C_i^0	Category C_i^+
Treatment group 1	n_1^-	n_1^0	n_1^+
...	...	...	...
Treatment group m	n_m^-	n_m^0	n_m^+

The likelihood-ratio test for association in Table 3.5 is easy to implement in PROC FREQ, which supports both asymptotic and exact versions of this test. Program 3.20 fits the trinomial model (3.5) to the paired binary data in Table 3.4 and estimates the α and β parameters in the two groups (note that the normal outcomes in the ECGEVAL data set are coded as 0 and abnormal outcomes are coded as 1). The program also computes p-values produced by the asymptotic and exact likelihood-ratio tests for the equality of change patterns in Treatment group 1 and Treatment group 2.

Program 3.20 Trinomial model for the changes in the overall ECG evaluations from baseline to endpoint

```
data ecgeval;
    input therapy $ baseline endpoint count @@;
    datalines;
```

```
      DrugA 0 0 83 DrugA 1 0 1 DrugA 0 1 1 DrugA 1 1 18
      DrugB 0 0 80 DrugB 1 0 8 DrugB 0 1 7 DrugB 1 1  7
      ;
data transform;
    set ecgeval;
    if baseline+endpoint^=1 then change="Same";
    if baseline=0 and endpoint=1 then change="Up";
    if baseline=1 and endpoint=0 then change="Down";
proc sort data=transform;
    by therapy change;
proc means data=transform noprint;
    by therapy change;
    var count;
    output out=sum sum=sum;
data estimate;
    set sum;
    by therapy;
    retain nminus nzero nplus;
    if change="Same" then nzero=sum;
    if change="Up" then nplus=sum;
    if change="Down" then nminus=sum;
    alpha=(nminus+nplus)/(nminus+nzero+nplus);
    if nminus+nplus>0 then beta=nplus/(nminus+nplus); else beta=1;
    if last.therapy=1;
    keep therapy beta alpha;
proc print data=estimate noobs;
proc freq data=sum;
    ods select LRChiSq;
    table therapy*change;
    exact lrchi;
    weight sum;
    run;
```

Output from Program 3.20

```
therapy    alpha       beta

DrugA    0.01942    0.50000
DrugB    0.14706    0.46667


 Likelihood Ratio Chi-Square Test

Chi-Square                 12.2983
DF                               2
Asymptotic Pr >  ChiSq     0.0021
Exact      Pr >= ChiSq     0.0057
```

Output 3.20 lists the estimated α and β parameters in the two treatment groups accompanied by the asymptotic and exact likelihood ratio p-values. We see that there is little separation between the β parameters, which indicates that the magnitudes of marginal changes are in close agreement in the two treatment groups. However, the discordance rate in Treatment group 1 is much smaller than that in Treatment group 2 ($\alpha_1 = 0.019$ and $\alpha_2 = 0.147$, respectively). The asymptotic test statistic for the homogeneity of treatment-induced changes is equal to 12.2983 with 2 degrees of freedom and is highly significant ($p = 0.0021$). The exact likelihood-ratio p-value, which is more reliable in this situation, is also highly significant ($p = 0.0057$). Both the asymptotic and exact tests clearly indicate that different patterns of change in the overall ECG evaluation are observed in the two treatment groups.

3.3.4 Summary

This section reviewed methods for the analysis of repeated categorical outcomes. Although the focus of the section was on responses derived from quantitative safety and diagnostic measures, the described methods can be successfully used in any statistical problem involving repeated categorical responses, such as in longitudinal efficacy analyses.

The two most popular approaches to the analysis of categorical data in a longitudinal setting are based on generalized estimating equations and random effects models. We demonstrated in this section how to perform GEE inferences using PROC GENMOD both in the case of binary and ordinal responses. GEE methods produce consistent estimates of the regression parameters that are robust with respect to the working covariance matrix. Although regression estimates become less efficient if the selected correlation structure substantially differs from the true correlation structure, their consistency is not affected by the wrong choice of the working covariance matrix. GEE methods are attractive in clinical applications because they allow the statistician to consistently estimate the model parameters when no prior information is available to aid in the selection of a correlation structure.

GEE models are commonly referred to as population-averaged models because they describe an average of responses in the underlying population at each particular time point. Population-averaged inferences need to be carefully interpreted in a clinical trial setting because they do not adequately account for the between-subject heterogeneity. It is well known that samples of patients recruited in clinical trials are not randomly selected from a larger population of patients. When the resulting sample is highly heterogeneous, response profiles produced by GEE methods may not correspond to any possible patient and therefore can sometimes be misleading.

The other widely used analysis method relies on random effects models for repeated categorical measurements. The random effects models include a subject-specific random term and thus account for the heterogeneity of subjects' response profiles. Parameter estimation in the random effects models is typically performed based on marginal likelihood and requires a substantial amount of numerical integration. PROC NLMIXED helps the statistician solve the computational problem and make inferences in a wide class of nonlinear random effects models.

Finally, this section discussed analysis of paired categorical variables based on direct models for cell probabilities in shift tables. This modeling approach complements the GEE and logistic random effects methods in the analysis of shift tables with identical or virtually identical marginal distributions.

Interim Data Monitoring

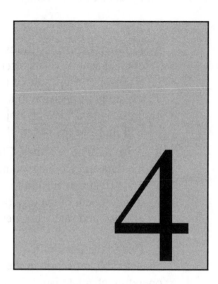

This chapter reviews sequential data monitoring strategies in clinical trials. It introduces a class of group sequential tests (known as repeated significance tests) that are widely used in the assessment of interim findings in clinical applications. The first part of the chapter provides a detailed review of the process of designing group sequential trials and also discusses flexible procedures for monitoring clinical trial data. The second part of the chapter reviews popular approaches to constructing futility-testing procedures in clinical trials. These approaches are based on frequentist (conditional power), mixed Bayesian-frequentist (predictive power) and fully Bayesian (predictive probability) methods.

4.1 Introduction

Sequential monitoring of safety and efficacy data has become an integral part of modern clinical trials. Although in theory one can consider continuous monitoring strategies, practical considerations dictate that interim monitoring be performed in a *group sequential* manner; i.e., interim data looks should be taken after groups of patients have completed the study. Within a sequential testing framework, a clinical tial is stopped as soon as enough information is accumulated to reach a conclusion about the properties of a new drug, such as whether the drug is superior or inferior to the control.

In general, interim assessments of efficacy and safety data in clinical trials are motivated by the following considerations (Enas et al., 1989; Jennison and Turnbull, 1990; Ellenberg, Fleming and DeMets, 2002):

- **Ethical requirements.** It is imperative to ensure that patients are not exposed to harmful therapies, and thus a clinical trial must be stopped as soon as the experimental therapy is found to cause serious side effects. Interim safety evaluations are generally mandated in clinical trials with nonreversible outcomes, such as mortality trials.

- **Financial considerations.** In order to make the optimal use of research and development dollars, clinical trial sponsors often introduce interim analyses of efficacy endpoints in early proof-of-concept studies (as well as larger Phase II and III trials) to help predict the final outcome of the study. A decision to terminate the study may be reached if it becomes evident that the study is unlikely to achieve its objectives at the planned end; e.g., there is very little evidence that the drug will improve the patients' condition.

- **Administrative issues.** Clinical researchers often rely on interim data to judge the overall quality of the data and facilitate administrative or business decisions. For example, early evidence of efficacy may trigger a decision to increase manufacturing spending in order to support continuing development of the experimental drug. The trial may still be continued to help better characterize the efficacy and safety profiles of the drug.

Due to the possibility of early stopping, use of sequential data monitoring strategies leads to a considerable reduction in the average size of the trial compared to a fixed-sample trial with the same operating characteristics. To illustrate this attractive feature of group sequential designs, consider the following hypothetical example.

EXAMPLE: Comparison of Group Sequential and Fixed-Sample Designs

A two-arm clinical trial with a continuous primary endpoint has been designed to compare an experimental drug to a placebo. The trial has been sized to achieve 80% power at a two-sided 0.05 significance level under the assumption that the mean difference is equal to 0.2 standard deviations (effect size of 0.2). Figures 4.1 and 4.2 show how much savings in terms of the total number of patients one should expect with popular group sequential designs proposed by Pocock (1977) and O'Brien and Fleming (1979).

Figure 4.1 demonstrates that, with only one interim analysis that occurs halfway into the trial, the average number of patients required by the O'Brien-Fleming sequential design is 10% smaller than that of a fixed-sample design when the effect size is truly equal to 0.2. An application of the Pocock group sequential plan results in a 15% savings. The average sample-size reduction increases with the true effect size; for example, it is equal to 28% (O'Brien-Fleming plan) and 35% (Pocock plan) when the true effect size is 0.3. On the other hand, sequential testing can potentially increase the average sample size. For example, we can see from Figure 4.1 that the average number of patients required by the Pocock design is greater than that of the fixed-sample design when the treatment difference is close to 0.

Figure 4.1 Average sample size reduction associated with the O'Brien-Fleming (—) and Pocock (- - -) group sequential designs compared to a fixed-sample design (one interim analysis)

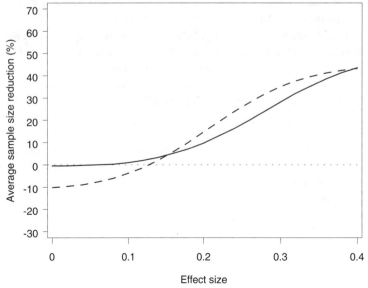

Figure 4.2 Average sample size reduction associated with the O'Brien-Fleming (—) and Pocock (- - -) group sequential designs compared to a fixed-sample design (four equally spaced interim analyses)

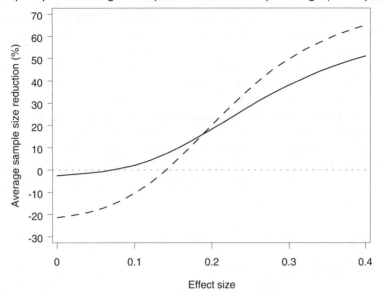

It is interesting to note that one should expect a more substantial reduction in the average sample size with more frequent interim looks. Figure 4.2 shows that the O'Brien-Fleming and Pocock designs with four equally spaced interim analyses offer an 18% and 20% reduction in the number of patients, respectively, compared to a nonsequential design (the true effect size is assumed to be 0.2).

A variety of methods have been proposed in the literature for designing group sequential trials and monitoring trial data to help detect early evidence of an overwhelming treatment effect or lack of therapeutic benefit. The most popular ones are the repeated significance and boundaries approaches:

- Repeated significance testing goes back to group sequential procedures with prespecified equally spaced looks (Pocock, 1977; O'Brien and Fleming, 1979) which were subsequently generalized to allow flexible sequential monitoring.

- The boundaries approach (triangular and related tests) represents an extension of sequential procedures for continuous data monitoring (e.g., Wald's sequential probability ratio test) which were suitably modified to be used in a group sequential manner.

Repeated significance testing is currently the most widely used approach and will be the focus of this section. For a comprehensive review of the boundaries approach, see Whitehead (1997) and other publications by John Whitehead and his colleagues, such as Whitehead and Stratton (1983) and Whitehead (1999).

To illustrate repeated significance tests, we will use examples from clinical trials with continuous, normally distributed or binary endpoints. As always, the case of normally distributed outcome variables is generally applicable to the analysis of test statistics computed from nonnormal data. Group sequential tests for time-to-event endpoints are conceptually similar to those discussed in the following section.[1]

The following two examples will be used throughout the section.

---

[1] As shown by Jennison and Turnbull (2000, Chapter 13), the group sequential designs and sequential monitoring strategies discussed later in this section are easily extended to the case of time-to-event variables. An interesting feature of group sequential tests in clinical trials with time-to-event endpoints that differentiates them from normally distributed and binary endpoints is a repeated use of data collected from the same patient. For example, in survival trials, the test statistic at each interim look is computed from all survival times (either observed or censored) and thus any patient who survives to the end of the study contributes to every interim test statistic.

EXAMPLE: Trial in Patients with Clinical Depression

A clinical trial was conducted to test a single dose of a new drug for treating disorders of the central nervous system. The trial's primary objective was to demonstrate that the chosen dose of the drug was superior to a placebo in the acute treatment of subjects who meet criteria for major depression. The efficacy of the experimental drug was evaluated using the mean reduction from baseline to the end of the 8-week study period in the total score of the 17-item Hamilton Depression Rating Scale (HAMD17).

To determine the size of the trial, clinical researchers wanted to have adequate power to detect a treatment difference in the mean reduction in the HAMD17 total score when this difference is 3 with a standard deviation of 8. With a fixed-sample design, a sample size of 150 patients per group provides a 90% power to detect a statistically significant difference at a two-sided 0.05 level.

The clinical trial employed two interim analyses and a final analysis. The analyses were planned to take place after approximately 50% and 75% of the patients had completed the study. The patient enrollment was to be terminated in the presence of overwhelming efficacy at either analysis. The data collected in the trial are summarized in Table 4.1.

Table 4.1 Summary of HAMD17 data collected in the depression trial

Analysis	Experimental group		Placebo group	
	n	Mean improvement in HAMD17 total score (SD)	n	Mean improvement in HAMD17 total score (SD)
Interim analysis 1	78	8.3 (6.2)	78	5.9 (6.5)
Interim analysis 2	122	8.0 (6.3)	120	6.3 (5.9)
Final analysis	150	8.2 (5.9)	152	6.1 (5.8)

EXAMPLE: Trial in Patients with Severe Sepsis

A placebo-controlled clinical trial was designed to study the effect of an experimental drug on 28-day all-cause mortality in patients with severe sepsis. The objective of the trial was to assess whether the experimental drug had superior efficacy compared to the placebo.

It was assumed that the 28-day placebo mortality was 30% and administration of the experimental drug reduced the mortality rate to 24%. Using a fixed-sample design with a two-sided significance level of 0.05, 859 patients would need to be enrolled in each of the two treatment groups to achieve 80% power of detecting an absolute mortality reduction of 6%.

The mortality data were examined at two interim analyses. These analyses were scheduled to occur after approximately 20 and 66 percent of the patients completed the study. The first interim analysis was introduced mainly to assess the futility of the drug. The trial was to be terminated early for efficacy only in the presence of an extremely beneficial treatment effect. The objective of the second interim analysis was to examine both efficacy and futility.

The 28-day survival data collected at the two interim analyses are presented in Table 4.2.

Table 4.2 Summary of 28-day survival data collected in the sepsis trial

Analysis	Experimental group			Placebo group		
	Total	Alive	Survival	Total	Alive	Survival
Interim analysis 1	220	164	74.5%	216	152	70.4%
Interim analysis 2	715	538	75.2%	715	526	73.6%

Overview

Section 4.2 provides a detailed review of group sequential plans, including the O'Brien-Fleming and Pocock plans, and describes a rich family of designs introduced by Wang and Tsiatis (1987). We will show how to calculate sample size and stopping boundaries in group sequential trials for assessing efficacy or both efficacy and futility of an experimental drug. The section also discusses flexible data monitoring strategies based on the powerful error spending approach proposed by Lan and DeMets (1983) and demonstrates how to calculate repeated confidence intervals for the treatment difference at each look as well as bias-adjusted point estimates and confidence intervals at the last analysis. Lastly, we briefly review validation work that was done to ensure the SAS macros introduced in this section are reliable and can be used in clinical trial applications.

Section 4.3 introduces an alternative approach to interim monitoring of clinical trials known as the *stochastic curtailment approach*. It is shown how to apply stochastic curtailment methods to develop futility rules for determining whether or not it is fruitful to continue the trial to the planned end. The section introduces three families of futility tests with applications to clinical trials with normally distributed and binary primary endpoints:

- conditional power tests (frequentist approach)
- predictive power tests (mixed Bayesian-frequentist approach)
- predictive probability tests (Bayesian approach).

Finally, it is important to remind the reader that this chapter deals with *statistical* rules for examining efficacy and futility in group sequential clinical trials. Other considerations that play an important role in the decision making process cannot be fully addressed within the statistical sequential testing framework. It is widely recognized that a data monitoring committee is authorized to terminate a clinical trial or modify its design for a variety of reasons, such as safety concerns, secondary findings, consistency of results across subsets and convincing findings from similarly designed studies; see Ellenberg, Fleming and DeMets (2002, Chapter 8) for more details. As stated by DeMets and Lan (1984), "Just as good statistical inference is more than computing a *p*-value, so also is decision making in terminating a clinical trial."

4.2 Repeated Significance Tests

Consider a clinical trial comparing an experimental therapy to a control and assume that the following group sequential plan with m interim analyses will be adopted in the trial. Let N denote the maximum sample size per treatment group. Further, $X_{i1}, \ldots, X_{iN}$ will denote the independent, identically distributed measurements in the ith group, $i = 1, 2$. The measurements can be either continuous or binary. In the case of a continuous outcome variable, the treatment effect δ is equal to the difference between the treatment means. In the binary case, δ is the difference between the proportions of patients who experienced the event of interest in the two treatment groups.

Assume that $2n$ patients complete the trial between successive looks (n patients per treatment group). The null hypothesis of no treatment effect will be tested at the kth interim analysis using the test statistic

$$Z_k = \sqrt{\frac{kn}{2s^2}} \left(\frac{1}{kn} \sum_{j=1}^{kn} X_{1j} - \frac{1}{kn} \sum_{j=1}^{kn} X_{2j} \right),$$

where s denotes the pooled sample standard deviation.

The objective of the trial is to test the null hypothesis of no treatment effect

$$H_0: \quad \delta = \delta_0 = 0$$

against a one-sided alternative

$$H_1: \quad \delta = \delta_1 > 0.$$

Here δ_1 denotes a clinically meaningful treatment difference.

We will now consider the problem of setting up group sequential designs for evaluating evidence in favor of the one-sided alternative or null hypotheses. Although this chapter focuses on one-sided testing problems, group sequential tests introduced in the following sections are easily generalized to a two-sided setting. This is accomplished by adding symmetric stopping boundaries. For example, a group sequential design with a two-sided alternative relies on two symmetric boundaries. Similarly, simultaneous efficacy/futility testing with a two-sided alternative hypothesis requires two sets of two symmetric boundaries.

Group Sequential Plan for Detecting Superior Efficacy

The null hypothesis is tested by sequentially comparing the test statistics $Z_1, \ldots, Z_m$ to adjusted critical values $u_1(\alpha), \ldots, u_m(\alpha)$ forming an upper stopping boundary. The adjusted critical values $u_1(\alpha), \ldots, u_m(\alpha)$ are selected to preserve the overall Type I error rate α. The following decision rule is used at the kth interim look:

1. Stop the trial and conclude that the experimental drug is superior to placebo if $Z_k > u_k(\alpha)$.

2. Continue the trial if $Z_k \leq u_k(\alpha)$.

In other words, a clinical trial designed to study the efficacy of a drug is discontinued when the test statistic crosses the upper stopping boundary. For example, Figure 4.3 depicts the results observed in a hypothetical clinical trial, which is stopped at the third interim look due to overwhelming evidence of therapeutic benefit.

Figure 4.3 Group sequential plan for detecting superior efficacy

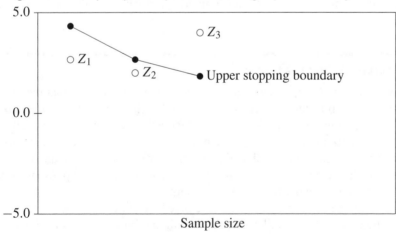

Group Sequential Plan for Detecting Futility

Futility testing relies on comparing the statistics $Z_1, \ldots, Z_m$ to critical values $l_1(\beta), \ldots, l_m(\beta)$ forming a lower stopping boundary (the critical values are chosen to maintain the nominal Type II error rate). The experimental drug is declared futile at the kth interim analysis if the accumulated evidence suggests that the alternative hypothesis is false, i.e.,

$$Z_k < l_k(\beta),$$

Figure 4.4 Group sequential plan for detecting futility

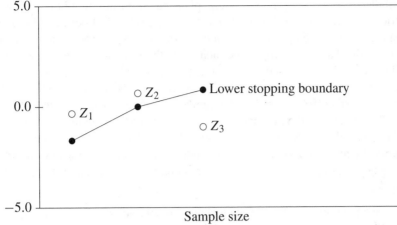

and the trial is continued otherwise. To illustrate this decision rule, Figure 4.4 presents a scenario in which a clinical trial is terminated at the third interim look due to futility.

Group Sequential Plan for Simultaneous Efficacy and Futility Testing

Finally, a clinical trial that assesses both the efficacy and futility profiles of the experimental drug is stopped when the test statistic crosses either the lower or upper boundary. In this case, the decision rule at the kth interim analysis looks like this:

1. Stop the trial for efficacy if $Z_k > u_k(\alpha, \beta)$.
2. Continue the trial if $l_k(\alpha, \beta) \leq Z_k \leq u_k(\alpha, \beta)$.
3. Stop the trial for futility if $Z_k < l_k(\alpha, \beta)$.

Note that the stopping boundaries are selected to protect both the Type I and Type II error probabilities α and β. See Figure 4.5 for an example of a clinical trial terminated at the third interim look because the test statistic crossed the lower stopping boundary.

Figure 4.5 Group sequential plan for simultaneous efficacy and futility testing

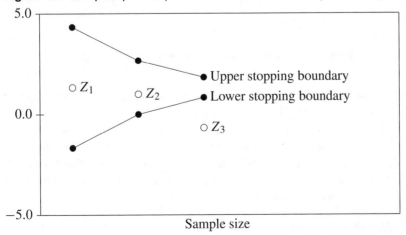

Popular Group Sequential Designs

In this section we will discuss popular group sequential plans based on stopping boundaries proposed by Pocock (1977), O'Brien and Fleming (1979) and Wang and Tsiatis (1987). Pocock and O'Brien and Fleming were among the first to develop statistical methods for designing group sequential clinical trials. Pocock (1977) described a set of stopping boundaries with the same critical value at each interim look. O'Brien and Fleming (1979) proposed a sequential plan under which earlier analyses are performed in a conservative manner and the later tests are carried out at significance levels close to the nominal level. Wang and Tsiatis (1987) introduced a family of group sequential plans indexed by the ρ parameter that ranges between 0 and 0.5 and determines the shape of the stopping boundaries. The Wang-Tsiatis family includes the Pocock ($\rho = 1/2$) and O'Brien-Fleming ($\rho = 0$) plans.

The Pocock, O'Brien-Fleming and Wang-Tsiatis boundaries for efficacy clinical trials are shown in Table 4.3. The corresponding stopping boundaries for simultaneous efficacy and futility testing will be introduced in Section 4.2.2.

Table 4.3 Popular stopping boundaries for efficacy testing (the constants $c_P(\alpha, m)$, $c_{OF}(\alpha, m)$ and $c_{WT}(\alpha, \rho, m)$ are chosen to protect the overall Type I error rate)

Adjusted critical value $u_k(\alpha)$	Reference
$c_P(\alpha, m)$	Pocock (1977)
$c_{OF}(\alpha, m)k^{-1/2}$	O'Brien and Fleming (1979)
$c_{WT}(\alpha, \rho, m)k^{\rho-1/2}, 0 \leq \rho \leq 1/2$	Wang and Tsiatis (1987)

Any group sequential test is uniquely defined by a set of *stopping probabilities* (or *exit probabilities*)

$$P_1(\delta), \ldots, P_m(\delta).$$

They are defined as the likelihood of crossing the stopping boundary (or boundaries) at the kth interim look assuming the true value of the treatment effect is δ. Examining stopping probabilities for the upper boundary under H_0 helps us understand how a group sequential plan "spends" the overall Type I error rate α throughout the course of a trial. For example, it will be shown in Section 4.2.1 that, under the Pocock plan, the chances of stopping the trial well before its planned termination are quite high. By contrast, the O'Brien-Fleming test "spends" very small amounts of α at early interim looks.

Another important characteristic of a sequential test is the *expected sample size* (also known as the *average sample number*). The expected sample size provides information on the number of patients anticipated in a group sequential trial in order to reach a decision point. The expected number of patients per group is easy to compute once we have calculated the probability of stopping at each interim analysis:

$$\text{Expected sample size}(\delta) = n \sum_{k=1}^{m-1} k P_k(\delta) + nm \left(1 - \sum_{k=1}^{m-1} P_k(\delta) \right).$$

Since the expected sample size is a function of stopping probabilities, it depends on the number and timing of interim looks as well as the selected stopping boundaries. As was shown in the introduction to this chapter, sequential testing strategies are often compared with respect to their expected sample size.

Although we have talked only about group sequential plans with equally spaced looks, the described group sequential procedures are easily extended to the case of unequal spacings. The SAS macros introduced later in this section allow the user to set up Pocock and O'Brien-Fleming group sequential plans with equally or unequally spaced interim looks.

Design and Data Monitoring Stages

The following is a brief description of steps one needs to go through to design a group sequential trial and perform interim monitoring (it also serves as an outline of this section).

Design stage

1. Choose the group sequential plan that reflects the objectives of the clinical trial: early stopping in favor of the one-sided alternative hypothesis (Section 4.2.1) or early stopping in favor of either the null or alternative hypothesis (Section 4.2.2). Note that group sequential plans for detecting early evidence of futility (i.e., early termination in favor of the null hypothesis only) are not discussed in this section; see Section 4.3 for a detailed review of *stochastic curtailment* futility tests.

2. Specify the stopping boundaries (O'Brien-Fleming, Pocock or other boundaries from the Wang-Tsiatis family). This decision is driven by a variety of factors that will be discussed in Section 4.2.1.

3. Design a group sequential plan: generate stopping boundaries on test statistic or p-value scales (statisticians often favor the test statistic scale whereas their clinical colleagues prefer the p-value scale), and compute the maximum number of patients, average sample size and power as a function of an anticipated treatment difference.

Monitoring stage

1. Implement a flexible data monitoring scheme based on the Lan-DeMets error spending approach (Section 4.2.3). Select an error spending function and compute adjusted critical values and p-value cutoff points at each interim analysis (Sections 4.2.4 and 4.2.5). The advantage of the error spending approach is that it provides the trial's sponsor or independent data monitoring committee with flexibility by allowing them to deviate from the prespecified sequential plan in the number or timing of interim looks.

2. Compute repeated confidence limits for the true treatment difference at each interim look (Section 4.2.6) and a bias-adjusted estimate of the treatment difference and confidence limits at the last analysis (Section 4.2.7).

4.2.1   Design Stage: Interim Efficacy Assessments

To illustrate the process of setting a group sequential plan for detecting early evidence of superior efficacy, consider the clinical trial in patients with clinical depression described in the introduction to this chapter. Recall that the two interim analyses in this trial took place after 50 and 75 percent of the patients had completed the study and both analyses tested superior efficacy of the experimental drug compared to a placebo.

In order to construct and compare alternative group sequential plans for this clinical trial example, we will utilize the %EffDesign macro given in the Appendix. This powerful macro can be used to design a wide variety of group sequential trials for early detection of superior efficacy based on stopping boundaries from the Wang-Tsiatis family.

%EffDesign Macro

The %EffDesign macro has the following arguments:

- FRACTION is the name of the input data set that contains fractions of the total sample size at successive analyses.

- EFFSIZE is the hypothesized effect size (i.e., the treatment difference divided by the standard deviation).

- POWER is the power of the group sequential plan to detect the hypothesized effect size.

- ALPHA is the one-sided Type I error probability (the treatment difference is assumed to be positive under the alternative hypothesis).

- RHO is the shape parameter in the Wang-Tsiatis family of stopping boundaries (let RHO=0.5 to request Pocock boundaries and RHO=0 to request O'Brien-Fleming boundaries).

- BOUNDARY is the name of the data set that will contain stopping boundaries and probabilities at the scheduled interim looks. This data set will be generated by the macro and includes the following variables:
  - ANALYSIS is the analysis number.
  - SIZE is the sample size per group.
  - TESTSTBOUNDARY is the one-sided stopping boundary on the test statistic scale, i.e., the stopping boundary for z statistics.
  - PVALBOUNDARY is the one-sided stopping boundary on the p-value scale, i.e., the stopping boundary for one-sided p-values.
  - PROBH0 is the probability of stopping at the current analysis under the null hypothesis of no treatment effect.
  - CUMPROBH0 is the probability of stopping at the current or earlier analysis under the null hypothesis of no treatment effect.
  - PROBH1 is the probability of stopping at the current analysis under the alternative hypothesis associated with the specified effect size.
  - CUMPROBH1 is the probability of stopping at the current or earlier analysis under the alternative hypothesis associated with the specified effect size.
- SIZEPOWER is the name of the data set with the power and average sample size of the sequential test for selected effect sizes. This data set will also be generated by the macro and includes the following variables:
  - EFFSIZE is the effect size.
  - AVESIZE is the average sample size of the sequential test per group for the specified effect size.
  - POWER is the power of the sequential test assuming the specified effect size.

The %EffDesign macro prints a brief summary of the plan's characteristics and creates two SAS data sets containing stopping boundaries and data on power and average sample size.

The macro achieves computational efficiency in complex group sequential designs by relying on two powerful SAS/IML functions. The SEQ function is used for computing stopping probabilities and the overall Type I error rate associated with an arbitrary set of stopping boundaries. This calculation is based on the recursive integration algorithm of Armitage, McPherson and Rowe (1969). Further, in order to ensure that the overall error rate is equal to its nominal value, the %EffDesign macro scales the specified boundaries by invoking the SEQSCALE function. The reader is referred to Section 4.2.8 for a more detailed description of the SEQ and SEQSCALE functions.

O'Brien-Fleming Group Sequential Design in the Depression Trial

Program 4.1 shown below demonstrates how the %EffDesign macro can help us set up a group sequential design proposed by O'Brien and Fleming (1979) in the depression trial example. In order to call the macro, we need to specify the following parameters:

- FRACTION parameter. The two interim analyses are planned to occur after 50% and 75% of the patients have completed the study and therefore we will need set up a data set with a single variable that assumes three values: 0.5, 0.75 and 1. For example,

```
data DepTrial;
    input fraction @@;
    datalines;
    0.5 0.75 1
    ;
```

In order to pass the name of this data set to the %EffDesign macro, let FRACTION=DEPTRIAL.

- EFFSIZE parameter. The mean treatment difference is assumed to equal 3 with a standard deviation of 8, the effect size is $3/8 = 0.375$ and thus EFFSIZE=0.375.

- POWER parameter is set to 0.9.

- ALPHA parameter. Recall that the primary analysis is performed at a two-sided significance level of 0.05 and therefore the one-sided ALPHA needs to be set to 0.025.

- RHO parameter. In order to request the O'Brien-Fleming test, we need to set the shape parameter RHO to 0.

- BOUNDARY parameter. When we set BOUNDARY=OFBOUNDARY, the %EffDesign macro will store the one-sided stopping boundary of the sequential plan in the OFBOUNDARY data set.

- SIZEPOWER parameter. Similarly, setting SIZEPOWER=OFPOWER tells the macro to write the power and average sample size data to the OFPOWER data set.

Program 4.1 Group sequential test with the O'Brien-Fleming stopping boundary (RHO=0)

```
data DepTrial;
    input fraction @@;
    datalines;
    0.50 0.75 1
    ;
%EffDesign(fraction=DepTrial,effsize=0.375,power=0.9,alpha=0.025,
    rho=0,boundary=OFBoundary,sizepower=OFPower);
proc print data=OFBoundary noobs label;
    var Analysis Size TestStBoundary PValBoundary;
proc print data=OFBoundary noobs label;
    var Analysis ProbH0 CumProbH0 ProbH1 CumProbH1;
* Stopping boundary on a test statistic scale;
axis1 minor=none label=(angle=90 "Test statistic") order=(1 to 3 by 1);
axis2 minor=none label=("Sample size per group") order=(0 to 200 by 50);
symbol1 value=dot color=black i=join line=1;
symbol2 value=circle color=black i=none;
data plot1;
    set OFBoundary;
    format TestStBoundary 1.0;
    group=1;
data plot2;
    size=150; TestStBoundary=1.96; group=2;
data plot;
    set plot1 plot2;
proc gplot data=plot;
    plot TestStBoundary*Size=group/frame nolegend haxis=axis2 vaxis=axis1;
    run;
* Stopping boundary on a p-value scale;
axis1 minor=none label=(angle=90 "P-value") order=(0 to 0.03 by 0.01);
axis2 minor=none label=("Sample size per group") order=(0 to 200 by 50);
symbol1 value=dot color=black i=join line=1;
symbol2 value=circle color=black i=none;
data plot1;
    set OFBoundary;
    format PValBoundary 4.2;
    group=1;
data plot2;
    size=150; PValBoundary=0.025; group=2;
data plot;
    set plot1 plot2;
```

```
proc gplot data=plot;
    plot PValBoundary*Size=group/frame nolegend haxis=axis2 vaxis=axis1;
    run;
* Power function;
axis1 minor=none label=(angle=90 "Power") order=(0 to 1 by 0.2);
axis2 minor=none label=("True effect size") order=(0 to 0.6 by 0.1);
symbol1 value=none color=black i=join line=1;
symbol2 value=none color=black i=join line=34;
data plot;
    set OFPower;
    format Power FixedSamplePower 3.1;
    FixedSampleSize=150;
    alpha=0.025;
    FixedSamplePower=probnorm(sqrt(FixedSampleSize/2)*EffSize
    -probit(1-alpha));
proc gplot data=plot;
    plot Power*EffSize FixedSamplePower*EffSize/frame overlay nolegend
    haxis=axis2 vaxis=axis1;
    run;
* Average sample size;
axis1 minor=none label=(angle=90 "Average sample size per group")
    order=(0 to 200 by 50);
axis2 minor=none label=("True effect size") order=(0 to 0.6 by 0.1);
symbol1 value=none color=black i=join line=1;
data plot;
    set OFPower;
    format AveSize 4.0;
proc gplot data=plot;
    plot AveSize*EffSize/frame nolegend haxis=axis2 vaxis=axis1
        vref=150 lvref=34;
    run;
```

Output from Program 4.1

Summary	Value
One-sided Type I error probability	0.025
Power	0.9
True effect size	0.375
Stopping boundary parameter	0
Maximum sample size per group	153
Average sample size per group under H0	153
Average sample size per group under H1	115
Fixed sample size per group	150

Analysis	Sample size per group	Stopping boundary (test statistic scale)	Stopping boundary (p-value scale)
1	77	2.8626	0.0021
2	115	2.3373	0.0097
3	153	2.0242	0.0215

Analysis	Stopping probability under H0	Cumulative stopping probability under H0	Stopping probability under H1	Cumulative stopping probability under H1
1	0.0021	0.0021	0.2928	0.2928
2	0.0084	0.0105	0.4033	0.6960
3	0.0145	0.0250	0.2040	0.9000

Program 4.1 computes several important operating characteristics of the O'Brien-Fleming sequential plan. First, the top part of Output 4.1 shows that the maximum number of patients per treatment group that might be required by the sequential test is 153 and the average sample sizes under the null and alternative hypotheses are 153 and 115, respectively. The corresponding sample size for the fixed-sample design is 150. This sample size is computed using the well-known formula with a one-sided Type I error rate α and Type I error rate β:

$$n = \frac{2(z_{1-\alpha} + z_{1-\beta})^2}{\theta^2},$$

where $z_{1-\alpha}$ and $z_{1-\beta}$ are the $100(1 - \alpha)$th and $100(1 - \beta)$th percentiles of the standard normal distribution and θ is the hypothesized effect size. Although the maximum sample size for the O'Brien-Fleming sequential test is slightly larger than the fixed-sample size, we should on average see a 23% reduction in the sample size if the effect size is truly equal to 0.375.

The bottom part of Output 4.1 presents the one-sided O'Brien-Fleming stopping boundary and probabilities of crossing the boundary at each of the 3 analyses. These quantities come from the OFBOUNDARY data set produced by the %EffDesign macro. Note that, with the O'Brien-Fleming plan, early stopping is fairly unlikely. If we assume that the true treatment difference on the HAMD17 scale is 3 points, there is only a 29% chance that the trial will be terminated at the first interim analysis.

Using the output of Program 4.1, it is easy to express the O'Brien-Fleming decision rules in terms of observed mean treatment differences at each of the two interim analyses and the final analysis. The latter can be included in the data monitoring committee interim analysis guidelines (also known as the *data monitoring committee charter*). The following is an example of such guidelines:

- The first interim analysis will be conducted after approximately 77 patients have completed the study in each treatment group. The trial will be stopped for efficacy if the z statistic for the treatment effect is greater than 2.8626 (i.e., the one-sided p-value is less than 0.0021). Assuming that the standard deviation of changes in the HAMD17 total score is 8, the trial will be terminated at the first interim analysis provided the mean treatment difference exceeds 3.69 points.[2]

- The second interim analysis will occur after approximately 115 patients have completed the study in each treatment group. The trial will be stopped for efficacy if the one-sided p-value for the treatment effect is less than 0.0097. The trial will be terminated at the second interim analysis provided the mean treatment difference is greater than 2.47 points (under the assumption that the standard deviation of HAMD17 changes equals 8).

- The experimental drug will be declared superior to placebo at the final analysis if the one-sided p-value is significant at the 0.0215 level. A significant p-value will be observed if the mean treatment difference exceeds 1.85 (assuming that the standard deviation of HAMD17 changes is 8).

---

[2]This treatment difference is equal to $c\sigma\sqrt{2/n}$, where c is the adjusted critical value, σ is the common standard deviation, and n is the sample size per group. In this case, $c = 2.8626$, $\sigma = 8$, and $n = 77$. Therefore, the detectable treatment difference is 3.69.

To better understand the principles underlying the constructed sequential test, it is helpful to plot the stopping boundary shown in Output 4.1 against the sample size. Figures 4.6 and 4.7 display the O'Brien-Fleming boundary on the test statistic and *p*-value scales. Although the stopping boundary appears to be continuous, it is important to remember that this is not really the case. The actual boundary is discrete (it is represented by the three dots) and the lines connecting the dots are introduced to help visualize the effect of repeated significant testing on adjusted critical values. Also, to emphasize that only one analysis is performed under a fixed-sample design, the fixed-sample case is represented by a single circle.

It was pointed out earlier in this section that, under the group sequential plan proposed by O'Brien and Fleming (1979), early analyses are performed in a very conservative fashion, which gives us an ability to conduct the final analysis at a significance level close to the nominal level. Indeed, it is clear

Figure 4.6 Stopping boundary of the O'Brien-Fleming design (•) and critical value of the fixed-sample design (○) on a test statistic scale in the depression trial example

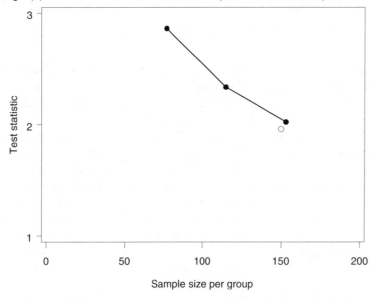

Figure 4.7 Stopping boundary of the O'Brien-Fleming design (•) and critical value of the fixed-sample design (○) on a *p*-value scale in the depression trial example

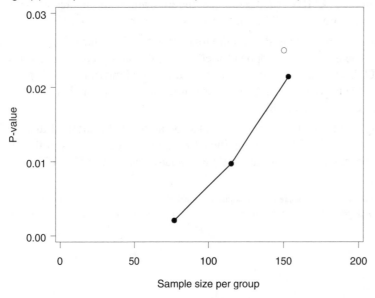

from Figure 4.6 that the adjusted critical values at the first two looks are well above the open circle corresponding to the unadjusted critical value of 1.96; however, the difference between the adjusted and unadjusted critical values at the final analysis is rather small. The same is true for the O'Brien-Fleming stopping boundary on the *p*-value scale in Figure 4.7.

Further, it is instructive to examine the power and average sample size of the O'Brien-Fleming sequential test included in the OFPOWER data set created by the %EffDesign macro. Figures 4.8 and 4.9 depict the power and average sample size of the sequential test as a function of the true effect size.

Figure 4.8 demonstrates that the power of the O'Brien-Fleming sequential test is identical to the power of the corresponding fixed-sample test and remains above 80% if the true effect size is greater than 0.3375 (this corresponds to the mean treatment difference of 2.7 points on the HAMD17 scale).

Figure 4.8 Power of the O'Brien-Fleming (—) and fixed-sample ($\cdots$) tests in the depression trial example

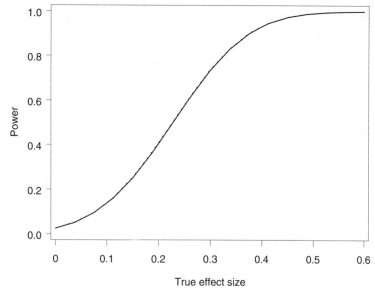

Figure 4.9 Average sample size of the O'Brien-Fleming (—) and fixed-sample ($\cdots$) tests in the depression trial example

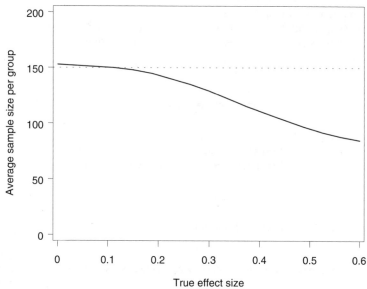

Figure 4.9 indicates that the average sample size of the sequential test is less than the sample size of 150 patients per group associated with the fixed-sample design except for effect sizes in a small neighborhood of H_0. Use of the O'Brien-Fleming plan results in appreciable savings in terms of the expected size of the trial when the treatment effect is large. In the extreme case when the true effect size equals 0.6, the trial will on average be terminated after 85 patients have been enrolled in each treatment group, which translates into a 43% reduction compared to the fixed-sample case.

Pocock Group Sequential Design in the Depression Trial

The O'Brien-Fleming sequential design we have just set up represents one extreme of the Wang-Tsiatis family of group sequential plans. The other extreme corresponds to the Pocock plan with the shape parameter $\rho = 0.5$. Program 4.2 shows how we can utilize the %EffDesign macro to construct the Pocock sequential test in the depression trial. The macro has the same arguments as in Program 4.1 with the exception of the shape parameter RHO, which is now set to 0.5.

Program 4.2 Group sequential test with the Pocock stopping boundary (RHO=0.5)

```
data DepTrial;
    input fraction @@;
    datalines;
    0.5 0.75 1
    ;
%EffDesign(fraction=DepTrial,effsize=0.375,power=0.9,alpha=0.025,
    rho=0.5,boundary=PBoundary,sizepower=PPower);
proc print data=PBoundary noobs label;
    var Analysis Size TestStBoundary PValBoundary;
proc print data=PBoundary noobs label;
    var Analysis ProbH0 CumProbH0 ProbH1 CumProbH1;
* Compare with the O'Brien-Fleming sequential plan;
%EffDesign(fraction=DepTrial,effsize=0.375,power=0.9,alpha=0.025,
    rho=0,boundary=OFBoundary,sizepower=OFPower);
data plot1;
    set OFBoundary; group=1;
data plot2;
    set PBoundary; group=2;
data plot3;
    set plot1 plot2;
    format TestStBoundary 1.0 PValBoundary 4.2;
* Stopping boundaries on a test statistic scale;
axis1 minor=none label=(angle=90 "Test statistic") order=(1 to 3 by 1);
axis2 minor=none label=("Sample size per group") order=(0 to 200 by 50);
symbol1 value=dot color=black i=join line=1;
symbol2 value=dot color=black i=join line=20;
proc gplot data=plot3;
    plot TestStBoundary*Size=group/frame haxis=axis2 vaxis=axis1 nolegend;
    run;
* Stopping boundaries on a p-value scale;
axis1 minor=none label=(angle=90 "P-value") order=(0 to 0.03 by 0.01);
axis2 minor=none label=("Sample size per group") order=(0 to 200 by 50);
symbol1 value=dot color=black i=join line=1;
symbol2 value=dot color=black i=join line=20;
proc gplot data=plot3;
    plot PValBoundary*Size=group/frame nolegend;
data plot1;
    set OFPower; group=1;
```

```
data plot2;
    set PPower; group=2;
data plot3;
    set plot1 plot2;
    format Power 3.1 AveSize 4.0;
    run;
* Power functions;
axis1 minor=none label=(angle=90 "Power") order=(0 to 1 by 0.2);
axis2 minor=none label=("True effect size") order=(0 to 0.6 by 0.1);
symbol1 value=none color=black i=join line=1;
symbol2 value=none color=black i=join line=20;
proc gplot data=plot3;
    plot Power*EffSize=group/frame haxis=axis2 vaxis=axis1 nolegend;
    run;
* Average sample size;
axis1 minor=none label=(angle=90 "Average sample size per group")
    order=(0 to 200 by 50);
axis2 minor=none label=("True effect size") order=(0 to 0.6 by 0.1);
symbol1 value=none color=black i=join line=1;
symbol2 value=none color=black i=join line=20;
proc gplot data=plot3;
    plot AveSize*EffSize=group/frame haxis=axis2 vaxis=axis1 nolegend;
    run;
```

Output from Program 4.2

Summary	Value
One-sided Type I error probability	0.025
Power	0.9
True effect size	0.375
Stopping boundary parameter	0.5
Maximum sample size per group	167
Average sample size per group under H0	166
Average sample size per group under H1	111
Fixed sample size per group	150

Analysis	Sample size per group	Stopping boundary (test statistic scale)	Stopping boundary (p-value scale)
1	84	2.2497	0.0122
2	126	2.2497	0.0122
3	167	2.2497	0.0122

Analysis	Stopping probability under H0	Cumulative stopping probability under H0	Stopping probability under H1	Cumulative stopping probability under H1
1	0.0122	0.0122	0.5688	0.5688
2	0.0072	0.0194	0.2173	0.7861
3	0.0056	0.0250	0.1139	0.9000

Output 4.2 summarizes the key characteristics of the Pocock sequential test. A quick comparison with Output 4.1 reveals that the use of the Pocock stopping boundary results in an approximately 10% increase in the maximum sample size (from 153 to 167). The same is also true for the average sample size under the null hypothesis of no treatment effect. On the other hand, we can see from Output 4.1 and Output 4.2 that, under the alternative hypothesis, the average sample sizes per group associated with the O'Brien-Fleming and Pocock plans are 115 and 111, respectively. This means that one should expect to enroll fewer patients in a group sequential trial with the Pocock stopping boundaries when the experimental drug is truly efficacious.

To see why this happens, note from the bottom part of Output 4.2 that the Pocock stopping boundary offers a higher likelihood of early stopping under the alternative hypothesis. The probability of stopping at the first interim analysis equals 57% and is almost twice as high as the one associated with the O'Brien-Fleming stopping boundary (see Output 4.1). As a consequence, group sequential trials with a Pocock boundary are likely to be shorter in duration under H_1.

Figure 4.10 Stopping boundaries of the O'Brien-Fleming (—) and Pocock (- - -) designs on a test statistic scale in the depression trial example

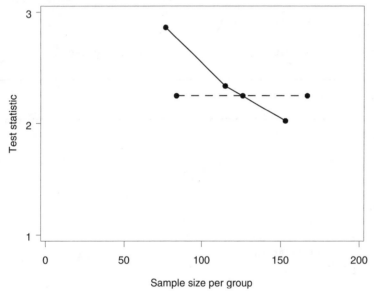

Figure 4.10 shows that the Pocock sequential test relies on adjusted critical values which are constant across the three analyses. An important implication of this property of the Pocock plan is that the Pocock-adjusted critical values are smaller than the O'Brien-Fleming-adjusted critical values early in the trial. This also implies that the Pocock test has less power to detect a significant difference at the final analysis. We can see from Figure 4.11 that, with the Pocock boundary, a one-sided p-value will be declared significant at the scheduled termination point if it is less than 0.0122. The corresponding p-value threshold for the O'Brien-Fleming test is substantially higher, i.e., 0.0215.

Figures 4.12 and 4.13 compare the power and average sample size of the O'Brien-Fleming and Pocock sequential tests. The power curves of the two tests are virtually superimposed and sample size curves are also fairly close to each other. As we have noticed before, the Pocock test requires more patients when the treatment difference is equal to zero compared to the O'Brien-Fleming test and has a slight sample size advantage under the alternative hypothesis (i.e., when the true effect size is 0.375). Overall, the magnitude of this advantage is quite small and one can argue that the Pocock test is generally inferior to the O'Brien-Fleming test in terms of the average sample size when the true effect size is less than its hypothesized value.

Figure 4.11 Stopping boundaries of the O'Brien-Fleming (—) and Pocock (- - -) designs on a *p*-value scale in the depression trial example

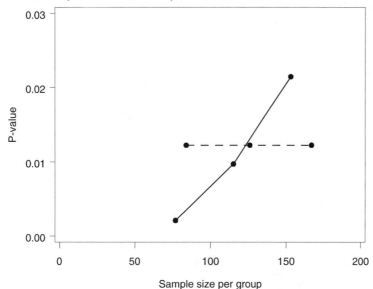

Figure 4.12 Power of the O'Brien-Fleming (—) and Pocock (- - -) tests in the depression trial example

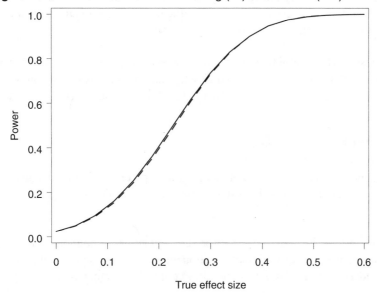

Comparison of Stopping Boundaries

After we have reviewed group sequential plans with Pocock and O'Brien-Fleming stopping boundaries, it is natural to ask for recommendations or rules of thumb on how to pick a set of stopping boundaries for a particular trial. There is really no hard-and-fast rule, and the answer to this question depends heavily on the objectives of the trial. The following is a set of general guidelines that can help us select an appropriate set of stopping boundaries in most clinical trials.

- **Clinical considerations.** The magnitude of the treatment effect observed in a clinical trial needs to be balanced against the size of the sample it was estimated from. Only an absolutely overwhelming treatment difference can justify the termination of a clinical trial after a quarter or a third of the patients have been enrolled. Additionally, as was pointed out in the introduction to this chapter, early stopping of a trial complicates a full characterization of the safety profile of the drug. A decision to

Figure 4.13 Average sample size of the O'Brien-Fleming (—) and Pocock (- - -) tests in the depression trial example

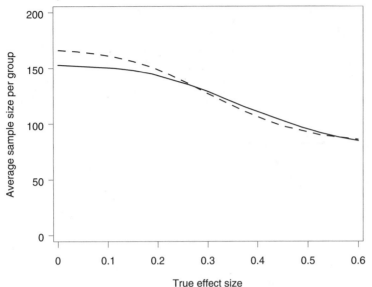

terminate a trial prematurely is clearly undesirable when one wishes to examine the effect of an experimental therapy on multiple safety and secondary efficacy variables in an adequately sized study. To stress this point, Emerson and Fleming (1989) noted that

> A design that suggests early termination only in the presence of extreme evidence for one treatment over another will allow greatest flexibility to examine other response variables or long-term effects while maintaining adequate treatment of the ethical concerns in clinical trials.

Along the same line, O'Brien (1990) indicated that

> One of the disadvantages of early termination is that it may preclude obtaining satisfactory answers to secondary (but nonetheless important) questions pertaining to drug safety and efficacy.

In view of these considerations, it should not be surprising that stopping boundaries are typically chosen to minimize the chances of early trial termination and thus group sequential plans with O'Brien-Fleming boundaries are used more frequently in clinical trials than plans with Pocock boundaries.

- **Sample size considerations.** Another important consideration in a group sequential setting is the average and maximum number of patients that will be enrolled into the trial. It is known that sequential plans based on Pocock boundaries have a smaller average sample size when the true treatment difference is large. Using O'Brien-Fleming boundaries results in a smaller maximum sample size and smaller average sample size under the null hypothesis of no treatment difference. A smaller expected sample size is easily achieved by increasing the probability of early termination. For example, Wang and Tsiatis (1987) studied group sequential tests that minimize the expected sample size under the alternative hypothesis and concluded that the Pocock test is nearly optimal in most practical situations (e.g., in clinical trials powered at 80% and 90%). However, in general, mathematical considerations such as optimization of the average sample size in a group sequential procedure are less important than clinical considerations outlined above.

- **Data management considerations.** Quite often, the first interim analysis is conducted to test the data management process, check compliance and protocol violations, and ensure the quality of the data received by a data monitoring committee. Once it has been verified that the interim data are reliable, a data monitoring committee will have more confidence in the data reported at subsequent interim analyses. In order to avoid early stopping for efficacy at the first interim analysis, one can use the O'Brien-Fleming or similar boundary. Later interim analyses may be designed to detect early evidence of efficacy, in which case the O'Brien-Fleming boundary is again preferable to the Pocock boundary because it maximizes the probability of stopping in the second half of the study if the experimental drug is truly efficacious.

There may be other considerations that determine the choice of a sequential testing plan. For example, in clinical trials with a futility stopping boundary the trial's sponsor would generally hesitate to go for an "early kill" of a drug with a new mechanism of action because it will have negative implications for all drugs in the same class. Because of this, the sponsor will most likely vote for an O'Brien-Fleming-type stopping boundary. On the other hand, it takes less evidence in order to convince clinical researchers to stop developing a drug with a well-understood mechanism of action.

4.2.2 Design Stage: Interim Efficacy and Futility Assessments

Thus far, we have considered group sequential tests for detecting early signs of superior efficacy. A key feature of sequential plans discussed in this section is an option to terminate the trial before its planned end due to apparent futility of the experimental therapy.

Futility monitoring plays a very important role in clinical trials. In a nutshell, a futility test causes the clinical trial to be stopped as soon as it becomes clear that a negative outcome is inevitable and thus it is no longer worthwhile continuing the trial to its completion. As pointed out by Ware, Muller and Braunwald (1985),

> ... early termination for futility could reduce the enormous expenditures of resources, human and financial, involved in the conduct of trials that ultimately provide a negative answer regarding the value of a medical innovation.

For this reason, group sequential plans for assessing the strength of evidence against the alternative hypothesis are used throughout the drug development cycle. They help quickly eliminate weak candidates in early proof-of-concepts studies and minimize the number of patients exposed to ineffective drugs for treating conditions that may be fatal or have irreversible outcomes.

%EffFutDesign Macro

Unlike group sequential plans considered in Section 4.2.1, simultaneous testing of the null and alternative hypotheses requires a specification of a lower boundary that is used for futility assessments. At each interim analysis the test statistic is compared to both the lower and upper boundaries. The trial is terminated if the statistic falls above the upper boundary (the null hypothesis H_0 is rejected) or below the lower boundary (the one-sided alternative hypothesis H_1 is rejected) and continues to the next look otherwise. The stopping boundaries meet at the last look in order to exclude the option to continue the trial.

The lower and upper stopping boundaries are chosen to ensure that the Type I and Type II error probabilities of the group sequential plan are equal to their nominal values α and β. Mathematically, this requirement can be stated as follows. Let δ_1 denote the value of a positive treatment difference δ under the alternative hypothesis. Then

$$P\{\text{Crossing the upper boundary if } \delta = 0\} = \alpha$$

and

$$P\{\text{Crossing the lower boundary if } \delta = \delta_1\} = \beta.$$

If we assume that the lower and upper boundaries belong to the Wang-Tsiatis family of stopping boundaries, it can be shown that these conditions translate into a system of two nonlinear equations for two multiplicative factors (denoted by c_{WT} in Table 4.3). The equations can be solved by performing a search in the two-dimensional space, which can be greatly facilitated by using powerful numerical optimization functions in the SAS/IML library. Once the multiplicative factors have been found, it is easy to determine other characteristics of the group sequential plan, including stopping probabilities, maximum sample size and expected number of patients under the null and alternative hypotheses. See Section 4.2.8 for more details.

The described algorithm is implemented in the %EffFutDesign macro given in the Appendix. The macro supports group sequential designs for testing efficacy and futility of experimental therapies using stopping boundaries from the Wang-Tsiatis family. The %EffFutDesign macro has the same arguments as the %EffDesign macro with the exception of the RHO parameter which is replaced by the following two parameters:

- RHOEFF is the shape parameter of the upper stopping boundary for efficacy testing.
- RHOFUT is the shape parameter of the lower stopping boundary for futility testing.

The RHOFUT parameter is introduced to provide clinical researchers with an ability to independently minimize or maximize the probability of early termination due to futility.

Group Sequential Design for Efficacy and Futility Testing in the Severe Sepsis Trial

Now that we have introduced a tool for implementing simultaneous efficacy/futility testing strategies, we will show how to construct a group sequential plan with efficacy and futility stopping boundaries in the severe sepsis trial. Recall from the introduction to this chapter that the first analysis was intended to be used primarily for futility testing. The trial was to be stopped for efficacy only in the presence of an overwhelming treatment difference. The second analysis was to involve efficacy and futility assessments. A group sequential plan that meets both of these objectives can be set up by using an O'Brien-Fleming stopping boundary for testing the efficacy of the experimental drug and a Pocock boundary for futility analyses. As we showed in Section 4.2.1, it is very difficult to exceed O'Brien-Fleming critical values early in the trial and thus using the O'Brien-Fleming boundary will minimize the chances of establishing superior efficacy at the first interim inspection. Furthermore, this boundary will improve the power of treatment comparisons at the second interim look and the final analysis. On the other hand, using a Pocock stopping boundary for futility assessments ensures that the trial can be terminated early if the observed treatment difference is negative or too small. The described group sequential design is consistent with the principle of futility testing outlined by DeMets and Ware (1980):

> When early evidence suggests the new therapy may be inferior, study termination and acceptance of [the null hypothesis] may be indicated before the statistic reaches a value as extreme as that required to reject [the null hypothesis] in favour of [the alternative hypothesis]. In other words, we are willing to terminate and accept [the null hypothesis] with less evidence that treatment could be harmful than we would require to claim a benefit.

Program 4.3 computes the key characteristics of the described sequential plan by invoking the %EffFutDesign macro. As in the case of sequential designs for testing efficacy, we need to specify design parameters such as the effect size, Type I error rate, power and shape parameters of the stopping boundaries.

First, the two interim analyses were planned to occur after 20% and 66% of the patients had completed the 28-day study period. To pass this information to the %EffFutDesign macro, we will create the SEPTRIAL data set with a single variable that assumes the values 0.2, 0.66 and 1.0:

```
data SepTrial;
    input fraction @@;
    datalines;
    0.2 0.66 1
    ;
```

In order to compute the effect size, let p_1 and p_2 denote the assumed 28-day survival rates in the experimental and placebo groups. In the binary case the effect size θ is given by

$$\theta = \frac{p_1 - p_2}{\sqrt{\overline{p}(1 - \overline{p})}},$$

where $\overline{p} = (p_1 + p_2)/2$. Since $p_1 = 0.76$ and $p_2 = 0.7$, the EFFSIZE parameter will be set to 0.1352. Further, the comparison of survival rates was to be performed at a two-sided significance level of 0.05 with 80% power and therefore we will set the one-sided ALPHA to 0.025 and POWER to 0.8. Finally, we will let RHOEFF=0 to specify an O'Brien-Fleming stopping boundary for efficacy testing and RHOFUT=0.5 to request a Pocock stopping boundary for futility analyses. The %EffFutDesign macro's output will be written to two data sets: BOUNDARY data set (stopping boundaries) and POWER data set (power and average sample size data).

Program 4.3 Group sequential plan for efficacy and futility testing in the severe sepsis trial

```
data SepTrial;
    input fraction @@;
    datalines;
    0.2 0.66 1
    ;
%EffFutDesign(fraction=SepTrial,effsize=0.1352,power=0.8,alpha=0.025,
    rhoeff=0,rhofut=0.5,boundary=Boundary,sizepower=Power);
proc print data=Boundary noobs label;
    var Analysis Size LowerTestStBoundary UpperTestStBoundary
        LowerPValBoundary UpperPValBoundary;
proc print data=Boundary noobs label;
    var Analysis ProbH0 CumProbH0 ProbH1 CumProbH1;
    run;
* Stopping boundaries on a test statistic scale;
axis1 minor=none label=(angle=90 "Test statistic") order=(0 to 5 by 1);
axis2 minor=none label=("Sample size per group") order=(0 to 1200 by 200);
symbol1 value=dot color=black i=join line=1;
symbol2 value=dot color=black i=join line=1;
symbol3 value=circle color=black i=none;
data plot1;
    set Boundary;
    boundary=LowerTestStBoundary;
    group=1;
    keep size boundary group;
data plot2;
    set Boundary;
    boundary=UpperTestStBoundary;
    group=2;
    keep size boundary group;
data plot3;
    size=859; boundary=1.96; group=3;
data plot;
    format boundary 1.0;
    set plot1 plot2 plot3;
```

```
proc gplot data=plot;
    plot boundary*size=group/frame nolegend haxis=axis2 vaxis=axis1;
    run;
* Stopping boundaries on a p-value scale;
axis1 minor=none label=(angle=90 "P-value") order=(0 to 0.5 by 0.1);
axis2 minor=none label=("Sample size per group") order=(0 to 1200 by 200);
symbol1 value=dot color=black i=join line=1;
symbol2 value=dot color=black i=join line=1;
symbol3 value=circle color=black i=none;
data plot1;
    set Boundary;
    boundary=LowerPValBoundary;
    group=1;
    keep size boundary group;
data plot2;
    set Boundary;
    boundary=UpperPValBoundary;
    group=2;
    keep size boundary group;
data plot3;
    size=859; boundary=0.025; group=3;
data plot;
    format boundary 3.1;
    set plot1 plot2 plot3;
proc gplot data=plot;
    plot boundary*size=group/frame nolegend haxis=axis2 vaxis=axis1;
    run;
* Power function;
axis1 minor=none label=(angle=90 "Power") order=(0 to 1 by 0.2);
axis2 minor=none label=("True effect size") order=(0 to 0.25 by 0.05);
symbol1 value=none color=black i=join line=1;
symbol2 value=none color=black i=join line=34;
data plot;
    set Power;
    format Power FixedSamplePower 3.1;
    FixedSampleSize=859; alpha=0.025;
    FixedSamplePower=probnorm(sqrt(FixedSampleSize/2)*EffSize
    -probit(1-alpha));
proc gplot data=plot;
    plot Power*EffSize FixedSamplePower*EffSize/frame overlay
    nolegend haxis=axis2 vaxis=axis1;
    run;
* Average sample size;
axis1 minor=none label=(angle=90 "Average sample size per group")
    order=(0 to 900 by 300);
axis2 minor=none label=("True effect size") order=(0 to 0.25 by 0.05);
symbol1 value=none color=black i=join line=1;
data plot;
    set Power;
    format AveSize 4.0;
proc gplot data=plot;
    plot AveSize*EffSize/frame nolegend haxis=axis2 vaxis=axis1
        vref=859 lvref=34;
    run;
```

Output from Program 4.3

Summary	Value
One-sided Type I error probability	0.025
Power	0.8
True effect size	0.1352
Shape parameter of upper boundary	0
Shape parameter of lower boundary	0.5
Maximum sample size per group	1078
Average sample size per group under H0	464
Average sample size per group under H1	753
Fixed sample size per group	859

Analysis	Sample size per group	Lower stopping boundary (test statistic scale)	Upper stopping boundary (test statistic scale)	Lower stopping boundary (p-value scale)	Upper stopping boundary (p-value scale)
1	216	0.1335	4.1766	0.4469	0.0000
2	711	1.2792	2.2991	0.1004	0.0107
3	1078	1.8678	1.8678	0.0309	0.0309

Analysis	Stopping probability under H0	Cumulative stopping probability under H0	Stopping probability under H1	Cumulative stopping probability under H1
1	0.5531	0.5531	0.1049	0.1049
2	0.3735	0.9266	0.6403	0.7452
3	0.0734	1.0000	0.2548	1.0000

Output 4.3 displays the main characteristics of the group sequential design in the severe sepsis trial. First, let us examine the effect of the futility boundary on the expected sample size under the null and alternative hypotheses. Recall from Output 4.1 that group sequential designs with an O'Brien-Fleming boundary require on average fewer patients than fixed-sample designs when the experimental drug is truly efficacious. This advantage, however, is lost under the null hypothesis. The top panel of Output 4.3 demonstrates that adding a lower stopping boundary completely changes the behavior of O'Brien-Fleming group sequential plans. Because of the possibility of early termination due to futility, the average sample size of the constructed plan equals 464 patients per group under H_0 and is substantially smaller than the fixed-sample size of 859 patients per group. The sequential plan is also superior to the fixed-sample plan under H_1. The only downside of simultaneous efficacy/futility testing strategies is an increased maximum sample size. We see from Output 4.3 that the sequential plan can potentially require 25% more patients than the fixed-sample design (1078 patients per group versus 859 patients per group).

The bottom panel of Output 4.3 (see also Figures 4.14 and 4.15) presents the lower and upper adjusted critical values at the two interim looks and final analysis. As expected, the upper critical value at the first interim inspection is extremely large ($z = 4.1766$) and will be exceeded only if the treatment difference is absolutely phenomenal. The corresponding lower critical value is positive ($z = 0.1335$) and thus the trial will be terminated at the first look with a rejection of H_1 unless the experimental drug demonstrates some degree of efficacy. Due to this choice of the lower critical value, there is a 55.3% chance that the trial will be terminated at this point if the drug does not improve patients' survival. The stringent futility rule is well justified in the sepsis trial because it is ethically unacceptable to expose patients with severe conditions to ineffective therapies. Moving on to the second look, we see that the continuation interval has become much narrower. The experimental drug will be declared futile if it does not meet minimum efficacy requirements (i.e., $z < 1.2792$) or superior to the placebo if the test statistic is greater than 2.2991. Finally, the trial will end with a positive outcome if the final test statistic exceeds 1.8678 or, equivalently, the final p-value is less than 0.0309. Note that this p-value cutoff is greater than the 0.025 cutoff that would have been used in a fixed-sample setting. This happens because early stopping due to futility deflates the overall Type I error probability, and the critical value at the final analysis has to be adjusted upward to keep the one-sided Type I error rate at the 0.025 level. See Chang and Chuang-Stein (2004) for a detailed discussion of this phenomenon.

Figure 4.14 Stopping boundaries of the group sequential design (●) and critical value of the fixed-sample design (○) on a test statistic scale in the severe sepsis trial example

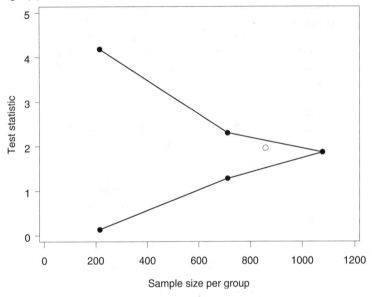

Figure 4.15 Stopping boundaries of the group sequential design (●) and critical value of the fixed-sample design (○) on a p-value scale in the severe sepsis trial example

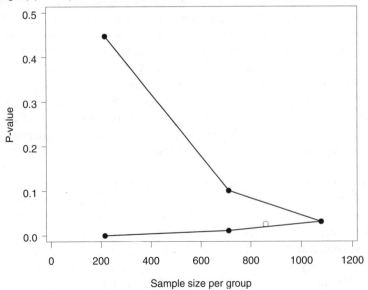

Figures 4.16 and 4.17 depict the relationship between the true effect size and the power and expected sample size (per treatment group) of the group sequential plan in the severe sepsis trial. As in the case of the O'Brien-Fleming plan for detecting superior efficacy, the power function of the constructed sequential plan is virtually identical to the power function of the fixed-sample design. Further, Figure 4.17 shows that the expected sample size of the sequential plan achieves its maximum (754 patients per group) when the effect size is equal to 0.12 and begins to decrease slowly with increasing treatment difference.

Figure 4.16 Power of the group sequential (—) and fixed-sample (···) tests in the severe sepsis trial example

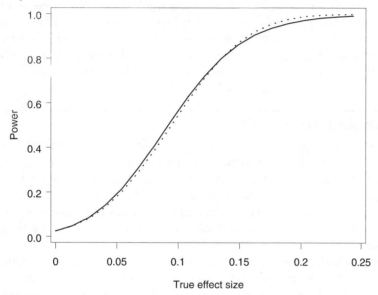

Figure 4.17 Average sample size of the group sequential (—) and fixed-sample (···) tests in the severe sepsis trial example

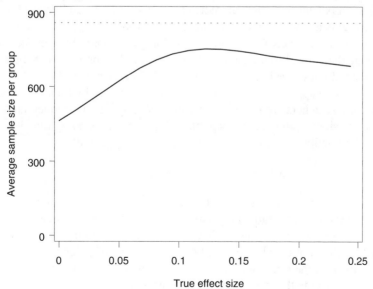

Group Sequential Designs for Efficacy and Futility Testing: Alternative Approaches

As pointed out by Dr. Gordon Lan, the described group sequential approach to simultaneous efficacy and futility testing may have serious fundamental flaws in practice. It was explained in the beginning of this section that the lower stopping boundary for futility testing is driven by the Type II error probability under the alternative hypothesis and thus depends heavily on the assumed value of the effect size, say $\theta = \theta_1$. For example, the lower boundary in the severe sepsis example was computed assuming the effect size was $\theta_1 = 0.1352$ and the boundary's shape will change if a smaller or larger value of θ_1 is used in calculations.

When the experimental drug appears futile and the trial sponsor or members of the data monitoring committee consider early termination due to lack of efficacy, is it still reasonable to assume that the true effect size is θ_1 and is it still reasonable to rely on the futility boundary determined from θ_1? Since the estimated effect size $\widehat{\theta}$ is no longer consistent with θ_1, it is prudent to consider a range of alternatives from $\theta = 0$ to $\theta = \widehat{\theta}$ in order to predict the final outcome of the trial. This approach appears to be more robust than the traditionally used group sequential approach and is closely related to adaptive stochastic curtailment tests that will be introduced in Section 4.3.

4.2.3 Error Spending Approach

There are two approaches to sequential data monitoring in clinical trials. The first one relies on a set of prespecified time points at which the data are reviewed. The Pocock and O'Brien-Fleming stopping boundaries were originally proposed for this type of inspection scheme. An alternative approach was introduced by Lan and DeMets (1983). It is based on an error spending strategy and enables the study sponsor or data monitoring committee to change the timing and frequency of interim looks. Within the error spending framework, interim monitoring follows the philosophical rationale of the design thinking while allowing considerable flexibility.

Why do we need flexibility with respect to timing and frequency of analyses? It is sometimes convenient to tie interim looks to *calendar time* rather than *information time* related to the sample size. Nonpharmaceutical studies often employ interim analyses performed at regular intervals, such as every 3 or 6 months; see, for example, Van Den Berghe et al. (2001). Flexible strategies are also preferable in futility monitoring. From a logistical perspective, it is more convenient to perform futility analyses on a monthly or quarterly basis rather than after a prespecified number of patients have been enrolled into the trial. In this case the number of patients changes unpredictably between looks and one needs to find a way to deal with random increments of information in the data analysis.

This section provides a review of the error spending methodology proposed by Lan and DeMets (1983) and illustrates it using the clinical trial examples from the introduction to this chapter. For a further discussion of the methodology, see Jennison and Turnbull (2000, Chapter 7).

To introduce the error spending approach, consider a two-arm clinical trial with n patients in each treatment group. The clinical researchers are interested in implementing a group sequential design to facilitate the detection of early signs of therapeutic benefit. A Type I error spending function $\alpha(t)$ is a nondecreasing function of the fraction of the total sample size t ($0 \leq t \leq 1$) with

$$\alpha(0) = 0 \text{ and } \alpha(1) = \alpha,$$

where α is the prespecified Type I error rate. Suppose that analyses are performed after $n_1, \ldots, n_m$ patients have been accrued in each of the treatment groups ($n_m = n$ is the total number of patients in each group). It is important to emphasize that interim looks can occur at arbitrary time points and thus $n_1, \ldots, n_m$ are neither prespecified nor equally spaced. Let $t_k = n_k/n$ and Z_k denote the fraction of the total sample size and test statistic at the kth look. The joint distribution of the test statistics is assumed to be multivariate normal. Finally, denote the true treatment difference by δ.

Put simply, the selected error spending function determines the rate at which the overall Type I error probability is spent during the trial. To see how it works, suppose that the first interim look is taken when the sample size in each treatment group is equal to n_1 patients. An upper one-sided critical value, denoted by u_1, is determined in such a way that the amount of Type I error spent equals $\alpha(n_1/n)$, which is equal to $\alpha(t_1)$. In other words, choose u_1 to satisfy the following criterion:

$$P\{Z_1 > u_1 \text{ if } \delta = 0\} = \alpha(t_1).$$

The trial is stopped at the first interim analysis if Z_1 is greater than u_1 and a decision to continue the trial is made otherwise.

Since we have already spent a certain fraction of the overall Type I error at the first analysis, the amount we have left for the second analysis is

$$\alpha(n_2/n) - \alpha(n_1/n) = \alpha(t_2) - \alpha(t_1).$$

Therefore, at the time of the second interim look, the critical value u_2 is obtained by solving the following equation:

$$P\{Z_1 \leq u_1, Z_2 > u_2 \text{ if } \delta = 0\} = \alpha(t_2) - \alpha(t_1).$$

Again, compare Z_2 to u_2 and proceed to the next analysis if Z_2 does not exceed u_2.

Likewise, the critical value u_3 used at the third interim analysis is defined in such a way that

$$P\{Z_1 \leq u_1, Z_2 \leq u_2, Z_3 > u_3 \text{ if } \delta = 0\} = \alpha(t_3) - \alpha(t_2),$$

and a similar argument is applied in order to compute how much Type I error can be spent at each of the subsequent analyses and determine the corresponding critical values $u_4, \ldots, u_m$. It is easy to verify that the overall Type I error associated with the constructed group sequential test is equal to

$$\alpha(t_1) + [\alpha(t_2) - \alpha(t_1)] + [\alpha(t_3) - \alpha(t_2)] + \ldots + [\alpha(t_m) - \alpha(t_{m-1})] = \alpha(t_m),$$

and, by the definition of an α-spending function,

$$\alpha(t_m) = \alpha(1) = \alpha.$$

The described sequential monitoring strategy preserves the overall Type I error rate regardless of the timing and frequency of interim looks.

To reiterate, the Lan-DeMets error spending approach allows for flexible interim monitoring without sacrificing the overall Type I error probability. However, the power of a group sequential trial may be dependent on the chosen monitoring strategy. As demonstrated by Jennison and Turnbull (2000, Section 7.2), the power is generally lower than the target value when the looks are more frequent than anticipated and greater than the target value otherwise. In the extreme cases examined by Jennison and Turnbull, the attained power differed from its nominal value by about 15%.

As shown by Pampallona and Tsiatis (1994) and Pampallona, Tsiatis and Kim (2001),[3] the outlined Type I error spending approach is easily extended to group sequential trials for futility monitoring, in which case a Type II error spending function is introduced, or to simultaneous efficacy and futility monitoring, which requires specification of both Type I and Type II error spending functions.

Finally, it is worth reminding the reader about an important property of the error spending approach. The theoretical properties of this approach hold under the assumption that the timing of future looks is independent of what has been observed in the past. In theory, the overall probability of Type I errors may no longer be preserved if one modifies the sequential testing scheme due to promising findings at one of the interim looks. Several authors have studied the overall Type I error rate of sequential plans in which this assumption is violated. For example, Lan and DeMets (1989) described a realistic scenario in which a large but nonsignificant test statistic at an interim look causes the data monitoring committee to request additional looks at the data. Lan and DeMets showed via simulations that data-dependent changes in the frequency of interim analyses generally have a minimal effect on the overall α level. Further, as pointed

---

[3] Although the paper by Pampallona, Tsiatis and Kim was published in 2001, it was actually written prior to 1994.

out by Proschan, Follman and Waclawiw (1992), the error spending approach provides a certain degree of protection against very frequent looks at the data. The amount of Type I error rate that can be spent at each analysis is roughly proportional to the amount of information accrued since the last look. Even though test statistic is close to the stopping boundary at the current look, there is a good chance it will not cross the boundary at the next look if that is taken immediately after the current one.

Choice of an Error Spending Function

Now that we have introduced the flexible error spending approach developed by Lan and DeMets (1983), we will describe error spending functions commonly used in clinical trial monitoring. We will concentrate on error spending functions for the Type I error (α-spending functions). Type II error spending functions (also known as β-spending functions) are defined in a similar manner.

We will define an exact design-based α-spending function described by Pampallona, Tsiatis and Kim (2001) and, in addition, introduce popular α-spending functions such as a ten-look function and functions proposed by Lan and DeMets (1983), Jennison and Turnbull (1990, 2000) and Hwang, Shih and DeCani (1990). In this section, we will focus mainly on design-based error spending functions. The ten-look, Lan-DeMets, Jennison-Turnbull and Hwang-Shih-DeCani functions are included in the interim monitoring SAS macros defined below in order to enable the reader to reproduce and better understand the results published in the literature.

Design-Based Error Spending Functions

The idea behind a design-based error spending function is that monitoring stopping boundaries should be derived from the same formula as the boundaries used in the design of a group sequential trial. For this reason, it is helpful to think of the monitoring boundaries as an extension of the design boundaries. When designing a group sequential trial, we select the number and timing of interim looks and evaluate the stopping boundaries at the appropriate time points. The resulting boundary is discrete and, to be flexible, a monitoring scheme requires a set of continuous stopping boundaries. To derive continuous boundaries, we convert the stopping boundary specified at the design stage into an error spending function and then use this function to generate adjusted critical values at arbitrary time points.[4]

As an illustration, consider the clinical depression trial example. This example was used in Section 4.2.1 to introduce O'Brien-Fleming and Pocock group sequential designs. It is easy to compute error spending functions associated with the O'Brien-Fleming and Pocock stopping boundaries. As shown in Output 4.1, the cumulative stopping probabilities under H_0 of an O'Brien-Fleming group sequential design are equal to 0.0021, 0.0105 and 0.025. This means that the O'Brien-Fleming test spends 8.4% (= 0.0021/0.025) of the overall Type I error by the first analysis and 42.0% (= 0.0105/0.025) by the second analysis. All of the Type I error is spent by the time the trial reaches the final analysis. The three percentages (8.4%, 42.0% and 100%) define the α-spending function for this particular design. Similar calculations show that the design-based α-spending function for the Pocock design is defined by 48.8%, 77.6% and 100%. The two α-spending functions are plotted in Figure 4.18.

Ten-Look Error Spending Functions

While a design-based error spending function is specific to each particular sequential plan, a ten-look function is derived from a sequential plan with ten equally spaced interim analyses (this number is fixed) and the stopping boundary that was used in the original group sequential plan (Pampallona, Tsiatis and Kim, 2001). For example, if we size a group sequential trial using a Pocock boundary, the ten-look method will generate an error spending function associated with a ten-look Pocock plan.

Figure 4.19 compares the α-spending functions generated by the design-based and ten-look methods in the clinical depression trial example. We can see from the figure that the two methods generate similar error spending functions under an O'Brien-Fleming design but the ten-look function is quite different from the design-based function in the case of a Pocock design. If we are interested in implementing a Pocock design, the ten-look method will lead to a much faster spending of the Type I error rate

---

[4]In the case of simultaneous monitoring of efficacy and futility, the prespecified stopping boundaries are converted into α- and β-spending functions.

Figure 4.18 Design-based α-spending functions in the depression trial example, O'Brien-Fleming plan (—), Pocock plan (- - -)

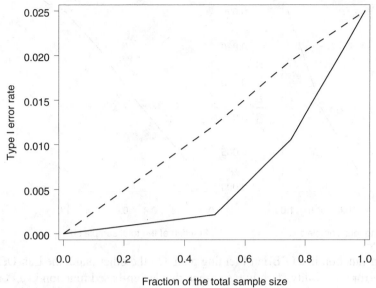

Figure 4.19 Design-based (—) and ten-look ($\cdots$) α-spending functions in the depression trial example. Left-hand panel: O'Brien-Fleming plan; right-hand panel: Pocock plan

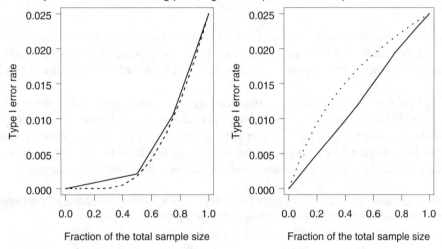

compared to the design-based method. In other words, in the depression trial example the ten-look approach will be more likely to trigger an early trial termination than the design-based approach.

Lan-DeMets Family of Error Spending Functions

Lan and DeMets (1983) introduced two functions that approximate the α-spending functions associated with the O'Brien-Fleming and Pocock sequential plans. For any prespecified overall Type I error probability α, the functions are given by

$$\alpha(t) = 2 - 2\Phi(z_{1-\alpha/2}/\sqrt{t}) \text{ (O'Brien-Fleming test),}$$

$$\alpha(t) = \alpha \ln(1 + (e - 1)t) \text{ (Pocock test),}$$

where $\Phi(x)$ is the cumulative probability function of the standard normal distribution. The two functions are depicted in Figure 4.20. It is evident from Figure 4.20 that the use of the Lan-DeMets α-spending function will result in less Type I error probability spent early in the trial compared to the

Figure 4.20 Design-based (—) and Lan-DeMets (· · ·) α-spending functions in the depression trial example. Left-hand panel: O'Brien-Fleming plan; right-hand panel: Pocock plan

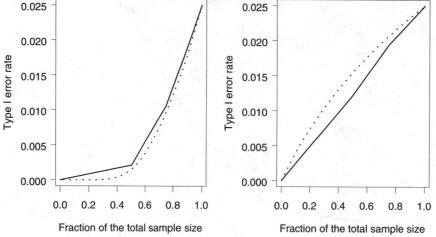

design-based α-spending function in a O'Brien-Fleming plan. On the other hand, the Lan-DeMets function spends Type I error probability slightly faster than the design-based function in a Pocock plan.

Jennison-Turnbull Family of Error Spending Functions

Jennison and Turnbull (1990, 2000)[5] studied a family of α-spending functions given by

$$\alpha(t) = \alpha t^\rho,$$

where ρ is a positive number. Larger values of the ρ parameter correspond to functions with a lower Type I error spending rate in the beginning of the trial. Conversely, selecting a small ρ results in a function that spends a significant amount of the overall Type I error early in the trial and quickly plateaus.

Jennison and Turnbull (1990) pointed out that stopping boundaries generated by the α-spending function with $\rho = 3$ closely mimic O'Brien-Fleming boundaries. A good approximation to Pocock boundaries is obtained when ρ is set to 1. A plot of the Jennison and Turnbull α-spending functions with $\rho = 1$ and $\rho = 3$ (see Figure 4.21) reveals that these spending functions provide a very good approximation to the design-based α-spending functions in the depression trial example.

Figure 4.21 Design-based (—) and Jennison-Turnbull (· · ·) α-spending functions in the depression trial example. Left-hand panel: O'Brien-Fleming plan; right-hand panel: Pocock plan

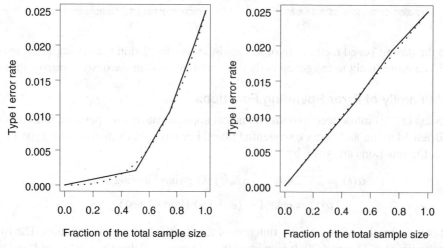

---

[5]Dr. KyungMann Kim introduced this family in his Ph.D. dissertation in 1986 at the University of Wisconsin at Madison.

Hwang-Shih-DeCani Family of Error Spending Functions

Another popular family of α-spending functions was introduced by Hwang, Shih and DeCani (1990). This family is based on truncated exponential distributions and is defined as follows:

$$\alpha(t) = \frac{\alpha(1 - e^{-\rho t})}{(1 - e^{-\rho})} \text{ if } \rho \neq 0,$$
$$= \alpha t \text{ if } \rho = 0.$$

Hwang, Shih and DeCani (1990) showed that two members of the family provide a close approximation to the α-spending functions for the O'Brien-Fleming and Pocock sequential plans. O'Brien-Fleming stopping boundaries are best approximated when $\rho = -4$ or $\rho = -5$ and the ρ parameter of 1 generates stopping boundaries that are similar to Pocock boundaries. Figure 4.22 depicts the design-based and Hwang-Shih-DeCani α-spending functions with $\rho = -4$ and $\rho = 1$.

Figure 4.22 Design-based (—) and Hwang-Shih-DeCani ($\cdots$) α-spending functions in the depression trial example. Left-hand panel: O'Brien-Fleming plan; right-hand panel: Pocock plan

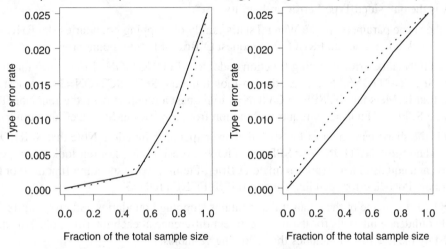

Comparison of Error Spending Functions

When comparing error spending functions available to clinical researchers, it is important to keep in mind that an error spending function used at the monitoring stage needs to be consistent with the group sequential plan chosen at the design stage.

To illustrate this point, recall from Output 4.2 that the Pocock critical value at the first interim look in the depression trial example is 2.2497. The corresponding critical value from the Lan-DeMets error spending function equals 2.1570 and is clearly inconsistent with the critical value specified in the original trial design. Although the likelihood of this outcome is rather small, it is conceivable that a test statistic computed at the first look is not significant with respect to the prespecified Pocock stopping boundary but exceeds the critical value computed from the Lan-DeMets error spending function. This discrepancy can potentially undermine the credibility of sequential inferences in a clinical trial. In order to avoid discrepancies of this kind, it is advisable to implement sequential monitoring using a design-based error spending function.

4.2.4   Monitoring Stage: Interim Efficacy Assessments

%EffMonitor Macro

The %EffMonitor macro, provided in the Appendix, has been developed to facilitate group sequential monitoring of clinical trials designed for early detection of a superior treatment effect. The macro supports the five types of α-spending functions defined in the previous subsection and a variety of other useful features, including repeated confidence intervals and bias-adjusted point estimates that will be described later in Sections 4.2.6 and 4.2.7.

The %EffMonitor macro has the following arguments (most of the arguments are identical to those in the %EffDesign and %EffFutDesign macros defined in Sections 4.2.1 and 4.2.2):

- FRACTION is the name of the input data set that contains fractions of the total sample size accrued at successive analyses.
- DATA is the name of the input data set containing summary statistics computed at each analysis (with one record per analysis). The %EffMonitor macro requires that this data set include the following two variables:
  - N is the number of patients in each treatment group (or the average of the numbers of patients if they are not the same).
  - STAT is the value of a normally distributed test statistic.
- EFFSIZE is the hypothesized effect size (the treatment difference divided by the standard deviation).
- POWER is the power of the group sequential plan.
- ALPHA is the one-sided Type I error probability.
- RHO is the shape parameter in the Wang-Tsiatis family of stopping boundaries (let RHO=0.5 to request Pocock boundaries and RHO=0 to request O'Brien-Fleming boundaries).
- SPFUNCTION is the error spending function code (let SPFUNCTION=1 to request the design-based function, SPFUNCTION=2 to request the ten-look function, SPFUNCTION=3 to request a function from the Lan-DeMets family, SPFUNCTION=4 to request a function from the Jennison-Turnbull family, and SPFUNCTION=5 to request a function from the Hwang-Shih-DeCani family).
- SPRHO is the shape parameter of the specified error spending function. Note that SPRHO is not required when SPFUNCTION=1 or SPFUNCTION=2 (design-based or ten-look error spending functions) and equals either 0 (approximate O'Brien-Fleming error spending function) or 0.5 (approximate Pocock error spending function) if SPFUNCTION=3.
- DECISION is the name of the data set that contains stopping boundaries and probabilities as well as repeated confidence intervals for the true treatment difference at each interim look. This data set is generated by the macro and includes the following variables:
  - ANALYSIS is the analysis number.
  - SIZE is the sample size per group.
  - FRACTION is the fraction of the total sample size.
  - TESTSTATISTIC is the computed test statistic.
  - PVALUE is the associated *p*-value.
  - TESTSTBOUNDARY is the stopping boundary on the test statistic scale.
  - PVALBOUNDARY is the stopping boundary on the *p*-value scale.
  - LOWERLIMIT is the lower limit of a one-sided repeated confidence interval for the standardized treatment difference (see Section 4.2.6 for more details).
  - DECISION is the decision reached at the current analysis ('Continue' or 'Reject H0').
- INFERENCE is the name of the data set containing the bias-adjusted estimate of the treatment effect with associated confidence limits computed at the last look (bias-adjusted estimates and confidence limits will be introduced in Section 4.2.7). This data set is generated by the macro.

Efficacy Monitoring in the Depression Trial Using an O'Brien-Fleming Plan

Having defined the %EffMonitor macro, we are now ready to discuss group sequential monitoring of the clinical trial in patients with clinical depression. Since stopping boundaries are defined on either a test statistic or *p*-value scale, we will begin with computing a normally distributed statistic and associated *p*-value at each of the interim looks.

Consider the following z statistic for testing the null hypothesis of no treatment difference

$$Z_k = \frac{(\overline{X}_{1k} - \overline{X}_{2k})}{s_k \sqrt{1/n_{1k} + 1/n_{2k}}},$$

where n_{1k} and $\overline{X}_{1k}$ (n_{2k} and $\overline{X}_{2k}$) denote the number of patients and sample mean in the experimental (placebo) group at the kth interim look. Also, s_k is the pooled standard deviation, i.e.,

$$s_k = \sqrt{\frac{(n_{1k} - 1)s_{1k}^2 + (n_{2k} - 1)s_{2k}^2}{n_{1k} + n_{2k} - 2}},$$

with s_{1k} and s_{2k} denoting the standard deviations of HAMD17 changes from baseline in the experimental and placebo groups, respectively, at the kth interim analysis.

It is important to note that we are by no means restricted to statistics from the two-sample z-test. The decision-making process described below can be used with any normally or nearly normally distributed test statistic, such as a test statistic from an ANOVA model with multiple terms representing important prognostic factors.

Since Z_k is normally distributed, a one-sided p-value for testing the superiority of the experimental drug to the placebo at the kth look is given by

$$p_k = 1 - \Phi(Z_k).$$

Program 4.4 uses the formulas displayed above to compute the z statistics and p-values from the mean HAMD17 changes and associated standard deviations presented in Table 4.1.

Program 4.4 Test statistics and associated p-values in the depression trial example

```
data DepTrialData;
    input n1 mean1 sd1 n2 mean2 sd2;
    datalines;
     78 8.3 6.2  78 5.9 6.5
    122 8.0 6.3 120 6.3 5.9
    150 8.2 5.9 152 6.1 5.8
    ;
data teststat;
    set DepTrialData;
    format stat p 6.4;
    n=(n1+n2)/2;
    s=sqrt(((n1-1)*sd1*sd1+(n2-1)*sd2*sd2)/(n1+n2-2));
    stat=(mean1-mean2)/(s*sqrt(1/n1+1/n2));
    p=1-probnorm(stat);
    label n="Sample size"
          stat="Z statistic"
          p="P-value";
    keep n stat p;
proc print data=teststat noobs label;
    var n stat p;
    run;
```

Output from Program 4.4

Sample size	Z statistic	P-value
78	2.3597	0.0091
121	2.1659	0.0152
151	3.1192	0.0009

Output 4.4 displays the sample sizes, test statistics and associated *p*-values at the three looks in the depression trial. The test statistics are highly significant at any of the three inspections; however, it remains to be seen whether or not the *z* statistics will stay significant after a proper adjustment for multiple analyses. In what follows we will examine adjustments based on the O'Brien-Fleming and Pocock group sequential plans.

Program 4.5 performs group sequential monitoring of the depression trial using an O'Brien-Fleming approach. The program relies on the %EffMonitor macro and, in order to call this macro, we will need to provide information about the trial design, chosen group sequential plan and interim monitoring strategy.

First, the FRACTION parameter will be set to the DEPTRIAL data set used in Program 4.1. This data set contains fractions of the total sample size corresponding to the three looks specified in the O'Brien-Fleming group sequential plan. Note that we don't have to perform interim analyses at the scheduled times. The error spending methodology enables us to examine the data at arbitrary time points and the information about the scheduled looks will be used only for computing the design-based α-spending function and maximum sample size.

Program 4.5 Efficacy monitoring in the depression trial using an O'Brien-Fleming group sequential plan

```
data DepTrial;
    input fraction @@;
    datalines;
    0.5 0.75 1
    ;

* First interim analysis;
data stat;
    set teststat;
    if _n_=1;
    keep n stat;
%EffMonitor(fraction=DepTrial,data=stat,effsize=0.375,power=0.9,
    alpha=0.025,rho=0,spfunction=1,sprho=0,decision=OFdecision,
    inference=OFinference);
proc print data=OFdecision noobs label;
    var Analysis TestStatistic Pvalue TestStBoundary PValBoundary Decision;

* Second interim analysis;
data stat;
    set teststat;
    if _n_<=2;
    keep n stat;
%EffMonitor(fraction=DepTrial,data=stat,effsize=0.375,power=0.9,
    alpha=0.025,rho=0,spfunction=1,sprho=0,decision=OFdecision,
    inference=OFinference);
proc print data=OFdecision noobs label;
    var Analysis TestStatistic Pvalue TestStBoundary PValBoundary Decision;

* Final analysis;
data stat;
    set teststat;
    keep n stat;
%EffMonitor(fraction=DepTrial,data=stat,effsize=0.375,power=0.9,
    alpha=0.025,rho=0,spfunction=1,sprho=0,decision=OFdecision,
    inference=OFinference);
proc print data=OFdecision noobs label;
    var Analysis TestStatistic Pvalue TestStBoundary PValBoundary Decision;
    run;
```

The %EffMonitor macro also requires a data set containing the test statistics and average sample sizes at each interim look. This information will be passed to the macro in the TESTSTAT data set created by Program 4.4. After that, we need to set the EFFSIZE, POWER and ALPHA parameters, referring to the effect size, power and one-sided significance level, to 0.375, 0.9 and 0.025, respectively. The RHO parameter will be set to 0 in order to request an O'Brien-Fleming design boundary.

The SPFUNCTION and SPRHO parameters describe the α-spending function that will be used to generate stopping boundaries during sequential monitoring. To save space, we will concentrate on the design-based error spending function and let SPFUNCTION=1 (note that the SPRHO parameter is not used in the computation of the design-based function and will be set to an arbitrary value).[6]

Lastly, we will let DECISION=OFDECISION and INFERENCE=OFINFERENCE to save the stopping boundaries and repeated confidence intervals for the true treatment difference at each interim look in the OFDECISION data set and the bias-adjusted estimate of the treatment difference in the OFINFERENCE data set. The repeated confidence intervals and bias-adjusted estimate of the treatment effect will be discussed later in Sections 4.2.6 and 4.2.7.

Output from Program 4.5 (First interim analysis)

Analysis	Test statistic	P-value	Stopping boundary (test statistic scale)	Stopping boundary (p-value scale)	Decision
1	2.3597	0.0091	2.8127	0.0025	Continue

Output 4.5 (First interim analysis) lists the observed z statistic and p-value along with the adjusted critical value and adjusted p-value cutoff computed from the design-based error spending function at the first interim look. The z statistic (2.3597) clearly lies below the stopping boundary (2.8127), which indicates that the design-based stopping boundary has not been crossed. As a result, the trial will continue to the next interim look.

Output from Program 4.5 (Second interim analysis)

Analysis	Test statistic	P-value	Stopping boundary (test statistic scale)	Stopping boundary (p-value scale)	Decision
1	2.3597	0.0091	2.8127	0.0025	Continue
2	2.1659	0.0152	2.2561	0.0120	Continue

Output 4.5 (Second interim analysis) displays the stopping boundaries computed at the first and second interim looks. The stopping boundary at the second look is 2.2561. Again, although the z statistic (which is equal to 2.1659) is clearly significant at a one-sided 0.025 level, it is not large enough to cross the stopping boundary. This implies that more evidence needs to be gathered before the experimental drug can be declared superior to placebo with respect to its effect on the HAMD17 total score, and the trial will be continued to the final analysis.

---

[6]Other error spending functions corresponding to the O'Brien-Fleming plan can be requested in a similar manner. For example, let SPFUNCTION=3 and SPRHO=0 to specify a Lan-DeMets error spending function or let SPFUNCTION=4 and SPRHO=3 to request a Jennison-Turnbull error spending function.

Output from Program 4.5 (Final analysis)

Analysis	Test statistic	P-value	Stopping boundary (test statistic scale)	Stopping boundary (p-value scale)	Decision
1	2.3597	0.0091	2.8127	0.0025	Continue
2	2.1659	0.0152	2.2561	0.0120	Continue
3	3.1192	0.0009	2.0546	0.0200	Reject H0

Output 4.5 (Final analysis) shows that the stopping boundary has been crossed at the final analysis and therefore we conclude that the mean treatment difference in HAMD17 changes is significantly different from zero at a one-sided 0.025 level.

As was noted before, one of the attractive features of O'Brien-Fleming sequential plans is that they spend very little Type I error probability early in the trial and thus the final analysis is performed at a significance level that is only marginally smaller than the corresponding unadjusted significance level. Indeed, we can see from Output 4.5 that the *p*-value cutoff at the final look (0.02) is only 20% lower than the cutoff of 0.025 that would have been used in a nonsequential setting. With a Pocock boundary, we should normally expect a much larger difference between the adjusted and unadjusted cutoff values.

Figure 4.23 depicts the O'Brien-Fleming monitoring boundary on a test statistic scale. The patient enrollment continues as long as the dots representing the observed *z* statistics lie below the monitoring boundary (solid curve). The dashed curve is the O'Brien-Fleming stopping boundary that was computed at the design stage (it is the same boundary that was depicted in Figure 4.6). Although the monitoring boundary was derived from the O'Brien-Fleming plan selected at the design stage, this boundary is not identical to the design boundary. The monitoring boundary has been adjusted to account for deviations from the inspection times specified in the original sequential plan.

Figure 4.23 Efficacy monitoring in the depression trial using an O'Brien-Fleming group sequential plan, observed *z* statistics (●), design stopping boundary (- - -), monitoring stopping boundary (—)

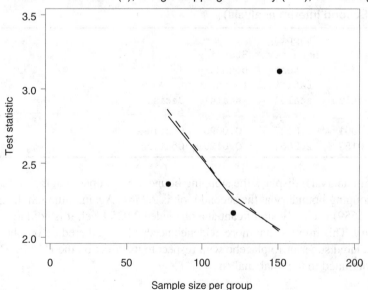

Efficacy Monitoring in the Depression Trial Using a Pocock Plan

It will be interesting to compare the O'Brien-Fleming monitoring strategy we considered in the preceding subsection to a strategy based on a Pocock group sequential plan. In order to request the

Pocock plan, one needs to change the RHO parameter in Program 4.5 to 0.5.[7] Program 4.6 performs sequential monitoring of the depression trial using a Pocock stopping boundary.

Program 4.6 Efficacy monitoring in the depression trial using a Pocock group sequential plan

```
* First interim analysis;
data stat;
    set teststat;
    if _n_=1;
    keep n stat;
%EffMonitor(fraction=DepTrial,data=stat,effsize=0.375,power=0.9,
    alpha=0.025,rho=0.5,spfunction=1,sprho=0,decision=OFdecision,
    inference=OFinference);
proc print data=OFdecision noobs label;
    var Analysis TestStatistic Pvalue TestStBoundary PValBoundary Decision;
    run;
```

Output from Program 4.6

Analysis	Test statistic	P-value	Stopping boundary (test statistic scale)	Stopping boundary (p-value scale)	Decision
1	2.3597	0.0091	2.2758	0.0114	Reject H0

Output 4.6 shows that the treatment difference turns out to be significant after only 156 patients have completed the trial. The z statistic at the first interim look equals 2.3597 and therefore exceeds the adjusted critical value generated by the design-based error spending function (2.2758). The observed inconsistency between the O'Brien-Fleming and Pocock decision functions is not completely unexpected. Pocock stopping boundaries are known to be anti-conservative at the early interim looks and are likely to lead to a rejection of the null hypothesis as soon as the raw p-value falls below 0.01.

4.2.5   Monitoring Stage: Interim Efficacy and Futility Assessments

In this section we will show how to extend the error spending methodology introduced in Section 4.2.4 to the case of simultaneous efficacy/futility monitoring. The extension is based on the ideas presented by Pampallona and Tsiatis (1994) and Pampallona, Tsiatis and Kim (2001). Recall that the efficacy-monitoring strategies of Section 4.2.4 rely on the original Lan-DeMets method of a flexible control of the Type I error rate. To successfully implement sequential monitoring in trials with early stopping in favor of H_0 or H_1, one needs to find a mechanism for controlling the probability of both false-positive and false-negative outcomes. It seems natural to introduce two types of error spending functions. An α-spending function determines what fraction of the overall Type I error probability can be "consumed" at an interim analysis, whereas a β-spending function controls the rate at which the Type II error probability is spent. The lower and upper critical values are computed at each interim look from the prespecified α- and β-spending functions using a method similar to that described in the beginning of Section 4.2.4.

The described Type I and Type II error spending approach is implemented in the %EffFutMonitor macro provided in the Appendix. In order to call this macro, one needs to specify the same parameters

---

[7]The SPRHO parameter may need to be changed as well when using Lan-DeMets, Jennison-Turnbull or Hwang-Shih-DeCani error spending functions. For example, to specify a Lan-DeMets error spending function corresponding to the Pocock plan, let SPFUNCTION=3 and SPRHO=0.5.

as in the %EffMonitor macro. The only difference between the two macros is that %EffFutMonitor requires two shape parameters to define the lower and upper stopping boundaries. The RHOEFF parameter determines the shape of the upper stopping boundary for efficacy testing and RHOFUT is the shape parameter of the lower stopping boundary for futility testing.

Efficacy and Futility Monitoring in the Severe Sepsis Trial

To illustrate simultaneous efficacy/futility monitoring in a clinical trial setting, we will come back to the severe sepsis example. First, we will need to compute the unadjusted z statistics (as well as associated p-values) for testing the null hypothesis of no drug effect at each of the two interim analyses. The z statistic for the comparison of survival rates p_{1k} (experimental group) and p_{2k} (placebo group) at the kth analysis is given by

$$Z_k = \frac{p_{1k} - p_{2k}}{\sqrt{\overline{p}_k(1 - \overline{p}_k)(1/n_{1k} + 1/n_{2k})}},$$

where $\overline{p}_k = (p_{1k} + p_{2k})/2$. The associated p-value is $p_k = 1 - \Phi(Z_k)$.

Program 4.7 computes the unadjusted z statistics and p-values from the 28-day survival data summarized in Table 4.2.

Program 4.7 Test statistics and associated p-values in the severe sepsis trial example

```
data SepTrialData;
    input n1 alive1 n2 alive2;
    datalines;
    220 164 216 152
    715 538 715 526
    ;
data teststat;
    set SepTrialData;
    format stat p 6.4;
    n=(n1+n2)/2;
    p1=alive1/n1; p2=alive2/n2;
    pave=(p1+p2)/2;
    s=sqrt(pave*(1-pave)*(1/n1+1/n2));
    stat=(p1-p2)/s;
    p=1-probnorm(stat);
    label n="Sample size"
          stat="Z statistic"
          p="P-value";
    keep n stat p;
proc print data=teststat noobs label;
    var n stat p;
    run;
```

Output from Program 4.7

Sample size	Z statistic	P-value
218	0.9757	0.1646
715	0.7272	0.2336

Output 4.7 demonstrates that the test statistics are far from being significant at either of the two analyses and suggests that the experimental drug may be futile. To see whether these findings warrant an early termination due to lack of treatment benefit, we will perform group sequential monitoring based on the design considered in Section 4.2.2.

The process of efficacy/futility monitoring is illustrated in Program 4.8. The program calls the %EffFutMonitor macro with the following parameters:

- FRACTION parameter specifies the name of the data set containing fractions of the total sample size corresponding to the three looks specified in the original group sequential plan. We will set this parameter to the SEPTRIAL data set used in Program 4.3. Just as in the case of efficacy monitoring, this information will be used only for computing the design-based α- and β-spending functions and maximum sample size of the group sequential plan.

- DATA parameter will be set to the name of the data set containing z statistics and p-values computed at the two interim looks.

- EFFSIZE, POWER and ALPHA parameters are set to 0.1352, 0.8 and 0.025, respectively.

- RHOEFF parameter will be set to 0 to request an O'Brien-Fleming boundary for efficacy analyses.

- RHOFUT parameter will be set to 0.5 to tell the macro that a Pocock boundary will be used in futility tests.

- SPFUNCTION and SPRHO parameters. We will use SPFUNCTION=1 to request design-based Type I and Type II error spending functions. As before, the SPRHO parameter is set to an arbitrary value because it is not used in the computation of design-based functions.

- DECISION and INFERENCE parameters. Let DECISION=DECISION and INFERENCE=INFERENCE to save the monitoring boundaries and repeated confidence intervals in the DECISION data set and the bias-adjusted estimate of the treatment difference in the INFERENCE data set.

Program 4.8 Efficacy and futility monitoring in the severe sepsis trial

```
data SepTrial;
    input fraction @@;
    datalines;
    0.2 0.66 1
    ;

* First interim analysis;
data stat;
    set teststat;
    if _n_=1;
    keep n stat;
%EffFutMonitor(fraction=SepTrial,data=stat,effsize=0.1352,power=0.8,
    alpha=0.025,rhoeff=0,rhofut=0.5,spfunction=1,sprho=1,
    decision=decision,inference=inference);
proc print data=decision noobs label;
    var Analysis TestStatistic LowerTestStBoundary UpperTestStBoundary
    Decision;
proc print data=decision noobs label;
    var Analysis PValue LowerPValBoundary UpperPValBoundary Decision;

* Second interim analysis;
data stat;
    set teststat;
    if _n_=2;
    keep n stat;
%EffFutMonitor(fraction=SepTrial,data=stat,effsize=0.1352,power=0.8,
    alpha=0.025,rhoeff=0,rhofut=0.5,spfunction=1,sprho=1,
    decision=decision,inference=inference);
```

```
proc print data=decision noobs label;
    var Analysis TestStatistic LowerTestStBoundary UpperTestStBoundary
    Decision;
proc print data=decision noobs label;
    var Analysis PValue LowerPValBoundary UpperPValBoundary Decision;
    run;
```

Output from Program 4.8 (First interim analysis)

Analysis	Test statistic	Lower stopping boundary (test statistic scale)	Upper stopping boundary (test statistic scale)	Decision
1	0.9757	0.1438	3.8162	Continue

Analysis	P-value	Lower stopping boundary (p-value scale)	Upper stopping boundary (p-value scale)	Decision
1	0.1646	0.4428	0.0001	Continue

Output 4.8 (First interim analysis) displays the z statistic and p-value computed at the first look as well as the lower and upper boundaries on the test statistic and p-value scales. We see that the test statistic falls between the lower and upper critical values (0.1438 and 3.8162) and thus the trial will need to continue to the second interim analysis.

Output from Program 4.8 (Second interim analysis)

Analysis	Test statistic	Lower stopping boundary (test statistic scale)	Upper stopping boundary (test statistic scale)	Decision
1	0.9757	0.1438	3.8162	Continue
2	0.7272	1.2884	2.2935	Reject H1

Analysis	P-value	Lower stopping boundary (p-value scale)	Upper stopping boundary (p-value scale)	Decision
1	0.1646	0.4428	0.0001	Continue
2	0.2336	0.0988	0.0109	Reject H1

Output 4.8 (Second interim analysis) shows the derived stopping boundaries at the first and second looks. As was noted in Section 4.2.2, the continuation interval at the second analysis is much narrower than that computed at the first analysis. It is evident that the z statistic (0.7272) is not large enough to

exceed the lower critical value at the second analysis (1.2884) and, as a consequence, the trial will be terminated at this point due to lack of therapeutic benefit.

4.2.6 Repeated Confidence Intervals

It has been pointed out before that an analysis of clinical trial data in a sequential manner is likely to greatly increase the overall Type I error rate and thus one needs to adjust the critical values upward at each interim look. For the same reason, one should avoid using naive (unadjusted) confidence intervals in group sequential trials. Mathematically, unadjusted confidence intervals are too narrow to achieve the nominal coverage probability at multiple interim analyses. In order to alleviate this problem, Jennison and Turnbull (1989) proposed a simple method for adjusting the width of confidence intervals to increase the joint coverage probability under any sequential monitoring scheme. The resulting confidence intervals are known as *repeated confidence intervals.*

To define repeated confidence intervals, consider a group sequential trial with m looks. Suppose that a study is conducted to test the two-sided hypothesis that the true treatment difference δ is equal to 0 (the treatment difference can be defined as a difference in means or a difference in proportions). Let $\widehat{\delta}_k$ and s_k denote the estimate of the treatment difference and its standard error at the kth look, respectively. In the repeated significance testing framework, the test statistic

$$Z_k = \widehat{\delta}_k / s_k$$

is compared to the lower and upper adjusted critical values l_k and u_k chosen in such a way that the probability of crossing the stopping boundaries does not exceed α under the null hypothesis of no treatment effect:

$$P\{Z_k < l_k \text{ or } Z_k > u_k \text{ for any } k = 1, \ldots, m \text{ if } \delta = 0\} = \alpha.$$

Jennison and Turnbull (1989) demonstrated that it is easy to invert this testing procedure in order to compute confidence intervals for the unknown treatment difference at each of the interim analyses. The repeated confidence intervals for δ are given by

$$CI_k = (\widehat{\delta}_k - u_k s_k, \widehat{\delta}_k - l_k s_k), \quad k = 1, \ldots, m,$$

and possess the following important property.[8] By the definition of the adjusted critical values, the *joint* coverage probability of the repeated confidence intervals is greater than or equal to $1 - \alpha$; i.e.,

$$P\{\widehat{\delta}_k - u_k s_k \le \delta \le \widehat{\delta}_k - l_k s_k \text{ for all } k = 1, \ldots, m\} \ge 1 - \alpha,$$

regardless of the choice of stopping boundaries or any other aspects of a sequential monitoring scheme. As pointed out by Jennison and Turnbull (2000, Chapter 9), this immediately implies that the constructed confidence intervals are valid under any group sequential plan. Indeed, for any random stopping time τ, the coverage probability is always maintained at the same level:

$$P\{\widehat{\delta}_\tau - u_\tau s_\tau \le \delta \le \widehat{\delta}_\tau - l_\tau s_\tau\} \ge 1 - \alpha.$$

Repeated confidence intervals in group sequential trials with a single upper boundary are defined in a similar manner. They are chosen to satisfy the following property:

$$P\{\widehat{\delta}_k - u_k s_k \le \delta \text{ for all } k = 1, \ldots, m\} \ge 1 - \alpha.$$

---

[8]To see why the *lower* limit of the confidence intervals is based on the *upper* stopping boundary and vice versa, note that the confidence intervals are defined to be consistent with the group sequential decision rule. For example, H_0 is rejected if $Z_k > u_k$, which implies that $\widehat{\delta}_k - u_k s_k > 0$. In other words, the lower confidence limit for the treatment difference excludes 0 when the group sequential test rejects the null hypothesis of no treatment difference. Likewise, $Z_k < l_k$ implies that the confidence interval lies completely below 0.

Repeated confidence intervals can be used in any group sequential design with both prespecified and flexible interim analyses. Unlike other types of confidence intervals which can be used only after the study has been stopped (see Section 4.2.7), repeated confidence intervals can be computed at each interim look and greatly facilitate the interpretation of interim findings.

Repeated confidence intervals are introduced to maintain the nominal coverage probability in group sequential trials and therefore they are wider than regular confidence intervals. The width of a repeated confidence interval depends on the selected sequential monitoring strategy. Jennison and Turnbull (1989) showed that in a clinical trial with five looks a 90% repeated confidence interval associated with the Pocock stopping boundary is 29% wider than a naive confidence interval with the same coverage probability. The width ratio is constant across the five looks because the Pocock-adjusted critical values are all the same. With the O'Brien-Fleming boundary, repeated confidence intervals computed at early looks are considerably wider than regular confidence intervals. However, the width ratio decreases very quickly. In a study with five analyses, a 90% repeated confidence interval computed at the last look is only 7% wider than an unadjusted 90% confidence interval.

Repeated confidence intervals are included in the DECISION data set created by the %EffMonitor and %EffFutMonitor macros. Both of the macros compute one-sided confidence intervals for the true treatment difference that are useful in assessing the efficacy profile of the experimental drug. Although, in theory, one can also set up confidence intervals for futility testing, it is seldom done in practice.

For computational convenience, the one-sided confidence intervals are contructed on a standardized treatment difference (effect size) scale. Since $Z_k = \widehat{\delta}_k/s_k$, the confidence interval for the effect size $\theta = \delta/\sigma$ is defined as

$$CI_k = \left((Z_k - u_k)\sqrt{\frac{2}{n_k}}, \infty \right), \quad k = 1, \ldots, m,$$

where n_k is the number of patients per treatment group included in the analysis at the kth interim look. In order to convert the obtained confidence interval into a confidence interval for the treatment difference δ, its lower limit needs to be multiplied by the pooled sample standard deviation—i.e., by

$$\sqrt{\frac{n_k}{2}} s_k, \quad k = 1, \ldots, m.$$

To demonstrate how to compute and interpret repeated confidence intervals in a group sequential setting, Program 4.9 generates the lower limits of one-sided 97.5% confidence intervals for the difference between the experimental drug and the placebo in the depression trial example. The limits are derived using the O'Brien-Fleming stopping boundary generated in Program 4.5.

Program 4.9 Repeated confidence intervals in the depression trial using an O'Brien-Fleming group sequential plan

```
data stat;
    set teststat;
    keep n stat;
%EffMonitor(fraction=fraction,data=stat,effsize=0.375,power=0.9,
    alpha=0.025,rho=0,spfunction=1,sprho=0,decision=OFdecision,
    inference=OFinference);
proc print data=OFdecision noobs label;
    var Analysis Size Fraction LowerLimit;
    run;
```

Output from Program 4.9

Analysis	Sample size per group	Sample size fraction	Lower 97.5% repeated confidence limit
1	78	0.5107	-.0725
2	121	0.7922	-.0116
3	151	0.9886	0.1225

Output 4.9 lists lower limits of one-sided repeated confidence intervals obtained at each of the three interim looks in the depression trial. The lower limit is negative at the first two analyses, indicating that the data were consistent with the null hypothesis of no treatment difference. However, the lower limit becomes positive at the third look, which means that, with a 97.5% probability, the treatment difference is greater than 0.

It was explained above that the limits in Output 4.9 are computed on an effect size scale. In order to derive one-sided confidence intervals for the mean treatment difference, we need to multiply the obtained lower limits by the pooled sample standard deviation. The resulting limits are displayed in Table 4.4. To facilitate the comparison with regular confidence intervals used in a nonsequential setting, the table also includes unadjusted lower limits.

Table 4.4 demonstrates an important feature of repeated confidence intervals. As we can see from the table, the repeated lower limits are consistent with the O'Brien-Fleming decision rule. A repeated confidence interval includes zero if the O'Brien-Fleming test fails to detect a significant treatment difference (which was the case at the first and second interim analyses) and excludes zero if the O'Brien-Fleming test rejects the null hypothesis. In contrast, the lower limits of regular confidence intervals are not properly adjusted for multiple looks and exclude zero at all three inspections. This conveys the wrong impression that the trial should have been stopped as early as the first interim look.

Table 4.4 Repeated and unadjusted confidence intervals for the mean treatment difference in the depression trial

Interim analysis	Sample size per group	Sample size fraction	Lower repeated confidence limit	Unadjusted lower confidence limit
1	78	0.5107	−0.4608	0.5120
2	121	0.7922	−0.0709	0.2117
3	151	0.9886	0.7167	1.0672

4.2.7 Estimation Following Sequential Testing

In the previous section we talked about repeated confidence intervals computed at each interim inspection as well as at the final analysis. This section shifts the focus to inferences performed upon the trial termination and covers adjustments to final estimates of the treatment effect and associated confidence limits.

An interesting feature of maximum likelihood estimates of population parameters (e.g., sample means in the normal case or sample proportions in the binary case) is their lack of sensitivity to the underlying data collection process. Identical maximum likelihood estimates are computed from samples with a prespecified size and samples obtained in a sequentially designed experiment. For example, under normal assumptions, the maximum likelihood estimate of the population mean is the sample mean, regardless of whether the sample size is fixed or random.

It has been shown that maximum likelihood estimates in a sequential setting possess the same asymptotic properties (e.g., consistency and asymptotic normality) as regular maximum likelihood estimates computed from fixed samples; see, for example, Dmitrienko and Govindarajulu (2000). However, the nonasymptotic case is a completely different story. The distribution of maximum likelihood estimates in group sequential trials is distinctly nonnormal and the estimates themselves are not centered around the population parameters. To see why this happens, recall that an estimate of the treatment difference is computed in a sequential setting only after the trial has been stopped. At this point, the test statistic is either larger or smaller than a prespecified threshold and therefore the obtained estimate is biased toward one of the two extremes. The estimate will overstate the treatment difference if the upper boundary is crossed and will have a negative bias if the lower boundary is crossed. It has been demonstrated in the literature that the bias can be quite large in magnitude and traditional estimates of the treatment effect (as well as associated confidence limits) become highly unreliable in a group sequential setting. Tsiatis, Rosner and Mehta (1984) and Emerson and Fleming (1990) showed via simulations that the coverage probability of confidence intervals computed after a group sequential test varies substantially depending on the magnitude of the treatment difference and can be far from its nominal value.

EXAMPLE: Group Sequential Trial in Critically Ill Patients

Van Den Berghe et al. (2001) reported the results of a clinical trial in critically ill patients that was stopped early due to a large difference in overall mortality between groups of patients treated with new and conventional therapies. The observed reduction in overall mortality was 42% with a 95% confidence interval of (22%, 62%). After a proper adjustment for sequential sampling, the estimate of the treatment effect was pulled toward 0. The adjusted reduction in overall mortality turned out to be 32% with a 95% confidence interval of (2%, 55%).

Several different approaches that account for the sequential nature of the testing procedure when computing point estimates or confidence intervals have been proposed over the last 20 years; see Siegmund (1978), Tsiatis, Rosner and Mehta (1984), Whitehead (1986), Kim and DeMets (1987), and Emerson and Fleming (1990). In what follows we will discuss the approach introduced by Tsiatis, Rosner and Mehta (1984) and extended by Kim and DeMets (1987). This method possesses a number of desirable properties; for example, it produces a true confidence interval without holes, which is consistent with the associated sequential test (i.e., the interval excludes the treatment difference of 0 if the null hypothesis was rejected by the test and vice versa). The Tsiatis-Rosner-Mehta point estimates and confidence intervals are also attractive from a computational perspective. Unlike some of its competitors, the method introduced below is based on a relatively simple algorithm that can be efficiently implemented in SAS.

The derivation of the Tsiatis-Rosner-Mehta point estimates and confidence limits is rather complicated and will not be discussed here. In short, the derivation requires that all possible observed outcomes of a group sequential test be ordered in some meaningful manner. Tsiatis, Rosner and Mehta (1984) considered the problem of sequential estimation of normal means and proposed to employ an ordering of the outcome space considered earlier by Siegmund (1978). Once the ordering has been specified, a bias-adjusted estimate (known as the *median unbiased estimate*) is chosen in such a way that it is less than the true treatment difference 50% of the time and greater 50% of the time. In other words, the median unbiased estimate of the true treatment difference δ is equal to $\widehat{\delta}$ satisfying the following requirement:

$$P\{\text{More extreme outcome than the observed outcome when } \delta = \widehat{\delta}\} = 1/2.$$

Bias-adjusted confidence limits are derived using the well-known duality of confidence intervals and significance tests. The upper limit of a $100(1 - \alpha)\%$ confidence interval is defined as the value δ_U such that

$$P\{\text{More extreme outcome than the observed outcome when } \delta = \delta_U\} = 1 - \alpha/2.$$

Similarly, the lower limit is the value δ_L such that

$$P\{\text{More extreme outcome than the observed outcome when } \delta = \delta_L\} = \alpha/2.$$

The introduced bias-adjusted confidence intervals are inherently different from repeated confidence intervals discussed in Section 4.2.6. As was stated in Section 4.2.6, repeated confidence intervals can be computed at any data look, including the last one. However, in general, repeated confidence intervals are best suited for assessing the size of the treatment effect at intermediate looks and are often inferior to bias-adjusted intervals constructed upon the trial termination. Recall that a repeated confidence interval is centered around the unadjusted estimate of the treatment effect and thus it implicitly assumes that the unadjusted estimate is reasonably close to the true population parameter and that its sample distribution is symmetric. Neither of the two assumptions holds when a group sequential trial is terminated early and thus a repeated confidence interval is less reliable than a bias-adjusted interval computed at the last look.

The difference between repeated and bias-adjusted confidence intervals becomes most pronounced when a decision to stop is reached very early in the trial. By the definition, repeated confidence intervals are made wide enough to ensure that intervals at *all* interim looks will contain the true treatment difference with a specified probability. If a clinical trial is terminated at the first interim analysis, the associated repeated confidence interval often turns out to be substantially wider than a bias-adjusted confidence interval, which is designed to be used at a single analysis. To stress this point, Jennison and Turnbull (1990) noted that

> it does appear unnecessarily conservative to use the final repeated confidence interval as a confidence interval on termination since this allows for any stopping rule whatsoever.

Both the %EffMonitor and %EffFutMonitor macros introduced earlier in this section support bias-adjusted inferences at the last analysis. The median unbiased estimate of the treatment effect and an adjusted one-sided confidence interval are included in the INFERENCE data set generated by the macros. It is important to mention that the estimate and confidence interval are computed only in those cases when the null hypothesis is rejected, i.e., the experimental drug is found to be efficacious. As in the case of repeated confidence intervals, it is theoretically possible to perform adjusted inferences after the futility stopping boundary has been crossed; however, these inferences might not be of much practical interest in a clinical trial setting.

As an illustration, Program 4.10 computes the bias-adjusted point estimate and the lower limit of a one-sided 97.5% confidence interval (both on an effect size scale) in the depression trial example. As in Program 4.9, the inferences are performed using the O'Brien-Fleming stopping boundary generated earlier in Program 4.5.

Program 4.10 Bias-adjusted estimate of the treatment effect and one-sided confidence interval in the depression trial using an O'Brien-Fleming group sequential plan

```
data stat;
    set teststat;
    keep n stat;
%EffMonitor(fraction=fraction,data=stat,effsize=0.375,power=0.9,
    alpha=0.025,rho=0,spfunction=1,sprho=0,decision=OFdecision,
    inference=OFinference);
proc print data=OFinference noobs label;
    run;
```

Output from Program 4.10

Parameter	Value
Median unbiased estimate	0.2889
Lower 97.5% confidence limit	0.035

Output 4.10 displays the median unbiased estimate of the treatment effect obtained at the last analysis in the depression trial as well as a one-sided confidence interval. It is instructive to compare the derived median unbiased estimate of the effect size to the unadjusted effect size computed at the final

analysis. Using the HAMD17 data from Table 4.1, it is easy to verify that the unadjusted effect size is 0.3590 and is more extreme than the adjusted effect size shown in Output 4.10 (0.2889). As expected, removing the bias caused by sequential sampling shifts the estimate of the treatment effect toward zero. Further, the lower confidence limit displayed in Output 4.10 (0.035) is less than the lower limit of the corresponding repeated confidence interval displayed in Output 4.9 (0.1225). As was explained above, the bias-adjusted limit is likely more reliable in this situation than its counterpart because it better accounts for the possibly nonnormal distribution of the treatment difference at the last look.

4.2.8 Implementation Details and Validation

This section provides a detailed description of SAS/IML functions used in the group sequential design and monitoring macros introduced in Sections 4.2.1, 4.2.2, 4.2.4 and 4.2.5. The functions implement the recursive integration algorithm developed by Armitage, McPherson and Rowe (1969) and are employed to compute most of the important characteristics of a group sequential test, including stopping boundaries and stopping probabilities. Additionally, we will provide examples of validation work that was done to ensure the group sequential macros (%EffDesign, %EffFutDesign, %EffMonitor and %EffFutMonitor) produce valid results and are suitable for real clinical trial applications. The validation was based on comparisons with the results published in the literature as well as numerous logical checks.

Computation of Design Stopping Boundaries

We will begin with a review of the design stage of group sequential trials. Consider a clinical trial comparing a single dose of an experimental drug to a placebo and employing $m - 1$ equally spaced interim analyses followed by a final analysis. Denote the total number of patients per treatment group by N and let $X_{i1}, \ldots, X_{iN}$ denote independent, normally distributed observations with mean μ_i and common standard deviation σ collected in treatment group i. The primary objective of the study is to test the null hypothesis of no treatment difference

$$H_0 : \mu_1 - \mu_2 = \delta_0 = 0$$

against the alternative hypothesis

$$H_1 : \mu_1 - \mu_2 = \delta_1 > 0.$$

Assuming that $2n$ patients complete the trial between successive interim looks, let S_k denote the cumulative sum statistic at the kth look:

$$S_k = \frac{1}{\sqrt{2\sigma^2}} \left(\sum_{j=1}^{kn} X_{1j} - \sum_{j=1}^{kn} X_{2j} \right).$$

The z statistic for testing the null hypothesis of no treatment difference at the kth look is equal to $Z_k = S_k/\sqrt{kn}$. The lower and upper Wang-Tsiatis stopping boundaries for S_k and Z_k are defined as

$$l_k = -ck^\rho, \quad u_k = ck^\rho \text{ (cumulative sum statistic)}, \tag{4.1}$$

$$l_k = -ck^{\rho-1/2}, \quad u_k = ck^{\rho-1/2} \text{ (z statistic)}.$$

Here ρ is a shape parameter ranging between 0 and 0.5. The Wang-Tsiatis boundaries simplify to the Pocock boundaries when $\rho = 0.5$ and to the O'Brien-Fleming boundaries when $\rho = 0$. The c constant in the equations (4.1) is chosen in such a way that the overall Type I error rate associated with the group sequential design is equal to α; i.e.,

$$P \left(S_k < l_k \text{ or } S_k > u_k \text{ for any } k = 1, \ldots, m \mid \mu_1 - \mu_2 = 0 \right) = \alpha. \tag{4.2}$$

The Type I error rate in equation (4.2) can be computed using the recursive integration algorithm introduced by Armitage, McPherson and Rowe (1969). The algorithm is implemented in the SEQ and

SEQSCALE functions included in the SAS/IML module. The SEQ function computes stopping probabilities for a specified set of stopping boundaries and the SEQSCALE function determines the c constant in the equations (4.1). The two functions can be applied to design group sequential clinical trials with an arbitrary number of interim looks (note that the looks do not need to be equally spaced).

Program 4.11 utilizes the SEQSCALE function to compute two-sided stopping boundaries as well as the adjusted significance level and the SEQ function to obtain stopping probabilities for the Pocock group sequential plan with five analyses. The overall Type I error rate is set at the 0.05 level and the interim looks are assumed equally spaced. The Pocock plan is requested in Program 4.11 by setting the shape parameter RHO to 0.5.

Program 4.11 Pocock group sequential plan with five analyses (two-sided 0.05 Type I error rate)

```
proc iml;
  * Two-sided Type I error probability;
  alpha=0.05;
  * Pocock plan;
  Rho=0.5;
  * Number of analyses;
  m=5;
  * Two-sided boundary on the cumulative sum scale;
  SBoundary=-(1:m)##Rho//(1:m)##Rho;
  call seqscale(prob,CritValue,SBoundary,1-alpha) eps=1e-8;
  * Two-sided boundary on the test statistic scale;
  ZBoundary=CritValue*(1:m)##(Rho-0.5);
  print ZBoundary[format=7.4];
  * Adjusted significance level;
  AdjAlpha=2*(1-probnorm(CritValue));
  print AdjAlpha[format=7.4];
  * Stopping probabilities under the null hypothesis;
  SBoundary=-CritValue*(1:m)##Rho//CritValue*(1:m)##Rho;
  call seq(prob0,SBoundary) eps=1e-8;
  StopProb=prob0[3,]-prob0[2,]+prob0[1,];
  print StopProb[format=7.4];
  run;
  quit;
```

Output from Program 4.11

```
               ZBOUNDARY

 2.4132   2.4132   2.4132   2.4132   2.4132

ADJALPHA

  0.0158

               STOPPROB

 0.0158   0.0117   0.0090   0.0073   0.0061
```

Output 4.11 displays the upper stopping boundary of the Pocock group sequential plan on the test statistic scale (ZBOUNDARY), corresponding adjusted significance level (ADJALPHA) and stopping probabilities under the null hypothesis (STOPPROB). The computed stopping boundary is equivalent to the stopping boundary derived by Pocock (1977, Page 193) (see Table 4.5). The adjusted significance level produced by the SEQSCALE function is identical to the adjusted significance level reported by

Table 4.5 Pocock and O'Brien-Fleming stopping boundaries in a clinical trial with five analyses

Analysis	Pocock upper stopping boundary		O'Brien-Fleming upper stopping boundary	
	Program 4.11	Pocock (1977)	Program 4.11	Pocock (1982)
1	2.4132	2.413	4.5617	4.562
2	2.4132	2.413	3.2256	3.226
3	2.4132	2.413	2.6337	2.634
4	2.4132	2.413	2.2809	2.281
5	2.4132	2.413	2.0401	2.040

Pocock (1982, Page 154). The stopping probabilities under the null hypothesis are computed from the PROB0 matrix generated by the SEQ function. The stopping probability at each interim look is computed by adding the probabilities of crossing the lower and upper boundaries.

It is easy to modify Program 4.11 to obtain the upper stopping boundary of the O'Brien-Fleming group sequential plan (let RHO=0 to request the O'Brien-Fleming plan). The resulting upper stopping boundary shown in Table 4.5 is equivalent to the stopping boundary computed by Pocock (1982, Page 158).

It is important to note that Program 4.11 utilizes the SEQSCALE and SEQ functions to compute stopping boundaries and probabilities for group sequential plans with equally spaced interim looks. The two functions also provide the user with an ability to specify an arbitrary interim monitoring schedule. This can be done using the TSCALE parameter of the SEQSCALE and SEQ functions.

Program 4.12 demonstrates how to set up a Pocock group sequential plan with interim analyses conducted after 20% and 50% of patients have completed the study. In order to pass the interim monitoring schedule to the SEQSCALE and SEQ functions, we will need to go through the following steps:

1. Introduce the FRACTION vector that captures the fractions of the total sample size at the three analyses, FRACTION={0.2,0.5,1}.

2. Compute standardized fractions (divide FRACTION by FRACTION[1]), STFRACTION={1,2.5,5}.

3. Define the INC vector containing increments of the standardized fractions, INC={1.5,2.5}.

4. Pass the INC vector to the SEQSCALE and SEQ functions using the TSCALE parameter.

The outlined algorithm is employed in the %EffDesign and %EffFutDesign macros for designing group sequential plans for interim efficacy and simultaneous efficacy/futility assessments.

Program 4.12 Pocock group sequential plan with interim analyses conducted after 20% and 50% of patients have completed the study (two-sided 0.05 Type I error rate)

```
proc iml;
    * Two-sided Type I error probability;
    alpha=0.05;
    * Pocock plan;
    Rho=0.5;
    * Fractions of the total sample size at three analyses;
    fraction={0.2,0.5,1};
    * Number of analyses;
    m=nrow(fraction);
    * Standardized fractions;
    StFraction=fraction/fraction[1];
    * Increments;
    inc=j(1,m-1,0);
```

```
     do i=1 to m-1;
          inc[i]=StFraction[i+1]-StFraction[i];
     end;
     * Two-sided boundary on the cumulative sum scale;
     SBoundary=-StFraction`##Rho//StFraction`##Rho;
     call seqscale(prob,CritValue,SBoundary,1-alpha) tscale=inc eps=1e-8;
     * Two-sided boundary on the test statistic scale;
     ZBoundary=CritValue*StFraction`##(Rho-0.5);
     print ZBoundary[format=7.4];
     * Adjusted significance level;
     AdjAlpha=2*(1-probnorm(CritValue));
     print AdjAlpha[format=7.4];
     * Stopping probabilities under the null hypothesis;
     SBoundary=-CritValue*StFraction`##Rho//CritValue*StFraction`##Rho;
     call seq(prob0,SBoundary) tscale=inc eps=1e-8;
     StopProb=prob0[3,]-prob0[2,]+prob0[1,];
     print StopProb[format=7.4];
     run;
     quit;
```

Output from Program 4.12

```
        ZBOUNDARY

 2.3227   2.3227   2.3227


ADJALPHA

  0.0202


        STOPPROB

 0.0202   0.0159   0.0139
```

Output 4.12 shows the upper Pocock stopping boundary (ZBOUNDARY), adjusted significance level (ADJALPHA) and stopping probabilities under the null hypothesis (STOPPROB) generated by Program 4.12.

Computation of Maximum Sample Size

To compute the power of the Pocock or O'Brien-Fleming group sequential tests, we need to evaluate the probability of early stopping under the alternative hypothesis. The obtained power function can then be used for computing the maximum sample size required to achieve the desirable Type II error probability β under the alternative hypothesis. Given the standard deviation of the observations σ and clinically significant treatment difference δ_1, the maximum number of patients per treatment group is given by

$$N = 2m \left(\frac{\sigma \, \psi}{\delta_1} \right)^2,$$

where ψ is the so-called *drift* parameter. The drift parameter is equal to the treatment difference $\mu_1 - \mu_2$ for which the power of the group sequential test equals $1 - \beta$; i.e.,

$$P\left(S_k < l_k \text{ or } S_k > u_k \text{ for any } k = 1, \ldots, m \mid \mu_1 - \mu_2 = \psi \right) = 1 - \beta. \tag{4.3}$$

This calculation is performed under the assumption that the effect size is 1 ($\delta_1 = \sigma$). The drift parameter is easily obtained from equation (4.3) using nonlinear optimization routines available in the SAS/IML module.

Program 4.13 computes the drift parameter ψ for Pocock group sequential trials with five analyses designed to achieve 90% power with a two-sided Type I error rate of 0.05. The four interim looks are assumed to be equally spaced. The computation relies heavily on the NLPDD function implementing the so-called *double dogleg* nonlinear optimization algorithm (see SAS/IML documentation for more details). The NLPDD function finds a solution of the equation (4.3) by minimizing the difference between the Type II error probability of the Pocock group sequential test and β (DRIFTSEARCH function). The starting value of the drift parameter (START variable) is obtained from the fixed-sample design with 90% power and a two-sided 0.05 confidence level. It is worth noting that slightly more advanced versions of the DRIFTSEARCH function and NLPDD optimization routine are included in the %EffDesign and %EffFutDesign macros to compute the maximum sample size in group sequential trials with an arbitrary number of analyses.

Program 4.13 Drift parameter for Pocock group sequential trials with five analyses (90% power, two-sided 0.05 Type I error rate)

```
proc iml;
    * Two-sided Type I error probability;
    alpha=0.05;
    * Type II error probability;
    beta=0.1;
    * Pocock plan;
    Rho=0.5;
    * Number of analyses;
    m=5;
    start DriftSearch(d) global(m,rho,critvalue,beta);
        lower=-critvalue*(1:m)##rho;
        upper=critvalue*(1:m)##rho;
        adjustment=d*(1:m);
        boundary=(lower-adjustment)//(upper-adjustment);
        call seq(p,boundary) eps=1e-8;
        diff=abs(beta-(p[2,]-p[1,])[m]);
        return(diff);
    finish;
    * Two-sided boundary on the cumulative sum scale;
    SBoundary=-(1:m)##rho//(1:m)##rho;
    call seqscale(prob,CritValue,SBoundary,1-alpha) eps=1e-8;
    * Starting value for the drift parameter search;
    start=(probit(1-beta)+probit(1-alpha))/sqrt(m);
    * Convergence parameters;
    tc=repeat(.,1,12);
    tc[1]=100;
    tc[3]=1e-5;
    call nlpdd(rc,drift,"DriftSearch",start) tc=tc;
    * Drift parameter;
    print drift[format=6.2];
    run;
    quit;
```

Output from Program 4.13

```
DRIFT

1.59
```

Output 4.13 displays the drift parameter ψ for the Pocock group sequential plan with five analyses. With this drift parameter, the maximum number of patients in the two treatment groups required to achieve 90% power with the effect size of 1 is

$$2N = 4m\psi^2 = 50.71.$$

The obtained maximum sample size is very close to the maximum sample size for the same group sequential plan reported by Wang and Tsiatis (1987, Page 196). Program 4.13 was re-run to compute maximum sample sizes for Pocock and O'Brien-Fleming group sequential tests under several scenarios. The results are summarized in Table 4.6. Table 4.6 shows that the difference between the maximum sample sizes generated by Program 4.13 and the results reported by Wang and Tsiatis (1987, Page 196) is insignificant. The relative error is less than 0.1%.

Table 4.6 Maximum sample size for Pocock and O'Brien-Fleming group sequential plans with the effect size of 1 (90% power, two-sided 0.05 Type I error rate)

Number of analyses	Pocock plan		O'Brien-Fleming plan	
	Program 4.13	Wang and Tsiatis (1987)	Program 4.13	Wang and Tsiatis (1987)
2	46.24	46.24	42.33	42.33
3	48.36	48.36	42.71	42.71
4	49.72	49.73	42.96	42.96
5	50.71	50.72	43.14	43.14

Computation of Expected Sample Size

Two important ingredients for computing the expected sample size of a group sequential plan under a certain hypothesis are the maximum sample size and stopping probabilities under the chosen hypothesis. Let N denote the maximum number of patients per treatment group and let $P_k(\delta)$ be the probability of stopping at the kth interim analysis when $\mu_1 - \mu_2 = \delta$, $k = 1, \ldots, m$. Then, assuming equally spaced looks, the expected sample size per group is given by

$$N^* = \frac{N}{m} \sum_{k=1}^{m-1} k P_k(\delta) + N \left(1 - \sum_{k=1}^{m-1} P_k(\delta)\right) \tag{4.4}$$

$$= \frac{N}{m} \left(m - \sum_{k=1}^{m} (m - k) P_k(\delta)\right).$$

The formula is easily extended to the case of unequally spaced analyses. The general version of this formula is used in the %EffDesign and %EffFutDesign macros for computing the expected sample size of Wang-Tsiatis group sequential plans.

Program 4.14 uses the formula (4.4) to compute the expected sample size under the alternative hypothesis for the Pocock group sequential plan considered in the previous subsection. The MAXIMUM variable is the maximum sample size and STOPPROB is the vector of stopping probabilities under the alternative hypothesis.

Program 4.14 Expected sample size under the alternative hypothesis for Pocock group sequential trials with five analyses (90% power, two-sided 0.05 Type I error rate)

```
proc iml;
    * Two-sided Type I error probability;
    alpha=0.05;
    * Type II error probability;
```

```
    beta=0.1;
    * Pocock plan;
    Rho=0.5;
    * Number of analyses;
    m=5;
    start DriftSearch(d) global(m,rho,critvalue,beta);
        lower=-critvalue*(1:m)##rho;
        upper=critvalue*(1:m)##rho;
        adjustment=d*(1:m);
        boundary=(lower-adjustment)//(upper-adjustment);
        call seq(p,boundary) eps=1e-8;
        diff=abs(beta-(p[2,]-p[1,])[m]);
        return(diff);
    finish;
    * Two-sided boundary on the cumulative sum scale;
    SBoundary=-(1:m)##rho//(1:m)##rho;
    call seqscale(prob,CritValue,SBoundary,1-alpha) eps=1e-8;
    * Starting value for the drift parameter search;
    start=(probit(1-beta)+probit(1-alpha))/sqrt(m);
    * Convergence parameters;
    tc=repeat(.,1,12);
    tc[1]=100;
    tc[3]=1e-5;
    call nlpdd(rc,drift,"DriftSearch",start) tc=tc;
    * Maximum sample size;
    maximum=2*m*drift*drift;
    * Expected sample size under the alternative hypothesis;
    lower=-critvalue*(1:m)##rho;
    upper=critvalue*(1:m)##rho;
    adjustment=drift*(1:m);
    boundary=(lower-adjustment)//(upper-adjustment);
    call seq(prob1,boundary) eps=1e-8;
    StopProb=prob1[3,]-prob1[2,]+prob1[1,];
    n=2*(maximum/m)*(m-(m-(1:m))*StopProb`);
    print n[format=6.2];
    run;
    quit;
```

For validation purposes, the algorithm implemented in Program 4.14 was carried out under several scenarios and the output was compared to the computations performed by Wang and Tsiatis (1987). The obtained results are displayed in Table 4.7. As in Table 4.6, the expected sample sizes generated by Program 4.14 are virtually identical to the expected sample sizes computed by Wang and Tsiatis (1987, Page 196).

Table 4.7 Expected sample size under the alternative hypothesis for Pocock and O'Brien-Fleming group sequential plans with the effect size of 1 (90% power, two-sided 0.05 Type I error rate)

Number of analyses	Pocock plan		O'Brien-Fleming plan	
	Program 4.14	Wang and Tsiatis (1987)	Program 4.14	Wang and Tsiatis (1987)
2	32.61	32.61	35.77	35.78
3	30.30	30.31	33.57	33.57
4	29.31	29.32	32.25	32.25
5	28.79	28.79	31.53	31.53

Computations in Group Sequential Designs for Efficacy/Futility Assessments

The computational algorithms discussed so far were related to efficacy interim monitoring and can be extended to set up group sequential plans for simultaneous efficacy/futility testing. Unlike efficacy group sequential plans with a single stopping boundary, group sequential plans for simultaneous efficacy/futility monitoring employ two stopping boundaries. The upper boundary is used for efficacy assessments, whereas the lower boundary is used for futility analyses. On the cumulative sum statistic scale, the two boundaries are defined as follows:

$$u_k = c_1 k^\rho, \quad l_k = \psi k - c_2 k^\rho,$$

where ψ is the drift parameter chosen in such a way that the two boundaries meet at the last analysis, i.e., $u_m = l_m$, and thus

$$\psi = (c_1 + c_2) m^{\rho-1}.$$

Further, c_1 and c_2 are constants determining the shape of the upper and lower boundaries, respectively. The two constants are selected to ensure that the Type I and Type II error rates of the group sequential plan are equal to the prespecified values α and β. In other words, c_1 and c_2 are found from the following equations:

$$P\left(S_k > u_k \text{ for any } k = 1, \ldots, m \,\middle|\, \mu_1 - \mu_2 = 0\right) = \alpha, \tag{4.5}$$

$$P\left(S_k < l_k \text{ for any } k = 1, \ldots, m \,\middle|\, \mu_1 - \mu_2 = \psi\right) = \beta.$$

In order to solve the two equations, the %EffFutDesign macro performs a search in the two-dimensional (c_1, c_2) space using the NLPDD nonlinear optimization routine (c_1 and c_2 are computed by minimizing the PARSEARCH function defined within the %EffFutDesign macro). Table 4.8 shows the obtained solutions to the equations (4.5) for Pocock and O'Brien-Fleming group sequential plans with equally spaced looks and compares them to the values reported by Pampallona and Tsiatis (1994, Page 23). The two sets of c_1 and c_2 values are virtually indistinguishable.

Table 4.8 Constants c_1 and c_2 for Pocock and O'Brien-Fleming group sequential plans for simultaneous efficacy/futility monitoring (90% power, one-sided 0.05 Type I error rate)

	Pocock plan		O'Brien-Fleming plan	
Number of analyses	%EffFutDesign macro	Pampallona and Tsiatis (1994)	%EffFutDesign macro	Pampallona and Tsiatis (1994)
2 analyses				
c_1	2.3101	2.3101	1.8078	1.8079
c_2	1.3324	1.3324	1.0460	1.0460
3 analyses				
c_1	2.8494	2.8493	1.9071	1.9071
c_2	1.6937	1.6936	1.1605	1.1605
4 analyses				
c_1	3.3118	3.3118	1.9756	1.9756
c_2	1.9987	1.9987	1.2383	1.2383
5 analyses				
c_1	3.7216	3.7217	2.0269	2.0268
c_2	2.2693	2.2693	1.2962	1.2962

Maximum and expected sample size calculations in group sequential plans for simultaneous efficacy/futility monitoring are based on the principles outlined above; for example, the expected sample size is computed from formula (4.4). Table 4.9 summarizes the expected sample sizes under the alternative hypothesis generated by the %EffFutDesign macro along with the values derived by Pampallona and Tsiatis (1994, Page 29). Again, the expected sample sizes generated by the macro are very close to those computed by Pampallona and Tsiatis.

Table 4.9 Expected sample size under the alternative hypothesis for Pocock and O'Brien-Fleming group sequential plans for simultaneous efficacy/futility monitoring with the effect size of 1 (90% power, one-sided 0.05 Type I error rate)

Number of analyses	Pocock plan		O'Brien-Fleming plan	
	%EffFutDesign macro	Pampallona and Tsiatis (1994)	%EffFutDesign macro	Pampallona and Tsiatis (1994)
2	21.17	21.18	20.67	20.67
3	20.00	20.00	19.16	19.16
4	19.29	19.29	18.37	18.37
5	18.86	18.86	17.89	17.88

Computation of Monitoring Stopping Boundaries

This subsection presents calculations that were performed to validate the method used to construct monitoring stopping boundaries from a given α-spending function or a set of α- and β-spending functions in the %EffMonitor and %EffFutMonitor macros. Since the two macros employ the same algorithm, we will focus on only one of them (%EffFutMonitor macro).

Consider the clinical trial example described by Pampallona, Tsiatis and Kim (2001). This example involves a two-arm trial with a normally distributed response variable designed to test an experimental drug versus a control. The trial was powered at 90% to detect a significant treatment difference at a one-sided 0.05 significance level assuming the effect size of 0.25. Three equally spaced interim analyses were included in the trial design to assess the efficacy and futility profiles of the experimental drug. O'Brien-Fleming stopping boundaries ($\rho = 0$) were chosen for both efficacy and futility assessments.

Program 4.15 calls the %EffFutDesign macro to compute important characteristics of the O'Brien-Fleming group sequential plan in the Pampallona-Tsiatis-Kim example. The PTKTRIAL data set passed to the macro indicates the number and timing of analyses in this trial. The EFFSIZE, POWER and ALPHA parameters specify the hypothesized effect size, power and one-sided significance level, respectively. Lastly, RHOEFF and RHOFUT are the shape parameters of the upper and lower stopping boundaries.

Program 4.15 O'Brien-Fleming group sequential plan for simultaneous efficacy/futility analyses in the clinical trial example described by Pampallona, Tsiatis and Kim (2001)

```
data PTKTrial;
    input fraction @@;
    datalines;
    0.25 0.5 0.75 1
    ;
%EffFutDesign(fraction=PTKTrial,effsize=0.25,power=0.9,alpha=0.05,
    rhoeff=0,rhofut=0,boundary=Boundary,sizepower=Power);
    run;
```

Output from Program 4.15

```
Summary                                         Value

One-sided Type I error probability              0.05
Power                                           0.9
True effect size                                0.25
Shape parameter of upper boundary               0
Shape parameter of lower boundary               0
Maximum sample size per group                   300
Average sample size per group under H0          180
Average sample size per group under H1          202
Fixed sample size per group                     275


                 Lower          Upper
                 stopping       stopping
                 boundary       boundary
                 (test          (test
                 statistic      statistic
Analysis         scale)         scale)


    1            -1.220         3.3721
    2             0.2197        2.3844
    3             1.0631        1.9469
    4             1.6860        1.6860
```

Output 4.15 displays the main characteristics of the O'Brien-Fleming plan as well as the lower and upper stopping boundaries on the test statistic scale. The maximum sample size per group (300 patients) and the boundaries computed by the %EffFutDesign macro are identical to the maximum sample size and stopping boundaries obtained by Pampallona, Tsiatis and Kim (2001, Page 1118):

- maximum sample size per group = 300 patients
- lower stopping boundary = $\{-1.220, 0.220, 1.063, 1.686\}$
- upper stopping boundary = $\{3.372, 2.384, 1.947, 1.686\}$.

Pampallona, Tsiatis and Kim (2001, Page 1120) also computed monitoring stopping boundaries derived from the ten-look α- and β-spending functions. The stopping boundaries along with the values of test statistics observed at two interim looks are displayed in Table 4.10.

Table 4.10 Test statistics and stopping boundaries in the clinical trial example described by Pampallona, Tsiatis and Kim (2001)

Interim analysis	Total number of patients	Test statistic	Lower boundary (test statistic scale)	Upper boundary (test statistic scale)
1	225	0.6	−0.396	2.767
2	374	1.2	0.69	2.119

Program 4.16 replicates the results shown in Table 4.10 by calling the %EffFutMonitor macro. The test statistics passed to the macro are included in the TESTSTAT data set. Note that a fractional sample size per group (112.5) is used at the first interim analysis to match the total sample size of 225 in the first row of Table 4.10. The SPFUNCTION parameter of the macro is set to 2 in order to request ten-look α- and β-spending functions. Ten-look spending functions do not require the SPRHO parameter and thus it can be set to an arbitrary value.

Program 4.16 Efficacy/futility monitoring in the clinical trial example described by Pampallona, Tsiatis and Kim (2001)

```
data PTKTrial;
    input fraction @@;
    datalines;
    0.25 0.5 0.75 1
    ;
data TestStat;
    input n stat;
    datalines;
    112.5 0.6
    187 1.2
    ;
%EffFutMonitor(fraction=PTKTrial,data=TestStat,effsize=0.25,power=0.9,
    alpha=0.05, rhoeff=0,rhofut=0,spfunction=2,sprho=1,decision=decision,
    inference=inference);
proc print data=decision noobs label;
    var Analysis TestStatistic LowerTestStBoundary UpperTestStBoundary;
    run;
```

Output from Program 4.16

Analysis	Test statistic	Lower stopping boundary (test statistic scale)	Upper stopping boundary (test statistic scale)
1	0.6000	-.3956	2.7669
2	1.2000	0.6920	2.1185

Output 4.16 lists the lower and upper adjusted critical values at the first and second interim looks computed by the %EffFutMonitor macro. The derived stopping boundaries are identical to the boundaries found by Pampallona, Tsiatis and Kim (2001) (see Table 4.10).

4.2.9 Summary

Sequential designs have long become part of the standard arsenal of statistical tools used in clinical trials. This section reviewed a popular approach to the design and monitoring of group sequential trials known as the *repeated significance testing* approach.

First, we provided a review of sequential plans from the Wang-Tsiatis family, which includes the popular O'Brien-Fleming and Pocock plans, and demonstrated how to design group sequential trials for testing efficacy or simultaneous testing of efficacy and futility of an experimental drug. These group sequential designs are supported by the %EffDesign and %EffFutDesign macros, respectively.

The section also discussed interim monitoring based on the flexible extension of the repeated significance testing methodology proposed by Lan and DeMets. The main advantage of the Lan-DeMets error spending approach is its ability to allow for unplanned and unequally spaced interim looks. Therefore, it should not be surprising that it has become the main tool for the sequential analysis of clinical trial data. It is important to keep the following two points in mind when applying the Lan-DeMets method in a clinical trial setting:

- The maximum sample size must be specified prior to the first interim analysis.
- The monitoring plan cannot be affected by the outcomes observed in the trial. Although it has been shown that the error spending approach is quite robust to data-dependent changes in the frequency of

interim analyses, clinical researchers need to avoid such practices. Requesting additional looks at the data after a nearly significant p-value was observed or after other data-driven decisions were made will inflate the overall Type I error rate.

The Lan-DeMets error spending approach is implemented in the %EffMonitor macro for monitoring trials for detecting early evidence of efficacy and the %EffFutMonitor macro for simultaneous efficacy and futility monitoring.

It is also critical to properly adjust measures of treatment effect such as point estimates and confidence intervals computed in group sequential trials. The adjustments reflect the fact that the trial was conducted in a sequential manner. The section reviewed two types of adjustment methods:

- **Repeated confidence intervals** provide a useful summary of the variability of the estimated treatment difference at each interim look. Repeated confidence intervals are defined to ensure that all confidence intervals will contain the true treatment difference with a specified probability. If a clinical trial is stopped early, a repeated confidence interval computed at the last analysis will be wider (and often substantially wider) than a confidence interval specifically designed to be used at the end of a group sequential trial.

- **Point estimates and confidence intervals at termination.** Naive estimates of the treatment effect and associated confidence intervals used in a fixed-sample analysis are misleading in sequentially designed trials because they tend to be biased toward more extreme values of the treatment difference. In order to alleviate this problem, point estimates and confidence limits following termination are constructed by removing the bias caused by sequential sampling. For instance, if an estimate of the treatment difference is biased upward, it will be shrunk toward zero using a suitable bias-adjustment procedure.

Repeated confidence intervals as well as point estimates and confidence limits at termination are easy to compute using the %EffMonitor and %EffFutMonitor macros introduced in this section.

Lastly, when conducting a group sequential trial, it is important to commit to the prespecified decision rules. Trial sponsors are sometimes hesitant to stop a trial early because the termination decision is driven by the primary endpoint, and there might be other endpoints to consider or the patient responses might be expected to change as recruitment progresses (the early patients recruited might not be similar to later patients due to a learning curve). However, if the futility boundary is crossed and the trial sponsor chooses to continue the trial, therapeutic benefit cannot be claimed under any circumstances. The upper and lower stopping boundaries were created assuming that crossing the lower boundary would require termination. See Lan, Lachin and Bautista (2003) for a further discussion of this problem.

4.3 Stochastic Curtailment Tests

We have pointed out repeatedly throughout the chapter that pivotal clinical trials are routinely monitored to find early evidence of beneficial or harmful effects. Section 4.2 introduced an approach to the design and analysis of group sequential trials based on repeated significance testing. This section looks at sequential testing procedures used in a slightly different context. Specifically, it reviews recent advances in the area of *stochastic curtailment* with emphasis on procedures for futility monitoring.

To help understand the difference between repeated significance and stochastic curtailment tests, recall that repeated significance testing is centered around the notion of error spending. The chosen error spending strategy determines the characteristics of a sequential test (e.g., the shape of stopping boundaries) and ultimately drives the decision-making process. In the stochastic curtailment framework, decision making is tied directly to the final trial outcome. A decision to continue the trial or curtail sampling at each interim look is based on the likelihood of observing a positive or negative treatment effect if the trial were to continue to the planned end. Another important distinction is that stochastic curtailment methods are aimed toward predictive inferences, whereas repeated significance tests focus on currently available data.

Stochastic curtailment procedures (especially futility rules) are often employed in clinical trials with a fixed-sample design without an explicit adjustment for repeated statistical analyses. It is not unusual to see a stochastic curtailment test used in a *post hoc* manner; for example, a futility rule may be adopted after the first patient visit.

This section reviews three popular types of stochastic curtailment tests with emphasis on constructing futility rules. Section 4.3.1 introduces frequentist methods commonly referred to as *conditional power* methods. We will discuss the conditional power test developed by Lan, Simon and Halperin (1982) and Halperin et al. (1982) as well as its adaptive versions proposed by Pepe and Anderson (1992) and Betensky (1997). Next, Sections 4.3.2 and 4.3.3 cover mixed Bayesian-frequentist and fully Bayesian methods considered, among others, by Herson (1979), Spiegelhalter, Freedman, and Blackburn (1986), Geisser (1992), Geisser and Johnson (1994), Johns and Anderson (1999) and Dmitrienko and Wang (2004).

The following two examples will be used to illustrate the methods for constructing futility rules reviewed in this section.

EXAMPLE: Generalized Anxiety Disorder Trial with a Continuous Endpoint

A small proof-of-concept trial in patients with generalized anxiety disorder will serve as an example of a trial with a continuous outcome variable. In this trial, patients were randomly assigned to receive an experimental drug or a placebo for 6 weeks. The efficacy profile of the drug was evaluated using the mean change from baseline in the Hamilton Anxiety Rating Scale (HAMA) total score. The total sample size was 82 patients (41 patients were to be enrolled in each of the two treatment arms). This sample size provides approximately 80% power to detect a treatment difference of 4 in the mean HAMA total score change. The power calculation is based on a one-sided test with an α-level of 0.1 and assumes a standard deviation of 8.5.

The trial was not intended to be stopped early in order to declare efficacy; however, HAMA total score data were monitored in this trial to detect early signs of futility or detrimental effects. Table 4.11 summarizes the results obtained at three interim looks. Note that the experimental drug improves the HAMA total score by decreasing it and thus negative changes in Table 4.11 indicate improvement.

Table 4.11 HAMA total score data in the generalized anxiety disorder trial

Interim analysis	Experimental group		Placebo group	
	n	Mean HAMA change (SD)	n	Mean HAMA change (SD)
1	10	−9.2 (7.3)	11	−8.4 (6.4)
2	20	−9.4 (6.7)	20	−8.1 (6.9)
3	31	−8.9 (7.4)	30	−9.1 (7.7)

EXAMPLE: Severe Sepsis Trial with a Binary Endpoint

Consider a two-arm clinical trial in patients with severe sepsis conducted to compare the effect of an experimental drug on 28-day all-cause mortality to that of a placebo. The trial design included a futility monitoring component based on monthly analyses of the treatment effect on survival. The total sample size of 424 patients was computed to achieve 80% power of detecting a 9% absolute improvement in the 28-day survival rate at a one-sided significance level of 0.1. This calculation was based on the assumption that the placebo survival rate is 70%.

The trial was discontinued after approximately 75% of the projected number of patients had completed the 28-day study period because the experimental drug was deemed unlikely to demonstrate superiority to the placebo at the scheduled termination point. Table 4.12 provides a summary of the mortality data at six interim analyses conducted prior to the trial's termination.

In both of these clinical trial examples we are interested in setting up a futility rule to help assess the likelihood of a positive trial outcome given the results observed at each of the interim looks.

Table 4.12 Survival data in the severe sepsis trial

Interim analysis	Experimental group			Placebo group		
	Total	Alive	Survival	Total	Alive	Survival
1	55	33	60.0%	45	29	64.4%
2	79	51	64.6%	74	49	66.2%
3	101	65	64.4%	95	62	65.3%
4	117	75	64.1%	115	77	67.0%
5	136	88	64.7%	134	88	65.7%
6	155	99	63.9%	151	99	65.6%

4.3.1   Futility Rules Based on Conditional Power

Lan-Simon-Halperin Conditional Power Test

To introduce the Lan-Simon-Halperin test, consider a two-arm clinical trial with N patients per treatment group and assume that we are planning to take an interim look at the data after n patients have completed the trial in each treatment group. Let Z_n be the test statistic computed at the interim look; i.e.,

$$Z_n = \frac{\widehat{\delta}_n}{\widehat{\sigma}\sqrt{2/n}},$$

where $\widehat{\delta}_n$ is the estimated treatment difference and $\widehat{\sigma}$ is the pooled sample standard deviation. Similarly, let Z_N denote the corresponding statistic at the end of the trial:

$$Z_N = \frac{\widehat{\delta}_N}{\widehat{\sigma}\sqrt{2/N}}.$$

Finally, δ and σ will denote the true treatment difference and common standard deviation of the response variable in the two treatment groups. This formulation of the problem can be used with both continuous and binary endpoints.

The conditional power test proposed by Lan, Simon and Halperin (1982) is based on an intuitively appealing idea of predicting the distribution of the final outcome given the data already observed in the trial. If the interim prediction indicates that the trial outcome is unlikely to be positive, ethical and financial considerations will suggest an early termination the trial. Mathematically, the decision rule can be expressed in terms of the probability of a statistically significant outcome—i.e., $Z_N > z_{1-\alpha}$, conditional on the interim test statistic Z_n. This conditional probability is denoted by $P_n(\delta)$ and is termed *conditional power*. The trial is stopped as soon as the conditional power falls below a prespecified value $1 - \gamma$, where γ is known as the *futility index* (Ware, Muller and Braunwald, 1985). Smaller values of γ are associated with a higher likelihood of early stopping and, most commonly, γ is set to a value between 0.8 and 1.

It was shown by Lan, Simon and Halperin (1982) that the outlined futility rule has a simple structure and is easy to apply in clinical trials with continuous or binary outcome variables (see Jennison and Turnbull (1990) for more details). Suppose that the test statistics Z_n and Z_N are jointly normally distributed and δ and σ are known. In this case, the conditional distribution of Z_N given Z_n is normal with

$$\text{mean} = \sqrt{\frac{n}{N}}Z_n + \frac{\delta(N-n)}{\sigma\sqrt{2N}} \text{ and variance} = \frac{N-n}{N}.$$

Therefore the conditional power function $P_n(\delta)$ is given by

$$P_n(\delta) = \Phi\left(\frac{\sigma\sqrt{n}Z_n + (N-n)\delta/\sqrt{2} - \sigma\sqrt{N}z_{1-\alpha}}{\sigma\sqrt{N-n}}\right).$$

As before, $z_{1-\alpha}$ denotes the $100(1 - \alpha)$th percentile of the standard normal distribution and $\Phi(x)$ is the cumulative probability function of the standard normal distribution.

A stopping rule can now be formulated in terms of the computed conditional power:

Terminate the trial due to lack of efficacy the first time $P_n(\delta) < 1 - \gamma$,

or in terms of the observed test statistic Z_n:

Terminate the trial due to lack of efficacy the first time $Z_n < l_n$,

where the adjusted critical value l_n is given by

$$l_n = \sqrt{\frac{N}{n}} z_{1-\alpha} + \sqrt{\frac{N-n}{n}} z_{1-\gamma} - \frac{\delta(N-n)}{\sigma\sqrt{2n}}.$$

It is clear that the introduced futility rule is heavily influenced by the assumed value of the treatment difference δ. The clinical trial will be stopped sooner if δ is small and vice versa. Lan, Simon and Halperin (1982) and Halperin et al. (1982) considered stochastic curtailment tests in which the conditional power function was evaluated at the value of δ corresponding to the alternative hypothesis. With this choice of δ, conditional power is computed assuming that future data are generated from the alternative hypothesis.

It is interesting to note that the resulting conditional power procedure is closely related to group sequential testing procedures discussed in Section 4.2. Jennison and Turnbull (1990) pointed out that a special case of the Lan-Simon-Halperin test is a continuous-time equivalent of the O'Brien-Fleming group sequential test. Davis and Hardy (1990) showed that the stopping boundary of the Lan-Simon-Halperin test for efficacy monitoring with $\gamma = 0.5$ is virtually equivalent to the stopping boundary of the O'Brien-Fleming test. Likewise, if one constructs the O'Brien-Fleming boundary for testing lack of treatment benefit, it will be very close to the stopping boundary of the Lan-Simon-Halperin test with $\gamma = 0.5$. Note, however, that the futility index γ is typically set at the 0.8 or higher level in clinical trials. Thus, the O'Brien-Fleming test for futility (and other repeated significance procedures) is more likely to trigger an early stopping due to lack of efficacy compared to the Lan-Simon-Halperin test.

%CondPowerLSH Macro

Program 4.17 applies the Lan-Simon-Halperin conditional power test to the analysis of the severe sepsis trial. The program computes the z statistics for the treatment effect at each of the 6 interim analyses and then calls the %CondPowerLSH macro provided in the Appendix to estimate the conditional probability of a positive trial outcome under the alternative hypothesis. The %CondPowerLSH macro has the following arguments:

- DATA is the name of the input data set with one record per interim look. The data set must include the following variables:
  - N is the number of patients per group included in the analysis data set at the current interim look. If the sample sizes are unequal in the two treatment groups, set N to the average of the two sample sizes.
  - TESTSTAT is the test statistic computed at the current interim look.
- EFFSIZE is the hypothesized effect size (i.e., the treatment effect divided by the standard deviation).
- ALPHA is the one-sided Type I error probability of the significance test carried out at the end of the trial.
- GAMMA is the futility index.
- NN is the projected number of patients per treatment group.

- PROB is the name of the data set containing the computed conditional power at each interim look. This data set is generated by the macro and includes the following variables:
  - ANALYSIS is the analysis number.
  - FRACTION is the fraction of the total sample size.
  - TESTSTAT is the test statistic from the input data set.
  - CONDPOWER is the computed conditional power.
- BOUNDARY is the name of the data set that contains the stopping boundary of the conditional power test. This data set is generated by the macro and includes the following variables:
  - FRACTION is the fraction of the total sample size.
  - STOPBOUNDARY is the stopping boundary on the test statistic scale.

In order to invoke the %CondPowerLSH macro, we need to specify the effect size under the alternative hypothesis. Assuming 28-day survival rates of 0.7 and 0.79 in the two treatment groups, the treatment difference δ is 0.09 and the pooled standard deviation σ is

$$\sqrt{0.745(1 - 0.745)} = 0.436,$$

where 0.745 is the average survival rate in the two treatment groups. Therefore, the effect size is equal to

$$\delta/\sigma = 0.09/0.436 = 0.2065$$

and we will let EFFSIZE=0.2065. From the severe sepsis trial example, the one-sided significance level ALPHA is 0.1 and the projected sample size per group NN is 212. Lastly, we will set the futility index GAMMA to 0.8 to avoid very early stopping. With this choice of the futility index, the trial will be stopped as soon as the conditional probability of detecting a statistically significant difference at the planned end falls below 0.2.

Program 4.17 Lan-Simon-Halperin conditional power test in the analysis of the severe sepsis trial

```
data sevsep;
    input ExpN ExpAlive PlacN PlacAlive;
    datalines;
     55  33  45  29
     79  51  74  49
    101  65  95  62
    117  75 115  77
    136  88 134  88
    155  99 151  99
    ;
data test;
    set sevsep;
    diff=ExpAlive/ExpN-PlacAlive/PlacN;
    ave=(ExpAlive/ExpN+PlacAlive/PlacN)/2;
    n=(ExpN+PlacN)/2;
    teststat=diff/sqrt(2*ave*(1-ave)/n);
    keep n teststat;
%CondPowerLSH(data=test,effsize=0.2065,alpha=0.1,gamma=0.8,nn=212,
    prob=p,boundary=boundary);
proc print data=p noobs label;
data test;
    set test;
    group=1;
    fraction=n/212;
    StopBoundary=teststat;
```

```
data boundary;
    set boundary;
    group=2;
data plot;
    set test boundary;
axis1 minor=none label=(angle=90 "Test statistic") order=(-3 to 1 by 1);
axis2 minor=none label=("Fraction of total sample size")
    order=(0 to 1 by 0.2);
symbol1 i=none v=dot color=black;
symbol2 i=join v=none color=black line=1;
proc gplot data=plot;
    plot StopBoundary*Fraction=group/frame nolegend
    haxis=axis2 vaxis=axis1 vref=0 lvref=34;
    run;
```

Output from Program 4.17

Analysis	Fraction of total sample size	Test statistic	Conditional power
1	0.24	-0.4583	0.5548
2	0.36	-0.2157	0.4739
3	0.46	-0.1329	0.3776
4	0.55	-0.4573	0.1644
5	0.64	-0.1666	0.1433
6	0.72	-0.3097	0.0354

Output 4.17 indicates that, despite a negative treatment difference at the first interim look, there is still a 55% chance that the trend will be reversed by the completion of the trial if the absolute treatment difference is truly equal to 9%. This probability is fairly high and suggests that the trial should be continued to the next interim analysis. However, we do not see any improvement in the conditional power over the next several looks. In fact, the conditional probability of a statistically significant outcome at the planned end of the trial decreases steadily over time and becomes exceedingly small by the last look. A close examination of the right-hand column in Output 4.17 reveals a notable drop in the conditional power approximately halfway into the trial (at the fourth interim look). Since the conditional power is below the prespecified 20% threshold, we conclude that the observed treatment difference is no longer consistent with the alternative hypothesis and the trial should have been terminated due to futility at the fourth interim analysis.

Figure 4.24 depicts the test statistics computed at the six interim analyses plotted along with the stopping boundary corresponding to the futility index of 0.8. The stopping boundary lies well below 0 at the time of the first look but catches up with the test statistics toward the midpoint of the trial. This confirms our conclusion that there is an early trend in favor of continuing the trial. Note that the stopping boundary crosses the dotted line drawn at $Z = 0$ when $n/N = 0.64$, which implies that any negative treatment difference observed beyond this point would cause the trial to be stopped due to lack of treatment benefit.

Program 4.18 produces an alternative graphical representation of the Lan-Simon-Halperin futility boundary in the severe sepsis trial. Instead of focusing on the z statistics computed at each of the six interim looks, the program plots stopping boundaries expressed in terms of observed survival rates. The stopping boundary is computed by fixing the survival rate in the experimental group and finding the smallest placebo survival rate for which the conditional probability of a statistically significant difference at the scheduled end of the trial is less than $1 - \gamma = 0.2$.

Figure 4.24 Stopping boundary of the Lan-Simon-Halperin test (—) and interim z statistics (•) in the severe sepsis trial example. The futility index γ is 0.8; the continuation region is above the stopping boundary.

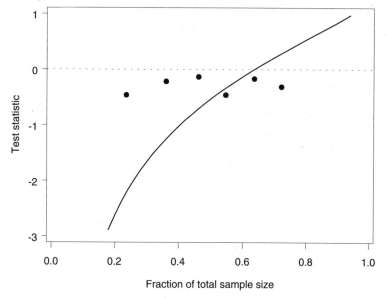

Program 4.18 Alternative representation of the Lan-Simon-Halperin futility boundaries in the severe sepsis trial

```
proc iml;
    expn={55, 79, 101, 117, 136, 155};
    placn={45, 74, 95, 115, 134, 151};
    lower=0.2;
    upper=0.8;
    nn=212;
    alpha=0.1;
    effsize=0.2065;
    gamma=0.8;
    boundary=j(1,3,.);
    do analysis=1 to 6;
    start=ceil(expn[analysis]*lower);
    end=floor(expn[analysis]*upper);
    temp=j(end-start+1,3,0);
    do i=start to end;
        p1=i/expn[analysis];
        j=ceil(placn[analysis]*lower)-1;
        prob=1;
        do while(prob>1-gamma & j<=placn[analysis]);
        j=j+1;
        p2=j/placn[analysis];
        ave=(p1+p2)/2;
        n=(expn[analysis]+placn[analysis])/2;
        teststat=(p1-p2)/sqrt(2*ave*(1-ave)/n);
        prob=1-probnorm((sqrt(nn)*probit(1-alpha)-sqrt(n)*teststat
        -(nn-n)*effsize/sqrt(2))/sqrt(nn-n));
        end;
        k=i-start+1;
        temp[k,1]=p1;
        temp[k,2]=p2;
        temp[k,3]=analysis;
```

```
      end;
      boundary=boundary//temp;
      end;
      varnames={"p1" "p2" "analysis"};
      create boundary from boundary[colname=varnames];
      append from boundary;
      quit;
 data points;
      p1=33/55; p2=29/45; analysis=7; output;
      p1=51/79; p2=49/74; analysis=8; output;
      p1=65/101; p2=62/95; analysis=9; output;
      p1=75/117; p2=77/115; analysis=10; output;
      p1=88/136; p2=88/134; analysis=11; output;
      p1=99/155; p2=99/151; analysis=12; output;
 data boundary;
      set boundary points;
 %macro BoundPlot(subset,analysis);
 axis1 minor=none label=(angle=90 "Observed survival rate (Placebo)")
      order=(0.5 to 0.8 by 0.1);
 axis2 minor=none label=("Observed survival rate (Exp drug)")
      order=(0.5 to 0.8 by 0.1);
 symbol1 i=j v=none color=black line=1;
 symbol2 i=none v=dot color=black;
 data annotate;
      xsys="1"; ysys="1"; hsys="4"; x=50; y=10; position="5";
      size=1; text="Interim analysis &analysis"; function="label";
 proc gplot data=boundary anno=annotate;
      where &subset;
      plot p2*p1=analysis/frame nolegend haxis=axis2 vaxis=axis1;
      run;
      quit;
 %mend BoundPlot;
 %BoundPlot(%str(analysis in (1,7)),1);
 %BoundPlot(%str(analysis in (2,8)),2);
 %BoundPlot(%str(analysis in (3,9)),3);
 %BoundPlot(%str(analysis in (4,10)),4);
 %BoundPlot(%str(analysis in (5,11)),5);
 %BoundPlot(%str(analysis in (6,12)),6);
```

Figure 4.25 displays the Lan-Simon-Halperin stopping boundaries with the futility index $\gamma = 0.8$ on an event rate scale. Since the Lan-Simon-Halperin test depends on the data through the Z_n statistic, the associated decision rule is driven mainly by the treatment difference and is not affected by the actual values of survival rates. As a consequence, the stopping boundaries in Figure 4.25 look like straight-line segments parallel to the identity line.

Stopping boundaries plotted on an event rate scale have a number of advantages that make them very appealing in a clinical trial setting. First, they facilitate the communication of interim findings to medical colleagues. Second, the stopping boundaries in Figure 4.25 help appreciate the effect of each additional death on the decision making process. Consider, for example, the fourth interim analysis. Figure 4.24 shows that the corresponding z statistic lies well below the stopping boundary and the survival rate in the experimental group is clearly too low to justify the continuation of the trial. However, Figure 4.25 demonstrates that the dot representing the observed survival rates sits right on the stopping boundary. Thus, instead of a clear-cut decision, we are likely dealing here with a borderline situation in which one additional death in the placebo group could easily change the conclusion. A simple sensitivity analysis proves that this is in fact the case. Assuming 75 survivors in the experimental group, one can check that an additional death in the placebo group would cause the dot at the fourth interim look to move into the continuation region.

Figure 4.25 Stopping boundary of the Lan-Simon-Halperin test (—) and interim survival rates (•) in the severe sepsis trial example. The futility index γ is 0.8; the continuation region is below the stopping boundary.

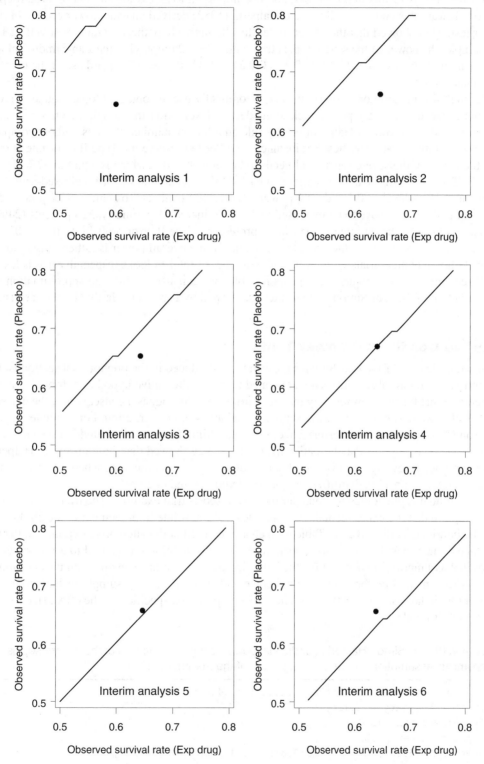

The last remark in this subsection is concerned with the effect of futility monitoring on the power of a clinical trial. Due to the possibility of early stopping in favor of the null hypothesis, any futility monitoring strategy results in power loss, and it is important to assess the amount of Type II error rate inflation. Toward this end, Lan, Simon and Halperin (1982) derived an exact lower bound for the power of their test. They showed that the power under the alternative hypothesis cannot be less than $1 - \beta/\gamma$. For example, the power of the severe sepsis trial with $\beta = 0.2$ employing the Lan-Simon-Halperin futility rule will always exceed 77.8% if $\gamma = 0.9$ and 71.4% if $\gamma = 0.7$, regardless of the number of interim analyses.

Although it is uncommon to do so, we can theoretically use the obtained lower bound to recalculate the sample size and bring the power back to the desired level. After the sample size has been adjusted, we can apply the Lan-Simon-Halperin futility rule an arbitrary number of times without compromising the trial's operating characteristics. For instance, in order to preserve the Type II error rate at the 0.2 level, the power of the severe sepsis trial needs to be set to $1 - \beta\gamma$, which is equal to 82% if $\gamma = 0.9$ and 86% if $\gamma = 0.7$. To see how this affects the trial's size, recall that the original fixed-sample design with a one-sided α-level of 0.1 and 80% power requires 424 patients. To achieve 82% power, the number of patients will have to be increased to 454 (7% increase). Similarly, 524 patients (24% increase) will need to be enrolled in the trial to protect the Type II error probability if $\gamma = 0.7$.

One should remember that the exact lower bound for the overall power is rather conservative and is achieved only in clinical trials with a very large number of interim looks (especially if γ is less than 0.7). If recomputing the sample size appears feasible, one can also consider an approximation to the power function of the Lan-Simon-Halperin test developed by Davis and Hardy (1990); see also Betensky (1997).

Adaptive Conditional Power Tests

An important feature of the Lan-Simon-Halperin test introduced in the previous subsection is the assumption that future observations are generated from the alternative hypothesis. It has been noted in the literature that this assumption may lead to spurious results and, as a consequence, the corresponding conditional power test does not always serve as a reliable stopping criterion. For example, Pepe and Anderson (1992) reviewed the performance of the Lan-Simon-Halperin test under a scenario when interim data do not support the alternative hypothesis. They showed that the Lan-Simon-Halperin test tends to produce an overly optimistic probability of a positive trial outcome when the observed treatment effect is substantially different from the hypothesized one.

To illustrate this phenomenon, consider the severe sepsis trial example. The trial was designed under the assumption that the experimental drug provides a 9% absolute improvement in the 28-day survival rate. The interim data displayed in Table 4.12 clearly contradict the alternative hypothesis: the treatment difference remains negative at all six interim looks. In this situation it is natural to ask whether adjusting the original assumptions to account for the emerging pattern will have an effect on the decision-making process. Program 4.19 performs conditional power calculations under assumptions that are more consistent with the interim data than the alternative hypothesis; specifically, the effect size for the future data is set to 0.1 and 0.

Program 4.19 Lan-Simon-Halperin conditional power test in the analysis of the severe sepsis trial under less optimistic assumptions about the magnitude of the treatment effect

```
%CondPowerLSH(data=test,effsize=0.1,alpha=0.1,gamma=0.8,nn=212,
    prob=p,boundary=boundary);
title "Effect size is 0.1";
proc print data=p noobs label;
%CondPowerLSH(data=test,effsize=0,alpha=0.1,gamma=0.8,nn=212,
    prob=p,boundary=boundary);
title "Effect size is 0";
proc print data=p noobs label;
run;
```

Output from Program 4.19

```
                    Effect size is 0.1
            Fraction of
            total sample     Test        Conditional
Analysis    size             statistic   power
   1        0.24             -0.4583      0.2059
   2        0.36             -0.2157      0.1731
   3        0.46             -0.1329      0.1322
   4        0.55             -0.4573      0.0432
   5        0.64             -0.1666      0.0421
   6        0.72             -0.3097      0.0085


                     Effect size is 0
            Fraction of
            total sample     Test        Conditional
Analysis    size             statistic   power
   1        0.24             -0.4583      0.0427
   2        0.36             -0.2157      0.0388
   3        0.46             -0.1329      0.0307
   4        0.55             -0.4573      0.0080
   5        0.64             -0.1666      0.0095
   6        0.72             -0.3097      0.0017
```

It is instructive to compare Output 4.19 with Output 4.17, in which the conditional power was computed under the alternative hypothesis and thus the effect size for the future data was set to 0.2065. The conditional power values in Output 4.19 are consistently lower than those in Output 4.17 with the conditional power estimates in the bottom half being extremely small right from the first futility analysis. This observation has a simple explanation. Since the true effect size for the future observations is assumed to be smaller in magnitude, there is a lower chance that the negative treatment difference will get reversed by the end of the trial and thus the conditional power of a positive trial outcome will also be lower. We can see from Output 4.19 that making an overly optimistic assumption about the size of the treatment effect delays the decision to terminate the trial and can potentially cause more patients to be exposed to an ineffective therapy. For this reason, in the absence of strong *a priori* evidence it may be inappropriate to use the alternative hypothesis for generating future data in conditional power calculations.

Since failure to account for emerging trends may undermine the utility of the simple conditional power method, Lan and Wittes (1988) proposed to evaluate the conditional power function at a data-driven value. Pepe and Anderson (1992) studied a conditional power test using the value of the treatment difference that is slightly more optimistic than the interim maximum likelihood estimate. This and similar adaptive approaches achieve greater efficiency than the simple conditional power method by "letting the data speak for themselves."

Using the Pepe-Anderson test as a starting point, Betensky (1997) introduced a family of adaptive conditional power tests in which the fixed value of δ is replaced in the decision rule with $\widehat{\delta}_n + cSE(\widehat{\delta}_n)$. Here $\widehat{\delta}_n$ is the maximum likelihood estimate of δ from the first $2n$ observations, $SE(\widehat{\delta}_n)$ denotes its standard error, and c is a positive parameter that determines the shape of the stopping boundary. The c parameter equals 1 in the Pepe-Anderson test, and Betensky (1997) recommended to let $c = 2.326$ (the 99th percentile of the standard normal distribution) to better control the amount of uncertainty about the final trial outcome.

Using our notation and assuming σ is known, it is easy to check that

$$\widehat{\delta}_n = \sigma\sqrt{2/n}\,Z_n$$

and

$$SE(\widehat{\delta}_n) = \sigma\sqrt{2/n}.$$

Therefore, the resulting Pepe-Anderson-Betensky decision rule is based on the conditional probability

$$P_n = \Phi \left(\frac{\sqrt{n}Z_n + (N-n)(Z_n+c)/\sqrt{n} - \sqrt{N}z_{1-\alpha}}{\sqrt{N-n}} \right),$$

and the trial is stopped the first time P_n is less than $1 - \gamma$. Note that this futility rule no longer depends on the standard deviation of the outcome variable (σ).

Equivalently, the Pepe-Anderson-Betensky rule can be formulated in terms of the test statistic Z_n. Specifically, the trial is terminated as soon as the test statistic drops below the adjusted critical value defined as follows:

$$l_n = \sqrt{\frac{n}{N}}z_{1-\alpha} + \sqrt{\frac{n(N-n)}{N^2}}z_{1-\gamma} - \frac{c(N-n)}{N}.$$

%CondPowerPAB Macro

Program 4.20 uses the Pepe-Anderson-Betensky test with $c = 1$ and $c = 2.326$ as the stopping criterion in the severe sepsis trial. The Pepe-Anderson-Betensky test is implemented in the %CondPowerPAB macro given in the Appendix. To call the %CondPowerPAB macro, we need to provide information similar to that required by the %CondPowerLSH macro:

- DATA is the name of the input data set with one record per interim look. The data set must include the N and TESTSTAT variables defined as in the %CondPowerLSH macro.

- ALPHA is the one-sided Type I error probability of the significance test carried out at the end of the trial.

- GAMMA is the futility index.

- C is the parameter determining the shape of the stopping boundary. Pepe and Anderson (1992) set C to 1 and Betensky (1997) recommended to set C to 2.326.

- NN is the projected number of patients per treatment group.

- PROB is the name of the data set containing the computed conditional power. This data set is generated by the macro and includes the ANALYSIS, FRACTION, TESTSTAT and CONDPOWER variables defined as in the %CondPowerLSH macro.

- BOUNDARY is the name of the data set that contains the stopping boundary of the conditional power test. This data set is generated by the macro and includes the FRACTION and STOPBOUNDARY variables defined as in the %CondPowerLSH macro.

The main difference between the %CondPowerLSH and %CondPowerPAB macros is that in order to generate future data the latter macro relies on a sample estimate of the effect size and thus it no longer requires the specification of the effect size under the alternative hypothesis.

Program 4.20 Pepe-Anderson-Betensky conditional power test in the analysis of the severe sepsis trial

```
%CondPowerPAB(data=test,alpha=0.1,gamma=0.8,c=1,nn=212,
    prob=p,boundary=boundary1);
title "Pepe-Anderson-Betensky test with c=1";
proc print data=p noobs label;
%CondPowerPAB(data=test,alpha=0.1,gamma=0.8,c=2.326,nn=212,
    prob=p,boundary=boundary2);
%CondPowerLSH(data=test,effsize=0.2065,alpha=0.1,gamma=0.8,nn=212,
    prob=p,boundary=boundary3);
title "Pepe-Anderson-Betensky test with c=2.326";
proc print data=p noobs label;
    run;
```

```
data test;
    set test;
    group=1;
    fraction=n/212;
    StopBoundary=teststat;
data boundary1;
    set boundary1;
    group=2;
data boundary2;
    set boundary2;
    group=3;
data boundary3;
    set boundary3;
    group=4;
data plot;
    set test boundary1 boundary2 boundary3;
axis1 minor=none label=(angle=90 "Test statistic") order=(-3 to 1 by 1);
axis2 minor=none label=("Fraction of total sample size")
    order=(0 to 1 by 0.2);
symbol1 i=none v=dot color=black;
symbol2 i=join v=none color=black line=20;
symbol3 i=join v=none color=black line=34;
symbol4 i=join v=none color=black line=1;
proc gplot data=plot;
    plot StopBoundary*Fraction=group/frame nolegend
    haxis=axis2 vaxis=axis1;
    run;
    quit;
```

Output from Program 4.20

Pepe-Anderson-Betensky test with c=1

Analysis	Fraction of total sample size	Test statistic	Conditional power
1	0.24	−0.4583	0.2279
2	0.36	−0.2157	0.2354
3	0.46	−0.1329	0.1747
4	0.55	−0.4573	0.0278
5	0.64	−0.1666	0.0429
6	0.72	−0.3097	0.0062

Pepe-Anderson-Betensky test with c=2.326

Analysis	Fraction of total sample size	Test statistic	Conditional power
1	0.24	−0.4583	0.9496
2	0.36	−0.2157	0.8516
3	0.46	−0.1329	0.6895
4	0.55	−0.4573	0.2397
5	0.64	−0.1666	0.2370
6	0.72	−0.3097	0.0469

Output 4.20 displays the conditional power estimates at the six interim looks produced by the Pepe-Anderson-Betensky test under two scenarios. Under the first scenario ($c = 1$), this test is more likely to lead to early termination than the Lan-Simon-Halperin test. The conditional power is very close to the 20% threshold at the very first interim analysis, suggesting that the alternative hypothesis is unlikely to be true. The conditional power falls below the threshold and the test rejects the alternative at the third analysis. The early rejection of the alternative hypothesis is consistent with the observation that the experimental drug is unlikely to improve survival and might even have a detrimental effect on patients' health.

In contrast, the Pepe-Anderson-Betensky test with $c = 2.326$ relies on a stopping boundary that virtually excludes the possibility of an early termination. The initial conditional power values are well above 50%. Although the conditional power decreases steadily, it remains above the 20% threshold at the fourth and fifth looks. The stopping criterion is not met until the last analysis.

Figure 4.26 depicts the Pepe-Anderson-Betensky stopping boundaries corresponding to $c = 1$ and $c = 2.326$ along with the stopping boundary of the Lan-Simon-Halperin test. The stopping boundary of the Pepe-Anderson-Betensky test with $c = 2.326$ is close to that of the Lan-Simon-Halperin test early in the trial. Although the Pepe-Anderson-Betensky test rejects the alternative hypothesis under both scenarios, it is clear that, with a large value of c, one runs a risk of missing an early negative trend.

Figure 4.26 Stopping boundaries of the Lan-Simon-Halperin test (—), Pepe-Anderson-Betensky test with $c = 1$ (- - -) and $c = 2.326$ ($\cdots$), and interim z statistics (•) in the severe sepsis trial example. The futility index γ is 0.8; the continuation region is above the stopping boundary.

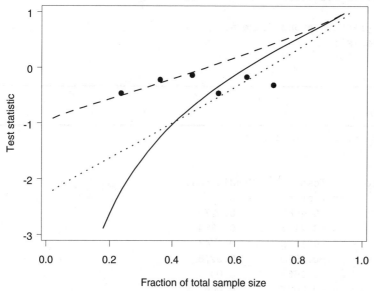

Figure 4.27 compares the Lan-Simon-Halperin and Pepe-Anderson-Betensky stopping boundaries with $\gamma = 0.8$ on an event rate scale. As in Figure 4.25, the resulting boundaries resemble straight-line segments parallel to the identity line. We can see from Figure 4.27 that the Lan-Simon-Halperin test is less likely to lead to early stopping at the first interim look compared to the Pepe-Anderson-Betensky tests with $c = 1$ and $c = 2.326$. However, the three stopping boundaries are pretty close to each other by the last look.

4.3.2 Futility Rules Based on Predictive Power

One of the important limitations of adaptive conditional power tests is that conditional power is computed assuming the observed treatment difference and standard deviation for the remainder of the trial. The observed treatment effect and its variability essentially serve as a prediction tool; however, no adjustment is made to account for the associated prediction error. This feature of the adaptive

Figure 4.27 Stopping boundaries of the Lan-Simon-Halperin test (—), Pepe-Anderson-Betensky test with $c = 1$ (- - -) and $c = 2.326$ ($\cdots$), and interim survival rates (•) in the severe sepsis trial example. The futility index γ is 0.8; the continuation region is below the stopping boundary.

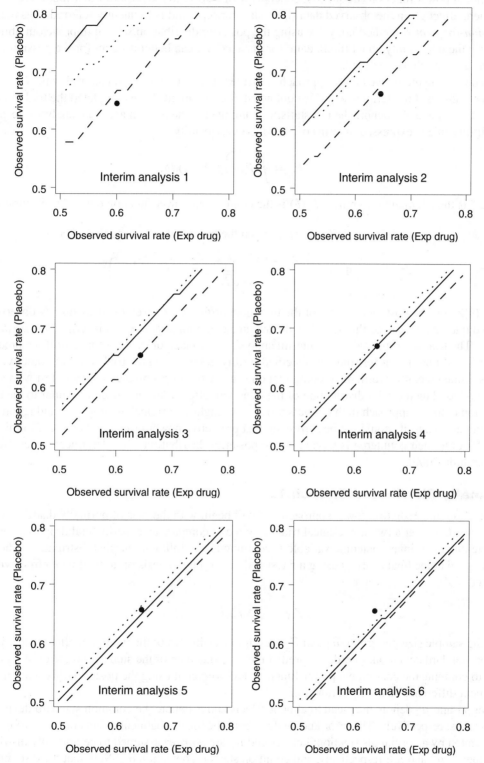

conditional power approach needs to be contrasted with corresponding features of *predictive power methods* discussed in this subsection. The predictive power methodology involves averaging the conditional power function (frequentist concept) with respect to the posterior distribution of the treatment effect given the observed data (Bayesian concept) and is frequently referred to as the *mixed Bayesian-frequentist* methodology. By using the posterior distribution we can improve our ability to quantify the uncertainty about future data; for instance, we can better account for the possibility that the current trend might be reversed.

To define the predictive power approach, consider again a two-arm clinical trial with N patients per treatment group. An interim analysis is conducted after n patients have completed the trial in each group. Let Z_n and Z_N denote the test statistics computed at the interim and final analyses, respectively. The futility rule is expressed in terms of the following quantity:

$$P_n = \int P_n(\delta) f(\delta | Z_n) d\delta,$$

where δ is the treatment difference, $P_n(\delta)$ is the conditional power function defined in Section 4.3.1, i.e.,

$$P_n(\delta) = P(Z_N > z_{1-\alpha} \text{ when the treatment effect equals } \delta | Z_n)$$

$$= \Phi\left(\frac{\sigma\sqrt{n}Z_n + (N-n)\delta/\sqrt{2} - \sigma\sqrt{N}z_{1-\alpha}}{\sigma\sqrt{N-n}}\right),$$

and $f(\delta | Z_n)$ is the posterior density of the treatment difference δ given the data already observed. The defined quantity P_n can be thought of as the average conditional power and is termed the *predictive power*. The trial is terminated at the interim analysis due to lack of treatment benefit if the predictive power is less than $1 - \gamma$ for some prespecified futility index γ, and the trial continues otherwise.

As a side note, it is worth mentioning that one can also set up a predictive power test with a weight function based on the prior distribution of the treatment effect. This approach is similar to the basic conditional power approach in that it puts too much weight on original assumptions and ignores the interim data. Thus, it should not be surprising that predictive power tests based on the prior distribution are inferior to their counterparts relying on the posterior distribution of the treatment effect (Bernardo and Ibrahim, 2000).

Normally Distributed Endpoints

To illustrate the predictive power approach, we will begin with the case of normally distributed endpoints. Consider a two-arm clinical trial designed to compare an experimental drug to a control, and assume that the primary outcome variable is continuous and follows a normal distribution. The data will be analyzed at the final analysis using a z test and the null hypothesis of no treatment effect will be rejected if $Z_N > z_{1-\alpha}$, where

$$Z_N = \sqrt{N/2}(\widehat{\mu}_1 - \widehat{\mu}_2)/s,$$

N is the sample size per group, $\widehat{\mu}_1$ and $\widehat{\mu}_2$ are sample estimates of the treatment effect, and s is the pooled standard deviation. In order to predict the final outcome of the study from the existing data, we need to compute the conditional power function and average it using the posterior distribution of the treatment difference as a weight function.

Let μ_1 and μ_2 denote the mean treatment effects and σ denote the common standard deviation in the two groups, respectively. The prior knowledge about the mean treatment effects in each group is represented by a normal distribution; i.e., μ_1 and μ_2 are *a priori* assumed to be normally distributed with means μ_1^* and μ_2^*, respectively, and common standard deviation σ^*. Note that the difference between μ_1^* and μ_2^* is equal to the mean treatment difference under the alternative hypothesis.

As shown by Dmitrienko and Wang (2004), the predictive power conditional upon the interim test statistic Z_n is given by

$$P_n = \Phi \left(\frac{\sqrt{N} Z_n (1 + a_n) + b_n/\sigma - \sqrt{n} z_{1-\alpha}}{\sqrt{\frac{N-n}{N} [(N - n)(1 - c_n) + n]}} \right),$$

where

$$a_n = \frac{n - N}{N} + \frac{N - n}{N} \left(1 + \frac{1}{n} \left(\frac{\sigma}{\sigma^*} \right)^2 \right)^{-1},$$

$$b_n = \sqrt{\frac{n}{2N}} (N - n)(\mu_1^* - \mu_2^*) \left(1 + n \left(\frac{\sigma^*}{\sigma} \right)^2 \right)^{-1},$$

$$c_n = \left(1 + n \left(\frac{\sigma^*}{\sigma} \right)^2 \right)^{-1}.$$

The trial will be stopped due to futility as soon as the computed predictive power falls below a prespecified threshold, i.e., as soon as $P_n < 1 - \gamma$. It is easy to invert this inequality and express the stopping rule in terms of the test statistic Z_n:

Discontinue the trial due to lack of efficacy the first time $Z_n < l_n$,

with the adjusted critical value given by

$$l_n = \frac{1}{\sqrt{N}(1 + a_n)} \left(\sqrt{n} z_{1-\alpha} + z_{1-\gamma} \sqrt{\frac{N-n}{N} [(N - n)(1 - c_n) + n]} - b_n/\sigma \right).$$

The derived formula for the predictive power involves the true standard deviation σ, which can be estimated by the pooled sample standard deviation. Also, the predictive power depends on the prior distributions of μ_1 and μ_2 only through the parameters a_n, b_n and c_n. These parameters measure the amount of prior information about the mean treatment difference and decrease in magnitude as the prior distributions of μ_1 and μ_2 become more spread out. In fact, it is easy to check that a_n, b_n and c_n approach zero as the common standard deviation of the priors increases in magnitude. Because of this, the formula for the predictive power simplifies significantly when we assume an improper uniform prior for both μ_1 and μ_2, i.e., let $\sigma^* \to \infty$. In this case, the predictive power P_n is equal to

$$\Phi \left(\frac{\sqrt{N} Z_n - \sqrt{n} z_{1-\alpha}}{\sqrt{(N - n)}} \right),$$

and the adjusted critical value l_n simplifies to

$$l_n = \sqrt{\frac{n}{N}} z_{1-\alpha} + \sqrt{\frac{N-n}{N}} z_{1-\gamma}.$$

Compared to the Lan-Simon-Halperin conditional power test introduced in Section 4.3.1, the unadjusted critical value $z_{1-\alpha}$ in the formula for the predictive power is multiplied by $\sqrt{n/(N-n)}$ instead of $\sqrt{N/(N-n)}$. As pointed out by Geisser (1992), this implies that the predictive power approach to futility monitoring can exhibit a counterintuitive behavior at the early interim looks. To see what happens, note that n is small relative to N early in the trial and therefore the predictive power becomes virtually independent of $z_{1-\alpha}$. Although the futility rule based on predictive power is designed to assess the likelihood of a statistically significant outcome at the end of the trial, it no longer depends on the significance level α. It might be difficult to interpret an early decision to stop a clinical trial due to lack of efficacy because it is unclear what definition of efficacy is used in the futility rule.

Now that we have talked about futility rules associated with uniform priors, let us look at the other extreme and assume that the common standard deviation of the prior distributions of μ_1 and μ_2 is small. It can be shown that in this case the predictive power asymptotically approaches the conditional power function evaluated at $\delta = \mu_1^* - \mu_2^*$. If we assume that the difference between μ_1^* and μ_2^* equals the clinically significant difference, the predictive power is asymptotically equivalent to the Lan-Simon-Halperin test. This should come as little surprise, because assuming that $\mu_1^* - \mu_2^*$ is very close to δ is another way of saying that the future data are generated from the alternative hypothesis.

We see that the choice of a prior distribution for the treatment difference can potentially impact predictive inferences, especially in small proof-of-concept trials; however, no consensus has been reached in the literature regarding a comprehensive prior selection strategy. For example, Spiegelhalter, Freedman and Blackburn (1986) recommended to use uniform prior distributions in clinical applications because they are quickly overwhelmed by the data and thus the associated predictive inferences are driven only by the observed data. Johns and Anderson (1999) also utilized decision rules based on a noninformative prior. In contrast, Herson (1979) stressed that a uniform prior is often undesirable because it assigns too much weight to extreme values of the treatment difference.

Elicitation of the prior distribution from clinical experts can be a complex and time-consuming activity; see Freedman and Spiegelhalter (1983) for a description of an elaborate interview of 18 physicians to quantify their prior beliefs about the size of the treatment effect in a clinical trial. Alternatively, one can utilize simple rules of thumb for selecting a prior distribution proposed in the literature. For example, Herson (1979) provided a set of guidelines for the selection of a prior distribution in the binary case. According to the guidelines, a beta prior with the coefficient of variation of 0.1 indicates a high degree of confidence, whereas the value of 0.5 corresponds to low confidence. A similar rule can be adopted to choose priors for the parameters of a normal distribution. For example, Table 4.13 presents two sets of parameters of normal priors in the generalized anxiety disorder trial. In both cases the means of the prior distributions are equal to the expected changes in the HAMA total score in the two treatment groups—i.e., -12 in the experimental group and -8 in the placebo group. The common standard deviation is chosen in such a way that the coefficient of variation with respect to the average HAMA change is equal to 0.1 or 1. The prior distributions in the experimental and placebo groups are displayed in Figure 4.28.

Table 4.13 Parameters of the normal prior for the mean changes in the HAMA score in the generalized anxiety disorder trial

	Experimental group		Placebo group	
Normal prior distribution	Mean	SD	Mean	SD
"Low confidence" prior (coefficient of variation=1)	−12	10	−8	10
"High confidence" prior (coefficient of variation=0.1)	−12	1	−8	1

%BayesFutilityCont Macro

The predictive power approach to futility monitoring in clinical trials with a normally distributed endpoint can be implemented using the %BayesFutilityCont macro provided in the Appendix. Note that the macro also supports the predictive probability approach introduced later in Section 4.3.3.

The %BayesFutilityCont macro has the following arguments:

- DATA is the name of the input data set with one record per interim look. The data set must include the following variables:
  - N1 and N2 are the numbers of patients in the experimental and placebo groups included in the analysis data set at the current interim look.

Figure 4.28 Low confidence (- - -) and high confidence (⋯) prior distributions of the mean change in the HAMA total score in the generalized anxiety disorder trial example. Upper panel: experimental group (Mean HAMA change is assumed to be −12); lower panel: placebo group (Mean HAMA change is assumed to be −8).

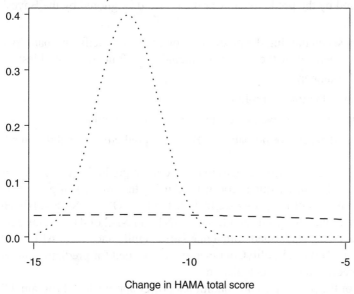

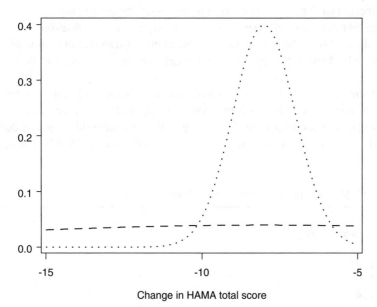

- MEAN1 and MEAN2 are the estimates of the mean treatment effects in the experimental and placebo groups at the current interim look.

- SD1 and SD2 are the sample standard deviations in the experimental and placebo groups at the current interim look.

- PAR is the name of the single-record input data set with the following variables:

  - NN1 and NN2 are the projected numbers of patients in the experimental and placebo groups.

  - MU1, MU2 and SIGMA are the means and common standard deviation of the prior distributions of the mean treatment effects in the experimental and placebo groups.

- DELTA is the clinically significant difference between the treatment groups. This parameter is required by the Bayesian predictive probability method and is ignored by the predictive power method.

- ETA is the confidence level of the Bayesian predictive probability method. This parameter is required by the Bayesian predictive probability method and is ignored by the predictive power method.
- ALPHA is the one-sided Type I error probability of the significance test carried out at the end of the trial. This parameter is required by the predictive power method and is ignored by the Bayesian predictive probability method.
- PROB is the name of the data set containing the predictive power and predictive probability at each interim look. This data set is generated by the macro and includes the following variables:
  - ANALYSIS is the analysis number.
  - FRACTION is the fraction of the total sample size.
  - PREDPOWER is the computed predictive power (predictive power method).
  - PREDPROB is the computed predictive probability (Bayesian predictive probability method).

Program 4.21 utilizes the %BayesFutilityCont macro to carry out the predictive power test in the generalized anxiety disorder trial. The futility rule is constructed using the two sets of prior distributions displayed in Table 4.13. The parameters of the priors are included in the LOWCONF and HIGHCONF data sets. The data sets also include the projected sample sizes NN1 and NN2 of 41 patients per treatment group. The futility analysis is performed with a one-sided significance level ALPHA=0.1. The DELTA and ETA parameters of the %BayesFutilityCont macro are intended for predictive probability inferences and are not used in predictive power calculations.

To facilitate the comparison of the predictive and conditional power approaches, Program 4.21 also carries out the Lan-Simon-Halperin test for the same set of interim results by calling the %CondPowerLSH macro. Note that the %CondPowerLSH macro requires the specification of the effect size under the alternative hypothesis. Since the treatment difference and the standard deviation of HAMA changes were assumed to be 4 and 8.5 in the sample size calculation, the effect size is $4/8.5 = 0.4706$.

Lastly, the %BayesFutilityCont macro, as well all other SAS macros introduced in this chapter, assumes that a positive treatment difference indicates improvement compared to the placebo. Since the experimental drug improves the HAMA total score by decreasing it, the treatment difference is defined in Program 4.21 as the mean HAMA change in the placebo group minus the mean HAMA change in the experimental group.

Program 4.21 Predictive power test in the generalized anxiety disorder trial

```
data genanx;
    input n1 mean1 sd1 n2 mean2 sd2;
    datalines;
    11 -8.4 6.4 10 -9.2 7.3
    20 -8.1 6.9 20 -9.4 6.7
    30 -9.1 7.7 31 -8.9 7.4
    ;
data lowconf;
    input nn1 nn2 mu1 mu2 sigma;
    datalines;
    41 41 -8 -12 10
    ;
data highconf;
    input nn1 nn2 mu1 mu2 sigma;
    datalines;
    41 41 -8 -12 1
    ;
%BayesFutilityCont(data=genanx,par=lowconf,delta=0,eta=0.9,alpha=0.1,
    prob=lowout);
```

```
%BayesFutilityCont(data=genanx,par=highconf,delta=0,eta=0.9,alpha=0.1,
    prob=highout);
proc print data=lowout noobs label;
    title "Predictive power test, Low confidence prior";
    var Analysis Fraction PredPower;
proc print data=highout noobs label;
    title "Predictive power test, High confidence prior";
    var Analysis Fraction PredPower;
data test;
    set genanx;
    s=sqrt(((n1-1)*sd1*sd1+(n2-1)*sd2*sd2)/(n1+n2-2));
    teststat=(mean1-mean2)/(s*sqrt(1/n1+1/n2));
    n=(n1+n2)/2;
    keep n teststat;
%CondPowerLSH(data=test,effsize=0.4706,alpha=0.1,gamma=0.8,nn=41,
    prob=out,boundary=boundary);
proc print data=out noobs label;
    title "Conditional power test";
    var Analysis Fraction CondPower;
    run;
```

Output from Program 4.21

```
Predictive power test, Low confidence prior

             Fraction of
             total sample    Predictive
Analysis        size           power
   1            0.26          0.3414
   2            0.49          0.3490
   3            0.74          0.0088


Predictive power test, High confidence prior

             Fraction of
             total sample    Predictive
Analysis        size           power
   1            0.26          0.6917
   2            0.49          0.6087
   3            0.74          0.0335


             Conditional power test

             Fraction of
             total sample    Conditional
Analysis        size           power
   1            0.26          0.6946
   2            0.49          0.6271
   3            0.74          0.0515
```

Output 4.21 displays the probabilities of a positive final outcome produced by the predictive and conditional power methods in the generalized anxiety disorder trial. Comparing the predictive power values associated with the low and high confidence priors, we see that the probability of observing a statistically significant result at the planned termination point is considerably higher when the variance of the prior is assumed to be small. This difference, however, does not affect the decision-making process. The predictive power is consistently above the 20% threshold at the first two looks, which suggests that the trial should continue, and falls below 5% at the third look. Given the low probability of success, it is prudent to discontinue the trial at the third interim inspection due to lack of efficacy.

The conditional power shown in the bottom part of Output 4.21 is quite close to the predictive power under the high confidence prior. This is because the predictive power method approximates the conditional power method as the prior information about the treatment difference becomes more precise. Since predictive power tests based on very strong priors assume that the future data are generated from the alternative hypothesis, they tend to produce an overly optimistic prediction about the final trial outcome.

Figure 4.29 displays the stopping boundaries of the predictive power test based on the low and high confidence priors as well as the boundary of the Lan-Simon-Halperin test. The boundaries have been generated by a program similar to Program 4.17. Figure 4.29 demonstrates the relationship between the amount of prior information about the treatment effect and the probability of early termination due to lack of benefit. An assumption of a weak prior increases the chances of an early termination. For example, with the low confidence prior, a trial will be stopped almost immediately if the observed z statistic is less than -0.5. In contrast, the test based on the high confidence prior (as well as the Lan-Simon-Halperin test) will consider this z statistic somewhat consistent with the alternative hypothesis in the first part of the trial. Clinical researchers need to keep this relationship in mind when selecting a futility rule based on predictive power.

Figure 4.29 Stopping boundaries of the Lan-Simon-Halperin test (—), predictive test based on a low confidence prior (- - -) and high confidence prior (· · ·) and interim z statistics (•) in the generalized anxiety disorder trial example. The futility index γ is 0.8; the continuation region is above the stopping boundary.

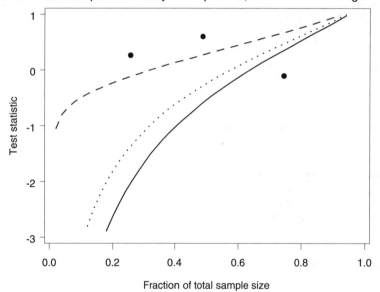

Binary Endpoints

In order to introduce predictive power futility rules for clinical trials with binary outcomes, we will return to the severe sepsis trial example. Before defining the predictive power test, it is instructive to point out an important difference between conditional and predictive power methods for binary data. Recall that conditional power tests in Section 4.3.1 rely on the asymptotic normality of z statistics and therefore can be applied to clinical trials with both continuous and binary variables. By contrast, the case of binary endpoints needs to be considered separately within the predictive power framework because predictive inferences are based on the Bayesian paradigm. Although a normal approximation can be used in the calculation of the conditional power function, one still needs to define prior distributions for event rates in the experimental and control groups. In this subsection we will derive an exact formula for the predictive power in the binary case that does not rely on a normal approximation; see Dmitrienko and Wang (2004) for more details.

Let π_1 and π_2 denote the survival rates in the experimental and placebo groups, and let B_i and A_i denote the number of patients who survived to the end of the 28-day study period in Treatment group i before and after the interim look, respectively. Efficacy of the experimental drug will be established at the final analysis if the test statistic

$$Z_N = (p_1 - p_2)/\sqrt{2\overline{p}(1 - \overline{p})/N}$$

is significant at a one-sided α level. Here p_1 and p_2 are estimated survival rates in the experimental and placebo groups and $\overline{p}$ is the average survival rate; i.e.,

$$p_i = \frac{B_i + A_i}{N}, \quad i = 1, 2, \quad \overline{p} = (p_1 + p_2)/2.$$

The event counts B_1 and B_2 are computed from the interim data; however, the future event counts A_1 and A_2 are unobservable and, in order to compute Z_N, we will need to rely on their predicted values. Assume that π_i follows a beta distribution with the parameters α_i and β_i. Given B_i, the predicted value of A_i follows a beta-binomial distribution; i.e.,

$$p_i(a|b) = P(A_i = a|B_i = b) = \frac{\Gamma(N - n + 1)B(b + a + \alpha_i, N - b - a + \beta_i)}{\Gamma(N - n - a + 1)\Gamma(a + 1)B(b + \alpha_i, n - b + \beta_i)},$$

where $0 \leq a \leq N - n$, and $\Gamma()$ and $B()$ are the gamma and beta functions.

Now that we have derived the predictive distribution of the future event counts A_1 and A_2, the predictive probability of a statistically significant difference at the planned end of the trial is given by

$$P_n = \sum_{j=0}^{N-n} \sum_{k=0}^{N-n} I(Z_N > z_{1-\alpha}|A_1 = j, A_2 = k)p_1(j|B_1)p_2(k|B_2).$$

Here $I()$ is the indicator function and thus the predictive probability P_n is computed by summing over the values of A_1 and A_2 that result in a significant test statistic Z_N. The trial is terminated at the interim analysis due to futility if the predictive probability of a positive trial outcome is sufficiently small.

Table 4.14 Prior distribution of 28-day survival rates in the severe sepsis trial

Beta prior distribution	Experimental group		Placebo group	
	α	β	α	β
"Low confidence" prior (uniform prior with coefficient of variation=0.58)	1	1	1	1
"High confidence" prior (coefficient of variation=0.025)	335	89	479	205

Table 4.14 shows two sets of prior distributions of 28-day survival corresponding to low and high confidence scenarios. The calculations assumed that the 28-day survival rates in the experimental and placebo groups are equal to 79% and 70%, respectively. The prior distributions were chosen using a version of the Herson rule. As was mentioned previously, Herson (1979) proposed a simple rule to facilitate the selection of prior distributions in clinical trials with a binary response variable:

- "Low confidence" prior: Beta distribution with the mean equal to the expected event rate (e.g., expected 28-day survival rate) and coefficient of variation equal to 0.5

- "Medium confidence" prior: Beta distribution with the mean equal to the expected event rate and coefficient of variation equal to 0.25
- "High confidence" prior: Beta distribution with the mean equal to the expected event rate and coefficient of variation equal to 0.1.

Once the mean m and coefficient of variation c of a beta distribution have been specified, its parameters are given by

$$\alpha = (1 - m)/c^2 - m, \quad \beta = \alpha(1 - m)/m.$$

In practice, one often needs to slightly modify the described rule. First, the Herson rule is applicable to event rates ranging from 0.3 to 0.7. Outside of this range, it may not be possible to achieve the coefficient of variation of 0.5, or even 0.25, with a bell-shaped beta distribution, and U-shaped priors are clearly undesirable in practice. For this reason, a uniform prior was selected to represent a low confidence scenario in the severe sepsis trial. Further, even prior distributions with the coefficient of variation around 0.1 are fairly weak and are completely dominated by the data in large trials. To specify high confidence priors in the severe sepsis trial, we set the coefficient of variation to 0.025. The obtained prior distributions are depicted in Figure 4.30.

%BayesFutilityBin Macro

Program 4.22 performs predictive power calculations in the severe sepsis trial by invoking the %BayesFutilityBin macro included in the Appendix. The macro implements the predictive power method based on the mixed Bayesian-frequentist approach as well as the fully Bayesian predictive method that will be described later in Section 4.3.3. Here we will focus on predictive power inferences to examine early evidence of futility in the severe sepsis trial.

The %BayesFutilityBin macro has the following arguments:

- DATA is the name of the input data set with one record per interim look. The data set must include the following variables:
  - N1 and N2 are the numbers of patients in the experimental and placebo groups included in the analysis data set at the current interim look.
  - COUNT1 and COUNT2 are the observed event counts in the experimental and placebo groups at the current interim look.
- PAR is the name of the single-record input data set with the following variables:
  - NN1 and NN2 are the projected numbers of patients in the experimental and placebo groups.
  - ALPHA1 and ALPHA2 are the α parameters of beta priors for event rates in the experimental and placebo groups.
  - BETA1 and BETA2 are the β parameters of beta priors for event rates in the experimental and placebo groups.
- DELTA is the clinically significant difference between the treatment groups. This parameter is required by the Bayesian predictive probability method and is ignored by the predictive power method.
- ETA is the confidence level of the Bayesian predictive probability method. This parameter is required by the Bayesian predictive probability method and is ignored by the predictive power method.
- ALPHA is the one-sided Type I error probability of the significance test carried out at the end of the trial. This parameter is required by the predictive power method and is ignored by the Bayesian predictive probability method.
- PROB is the name of the data set containing the predictive power and predictive probability at each interim look. This data set includes the same four variables as the output data set in the %BayesFutilityCont macro, i.e., ANALYSIS, FRACTION, PREDPOWER and PREDPROB.

Figure 4.30 Low confidence (- - -) and high confidence (· · ·) prior distributions of 28-day survival rates in the severe sepsis trial example. Upper panel: experimental group (28-day survival rate is assumed to be 79%); lower panel: placebo group (28-day survival rate is assumed to be 70%).

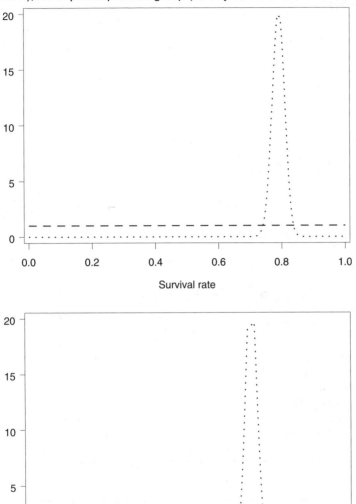

In order to assess the amount of evidence in favor of the experimental drug at each interim look, Program 4.22 computes the predictive power using the prior distributions of 28-day survival rates shown in Table 4.14. The parameters of these beta distributions, included in the LOWCONF and HIGHCONF data sets, are passed to the %BayesFutilityBin macro. The one-sided significance level ALPHA is 0.1 and the projected sample sizes NN1 and NN2 are set to 212 patients. The DELTA and ETA parameters are not used in predictive power calculations and are set to arbitrary values.

Output 4.22 summarizes the results of predictive power inferences performed at each of the six looks in the severe sepsis trial. As in the case of normally distributed endpoints, the use of less informative priors increases the chances to declare futility. Output 4.22 shows that, with the low confidence prior, the probability of eventual success is 11.1% at the first look, which is substantially less than 22.8% Pepe-Anderson-Betensky test with $c = 1$ in Output 4.20) or 55.5% (Lan-Simon-Halperin test in Output 4.17). As a result, the futility rule is met at the very first interim analysis.

Program 4.22 Predictive power test in the severe sepsis trial

```
data sevsep2;
    input n1 count1 n2 count2;
    datalines;
     55  33  45  29
     79  51  74  49
    101  65  95  62
    117  75 115  77
    136  88 134  88
    155  99 151  99
    ;
data LowConf;
    input nn1 nn2 alpha1 alpha2 beta1 beta2;
    datalines;
    212 212  1  1  1  1
    ;
data HighConf;
    input nn1 nn2 alpha1 alpha2 beta1 beta2;
    datalines;
    212 212 335 479 89 205
    ;
%BayesFutilityBin(data=sevsep2,par=LowConf,delta=0,eta=0.9,
    alpha=0.1,prob=LowProb);
%BayesFutilityBin(data=sevsep2,par=HighConf,delta=0,eta=0.9,
    alpha=0.1,prob=HighProb);
proc print data=LowProb noobs label;
    title "Low confidence prior";
    var Analysis Fraction PredPower;
proc print data=HighProb noobs label;
    title "High confidence prior";
    var Analysis Fraction PredPower;
    run;
```

Output from Program 4.22

```
              Low confidence prior

              Fraction of
              total sample    Predictive
    Analysis     size           power
       1         0.24          0.1107
       2         0.36          0.1091
       3         0.46          0.0864
       4         0.55          0.0183
       5         0.64          0.0243
       6         0.72          0.0041


              High confidence prior

              Fraction of
              total sample    Predictive
    Analysis     size           power
       1         0.24          0.3349
       2         0.36          0.3012
       3         0.46          0.2023
```

4	0.55	0.0652
5	0.64	0.0579
6	0.72	0.0087

Selecting a more informative prior increases the probability of success at the first interim analysis to 33.5% and brings the predictive power test closer to the Lan-Simon-Halperin conditional power test. However, even in this setting the predictive power drops below the 20% threshold at the fourth look, indicating that a decision to discontinue the patient enrollment should have been considered early in the trial.

4.3.3 Futility Rules Based on Predictive Probability

As we explained in the previous subsection, predictive power tests are derived by averaging the conditional power function with respect to the posterior distribution of the treatment difference given the already observed data. Several authors have indicated that predictive power tests are based on a mixture of Bayesian and frequentist methods and therefore "neither Bayesian nor frequentist statisticians may be satisfied [with them]" (Jennison and Turnbull, 1990), and "the result does not have an acceptable frequentist interpretation and, furthermore, this is not the kind of test a Bayesian would apply" (Geisser and Johnson, 1994).

This section introduces an alternative approach to Bayesian futility monitoring known as the *predictive probability* approach. Roughly speaking, predictive probability tests are constructed by replacing the frequentist component of predictive power tests (conditional power function) with a Bayesian one (posterior probability of a positive trial outcome). The predictive probability approach is illustrated below using examples from clinical trials with normally distributed and binary response variables.

Normally Distributed Endpoints

As we indicated above, a positive trial outcome is defined within the Bayesian predictive probability framework in terms of the posterior probability of a clinically important treatment effect rather than statistical significance. To see how this change affects futility testing in clinical applications, consider a trial comparing an experimental drug to a placebo and assume that its primary endpoint is a continuous, normally distributed variable.

The trial will be declared positive if one demonstrates that the posterior probability of a clinically important improvement is greater than a prespecified confidence level η; i.e.,

$$P(\mu_1 - \mu_2 > \delta | \text{observed data}) > \eta,$$

where μ_1 and μ_2 denote the mean treatment effects in the two treatment groups, δ is a clinically significant treatment difference, and $0 < \eta < 1$. Note that η is typically greater than 0.8, and choosing a larger value of the confidence level reduces the likelihood of a positive trial outcome. The treatment difference δ can either be a constant or be expressed in terms of the standard deviation, in which case the introduced criterion becomes a function of the effect size $(\mu_1 - \mu_2)/\sigma$ (here σ denotes the common standard deviation in the two treatment groups).

In order to predict the probability of a positive trial outcome from the data available at an interim analysis, we will employ a trick similar to the one we used in the derivation of the predictive power test for binary endpoints in Section 4.3.2. In broad strokes, the data collected before the interim analysis are used to predict future data, which are then combined with the observed data to estimate the posterior probability of a clinically significant treatment difference.

Assume that the mean treatment effects μ_1 and μ_2 are normally distributed with means μ_1^* and μ_2^* and standard deviation σ^*. As stated by Dmitrienko and Wang (2004), the predictive probability of observing a clinically significant treatment difference upon termination given the interim test statistic Z_n is equal to

$$P_n = \Phi \left(\frac{\sqrt{N} Z_n (1 - a_n) + b_n/\sigma - (\delta/\sigma)\sqrt{nN/2} - \sqrt{n} z_\eta (1 - c_N)}{\sqrt{\frac{N-n}{N} (1 - a_N)^2 [(N - n)(1 - a_n) + n]}} \right),$$

where

$$a_n = \left(1 + n \left(\frac{\sigma^*}{\sigma} \right)^2 \right)^{-1},$$

$$b_n = \sqrt{\frac{nN}{2}} (\mu_1^* - \mu_2^*) \left(1 + n \left(\frac{\sigma^*}{\sigma} \right)^2 \right)^{-1},$$

$$c_n = 1 - \left(1 + \frac{1}{n} \left(\frac{\sigma}{\sigma^*} \right)^2 \right)^{-1}.$$

The trial will be stopped in favor of the null hypothesis of no treatment effect as soon as the predictive probability falls below $1 - \gamma$.

As in Section 4.3.2, the unknown standard deviation σ can be estimated using the pooled sample standard deviation. The parameters a_n, b_n and c_n quantify the amount of prior information about the mean treatment effects μ_1 and μ_2. The three parameters converge to zero as $\sigma^* \to \infty$, i.e., as the prior information becomes less precise. The limiting value of the predictive probability corresponding to the case of uniform priors is given by

$$P_n = \Phi \left(\frac{\sqrt{N} Z_n - \sqrt{n} z_\eta - (\delta/\sigma)\sqrt{nN/2}}{\sqrt{(N - n)}} \right).$$

Comparing this formula to the formula for the predictive power derived in Section 4.3.2, we see that the predictive probability method can be thought of as a "mirror image" of the predictive power method when the clinically significant treatment difference δ is set to 0. Indeed, assuming a uniform prior and $\delta = 0$, it is easy to verify that the two methods become identical when $\eta = 1 - \alpha$. For example, a predictive probability test with a 90% confidence level ($\eta = 0.9$) is identical to a predictive power test with a one-sided 0.1 level ($\alpha = 0.1$).

Looking at the case of a small common variance of the prior distributions of μ_1 and μ_2, it is easy to demonstrate that the predictive probability test is asymptotically independent of the test statistic Z_n and thus it turns into a deterministic rule. Specifically, the predictive probability converges to 1 if $\mu_1^* - \mu_2^* > \delta$ and 0 otherwise. As a result, a predictive probability test will trigger an early termination of the trial regardless of the size of the treatment difference as long as the selected prior distributions meet the condition $\mu_1^* - \mu_2^* \leq \delta$. Due to this property, it is advisable to avoid strong prior distributions when setting up futility rules based on the predictive probability method.

Program 4.23 explores the relationship between the magnitude of the clinically significant treatment difference δ and predictive probability of a positive final outcome in the generalized anxiety disorder trial. To save space, we will focus on the low confidence priors for the mean HAMA changes displayed in Table 4.13. The calculations can be easily repeated for the high confidence priors or any other set of prior distributions.

The predictive probability is computed in Program 4.23 by invoking the %BayesFutilityCont macro with DELTA=1, 2 and 3 and ETA=0.9. The chosen value of the confidence level η corresponds to a one-sided significance level of 0.1 in the predictive power framework. Note that the ALPHA parameter will be ignored in predictive probability calculations.

Program 4.23 Predictive probability test in the generalized anxiety disorder trial

```
%BayesFutilityCont(data=genanx,par=lowconf,delta=1,eta=0.9,
    alpha=0.1,prob=delta1);
%BayesFutilityCont(data=genanx,par=lowconf,delta=2,eta=0.9,
    alpha=0.1,prob=delta2);
%BayesFutilityCont(data=genanx,par=lowconf,delta=3,eta=0.9,
    alpha=0.1,prob=delta3);
proc print data=delta1 noobs label;
    title "Delta=1";
    var Analysis Fraction PredProb;
proc print data=delta2 noobs label;
    title "Delta=2";
    var Analysis Fraction PredProb;
proc print data=delta3 noobs label;
    title "Delta=3";
    var Analysis Fraction PredProb;
    run;
```

Output from Program 4.23

```
          Delta=1

          Fraction of
          total sample    Predictive
Analysis     size         probability

   1         0.26           0.2135
   2         0.49           0.1523
   3         0.74           0.0004


          Delta=2

          Fraction of
          total sample    Predictive
Analysis     size         probability

   1         0.26           0.1164
   2         0.49           0.0458
   3         0.74           0.0000


          Delta=3

          Fraction of
          total sample    Predictive
Analysis     size         probability

   1         0.26           0.0556
   2         0.49           0.0094
   3         0.74           0.0000
```

Output 4.23 shows the predictive probability of observing a 1-, 2- and 3-point improvement (DELTA parameter) in the mean HAMA change compared to the placebo at each of the three interim looks. As expected, the predictive probability declines quickly with the increasing DELTA parameter. Consider, for example, the first interim analysis. The predictive probability of observing a 1-point mean treatment difference at the end of the trial is 21.4%, whereas the predictive probability for 2-and 3-point differences are equal to 11.6% and 5.6%, respectively. The findings suggest that it is no longer worthwhile continuing the trial to its planned end if one is interested in detecting a substantial amount of improvement over the placebo.

Binary Endpoints

The predictive probability framework introduced in the previous subsection is easily extended to the case of binary outcome variables. Consider again the severe sepsis trial example and let p_1 and p_2 denote the 28-day survival rates in the experimental and placebo groups. The trial will be declared successful at the final analysis if the probability of a clinically meaningful difference in survival rates exceeds a prespecified confidence level η; i.e.,

$$P(p_1 - p_2 > \delta | \text{observed data}) > \eta,$$

where δ denotes a clinically significant treatment difference.

As in the normal case, the posterior probability of $p_1 - p_2 > \delta$ depends both on the interim and future data. Let B_i and A_i denote the event counts in treatment group i at the interim analysis and between the interim and final analyses, respectively. Since the future event counts A_1 and A_2 are not available to the clinical researchers at the time the interim analysis is performed, they will be replaced by their predicted values. The predicted values of A_1 and A_2 are computed from B_1 and B_2 as well as prior distributions of the survival rates p_1 and p_2 and, as shown in Section 4.3.2, follow a beta-binomial distribution. Given the predicted values, it is easy to prove that the posterior distribution of the survival rates p_1 and p_2 is beta with the parameters

$$\alpha_i^* = B_i + A_i + \alpha_i, \quad \beta_i^* = N - B_i - A_i + \beta_i.$$

Now that all of the individual ingredients have been obtained, we can compute the predictive probability of a positive trial outcome given the data observed at the interim look (Dmitrienko and Wang, 2004):

$$P_n = \sum_{j=0}^{N-n} \sum_{k=0}^{N-n} I(P(p_1^* - p_2^* > \delta | A_1 = j, A_2 = k) > \eta) p_1(j|B_1) p_2(k|B_2),$$

where $I()$ is an indicator function and asterisks indicate that the probability is computed with respect to the posterior distribution of the survival rates p_1 and p_2. Put simply, the predictive probability is obtained by summing over all possible values of future event counts for which the posterior probability of $p_1 - p_2 > \delta$ is greater than the prespecified threshold η. Configurations of future event counts that do not lead to a positive trial outcome are automatically excluded from the calculation. The experimental drug will be considered futile and patient enrollment will be stopped as soon as $P_n < 1 - \gamma$.

The value of

$$P(p_1^* - p_2^* > \delta | A_1 = j, A_2 = k)$$

can be computed exactly by taking advantage of the fact that p_1^* and p_2^* are independent random variables with a beta distribution:

$$P(p_1^* - p_2^* > \delta | A_1 = j, A_2 = k)$$

$$= \frac{1}{B(\alpha_1^*, \beta_1^*)} \int_{\delta}^{1} p^{\alpha_1^* - 1} (1 - p)^{\beta_1^* - 1} F_{B(\alpha_2^*, \beta_2^*)}(p - \delta) dp,$$

where $F_{B(\alpha_2^*, \beta_2^*)}$ is the cumulative distribution function of a $B(\alpha_2^*, \beta_2^*)$ distribution. The integral in this formula can be computed using any numerical integration routine. The %BayesFutilityBin macro that implements the outlined futility testing method relies on the QUAD function in the SAS/IML library.

Program 4.24 performs predictive probability calculations in the severe sepsis trial by utilizing the %BayesFutilityBin macro. We are interested in computing the predictive probability of observing any improvement in 28-day survival as well as observing a 5% and 10% absolute increase in 28-day survival at the end of the trial. Therefore the DELTA parameter will be set to 0, 0.05 and 0.1. The confidence level of the Bayesian predictive probability test (ETA parameter) is equal to 0.9. The calculations will be performed for the set of low confidence priors shown in Table 4.14. Lastly, as in Program 4.23, the ALPHA parameter will be ignored in predictive probability calculations.

Program 4.24 Predictive probability test in the severe sepsis trial

```
%BayesFutilityBin(data=sevsep2,par=lowconf,delta=0,eta=0.9,
    alpha=0.1,prob=delta1);
%BayesFutilityBin(data=sevsep2,par=lowconf,delta=0.05,eta=0.9,
    alpha=0.1,prob=delta2);
%BayesFutilityBin(data=sevsep2,par=lowconf,delta=0.1,eta=0.9,
    alpha=0.1,prob=delta3);
proc print data=delta1 noobs label;
    title "Delta=0";
    var Analysis Fraction PredProb;
proc print data=delta2 noobs label;
    title "Delta=0.05";
    var Analysis Fraction PredProb;
proc print data=delta3 noobs label;
    title "Delta=0.1";
    var Analysis Fraction PredProb;
    run;
```

Output from Program 4.24

```
          Delta=0

          Fraction of
          total sample   Predictive
Analysis     size        probability

    1        0.24          0.1099
    2        0.36          0.1088
    3        0.46          0.0862
    4        0.55          0.0183
    5        0.64          0.0243
    6        0.72          0.0041


          Delta=0.05

          Fraction of
          total sample   Predictive
Analysis     size        probability

    1        0.24          0.0341
    2        0.36          0.0190
    3        0.46          0.0081
    4        0.55          0.0004
    5        0.64          0.0002
    6        0.72          0.0000
```

```
              Delta=0.1

              Fraction of
              total sample   Predictive
   Analysis       size       probability

      1           0.24         0.0074
      2           0.36         0.0019
      3           0.46         0.0003
      4           0.55         0.0000
      5           0.64         0.0000
      6           0.72         0.0000
```

Output 4.24 lists predictive probability values computed at each of the six interim looks under three choices of the DELTA parameter. Recall from the beginning of this section that, for normally distributed outcomes, the predictive probability test is closely related to the predictive power test when $\eta = 1 - \alpha$ and the clinically meaningful treatment difference δ is set to 0. A similar relationship is observed in the binary case as well. We see from Output 4.24 that the predictive probabilities with DELTA=0 are virtually equal to the predictive power values with $\alpha = 0.1$ shown under "Low confidence prior" in Output 4.22. Therefore, the constructed predictive probability test will roughly correspond to the predictive power test with a one-sided significance level of 0.1.

We also see from Output 4.24 that larger values of the clinically meaningful treatment difference δ are associated with lower predictive probabilities of a positive trial outcome. For example, if one would like to demonstrate with a 90% confidence that the experimental drug improves the 28-day survival rate by 5% or 10% (in absolute terms), the predictive probability of a positive trial outcome at the very first interim look drops to 3.4% and 0.7%, respectively. It appears prudent to suspend the patient enrollment at the first look, because the negative conclusion is unlikely to change even if the trial continued to the planned end.

4.3.4 Summary

This section reviewed three approaches to constructing futility testing procedures in clinical trials: frequentist conditional power methods, mixed Bayesian-frequentist methods based on predictive power, and Bayesian predictive probability methods. These futility tests are often collectively referred to as *stochastic curtailment tests* because they rely on stochastic arguments in order to decide when to curtail sampling. Specifically, a clinical trial is terminated at an interim analysis when the observed data indicate that it is highly unlikely that the experimental drug would separate from the control at the end of the study. The three families of futility tests differ in how they define separation between treatment arms:

- **Conditional power tests** reviewed in the section can be further subdivided into *basic* and *adaptive* conditional power tests. Both methods evaluate the probability of observing a statistically significant treatment difference at the planned end of the trial given the interim data. Basic conditional power procedures (e.g., Lan-Simon-Halperin test) rely heavily on the hypothesized value of the treatment effect, whereas adaptive conditional power procedures (e.g., Pepe-Anderson-Betensky test) are based on a sample estimate of the treatment difference to predict the distribution of the future data. For this reason, adaptive tests are generally more appealing in clinical trial applications than tests tied to an assumed value of the treatment difference. The basic and adaptive conditional power methods can be implemented using the %CondPowerLSH and %CondPowerPAB macros described in this section.

- **Predictive power tests** extend the adaptive approach further by incorporating more data-driven elements into the decision rule. This is achieved by averaging the conditional power function with respect to a posterior distribution of the treatment difference. The clinical trial is terminated as soon as the average conditional power (known as the *predictive power*) falls below a certain threshold. An assumed prior distribution of the mean treatment difference can have great influence on the resulting futility rule. Selecting a noninformative prior that is quickly dominated by the data increases the chances of early stopping due to futility. On the other hand, with a strong prior distribution, a predictive power test is asymptotically equivalent to a frequentist conditional power test and thus is generally less sensitive to negative trends in the data. The section introduced two SAS macros (%BayesFutilityCont and %BayesFutilityBin macros) for carrying out predictive power tests in clinical trials with normally distributed and binary endpoints.

- **Predictive probability tests** provide a fully Bayesian solution to the futility testing problem. Within the predictive probability framework, a positive trial outcome is defined in terms of the posterior probability of a clinically important treatment effect rather than statistical significance. Under a noninformative prior, predictive probability tests yield results similar to those produced by predictive power tests and turn into deterministic rules when the variance of the prior distribution is small. For this reason, it is advisable to avoid strong priors when setting up futility rules based on the predictive probability method. Bayesian predictive probability inferences can be performed using the %BayesFutilityCont and %BayesFutilityBin macros.

Although the Type II error rate of trial designs with futility monitoring is greater than the nominal value, adjustments are rarely done in practice. This is due mainly to the fact that stochastic curtailment tests minimize the probability of early termination compared to their group sequential counterparts.

Finally, due to their simplicity, futility tests reviewed in this section may be more appealing in practice than computationally complex futility monitoring strategies based on error spending functions. In addition, the futility boundary of a group sequential design depends heavily on the assumed value of the treatment difference, which may no longer be supported by the data. Therefore, the repeated significance approach is less robust than stochastic curtailment approaches such as the adaptive conditional power or Bayesian methods described in this section.

5 Analysis of Incomplete Data

A large number of empirical studies are prone to incompleteness. Over the last decades, a number of methods have been developed to handle incomplete data. Many of these methods are relatively simple, but their validity can be questioned. With increasing computational power and software tools available, more flexible methods have come within reach. This chapter sketches a general taxonomy within which incomplete data methods can be placed and then focuses on methods that can be implemented within the SAS environment, thereby commenting on their relative advantages and disadvantages. All methods are illustrated using practical examples, and sufficiently generic SAS code is provided. Both Gaussian and non-Gaussian outcomes are covered.

5.1 Introduction

In a longitudinal study, each unit is measured on several occasions. It is not unusual in practice for some sequences of measurements to terminate early for reasons outside the control of the investigator, and any unit so affected is called a dropout. It might therefore be necessary to accommodate dropouts in the modeling process.

Early work on missing values was largely concerned with algorithmic and computational solutions to the induced lack of balance or deviations from the intended study design (Afifi and Elashoff, 1966; Hartley and Hocking, 1971). More recently, general algorithms such as expectation-maximization (EM) (Dempster, Laird and Rubin, 1977) and data imputation and augmentation procedures (Rubin, 1987), combined with powerful computing resources, have largely provided a solution to this aspect of the problem. The very difficult and important question of assessing the impact of missing data on subsequent statistical inference remains.

When referring to the missing-value, or nonresponse, process we will use the terminology of Little and Rubin (1987, Chapter 6). A nonresponse process is said to be *missing completely at random* (MCAR) if the missingness is independent of both unobserved and observed data. It is said to be *missing at random* (MAR) if, conditional on the observed data, the missingness is independent of the unobserved measurements. A process that is neither MCAR nor MAR is termed *nonrandom*, or *missing not at random* (MNAR). In the context of likelihood inference, and when the parameters describing the measurement process are functionally independent of the parameters describing the missingness process, MCAR and MAR are *ignorable,* while a nonrandom process is nonignorable.

Many methods are formulated as selection models (Little and Rubin, 1987) as opposed to pattern-mixture modeling (PMM) (Little 1993, 1994). A selection model factors the joint distribution of the measurement and response mechanisms into the marginal measurement distribution and the response distribution, conditional on the measurements. This is intuitively appealing since the marginal measurement distribution would be of interest also with complete data. Little and Rubin's taxonomy is most easily developed in the selection setting. Parameterizing and making inference about the effect of treatment and its evolution over time is straightforward in the selection model context.

In the specific case of a clinical trial setting, standard methodology used to analyze longitudinal data subject to nonresponse is mostly based on such methods as *last observation carried forward* (LOCF), *complete case analysis* (CC), or simple forms of imputation. This is often done without questioning the possible influence of these assumptions on the final results, even though several authors have written about this topic. A relatively early account is given in Heyting, Tolboom and Essers (1992). Mallinckrodt et al. (2003a, 2003b) and Lavori, Dawson and Shera (1995) propose direct likelihood and multiple-imputation methods, respectively, to deal with incomplete longitudinal data. Siddiqui and Ali (1998) compare direct likelihood and LOCF methods.

As will be discussed in subsequent sections, it is unfortunate that there is such a strong emphasis on methods like LOCF and CC, because they are based on extremely strong assumptions. In particular, even the strong MCAR assumption does not suffice to guarantee an LOCF analysis is valid. On the other hand, under MAR, valid inference can be obtained through a likelihood-based analysis, without the need for modeling the dropout process. As a consequence, one can simply use, for example, linear or generalized linear mixed models (Verbeke and Molenberghs, 2000) without additional complication or effort. We will argue that such an analysis not only enjoys much wider validity than the simple methods but in addition is simple to conduct *without additional data manipulation* using such tools as, for example, the SAS procedures MIXED or NLMIXED. Thus, longitudinal data practice should shift away from the *ad hoc* methods and focus on likelihood-based ignorable analyses instead. As will be argued further, the cost involved in having to specify a model will arguably be mild to moderate in realistic longitudinal settings. Thus, we favor the use of direct likelihood ignorable methods over the use of the LOCF and CC approaches.

At the same time, we cannot avoid a reflection on the status of MNAR approaches. In realistic settings, the reasons for dropout are varied and it is therefore difficult to fully justify on *a priori* grounds the assumption of MAR.

Two case studies used throughout this chapter, a depression trial and orthodontic growth data, are introduced in Section 5.2. The general data setting is introduced in Section 5.3, as well as a formal framework for incomplete longitudinal data. An analysis of the complete GROWTH data set, stemming from Little and Rubin (1987), is given in Section 5.4. A discussion on the problems associated with simple methods is presented in Section 5.5. Available case methods are discussed in Section 5.6, while Section 5.7 is devoted to likelihood-based ignorable analysis. Multiple imputation and the expectation-maximization algorithm are the topics of Sections 5.8 and 5.9, respectively. While most of the chapter is devoted to continuous outcomes, categorical data are treated briefly in Section 5.10. A perspective on sensitivity analysis is sketched in Section 5.11.

5.2 Case Studies

EXAMPLE: Depression Trial

A first set of data comes from a clinical trial including 342 patients with post-baseline data. The Hamilton Depression Rating Scale (HAMD17) is used to measure the depression status of the patients. For each patient, a baseline assessment is available.

For blinding purposes, therapies are coded as A1 for the primary dose of the experimental drug, A2 for the secondary dose of the experimental drug, and B and C for nonexperimental drugs. Individual profiles and mean profiles of the changes from baseline in HAMD17 scores per treatment arm are shown in Figures 5.1 and 5.2 respectively.

Figure 5.1 Individual profiles for the depression trial data

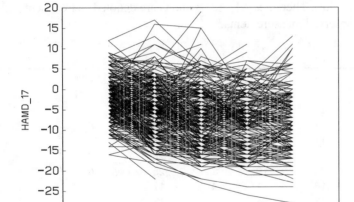

Figure 5.2 Mean profiles per treatment arm for the depression trial data

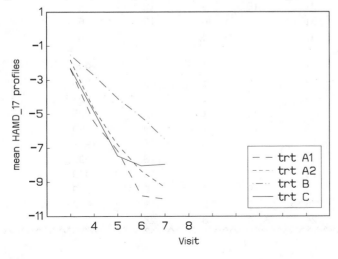

Figure 5.3 Evolution of dropout per treatment arm. Treatment arms 1 and 4 (A1 and C) are the ones of primary interest.

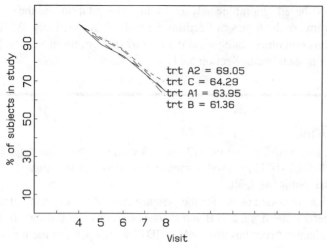

The primary contrast is between A1 and C. Emphasis is on the difference between arms at the end of the study. A graphical representation of the dropout per arm is given in Figure 5.3. Part of the DEPRESSION data set is given below. Therapies A1, A2, B and C are denoted as treatment 1, 2, 3 and 4 respectively. Dots represent unobserved measurements.

Depression trial data

Obs	PATIENT	VISIT	Y	CHANGE	TRT	BASVAL	INVEST
1	1501	4	18	-7	1	25	6
2	1501	5	11	-14	1	25	6
3	1501	6	11	-14	1	25	6
4	1501	7	8	-17	1	25	6
5	1501	8	6	-19	1	25	6
6	1502	4	16	-1	4	17	6
7	1502	5	13	-4	4	17	6
8	1502	6	13	-4	4	17	6
9	1502	7	12	-5	4	17	6
10	1502	8	9	-8	4	17	6
11	1504	4	21	9	4	12	6
12	1504	5	17	5	4	12	6
13	1504	6	31	19	4	12	6
14	1504	7	31	.	4	12	6
15	1504	8	31	.	4	12	6
...							
1696	4901	4	11	2	1	9	999
1697	4901	5	3	-6	1	9	999
1698	4901	6	3	.	1	9	999
1699	4901	7	3	.	1	9	999
1700	4901	8	3	.	1	9	999
1701	4907	4	15	-3	3	18	999
1702	4907	5	13	-5	3	18	999
1703	4907	6	15	-3	3	18	999
1704	4907	7	9	-9	3	18	999
1705	4907	8	6	-12	3	18	999
1706	4909	4	24	-4	3	28	999

1707	4909	5	34	6	3	28	999
1708	4909	6	28	0	3	28	999
1709	4909	7	33	5	3	28	999
1710	4909	8	33	.	3	28	999

EXAMPLE: Growth Data

These data, introduced by Pothoff and Roy (1964), contain growth measurements for 11 girls and 16 boys. For each subject, the distance from the center of the pituitary to the maxillary fissure was recorded at ages 8, 10, 12, and 14. The data were used by Jennrich and Schluchter (1986) to illustrate estimation methods for unbalanced data, where unbalancedness is to be interpreted in the sense of an unequal number of boys and girls.

Individual profiles and residual individual profiles are shown in Figure 5.4. Residual individual profiles result after subtracting the mean of the raw individual profiles.

Figure 5.4 Growth data. Raw and residual individual profiles. Solid lines for girls, dashed lines for boys.

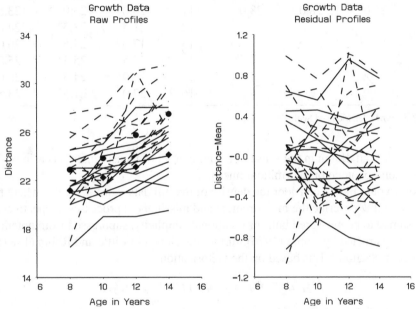

Little and Rubin (1987) deleted nine of the $[(11 + 16) \times 4]$ measurements, rendering nine incomplete subjects. Deletion is confined to the age 10 measurements. Little and Rubin describe the mechanism to be such that subjects with a low value at age 8 are more likely to have a missing value at age 10. The data are presented in Table 5.1. The measurements that were deleted are marked with an asterisk.

5.3   Data Setting and Modeling Framework

Assume that for subject $i = 1, \ldots, N$ in the study a sequence of responses Y_{ij} is designed to be measured at occasions $j = 1, \ldots, n$. The outcomes are grouped into a vector $Y_i = (Y_{i1}, \ldots, Y_{in})'$. In addition, define a dropout indicator D_i for the occasion at which dropout occurs and make the convention that $D_i = n + 1$ for a complete sequence. It is often necessary to split the vector Y_i into observed (Y_i^o) and missing (Y_i^m) components respectively. Note that dropout is a particular case of monotone missingness. In order to have a monotone pattern of missingness, there must be a permutation of the measurement components such that a measurement earlier in the permuted sequence is observed for at least those subjects that are observed at later measurements. For this definition to be meaningful,

Table 5.1 Growth data for 11 girls and 16 boys. Measurements marked with ∗ were deleted by Little and Rubin (1987).

Girl	Age (in years) 8	10	12	14	Boy	Age (in years) 8	10	12	14
1	21.0	20.0	21.5	23.0	1	26.0	25.0	29.0	31.0
2	21.0	21.5	24.0	25.5	2	21.5	22.5*	23.0	26.5
3	20.5	24.0*	24.5	26.0	3	23.0	22.5	24.0	27.5
4	23.5	24.5	25.0	26.5	4	25.5	27.5	26.5	27.0
5	21.5	23.0	22.5	23.5	5	20.0	23.5*	22.5	26.0
6	20.0	21.0*	21.0	22.5	6	24.5	25.5	27.0	28.5
7	21.5	22.5	23.0	25.0	7	22.0	22.0	24.5	26.5
8	23.0	23.0	23.5	24.0	8	24.0	21.5	24.5	25.5
9	20.0	21.0*	22.0	21.5	9	23.0	20.5	31.0	26.0
10	16.5	19.0*	19.0	19.5	10	27.5	28.0	31.0	31.5
11	24.5	25.0	28.0	28.0	11	23.0	23.0	23.5	25.0
					12	21.5	23.5*	24.0	28.0
					13	17.0	24.5*	26.0	29.5
					14	22.5	25.5	25.5	26.0
					15	23.0	24.5	26.0	30.0
					16	22.0	21.5*	23.5	25.0

Source: Pothoff and Roy (1964), Jennrich and Schluchter (1986).

we need to have a balanced design in the sense of a common set of measurement occasions. Other patterns are called nonmonotone or intermittent missingness.

In principle, one would like to consider the density of the full data $f(y_i, d_i | \theta, \psi)$, where the parameter vectors θ and ψ describe the measurement and missingness processes, respectively. Covariates are assumed to be measured but, for notational simplicity, suppressed from notation.

The taxonomy, constructed by Rubin (1976), further developed in Little and Rubin (1987), and informally sketched in Section 5.1, is based on the factorization

$$f(y_i, d_i | \theta, \psi) = f(y_i | \theta) f(d_i | y_i, \psi),$$ (5.1)

where the first factor is the marginal density of the measurement process and the second one is the density of the missingness process, conditional on the outcomes. Factorization (5.1) forms the basis of *selection modeling* because the second factor corresponds to the (self-)selection of individuals into *observed* and *missing* groups. An alternative taxonomy can be built based on so-called *pattern-mixture models* (Little, 1993, 1994). These are based on the factorization

$$f(y_i, d_i | \theta, \psi) = f(y_i | d_i, \theta) f(d_i | \psi).$$ (5.2)

Indeed, equation (5.2) can be seen as a mixture of different populations, characterized by the observed pattern of missingness.

In the selection modeling framework, let us first describe a measurement model and missingness model in turn, and then formally introduce and comment on ignorability.

Assume we want to perform a longitudinal analysis of the data. In that case, the choice of the measurement model depends on the nature of the outcome. For continuous outcomes as is the case in our case studies, one typically assumes a linear mixed effects model, perhaps with serial correlation:

$$Y_i = X_i \beta + Z_i b_i + \varepsilon_{(1)i} + \varepsilon_{(2)i},$$ (5.3)

(Verbeke and Molenberghs, 2000) where Y_i is the n dimensional response vector for subject i, $1 \leq i \leq N$, N is the number of subjects, X_i and Z_i are $(n \times p)$ and $(n \times q)$ known design matrices, β is the p dimensional vector containing the fixed effects, and $b_i \sim N(0, D)$ is the q dimensional vector containing the random effects. The residual components ε_i are decomposed as $\varepsilon_i = \varepsilon_{(1)i} + \varepsilon_{(2)i}$, in which $\varepsilon_{(2)i}$ is a component of serial correlation and $\varepsilon_{(1)i} \sim N(0, \sigma^2 I_{n_i})$ is an extra component of measurement error. Thus serial correlation is captured by the realization of a Gaussian stochastic process, $\varepsilon_{(2)i}$, which is assumed to follow a $N(0, \tau^2 H_i)$ law. The serial covariance matrix H_i depends on i only through the number n of observations and through the time points t_{ij} at which measurements are taken. The structure of the matrix H_i is determined through the autocorrelation function $\rho(t_{ij} - t_{ik})$. This function decreases such that $\rho(0) = 1$ and $\rho(+\infty) = 0$. Further, D is a general $(q \times q)$ covariance matrix with (i, j) element $d_{ij} = d_{ji}$. Finally, $b_1, \ldots, b_N, \varepsilon_{(1)1}, \ldots, \varepsilon_{(2)N}, \varepsilon_{(2)1}, \ldots, \varepsilon_{(2)N}$ are assumed to be independent. Inference is based on the marginal distribution of the response Y_i which, after integrating over random effects, can be expressed as

$$Y_i \sim N(X_i\beta, Z_i D Z_i' + \Sigma_i). \tag{5.4}$$

Here, $\Sigma_i = \sigma^2 I_{n_i} + \tau^2 H_i$ is a $(n \times n)$ covariance matrix grouping the measurement error and serial components. Further, we define $V_i = Z_i D Z_i' + \Sigma_i$ as the general covariance matrix of Y_i.

Assume that incompleteness is due to dropout only, and that the first measurement Y_{i1} is obtained for everyone. The model for the dropout process is based on, for example, a logistic regression for the probability of dropout at occasion j, given the subject is still in the study. We denote this probability by $g(h_{ij}, y_{ij})$ in which h_{ij} is a vector containing all responses observed up to but not including occasion j, as well as relevant covariates. We then assume that $g(h_{ij}, y_{ij})$ satisfies

$$\text{logit}[g(h_{ij}, y_{ij})] = \text{logit}\left[\text{pr}(D_i = j | D_i \geq j, y_i)\right] = h_{ij}\psi + \omega y_{ij}, \tag{5.5}$$

$i = 1, \ldots, N$. When ω equals zero, the dropout model is MAR, and all parameters can be estimated easily using SAS because the measurement model for which we use a linear mixed model and the dropout model, assumed to follow a logistic regression, can then be fitted separately. If $\omega \neq 0$, the posited dropout process is MNAR. Model (5.5) provides the building blocks for the dropout process $f(d_i | y_i, \psi)$.

Rubin (1976) and Little and Rubin (1987) have shown that, under MAR and mild regularity conditions (parameters θ and ψ are functionally independent), likelihood-based inference is valid when the missing data mechanism is ignored; see also Verbeke and Molenberghs (2000). Practically speaking, the likelihood of interest is then based upon the factor $f(y_i^o | \theta)$. This is called *ignorability*.

The practical implication is that a software module with likelihood estimation facilities and with the ability to handle incompletely observed subjects manipulates the correct likelihood, providing valid parameter estimates and likelihood ratio values. A few cautionary remarks are in order. First, when at least part of the scientific interest is directed towards the nonresponse process, obviously both processes need to be considered. Still, under MAR, both processes can be modeled and parameters estimated separately. Second, likelihood inference is often surrounded with references to the sampling distribution (e.g., to construct precision estimators and for statistical hypothesis tests (Kenward and Molenberghs, 1998)). However, the practical implication is that standard errors and associated tests, when based on the observed rather than the expected information matrix and given that the parametric assumptions are correct, are valid. Third, it may be hard to fully rule out the operation of an MNAR mechanism. This point was brought up in the introduction and will be discussed further in Section 5.11. Fourth, a full longitudinal analysis is necessary, even when interest lies, for example, in a comparison between the two treatment groups at the last occasion. In the latter case, the fitted model can be used as the basis for inference at the last occasion. A common criticism is that a model needs to be considered. However, it should be noted that in many clinical trial settings the repeated measures are balanced in the sense that a common (and often limited) set of measurement times is considered for all subjects, allowing the *a priori* specification of a saturated model (e.g., a full group-by-time interaction model for the fixed effects and unstructured variance-covariance matrix). Such an ignorable linear mixed model specification is given in Mallinckrodt et al. (2001a, 2001b).

5.4 Analysis of Complete Growth Data

Verbeke and Molenberghs (2000, Chapter 9) and Diggle et al. (2002) provide general guidelines to conduct model building. These will be reviewed in Section 5.4.1. They will be applied to the complete GROWTH data set in Section 5.4.2.

5.4.1 Model-Building Guidelines

Fitting linear mixed models implies that an appropriate mean structure as well as a covariance structure—i.e., both for random effects and error components—needs to be specified. These steps are not independent of each other.

First, unless robust inference is used, an appropriate covariance model is essential to obtain valid inferences for the parameters in the mean structure, which is usually of primary interest. This is especially so in the case of missing data, since robust inference then provides valid results only under often unrealistically strict assumptions about the missing data process. Too restrictive specifications invalidate inferences when the assumed structure does not hold, whereas overparameterization of the covariance structure leads to inefficient estimation and poor assessment of standard errors (Altham, 1984).

Further, the covariance structure itself may be of interest for understanding the random variation observed in the data. However, because it only explains the variability not explained by systematic trends, it is highly dependent on the specified mean structure.

Finally, note that an appropriate covariance structure also yields better predictions. For example, the prediction based on model (5.3) of a future observation y_i^* for individual i, to be taken at time point t_i^*, is given by

$$\widehat{y_i^*} = X_i^* \hat{\beta} + Z_i^* \hat{b}_i + \widehat{E}(\varepsilon_{(2)i}^* | y_i),$$

in which X_i^* and Z_i^* are the fixed effects and random effects covariates, respectively, and $\varepsilon_{(2)i}^*$ is the serial error, at time t_i^*. The estimation of the random effect b_i is $\hat{b}_i$. Chi and Reinsel (1989) have shown that if the components of $\varepsilon_{(2)i}^*$ follow an AR(1) process,

$$\widehat{E}(\varepsilon_{(2)i}^* | y_i) = \phi^{(t_i^* - t_{i,n_i})} \left[y_i - X_i \hat{\alpha} - Z_i \hat{b}_i \right]_{n_i},$$

for ϕ equal to the constant that determines the AR(1) process, $|\phi| < 1$. This means that the inclusion of serial correlation may improve the prediction because it exploits the correlation between the observation to be predicted and the last observed value y_{i,n_i}. We will now present some simple guidelines that can help the data analyst to select an appropriate linear mixed model for some specific data set at hand.

Since the covariance structure models all variability in the data that cannot be explained by the fixed effects, we start by first removing all systematic trends. As proposed by Diggle (1988) and Diggle et al. (2002), we use an overelaborate model for the mean response profile. When the data are from a designed experiment in which the only relevant explanatory variables are the treatment labels, it is a sensible strategy to use a *saturated model* for the mean structure. This incorporates a separate parameter for the mean response at each time point within each treatment group.

For data in which the times of measurement are not common to all individuals or when there are continuous covariates that are believed to affect the mean response, the concept of a saturated model breaks down and the choice of our most elaborate model becomes less obvious. In such cases, a plot of smoothed average trends or individual profiles often helps to select a candidate mean structure.

Once an appropriate mean structure $X_i\beta$ for $E(Y_i)$ has been selected, we use the ordinary least squares (OLS) method to estimate β, and we hereby ignore the fact that not all measurements are independent. It follows from the theory of generalized estimating equations (GEE) that this OLS estimator is consistent for β (Liang and Zeger, 1986).

In a second step, we select a set of random effects to be included in the covariance model. Note that random effects for time-independent covariates can be interpreted as subject-specific corrections to the overall mean structure. They are similar to random intercepts, but allow different corrections to different levels of the covariate. Generally, they are harder to distinguish from the random intercepts than are random effects associated with time-varying covariates.

A helpful tool for deciding which time-varying covariates should be included in the model is a plot of the OLS residual profiles versus time. When this plot shows constant variability over time, we assume stationarity and we do not include random effects other than intercepts. In cases where the variability varies over time and where there is still some remaining systematic structure in the residual profiles (i.e., where the between-subject variability is large in comparison to the overall variation), the following guidelines can be used to select one or more random effects additional to the random intercepts.

- Try to find a regression model for each residual profile in the above plot. Such models contain subject-specific parameters and are therefore perfect candidates as random effects in our general linear mixed model. For example, if the residual profiles can be approximated by straight lines, then only random intercepts and random slopes for time would be included.

- Since our model always assumes the random effects b_i to have mean zero, we only consider covariates Z_i which have already been included as covariates in the fixed part (i.e., in X_i) or which are linear combinations of columns of X_i.

- Morrell, Pearson and Brant (1997) have shown that Z_i should not include a polynomial effect if not all hierarchically inferior terms are also included, and similarly for interaction terms. This generalizes the well-known results from linear regression (see, e.g., Peixoto (1987, 1990)) to random effects models. It ensures that the model is invariant to coding transformations and avoids unanticipated covariance structures. This means that if, for example, we want to include quadratic random time effects, then also linear random time effects and random intercepts should be included.

- The choice of a set of random effects for the model automatically implies that the covariance matrix for Y_i is assumed to be of the general form $V_i = Z_i D Z_i' + \Sigma_i$. In the presence of random effects other than intercepts, it is often assumed (see, e.g., Diggle et al. (2002)) that the diagonal elements in Σ_i are all equal such that the variance of $Y_i(t)$ depends on time only through the component $Z_i(t) D Z_i'(t)$, where it is now explicitly indicated that the covariates Z_i depend on time. As an informal check for the appropriateness of the selected random effects, one can compare the fitted variance function based on a mixed effects model with $\Sigma_i = \sigma^2 I_{n_i}$ to the smoothed sample variance function of the residuals r_{ij}.

Conditional on our selected set of random effects, we now need to specify the covariance matrix Σ_i for the error components ε_i. Many possible covariance structures are available at this stage.

Unfortunately, apart from the use of information criteria such as the ones given in Table 5.2, there are no general simple techniques available to compare all these models. For highly unbalanced data with many repeated measurements per subject, one usually assumes that random effects can account for most of the variation in the data and that the remaining error components ε_i have a very simple covariance structure, leading to parsimonious models for V_i.

Based on the residual covariance structure specified in the previous step, we can now investigate whether the random effects which we included are really needed in the model. As discussed before, Z_i

Table 5.2 Overview of frequently used information criteria for comparing linear mixed models. We hereby define n^* equal to the total number $n = \sum_{i=1}^{N} n_i$ of observations, or equal to $n - p$, depending on whether ML or REML estimation was used in the calculations. Further, $\#\theta$ denotes the number of parameters.

Criterion	Definition of $\mathcal{F}(\cdot)$
Akaike (AIC)	$\mathcal{F}(\#\theta) = \#\theta$
Schwarz (SBC)	$\mathcal{F}(\#\theta) = (\#\theta \ln n^*)/2$
Hannan and Quinn (HQIC)	$\mathcal{F}(\#\theta) = \#\theta \ln(\ln n^*)$
Bozdogan (CAIC)	$\mathcal{F}(\#\theta) = \#\theta (\ln n^* + 1)/2$

should not contain a polynomial effect if not all hierarchically inferior terms are also included. Taking into account this hierarchy, one should test the significance of the highest-order random effects first. We emphasize that the need for random effects cannot be tested using classical likelihood ratio tests, because the null hypotheses of interest are on the boundary of the parameter space, which implies that the likelihood ratio statistic does not have the classical asymptotic chi-squared distribution. Indeed, the asymptotic null distribution for the likelihood ratio test statistic for testing the need for some of the random effects in the model is often a mixture of chi-squared distributions rather than the classical single chi-squared distribution (Self and Liang, 1987; Stram and Lee, 1994, 1995; Verbeke and Molenberghs, 2000).

Further, now that the final covariance structure for the model has been selected, the tests for the fixed effects in the preliminary mean structure become available. When the number of variance components is not excessive, the classical likelihood ratio test is a sensible choice. However, as indicated by many authors (Verbeke and Molenberghs, 2000; Pinheiro and Bates, 2000), such tests may be anticonservative, and then the approximate F tests could be used.

5.4.2 An Application to the GROWTH Data Set

Let us exemplify the ideas developed above using the GROWTH data set. First, we construct residuals, based on subtracting a saturated sex-by-time mean model from the measurements. When a satisfactory covariance model is found, attention then shifts to simplification of the mean structure. However, this insight is relatively recent and was certainly not the standard procedure in the mid-eighties. Jennrich and Schluchter (1986) constructed eight models, with the first three concentrating on the mean model, leaving the 4×4 covariance matrix of the repeated measurements completely unstructured. Once an adequate mean model is found, the remaining five models are fitted to enable simplification of the covariance structure. Jennrich and Schluchter primarily wanted to illustrate their estimation procedures and did not envisage a comprehensive data analysis. Moreover, since this procedure can be considered legitimate in small balanced studies and also for reasons of comparability, we will, at first, adopt the same eight models in the same order. In this section, these models will be fitted to the original data, referred to henceforth as the *complete data set*. The results of Jennrich and Schluchter (1986) will be recovered and additional insight will be given. In Section 5.7, these solutions will be compared to the results for the same eight models on the incomplete data. Jennrich and Schluchter used Newton-Raphson, Fisher scoring, and generalized expectation-maximization (EM) algorithms to maximize the log-likelihood. We will show that the data can be analyzed relatively easily using PROC MIXED.

The models of Jennrich and Schluchter (1986) can be expressed in the general linear mixed models family:

$$Y_i = X_i \beta + Z_i b_i + \varepsilon_i, \tag{5.6}$$

where

$$b_i \sim N(0, D),$$

$$\varepsilon_i \sim N(0, \Sigma),$$

and b_i and ε_i are statistically independent. As before, Y_i is the (4×1) response vector, X_i is a $(4 \times p)$ design matrix for the fixed effects, β is a vector of unknown fixed regression coefficients, Z_i is a $(4 \times q)$ design matrix for the random effects, b_i is a $(q \times 1)$ vector of normally distributed random parameters with covariance matrix D, and ε_i is a normally distributed (4×1) random error vector with covariance matrix Σ. Since every subject contributes exactly four measurements at exactly the same time points, it has been possible to drop the subscript i from the error covariance matrix Σ. The random error ε_i encompasses both measurement error (as in a cross-sectional study) and serial correlation. In this study, the design will be a function of age, sex, and/or the interaction between both. Let us indicate boys with $x_i = 0$, girls with $x_i = 1$, and age with $t_j = 8, 10, 12, 14$.

Table 5.3 Growth data. Set of models to be considered.

	Mean Structure	Covar	# par
0	unstructured	unstructured (different per sex)	28
1	unstructured	unstructured	18
2	$\neq$ slopes	unstructured	14
3	$=$ slopes	unstructured	13
4	$\neq$ slopes	Toeplitz	8
5	$\neq$ slopes	AR(1)	6
6	$\neq$ slopes	random int+slope	8
7	$\neq$ slopes	CS/random intercept	6
8	$\neq$ slopes	simple	5

A Set of Eight Plus One Models

In Table 5.3, we provide a parsimonious description of nine models, eight of which were considered by Jennrich and Schluchter (1986), with Model 0 added. The models are described in terms of the mean structure they assume, together with the variance-covariance structure. For ease of reference, the number of model parameters is listed as well.

In subsequent sections, we will discuss Models 1 through 8, highlighting key features, as well as how they can be fitted with the SAS procedure MIXED.

Model 1

The first model we will consider assumes a separate mean for each of the eight age$\times$sex combinations, together with an unstructured covariance. This is done by assuming that the covariance matrix Σ of the error vector ε_i is a completely general positive definite matrix and no random effects are included. This model can be expressed as

$$
\begin{aligned}
Y_{i1} &= \beta_0 + \beta_1(1 - x_i) + \beta_{0,8}(1 - x_i) + \beta_{1,8}x_i + \varepsilon_{i1}, \\
Y_{i2} &= \beta_0 + \beta_1(1 - x_i) + \beta_{0,10}(1 - x_i) + \beta_{1,10}x_i + \varepsilon_{i2}, \\
Y_{i3} &= \beta_0 + \beta_1(1 - x_i) + \beta_{0,12}(1 - x_i) + \beta_{1,12}x_i + \varepsilon_{i3}, \\
Y_{i4} &= \beta_0 + \beta_1(1 - x_i) + \varepsilon_{i4},
\end{aligned}
\tag{5.7}
$$

Thus, the mean parameters are $\beta = (\beta_0, \beta_1, \beta_{0,8}, \beta_{0,10}, \beta_{0,12}, \beta_{1,8}, \beta_{1,10}, \beta_{1,12})'$. With this parameterization, the means for girls are $\beta_0 + \beta_{1,8}$; $\beta_0 + \beta_{1,10}$; $\beta_0 + \beta_{1,12}$; and β_0 at ages 8, 10, 12, and 14, respectively. The corresponding means for boys are $\beta_0 + \beta_1 + \beta_{0,8}$; $\beta_0 + \beta_1 + \beta_{0,10}$; $\beta_0 + \beta_1 + \beta_{0,12}$; and $\beta_0 + \beta_1$, respectively. Of course, there are many equivalent ways to express the set of eight means in terms of eight linearly independent parameters.

This model can, for example, be fitted with the following SAS code:

Program 5.1 Growth data. Model 1.

```
proc mixed data = growth method = ml covtest;
    title "Growth Data, Model 1";
    class idnr sex age;
    model measure = sex age*sex / s;
    repeated / type = un subject = idnr r rcorr;
run;
```

Let us discuss the fit of the model. The deviance (minus twice the log-likelihood at maximum) equals 416.5093, and there are 18 model parameters (8 mean, 4 variance, and 6 covariance parameters). This deviance will serve as a reference to assess the goodness-of-fit of simpler models. Parameter estimates and standard errors are reproduced in Table 5.4. The deviances are listed in Table 5.6.

Table 5.4 Growth data. Maximum likelihood estimates and standard errors (model based and empirically corrected) for the fixed effects in Model 1 (complete-data set).

Parameter	MLE	(s.e.)[1]	(s.e.)[2]
β_0	24.0909	(0.6478)	(0.7007)
β_1	3.3778	(0.8415)	(0.8636)
$\beta_{0,8}$	−2.9091	(0.6475)	(0.3793)
$\beta_{0,10}$	−1.8636	(0.4620)	(0.3407)
$\beta_{0,12}$	−1.0000	(0.5174)	(0.2227)
$\beta_{1,8}$	−4.5938	(0.5369)	(0.6468)
$\beta_{1,10}$	−3.6563	(0.3831)	(0.4391)
$\beta_{1,12}$	−1.7500	(0.4290)	(0.5358)

[1] Default standard errors under Model 1.
[2] Sandwich standard errors, obtained from the EMPIRICAL option; also obtained under Model 0 (see further).

Table 5.5 Growth data. Predicted means.

Model	Age	Boys Estimate	Boys s.e.	Girls Estimate	Girls s.e.
1	8	22.88	0.56	21.18	0.68
	10	23.81	0.49	22.23	0.59
	12	25.72	0.61	23.09	0.74
	14	27.47	0.54	24.09	0.65
2	8	22.46	0.49	21.24	0.59
	10	24.11	0.45	22.19	0.55
	12	25.76	0.47	23.14	0.57
	14	27.42	0.54	24.10	0.65
3	8	22.82	0.48	20.77	0.57
	10	24.16	0.45	22.12	0.55
	12	25.51	0.47	23.47	0.56
	14	26.86	0.52	24.82	0.60
4	8	22.64	0.53	21.22	0.64
	10	24.23	0.48	22.17	0.57
	12	25.83	0.48	23.12	0.57
	14	27.42	0.53	24.07	0.64
5	8	22.75	0.54	21.19	0.66
	10	24.29	0.44	22.16	0.53
	12	25.83	0.44	23.13	0.53
	14	27.37	0.54	24.09	0.66
6	8	22.62	0.51	21.21	0.61
	10	24.18	0.47	22.17	0.56
	12	25.75	0.48	23.13	0.58
	14	27.32	0.55	24.09	0.67
7	8	22.62	0.52	21.21	0.63
	10	24.18	0.47	22.17	0.57
	12	25.75	0.47	23.13	0.57
	14	27.32	0.52	24.09	0.63
8	8	22.62	0.46	21.21	0.56
	10	24.18	0.30	22.17	0.37
	12	25.75	0.30	23.13	0.37
	14	27.32	0.46	24.09	0.56

Source: Jennrich and Schluchter (1986).

Table 5.6 Growth data. Model fit summary for the complete data set. The first column contains the model number, and a short description of the model is given in the second and third columns in terms of the mean and covariance structures, respectively. The number of parameters is given next, as well as the deviance (-2ℓ). The column labeled "Ref" displays one or more model numbers to which the current model is compared. The G^2 likelihood ratio statistic is the difference between -2ℓ of the current and the reference model. The final columns contain the number of degrees of freedom, and the p-value corresponds to the likelihood ratio test statistic.

	Mean	Covar	par	-2ℓ	Ref	G^2	df	p
1	unstr.	unstr.	18	416.509				
2	$\neq$ slopes	unstr.	14	419.477	1	2.968	4	0.5632
3	$=$ slopes	unstr.	13	426.153	2	6.676	1	0.0098
4	$\neq$ slopes	Toepl.	8	424.643	2	5.166	6	0.5227
5	$\neq$ slopes	AR(1)	6	440.681	2	21.204	8	0.0066
					4	16.038	2	0.0003
6	$\neq$ slopes	random	8	427.806	2	8.329	6	0.2150
7	$\neq$ slopes	CS	6	428.639	2	9.162	8	0.3288
					4	3.996	2	0.1356
					6	0.833	2	0.6594
					6	0.833	1:2	0.5104
8	$\neq$ slopes	simple	5	478.242	7	49.603	1	<0.0001
					7	49.603	0:1	<0.0001

The estimated covariance matrix $\widehat{\Sigma}$ of the error vector, based on this model, equals

$$\widehat{\Sigma} = \begin{pmatrix} 5.0143 & 2.5156 & 3.6206 & 2.5095 \\ 2.5156 & 3.8748 & 2.7103 & 3.0714 \\ 3.6206 & 2.7103 & 5.9775 & 3.8248 \\ 2.5095 & 3.0714 & 3.8248 & 4.6164 \end{pmatrix} \tag{5.8}$$

with the corresponding correlation matrix

$$\begin{pmatrix} 1.0000 & 0.5707 & 0.6613 & 0.5216 \\ 0.5707 & 1.0000 & 0.5632 & 0.7262 \\ 0.6613 & 0.5632 & 1.0000 & 0.7281 \\ 0.5216 & 0.7262 & 0.7281 & 1.0000 \end{pmatrix}. \tag{5.9}$$

These quantities are easily obtained in PROC MIXED by using the options R and RCORR in the REPEATED statement. Apparently, the variances are close to each other, and so are the correlations.

Even though we opted to follow closely the models discussed in Jennrich and Schluchter (1986), it is instructive to consider a more elaborate model, termed Model 0, where a separate unstructured covariance matrix is assumed for each of the two sex groups. This model has 10 extra parameters and can be fitted to the data using the following SAS code:

Program 5.2 Growth data. Model 0.

```
proc mixed data = growth method = ml covtest;
    title "Growth Data, Model 0";
    class idnr sex  age;
    model measure = sex age*sex / s;
    repeated / type = un subject = idnr
             r = 1,12 rcorr = 1,12 group = sex;
    run;
```

Since this model has individual-specific covariance matrices (although there are only two values, one for each gender), Σ has to be replaced by Σ_i.

These separate covariance matrices are requested by means of the GROUP=. option. These matrices and the corresponding correlation matrices are printed using the R=. and RCORR=. options. The estimated covariance matrix for girls is

$$\begin{pmatrix} 4.1033 & 3.0496 & 3.9380 & 3.9607 \\ 3.0496 & 3.2893 & 3.6612 & 3.7066 \\ 3.9380 & 3.6612 & 5.0826 & 4.9690 \\ 3.9607 & 3.7066 & 4.9690 & 5.4008 \end{pmatrix}$$

with the corresponding correlation matrix

$$\begin{pmatrix} 1.0000 & 0.8301 & 0.8623 & 0.8414 \\ 0.8301 & 1.0000 & 0.8954 & 0.8794 \\ 0.8623 & 0.8954 & 1.0000 & 0.9484 \\ 0.8414 & 0.8794 & 0.9484 & 1.0000 \end{pmatrix}.$$

The corresponding quantities for boys are

$$\begin{pmatrix} 5.6406 & 2.1484 & 3.4023 & 1.5117 \\ 2.1484 & 4.2773 & 2.0566 & 2.6348 \\ 3.4023 & 2.0566 & 6.5928 & 3.0381 \\ 1.5117 & 2.6348 & 3.0381 & 4.0771 \end{pmatrix}$$

and

$$\begin{pmatrix} 1.0000 & 0.4374 & 0.5579 & 0.3152 \\ 0.4374 & 1.0000 & 0.3873 & 0.6309 \\ 0.5579 & 0.3873 & 1.0000 & 0.5860 \\ 0.3152 & 0.6309 & 0.5860 & 1.0000 \end{pmatrix}.$$

From these, we suspect that there is a nonnegligible difference between the covariance structures for boys and girls, with, in particular, a weaker correlation among the boys' measurements. This is indeed supported by a deviance of 23.77 on 10 degrees of freedom ($p = 0.0082$). Nevertheless, the point estimates for the fixed effects coincide exactly with the ones obtained from Model 1 (see Table 5.4). However, even if attention is restricted to fixed effects inference, one still needs to address the quality of the estimates of precision. To this end, there are, in fact, two solutions. First, the more elaborate Model 0 can be fitted, as was done already. A drawback is that this model has 28 parameters altogether, which is quite a substantial number for such a small data set, implying that the asymptotic behavior of, for example, the deviance statistic becomes questionable. An alternative solution consists of retaining Model 1 and estimating the standard errors by means of the so-called robust estimator (equivalently termed the *sandwich* or *empirically corrected* estimator (Liang and Zeger, 1986)). To this end, the following code can be used:

Program 5.3 Growth data. Empirically corrected version of Model 1.

```
proc mixed data = growth method = ml covtest empirical;
    title "Growth Data, Model 1, Empirically Corrected";
    class idnr sex  age;
    model measure = sex age*sex / s;
    repeated / type = un subject = idnr r rcorr;
    run;
```

Here, the EMPIRICAL option is added to the PROC MIXED statement. This method yields a consistent estimator of precision, even if the covariance model is misspecified. In this particular case (a full factorial mean model), both methods (Model 0 on the one hand and the empirically corrected Model 1 on the other hand) lead to *exactly* the same standard errors. This illustrates that the robust method can be advantageous if correct standard errors are required, but finding an adequate covariance model is judged too involved. The robust standard errors are presented in Table 5.4 as the second entry in parentheses. It is seen that the naive standard errors are somewhat smaller than their robust counterparts, except for the parameters $\beta_{1,8}$, $\beta_{1,10}$, and $\beta_{1,12}$, where they are considerably larger. Even though the relation between the standard errors of the "correct model" (here, Model 0) and the empirically corrected "working model" (here, Model 1) will not always be a mathematical identity, the empirically corrected estimator option is a useful tool to compensate for misspecification in the covariance model.

Let us now return to our discussion of Model 1. It is instructive to consider the means for each of the eight categories explicitly. These means are presented in Table 5.5 for Models 1 through 8. The first panel of Figure 5.5 depicts the eight individual group means connected to form two profiles, one for each sex group.

Figure 5.5 Growth data. Profiles for the complete data from a selected set of models.

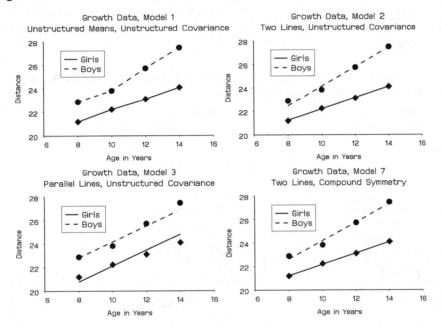

Clearly, there seems to be a linear trend in both profiles as well as a vague indication for diverging lines and hence different slopes. These hypotheses will be assessed on the basis of likelihood ratio tests, using the simpler Models 2 and 3.

Model 2

The first simplification occurs by assuming a linear trend within each sex group:

$$Y_{ij} = \beta_0 + \beta_{01}(1 - x_i) + \beta_{10}t_j(1 - x_i) + \beta_{11}t_jx_i + \varepsilon_{ij}. \tag{5.10}$$

Now, $\beta = (\beta_0, \beta_{01}, \beta_{10}, \beta_{11})'$.

The SAS code for Model 1 can be adapted simply by deleting age from the CLASS statement.

The likelihood ratio test comparing Model 2 to Model 1 does not reject the null hypothesis of linearity. A summary of model-fitting information for this and subsequent models as well as for comparisons between models is given in Table 5.6.

Model 3

The next step is to investigate whether the two profiles are parallel:

$$Y_{ij} = \beta_0 + \beta_{01}(1 - x_i) + \beta_1 t_j + \varepsilon_{ij}. \tag{5.11}$$

The parameter vector reduces to: $\beta = (\beta_0, \beta_{01}, \beta_1)'$.

Model 3 can be fitted in PROC MIXED by replacing the model statement in Model 2 with

```
model measure = sex age / s;
```

Table 5.6 reveals that the likelihood ratio test statistic (comparing Models 2 and 3) rejects the common slope hypothesis ($p = 0.0098$). This is consistent with the systematic deviation between observed and expected means in the third panel of Figure 5.5.

In line with the choice of Jennrich and Schluchter (1986), the mean structure of Model 2 will be kept. We will now turn our attention to simplifying the covariance structure.

Graphical Exploration

Figure 5.6 presents the 27 individual profiles. The left-hand panel shows the raw profiles, exhibiting the time trend found in the mean model. To obtain a rough idea about the covariance structure, it is useful to look at the right-hand panel, which gives the profiles after subtracting the means predicted by Model 2. Since these means agree closely with the observed means (see Figure 5.5), the corresponding sets of residuals are equivalent.

Figure 5.6 Growth data. Raw and residual profiles for the complete data set. (Girls are indicated with solid lines. Boys are indicated with dashed lines.)

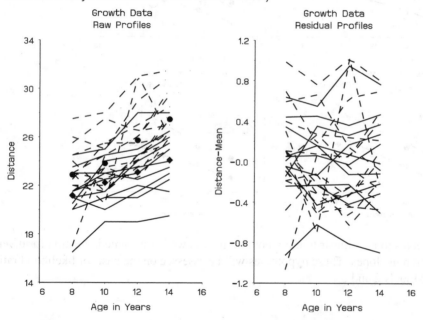

A noticeable though not fully general trend is that a profile tends to be high or low *as a whole*, which points to a random intercept. Apparently, the variance of the residuals is roughly constant over time, implying that the random effects structure is probably confined to the intercept. This observation is consistent with correlation matrix (5.9) of the unstructured Model 1. A more formal exploration can be done by means of the variogram (Diggle et al., 2002, Page 51) or its extensions (Verbeke, Lesaffre and Brant, 1998).

Jennrich and Schluchter (1986) considered several covariance structure models that are all included in PROC MIXED as standard options.

Model 4

The first covariance structure model is the so-called *Toeplitz* covariance matrix. Mean model formula (5.10) of Model 2 still applies, but the error vector ε_i is now assumed to follow a $\varepsilon_i \sim N(0, \Sigma)$ distribution, where Σ is constrained to $\sigma_{ij} = \alpha_{|i-j|}$; that is, the covariance depends on the measurement occasions through the lag between them only. In addition, Σ is assumed to be positive definite. For the growth data, there are only 4 free parameters, α_0, α_1, α_2, and α_3, instead of 10 in the unstructured case. The relationship among the α parameters is left unspecified. In the sequel, such additional constraints will lead to first-order autoregressive (Model 5) or exchangeable (Model 7) covariance structures.

To fit this model with **PROC MIXED**, the REPEATED statement needs to be changed, leading to the following program:

Program 5.4 Growth data. Model 4.

```
proc mixed data = growth method = ml covtest;
    title "Growth Data, Model 4";
    class sex idnr;
    model measure = sex age*sex / s;
    repeated / type = toep subject = idnr r rcorr;
    run;
```

Comparing the likelihood of this model to the one of the reference Model 2 shows that Model 4 is consistent with the data (see Table 5.6). At this point, Model 4 can replace Model 2 as the most parsimonious model consistent with the data found so far. Whether or not further simplifications are possible will be investigated next.

Model 5

A special case of the Toeplitz model is the first-order autoregressive model. This model is based on the assumption that the covariance between two measurements is a decreasing function of the time lag between them:

$$\sigma_{ij} = \sigma^2 \rho^{|i-j|}.$$

In other words, the variance of the measurements equals σ^2, and the covariance decreases with increasing time lag if $\rho > 0$. To fit this model with **PROC MIXED**, the REPEATED statement should include the option TYPE=AR(1).

Table 5.6 reveals that there is an apparent lack of fit for this model when compared to Model 2. Jennrich and Schluchter (1986) compared Model 5 to Model 2 as well. Alternatively, we might want to compare Model 5 to Model 4. This more parsimonious test (2 degrees of freedom) yields $p = 0.0003$, strongly rejecting the AR(1) structure.

Model 6

An alternative simplification of the unstructured covariance Model 2 is given by allowing the intercept and slope parameters to be random. While this model can be positioned within the sequence of models considered so far, it is conceptually somewhat different in the sense that it is generated from a hierarchical point of view. Indeed, assuming parameters to be random implicitly assumes a random effects structure to hold. Every such model implies a well-defined marginal model. The reverse is not true; i.e., when a particular marginal model produces an acceptable fit to the data, it is not necessarily correct to assert that a random effects model corresponding to it is consistent with the data as well. Model 6 is an example of model (5.6) with fixed effects design matrix X_i as in Model 2 (equation (5.10)), random effects design matrix

$$Z_i = \begin{pmatrix} 1 & 8 \\ 1 & 10 \\ 1 & 12 \\ 1 & 14 \end{pmatrix},$$

and measurement error structure $\Sigma = \sigma^2 I_4$.

An unstructured covariance matrix D for the random effects b_i will be assumed. The matrix D (requested by the G option in the RANDOM statement) is estimated to be

$$\hat{D} = \begin{pmatrix} 4.5569 & -0.1983 \\ -0.1983 & 0.0238 \end{pmatrix}.$$ (5.12)

One easily calculates the resulting covariance matrix of Y_i: $V_i = Z_i D Z_i' + \sigma^2 I_4$, which is estimated by

$$\hat{V}_i = Z_i \hat{D} Z_i' + \hat{\sigma}^2 I_4 = \begin{pmatrix} 4.6216 & 2.8891 & 2.8727 & 2.8563 \\ 2.8891 & 4.6839 & 3.0464 & 3.1251 \\ 2.8727 & 3.0464 & 4.9363 & 3.3938 \\ 2.8563 & 3.1251 & 3.3938 & 5.3788 \end{pmatrix},$$ (5.13)

where $\hat{\sigma}^2 = 1.7162$. Of course, this matrix can be requested by the V option in the REPEATED statement as well. Thus, this covariance matrix is a function of four parameters (three random effects parameters and one measurement error parameter). The corresponding estimated correlation matrix is

$$\begin{pmatrix} 1.0000 & 0.6209 & 0.6014 & 0.5729 \\ 0.6209 & 1.0000 & 0.6335 & 0.6226 \\ 0.6014 & 0.6335 & 1.0000 & 0.6586 \\ 0.5729 & 0.6226 & 0.6586 & 1.0000 \end{pmatrix}.$$ (5.14)

This model, approached from a marginal point of view, is a submodel of Model 2, but not of Model 4, because the correlations increase within each diagonal, albeit only moderately since the variance of the random slope is very modest. From Table 5.6, we observe that this model is a plausible simplification of Model 2. It has the same number of degrees of freedom as Model 4, although the latter one has a slightly smaller deviance.

Since the variance of the random slope is small, it is natural to explore whether a random intercept model is adequate.

Model 7

A hierarchical random intercepts model implies a compound symmetry model at the marginal level. However, not every compound symmetry model arises from such a random intercepts model; it happens only when the intraclass correlation is negative. The model is given by $Z_i = (1\ 1\ 1\ 1)'$, with variance of the random intercepts equal to d. The resulting covariance matrix of Y_i is

$$V_i = Z_i d Z_i' + \sigma^2 I_4 = d J_4 + \sigma^2 I_4,$$

where J_4 is a (4×4) matrix of ones. This covariance structure is called exchangeable or compound symmetry. All correlations are equal to $(d + \sigma^2)/\sigma^2$, implying that this model is a submodel of Models 4 and 6, as well as of Model 2. The marginal model implied by Model 7 can be fitted in PROC MIXED with two equivalent programs:

Program 5.5 Growth data. Model 7, using random effects modeling.

```
proc mixed data = growth method = ml covtest;
    title "Jennrich and Schluchter, Model 7";
    class sex idnr;
    model measure = sex age*sex / s;
    random intercept / type = un subject = idnr g;
    run;
```

and

Program 5.6 Growth data. Model 7, marginal point of view.

```
proc mixed data = growth method = ml covtest;
    title "Jennrich and Schluchter, Model 7";
    class sex idnr;
    model measure = sex age*sex / s;
    repeated / type = cs subject = idnr r rcorr;
    run;
```

The common variance is estimated to be 4.91, while the common correlation coefficient is estimated to be 0.62. Comparing this model to Model 2 yields $p = 0.3288$. Comparisons to Models 4 and 6 lead to the same conclusion. This implies that this model is currently the simplest one consistent with the data. It has to be noted that a comparison of Model 7 with Model 6 is slightly complicated by the fact that the null hypothesis implies that two of the three parameters in the D matrix of Model 6 are zero. For the variance of the random slope, this null value lies on the boundary of the parameter space. Stram and Lee (1994) show that the corresponding reference distribution is not χ_2^2, but a $50 : 50$ mixture of a χ_1^2 and a χ_2^2. Such a mixture is indicated by $\chi_{1:2}^2$, or simply by $1 : 2$. As a result, the corrected p-value would be 0.5104, thereby indicating no change in the conclusion. Similarly, comparing Models 2 and 6 as carried out earlier suffers from the same problem. Stram and Lee (1994) indicate that the asymptotic null distribution is even more complex and involves projections of random variables on curved surfaces. Therefore, the p-value is best determined by means of simulations. A simulation study of 500 samples yields $p = 0.046$, rather than $p = 0.215$, as reported in Table 5.6. To simulate the null distribution, we generated 500 samples of 270 individuals rather than 27 individuals to reduce small sample effects. Although this choice reflects the desire to perform asymptotic inference, it is debatable because one might rightly argue that generating samples of size 27 would reflect small-sample effects as well.

Although such a correction is clearly necessary, it is hard to use in general practice in its current form. Additional work in this area is certainly required.

Model 8

Finally, the independence model is considered in which the only source of variability is measurement error: $\Sigma = \sigma^2 I_4$. This model can be fitted in PROC MIXED using the TYPE=SIMPLE option in the REPEATED statement. Table 5.6 indicates that this model does not fit the data at all. Whether a χ_1^2 or a $\chi_{0:1}^2$ is used does not affect the conclusion.

In summary, among the models presented, Model 7 is preferred to summarize the data. In Sections 5.6 and 5.7, the trimmed version of the data will be analyzed, using frequentist available data methods and an ignorable likelihood-based analysis.

5.5   Simple Methods and MCAR

We will briefly review a number of relatively simple methods that have been and are still in extensive use. MCAR is required for a number of them, while for others, such as LOCF, this assumption is necessary but not sufficient. A detailed account is given in Verbeke and Molenberghs (1997, 2000). The case of clinical trials receives specific attention in Molenberghs et al. (2003). The focus will be on the complete case method, where data are removed, and on imputation strategies, where data are filled in. Regarding imputation, we distinguish between single and multiple imputation. In the first case, a single value is substituted for every "hole" in the data set and the resulting data set is analyzed as if it represented the true complete data. Multiple imputation properly acknowledges the uncertainty stemming from filling in missing values rather than observing them (Rubin, 1987; Schafer, 1997), and is deferred to Section 5.8. LOCF will be discussed within the context of imputation strategies, although not every author classifies the method as belonging to the imputation family.

5.5.1 Complete Case Analysis

A complete case analysis includes analyses of only those cases for which all n_i measurements were recorded. This method has obvious advantages. It is very simple to describe and, since the data structure is the same as what would have resulted from a complete experiment, standard statistical software can be used. Further, since the complete estimation is done on the same subset of completers, there is a common basis for inference, unlike with the available case methods.

Unfortunately, the method suffers from severe drawbacks. First, there is nearly always a substantial loss of information. For example, suppose there are 20 measurements, with 10% of missing data on each measurement. If we suppose further that missingness on the different measurements is independent, then the estimated percentage of incomplete observations is as high as 87%. The impact on precision and power is dramatic. Even though the reduction of the number of complete cases will be less dramatic in realistic settings where the missingness indicators R_i are correlated, the effect just sketched will undermine many complete case analyses. In addition, severe bias can result when the missingness mechanism is MAR but not MCAR. Indeed, should an estimator be consistent in the complete data problem, then the derived complete case analysis is consistent only if the missingness process is MCAR. Unfortunately, the MCAR assumption is much more restrictive than the MAR assumption.

Little and Rubin (1987) provide the following simple partial check on the MCAR assumption. Divide the observations on measurement j into two groups: (1) those subjects that are also observed on another measurement or set of measurements, (2) those missing on the other measurement(s). Should MCAR hold, then both groups should be random samples of the same population. Failure to reject equality of the distributional parameters of both samples increases the evidence for MCAR, but does not prove it.

EXAMPLE: Growth Data

In a complete case analysis of the growth data, the nine subjects that lack one measurement are deleted, resulting in a working data set with 18 subjects. This implies that 27 available measurements will not be used for analysis, a quite severe penalty on a relatively small data set.

Let us first consider the eight models described in Section 5.4. A summary of the model fit is given in Table 5.7.

Table 5.7 Growth data. Model fit summary for complete case analysis.

	Mean	Covar	par	-2ℓ	Ref	G^2	df	p
1	unstr.	unstr.	18	256.756				
2	$\neq$ slopes	unstr.	14	263.681	1	6.925	4	0.1399
3	$=$ slopes	unstr.	13	265.185	2	1.504	1	0.2201
4	$\neq$ slopes	banded	8	277.488	2	13.807	6	0.0319
5	$\neq$ slopes	AR(1)	6	288.063	2	24.382	8	0.0020
					4	10.575	2	0.0051
6	$\neq$ slopes	random	8	276.834	2	13.153	6	0.0407
7	$\neq$ slopes	CS	6	278.127	2	14.446	8	0.0709
					4	0.639	2	0.7265
					6	1.293	2	0.5239
					6	1.293	1:2	0.3897
8	$\neq$ slopes	simple	5	306.163	7	28.036	1	<0.0001
					7	28.036	0:1	<0.0001

There are a few striking features. On the one hand, the common slope Model 3 is not rejected. The banded correlation structure, on the other hand, is marginally rejected when compared to Model 2, whereas the compound symmetry Model 7 is at the other side of the nominal 5% level. The autoregressive structure is still not acceptable. The random slope and intercept Model 6 is marginally rejected. As before, Model 8 is strongly rejected. From this analysis we might conclude that Model 7 provides the most parsimonious description consistent with the data *among the eight models considered*, although this decision is less clear cut than in the analysis of the complete data set. Recall that we performed tests involving Model 6 with both the incorrect χ^2 null distributions and the asymptotic mixture null distributions (Stram and Lee, 1994) discussed on page 287.

Let us now study the influence of the restriction to completers on the analysis. From the fitted model (not shown) or from Figure 5.7, we observe that the separate slopes for boys and girls are closer to each other than in the analysis of the complete data set. This is true for both Models 2 and 7. Thus, the fact that Model 3 is not rejected is not only due to a reduced sample size, but also to convergence of the two profiles.

Figure 5.7 Growth data. Profiles for complete case analysis from a selected set of models. (The small dots are the observed group means for the complete data set. The large dots are the corresponding quantities for the incomplete data.)

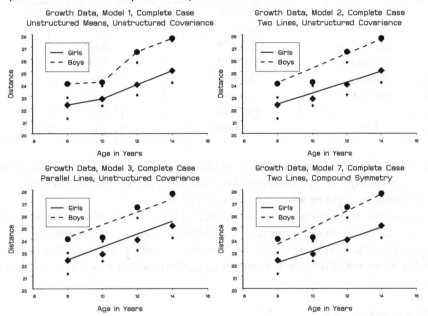

All observed group means have increased relative to the complete data set, but mostly so at age 8. This is to be expected, since the probability of missingness at age 10 was modeled by Little and Rubin (1987) to depend directly on the measurement at age 8, such that lower measurements led to more nonresponse. As a consequence, those subjects deleted had low values at age 8. There is only indirect dependence on the measurements at ages 10 and 12 through the correlation with the measurement at age 8. The net effect is that the profiles overestimate the average length and underestimate the difference in slopes between boys and girls. In addition, the average slope has decreased, leading to flattened profiles, especially for boys.

The covariance matrix, estimated under Model 1, is equal to

$$\begin{pmatrix} 2.2460 & 2.3155 & 2.3829 & 2.0754 \\ 2.3155 & 4.2763 & 2.0420 & 2.5741 \\ 2.3829 & 2.0420 & 5.4513 & 3.0752 \\ 2.0754 & 2.5741 & 3.0752 & 3.8806 \end{pmatrix}, \tag{5.15}$$

with the corresponding correlation matrix

$$\begin{pmatrix} 1.0000 & 0.7471 & 0.6810 & 0.7030 \\ 0.7471 & 1.0000 & 0.4229 & 0.6319 \\ 0.6810 & 0.4229 & 1.0000 & 0.6686 \\ 0.7030 & 0.6319 & 0.6686 & 1.0000 \end{pmatrix}. \tag{5.16}$$

Inspecting Table 5.7, it is clearly unsatisfactory that the unequal slopes model is carried along Models 4–8, even though the comparison of Models 2 and 3 does not reveal a departure from equality of the slopes. Alternatively, we might start simplifying the covariance structure from Model 3. A summary is presented in Table 5.8.

Table 5.8 Growth data. Model fit summary for additional models for complete case analysis.

	Mean	Covar	par	-2ℓ	Ref	G^2	df	p
1	unstr.	unstr.	18	256.756				
2	$\neq$ slopes	unstr.	14	263.681	1	6.925	4	0.1399
3	= slopes	unstr.	13	265.185	2	1.504	1	0.2201
4b	= slopes	banded	7	279.778	3	14.593	6	0.0237
5b	= slopes	AR(1)	5	288.670	3	23.485	8	0.0028
6b	= slopes	random	7	278.780	3	13.595	6	0.0345
7b	= slopes	CS	5	280.044	3	14.859	8	0.0619
8b	= slopes	simple	4	306.990	3	41.805	9	<0.0001

There is evidence for lack of fit in the Toeplitz (banded), AR(1), random, and simple (uncorrelated) models. While the compound symmetry model does exhibit a better fit, the evidence in favor of this model is not overwhelming. It might be wiser to stick to Model 3.

In conclusion, an analysis of the completers would lead to a linear profile with common slope but different intercepts (the difference in intercepts is 1.786 with standard error 0.717) and with an unstructured covariance matrix. This is in contrast with the analysis of the complete data set where we found a more complex mean model (different slopes) in conjunction with a very simple (exchangeable) covariance model.

EXAMPLE: Depression Trial

Since the difference between therapies A1 and C, or treatment arms 1 and 4, is of primary interest, we will only consider these in the analysis. In the depression trial, 170 patients received either therapy A1 or C, and 109 of these patients completed the study. This implies that measurements of 61 patients are deleted for a complete case analysis of the depression trial. The remaining data set is denoted as CC and can be obtained with the %CC macro. It requires four arguments. DATA is the data set to be analyzed. If this is not specified, the last data set is used. The name of the variable in the data set which contains the identification variable is ID. TIME specifies the variable indicating the time points, and RESPONSE is the response variable. The name of the data set, created with the macro, is given in OUT.

Program 5.7 Macro to prepare data for complete case analysis

```
%macro cc(data=,id=,time=,response=,out=);
%if %bquote(&data)= %then %let data=&syslast;
proc freq data=&data noprint;
    tables &id /out=freqsub;
    tables &time / out=freqtime;
    run;
proc iml;
    use freqsub;
```

```
    read all var {&id,count};
    nsub = nrow(&id);
    use freqtime;
    read all var {&time,count};
    ntime = nrow(&time);
    use &data;
    read all var {&id,&time,&response};
    n =  nrow(&response);
    complete = j(n,1,1);
    ind = 1;
    do while (ind <= nsub);
      if (&response[(ind-1)*ntime+ntime]=.) then
        complete[(ind-1)*ntime+1:(ind-1)*ntime+ntime]=0;
      ind = ind+1;
    end;
    create help var {&id &time &response complete};
    append;
    quit;
data &out;
    merge &data help;
    if complete=0 then delete;
    drop complete;
    run;
%mend;
```

Running the next statement will give us the complete case CC data set for the depression trial.

```
%cc(data=depression,id=patient,time=visit,response=change,out=cc);
```

Complete case data set

Obs	PATIENT	VISIT	CHANGE	TRT	BASVAL	INVEST
1	1501	4	-7	1	25	6
2	1501	5	-14	1	25	6
3	1501	6	-14	1	25	6
4	1501	7	-17	1	25	6
5	1501	8	-19	1	25	6
6	1502	4	-1	4	17	6
7	1502	5	-4	4	17	6
8	1502	6	-4	4	17	6
9	1502	7	-5	4	17	6
10	1502	8	-8	4	17	6
11	1510	4	3	1	18	6
12	1510	5	5	1	18	6
13	1510	6	0	1	18	6
14	1510	7	-9	1	18	6
15	1510	8	-9	1	18	6
...						
526	4706	4	-16	1	29	38
527	4706	5	-13	1	29	38
528	4706	6	-13	1	29	38
529	4706	7	-20	1	29	38
530	4706	8	-23	1	29	38
531	4710	4	-14	1	21	38

532	4710	5	−7	1	21	38
533	4710	6	−19	1	21	38
534	4710	7	−14	1	21	38
535	4710	8	−19	1	21	38
536	4712	4	−8	4	11	38
537	4712	5	−9	4	11	38
538	4712	6	−7	4	11	38
539	4712	7	−1	4	11	38
540	4712	8	11	4	11	38
541	4801	4	5	4	12	999
542	4801	5	−6	4	12	999
543	4801	6	−7	4	12	999
544	4801	7	−9	4	12	999
545	4801	8	−10	4	12	999

The primary null hypothesis (difference between the treatment and placebo in mean change of the HAMD17 total score at endpoint) will be tested by a likelihood-based, mixed effects repeated measures analysis.

Fitting linear mixed models implies that an appropriate mean structure as well as a covariance structure needs to be specified. They are not independent and some general guidelines for model building are given in Section 5.4.1.

PROC MIXED is used to perform this complete case analysis. The model we will fit will include the fixed categorical effects of treatment, investigator, visit and treatment-by-visit interaction, as well as the continuous, fixed covariates of baseline score and baseline score-by-visit interaction. These covariates are chosen beforehand. There are no random effects in the model and the serial correlation and the measurement error term have been combined into a single residual covariance term ε_i. Thus the model is $Y_i = X_i\beta + \varepsilon_i$, with $\varepsilon_i \sim \Sigma_i$. To keep the chance on errors as small as possible, we will use the most complex covariance structure, i.e., the unstructured one.

In the PROC MIXED statement in Program 5.8, the option METHOD=. specifies the estimation method. We specified METHOD=ML instead of the default METHOD=REML, requesting ML or REML estimation, respectively. The NOITPRINT option suppresses the display of the "Iteration History" table. The calculation of the information criteria, which can be used as a tool for model selection, can be requested by adding the option IC.

The CLASS statement specifies which variables should be considered as factors. Such classification variables can be either character or numeric. Internally, each of these factors will correspond to a set of dummy variables.

The MODEL statement names the response variable and all fixed effects, which determine the X_i matrices. The SOLUTION or S option is used to request the printing of the estimates for the fixed effects in the model, together with standard errors, t-statistics, and corresponding p-values for testing their significance. The estimation method for the degrees of freedom in the t- and F-approximations needed in tests for fixed effects estimates is specified in the DDFM=. option. Here, Satterthwaite's approximation was used, but other methods are also available within SAS.

To specify the Σ_i matrices in the mixed model, the REPEATED statement is used. The repeated effects define the ordering of the repeated measurements within each subject. These effects must be classification variables. In the example this variable is VISIT. The option SUBJECT=. identifies the subjects in the data set and complete independence is assumed across subjects. The variable PATIENT in SUBJECT=PATIENT is permitted to be continuous as well as categorical (specified in the CLASS statement). However, when PATIENT is continuous, PROC MIXED considers a record to be from a new subject whenever the value of PATIENT is different from a previous record. Hence, one then should first sort the data by the values of PATIENT. On the other hand, using a continuous PATIENT variable reduces execution times for models with a large number of subjects, since no large matrix of subject indicators needs to be manipulated. Further, the TYPE=. option specifies the covariance structure Σ_i for the error components ε_i.

Program 5.8 Complete case analysis for the depression trial

```
proc mixed data=cc method=ml noitprint ic;
    class patient visit invest trt;
    model change = trt invest visit trt*visit basval basval*visit
        / solution ddfm=satterth;
    repeated visit / subject=patient type=un;
    run;
```

Output from Program 5.8

```
                    Covariance Parameter Estimates

            Cov Parm     Subject       Estimate

            UN(1,1)      PATIENT        17.6909
            UN(2,1)      PATIENT         8.5695
            UN(2,2)      PATIENT        24.1209
            UN(3,1)      PATIENT         4.8799
            UN(3,2)      PATIENT        11.3321
            UN(3,3)      PATIENT        28.1113
            UN(4,1)      PATIENT         4.0338
            UN(4,2)      PATIENT        10.6874
            UN(4,3)      PATIENT        16.4904
            UN(4,4)      PATIENT        27.4436
            UN(5,1)      PATIENT         2.2028
            UN(5,2)      PATIENT         7.6408
            UN(5,3)      PATIENT        13.3963
            UN(5,4)      PATIENT        21.7397
            UN(5,5)      PATIENT        36.2240


                         Fit Statistics

            -2 Log Likelihood              3155.5
            AIC (smaller is better)        3247.5
            AICC (smaller is better)       3256.2
            BIC (smaller is better)        3371.3


               Null Model Likelihood Ratio Test

                 DF     Chi-Square      Pr > ChiSq

                 14       171.94          <.0001


                    Information Criteria

Neg2LogLike    Parms     AIC      AICC      HQIC      BIC      CAIC

   3155.5       46      3247.5    3256.2    3297.7    3371.3   3417.3
```

```
~~~~~~~~~~~~~~~~~~~~~~~~~~~~~~~~~~~~~~~~~~~~~~~~~~~~~~~~~~~~~~~~~~
                       Type 3 Tests of Fixed Effects

                         Num      Den
         Effect           DF       DF     F Value     Pr > F

         TRT               1      104        1.18      0.2794
         INVEST           16      109        4.80      <.0001
         VISIT             4      109        1.29      0.2787
         VISIT*TRT         4      109        0.82      0.5181
         BASVAL            1      113       36.78      <.0001
         BASVAL*VISIT      4      109        1.11      0.3568
```

From the output, we can deduce that the covariance matrix is given by

$$\begin{pmatrix} 17.6909 & 8.5695 & 4.8799 & 4.0338 & 2.2028 \\ 8.5695 & 24.1209 & 11.3321 & 10.6874 & 7.6408 \\ 4.8799 & 11.3321 & 28.1113 & 16.4904 & 13.3963 \\ 4.0338 & 10.6874 & 16.4904 & 27.4436 & 21.7397 \\ 2.2028 & 7.6408 & 13.3963 & 21.7397 & 36.2240 \end{pmatrix}.$$

Next in the output, the fit statistics are given, which are used to test the goodness-of-fit. The Type III tests of fixed effects show that neither treatment ($p = 0.2794$) nor the treatment-by-visit interaction ($p = 0.5181$) is significant.

5.5.2 Last Observation Carried Forward

An alternative way to obtain a data set on which complete data methods can be used is filling in the missing values, instead of deleting subjects with incomplete sequences. The principle of imputation is particularly easy. The observed values are used to impute values for the missing observations. There are several ways to use the observed information. First, one can use information on the same subject (e.g., last observation carried forward). Secondly, information can be borrowed from other subjects (e.g., mean imputation). Finally, both within- and between-subject information can be used (e.g., conditional mean imputation, hot deck imputation). Standard references are Little and Rubin (1987) and Rubin (1987). Imputation strategies have been very popular in sample survey methods.

However, great care has to be taken with imputation strategies. Dempster and Rubin (1983) write

> The idea of imputation is both seductive and dangerous. It is seductive because it can lull the user into the pleasurable state of believing that the data are complete after all, and it is dangerous because it lumps together situations where the problem is sufficiently minor that it can be legitimately handled in this way and situations where standard estimators applied to the real and imputed data have substantial biases.

For example, Little and Rubin (1987) show that the method could work for a linear model with one fixed effect and one error term, but that it generally does not work for hierarchical models, split-plot designs, repeated measures (with a complicated error structure), random effects models, and mixed effects models. At the very least, different imputations for different effects would be necessary.

The user of imputation strategies faces several dangers. First, the imputation model could be wrong and hence the point estimates would be biased. Secondly, even for a correct imputation model, the uncertainty resulting from incompleteness is masked. Indeed, even when one is reasonably sure about the mean value the unknown observation would have, the actual stochastic realization, depending on both the mean structure as well as on the error distribution, is still unknown.

Whenever a value is missing, the last observed value is substituted. It is typically applied to settings where incompleteness is due to attrition.

Very strong and often unrealistic assumptions have to be made to ensure validity of this method. First, when we consider a longitudinal analysis or when the scientific question is in terms of the last planned occasion, one has to believe that a subject's measurement stays at the same level from the moment of dropout onwards (or during the period they are unobserved in the case of intermittent missingness). In a clinical trial setting, one might believe that the response profile *changes* as soon as a patient goes off treatment and even that it would flatten. However, the constant profile assumption is even stronger. Second, this method shares with other single imputation methods the tendency to overestimate the precision by treating imputed and actually observed values as equal.

The situation in which the scientific question is in terms of the last observed measurement is often considered to be the real motivation for LOCF. However, in some cases the question, defined as such, has a very unrealistic and *ad hoc* flavor. Clearly, measurements at self-selected dropout times are lumped together with measurements made at the investigator-defined end of the study.

EXAMPLE: Growth Data

For this data set, the nine subjects that lack a measurement at age 10 are completed by imputing the age 8 value. It is clear that this procedure will affect the linear but nonconstant trend model discovered on the basis of the complete data set. We will also investigate the effect on the covariance model.

Let us first consider the eight models described in Section 5.4. A summary of the model fit is given in Table 5.9.

Table 5.9 Growth data. Model fit summary for last observation carried forward.

	Mean	Covar	par	-2ℓ	Ref	G^2	df	p
1	unstr.	unstr.	18	407.078				
2	$\neq$ slopes	unstr.	14	424.793	1	17.715	4	0.0014
3	$=$ slopes	unstr.	13	426.333	2	1.540	1	0.2146
4	$\neq$ slopes	banded	8	445.216	2	20.423	6	0.0023
5	$\neq$ slopes	AR(1)	6	449.640	2	24.847	8	0.0017
6	$\neq$ slopes	random	8	446.121	2	21.328	6	0.0016
7	$\neq$ slopes	CS	6	449.077	6	2.956	2	0.2281
					6	2.956	1:2	0.1568
8	$\neq$ slopes	simple	5	496.961	7	47.884	1	<0.0001
					7	47.884	0:1	<0.0001

Again, there are several noteworthy features. Both different (Model 2) and common (Model 3) slope profiles are inadequate. Inspecting Figure 5.8, the reason is immediately clear. The imputation procedure forces the means at ages 8 and 10 to be very similar, thereby destroying the linear relationship, as was anticipated.

There is more discrepancy between Models 2 and 7 here than in the complete data set. The slopes of Model 7 are considerably higher than those of Model 2; the slope for girls in Model 7 is almost as high as the slope for boys in Model 2. Of course, none of the models assuming a linear profile is consistent with these data, and either further modeling or restriction to the unstructured profiles of Model 1 seems necessary.

Let us consider the estimated correlation matrix of Model 1

$$\begin{pmatrix} 1.0000 & 0.9015 & 0.6613 & 0.5216 \\ 0.9015 & 1.0000 & 0.5567 & 0.5318 \\ 0.6613 & 0.5567 & 1.0000 & 0.7281 \\ 0.5216 & 0.5318 & 0.7281 & 1.0000 \end{pmatrix}.$$

This unstructured covariance matrix shows clearly the impact of the last observation carried forward (LOCF) approach. The measurements at ages 8 and 10 are made very similar, inducing a correlation as

Figure 5.8 Growth data. Profiles for last observation carried forward from a selected set of models. (The small dots are the observed group means for the complete data set. The large dots are the corresponding quantities for the incomplete data.)

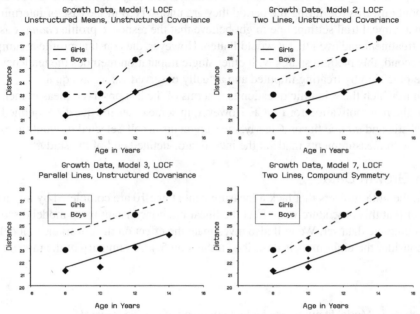

high as 0.9015, rather than 0.5707 in the complete data set. Thus, the three lag 1 correlations are more dissimilar, resulting in a bad fit for the Toeplitz model. Since Models 5, 6, and 7 simplify the Toeplitz structure, they show an equally bad fit. Let us take a closer look at the random effects Model 6. The covariance matrix D of random intercept and slope is estimated to be

$$\begin{pmatrix} 13.5992 & -0.7910 \\ -0.7910 & 0.0616 \end{pmatrix}.$$

Further, $\hat{\sigma}^2 = 1.8741$.

The resulting correlation matrix is

$$\begin{pmatrix} 1.0000 & 0.6842 & 0.6135 & 0.5126 \\ 0.6842 & 1.0000 & 0.6430 & 0.5782 \\ 0.6135 & 0.6430 & 1.0000 & 0.6288 \\ 0.5126 & 0.5782 & 0.6288 & 1.0000 \end{pmatrix}.$$

Comparison with Model 6 on the complete data set suggests the following interpretation. Carrying the observations from age 8 forward to age 10 increases the similarity and thus the correlation between this pair of outcomes. This implies an increased variance of the random intercept over the complete data set version (5.14). This is at the expense of the variance σ^2.

Next, we consider a few additional models. Their fit is presented in Table 5.10.

Table 5.10 Growth data. Model fit summary for additional models for last observation carried forward.

	Mean	Covar	par	-2ℓ	Ref	G^2	df	p
1	unstr.	unstr.	18	407.078				
2c	quadratic	unstr.	16	412.640	1	5.562	2	0.0620
4c	unstr.	banded	12	427.804	1	20.726	6	0.0021
5c	unstr.	AR(1)	10	433.714	1	26.636	8	0.0017
7c	unstr.	CS	10	437.394	1	30.216	8	0.0002

Figure 5.8 suggested that a linear profile is not appropriate, which was confirmed in the analysis. A quadratic time trend might seem more appropriate. Model 2c (Table 5.10) combines a quadratic time trend with an unstructured covariance matrix. It is marginally acceptable but it seems wiser to retain the unstructured Model 1. Simplifying the covariance structure (Toeplitz, AR(1), CS) does not seem possible.

In conclusion, the effect of an LOCF imputation is that both mean and covariance structure are severely distorted such that no obvious simplification is possible. Hence, a simple, intuitively appealing interpretation of the trends is rendered impossible. LOCF should be used with great caution. Of course, for the growth data there is a clear increasing trend over time. This is already seen from inspection of the completers. Therefore, LOCF seems particularly inappropriate. An alternative method, which might be better suited for intermittent missing data, would replace a missing observation with an average of the adjacent measurements. For example, a missing value at age 10 would be replaced with the average of the measurements at ages 8 and 12.

For unequally spaced measurements a weighted average might be more appropriate. In certain settings, the principle underlying LOCF might better reflect the true mechanism generating the data (e.g., in a randomized clinical trial). We have to reemphasize that even in such cases, imputing a single value for missing measurements would still result in overestimation of the precision.

The LOCF depends uniquely on the measurements of the individual for which an imputation has to be generated. As such, we could term it *horizontal* imputation.

EXAMPLE: Depression Trial

Instead of deleting the incomplete profiles, we complete them by filling in the missing measurements until the last planned visit by the last observed measurement of that patient. This is done in the %LOCF macro, which results in the LOCF data set. Again, TIME specifies the variable indication the time points, and RESPONSE is the original response variable. Further, LOCF is the response variable after completing the original variable RESPONSE.

Program 5.9 Macro to prepare for LOCF

```
%macro locf(data=,id=,time=,response=,out=);
%if %bquote(&data)= %then %let data=&syslast;
proc freq data=&data noprint;
    tables &id /out=freqsub;
    tables &time / out=freqtime;
    run;
proc iml;
    use freqsub;
    read all var {&id,count};
    nsub = nrow(&id);
    use freqtime;
    read all var {&time,count};
    ntime = nrow(&time);
    use &data;
    read all var {&id,&time,&response};
    n =  nrow(&response);
    locf = &response;
    ind = 1;
    do while (ind <= nsub);
      if (&response[(ind-1)*ntime+ntime]=.) then
        do;
          i = 1;
          do while (&response[(ind-1)*ntime+i]^=.);
            i = i+1;
          end;
```

```
            lastobserved = i-1;
            locf[(ind-1)*ntime+lastobserved+1:(ind-1)*ntime+ntime]
               = locf[(ind-1)*ntime+lastobserved];
         end;
      ind = ind+1;
   end;
   create help var {&id &time &response locf};
   append;
   quit;
data &out;
   merge &data help;
   run;
%mend;
```

Running the next statement gives us the data set we need for the LOCF analysis.

```
%locf(data=depression,id=patient,time=visit,response=change,out=locf);
```

LOCF data set

Obs	PATIENT	VISIT	CHANGE	LOCF	TRT	BASVAL	INVEST
1	1501	4	-7	-7	1	25	6
2	1501	5	-14	-14	1	25	6
3	1501	6	-14	-14	1	25	6
4	1501	7	-17	-17	1	25	6
5	1501	8	-19	-19	1	25	6
6	1502	4	-1	-1	4	17	6
7	1502	5	-4	-4	4	17	6
8	1502	6	-4	-4	4	17	6
9	1502	7	-5	-5	4	17	6
10	1502	8	-8	-8	4	17	6
11	1504	4	9	9	4	12	6
12	1504	5	5	5	4	12	6
13	1504	6	19	19	4	12	6
14	1504	7	.	19	4	12	6
15	1504	8	.	19	4	12	6
...							
836	4801	4	5	5	4	12	999
837	4801	5	-6	-6	4	12	999
838	4801	6	-7	-7	4	12	999
839	4801	7	-9	-9	4	12	999
840	4801	8	-10	-10	4	12	999
841	4803	4	-6	-6	1	16	999
842	4803	5	-8	-8	1	16	999
843	4803	6	-8	-8	1	16	999
844	4803	7	-10	-10	1	16	999
845	4803	8	.	-10	1	16	999
846	4901	4	2	2	1	9	999
847	4901	5	-6	-6	1	9	999
848	4901	6	.	-6	1	9	999
849	4901	7	.	-6	1	9	999
850	4901	8	.	-6	1	9	999

Again a likelihood-based, mixed effects repeated measures analysis will be done, including the same fixed categorical and continuous effects as in the complete case analysis.

Program 5.10 Last observation carried forward analysis for the depression trial

```
proc mixed data=locf method=ml noclprint noitprint;
    class patient visit invest trt;
    model locf = trt invest visit trt*visit basval basval*visit
        / solution ddfm=satterth;
    repeated visit / subject=patient type=un;
    run;
```

Output from Program 5.10

Cov Parm	Subject	Estimate
UN(1,1)	PATIENT	16.9671
UN(2,1)	PATIENT	9.2454
UN(2,2)	PATIENT	26.9981
UN(3,1)	PATIENT	8.5925
UN(3,2)	PATIENT	20.1808
UN(3,3)	PATIENT	40.7395
UN(4,1)	PATIENT	8.7862
UN(4,2)	PATIENT	20.5298
UN(4,3)	PATIENT	32.7794
UN(4,4)	PATIENT	44.0631
UN(5,1)	PATIENT	7.4426
UN(5,2)	PATIENT	18.3357
UN(5,3)	PATIENT	30.4906
UN(5,4)	PATIENT	39.9523
UN(5,5)	PATIENT	48.9177

Fit Statistics

-2 Log Likelihood	4877.3
AIC (smaller is better)	4969.3
AICC (smaller is better)	4974.7
BIC (smaller is better)	5113.6

Null Model Likelihood Ratio Test

DF	Chi-Square	Pr > ChiSq
14	545.40	<.0001

Information Criteria

Neg2LogLike	Parms	AIC	AICC	HQIC	BIC	CAIC
4877.3	46	4969.3	4974.7	5027.9	5113.6	5159.6

```
╲╱╲╱╲╱╲╱╲╱╲╱╲╱╲╱╲╱╲╱╲╱╲╱╲╱╲╱╲╱╲╱╲╱╲╱╲╱╲╱╲╱╲╱╲╱╲╱╲╱╲╱
                      Type 3 Tests of Fixed Effects


                        Num      Den
         Effect          DF       DF    F Value    Pr > F

         TRT              1      161      0.70      0.4042
         INVEST          16      170      4.41      <.0001
         VISIT            4      170      1.31      0.2686
         VISIT*TRT        4      170      1.51      0.2005
         BASVAL           1      187     24.54      <.0001
         BASVAL*VISIT     4      170      0.94      0.4422
```

From the output, we can calculate the covariance matrix, which results in

$$\begin{pmatrix} 16.9671 & 9.2454 & 8.5925 & 8.7862 & 7.4426 \\ 9.2454 & 26.9981 & 20.1808 & 20.5298 & 18.3357 \\ 8.5925 & 20.1808 & 40.7395 & 32.7794 & 30.4906 \\ 8.7862 & 20.5298 & 32.7794 & 44.0631 & 39.9523 \\ 7.4426 & 18.3357 & 30.4906 & 39.9523 & 48.9177 \end{pmatrix}.$$

Again, neither treatment ($p = 0.4042$) nor treatment-by-visit interaction ($p = 0.2005$) is significant.

5.6 Available Case Methods

Available case methods (Little and Rubin, 1987) use as much of the data as possible. Let us restrict attention to the estimation of the mean vector μ and the covariance matrix Σ. The jth component μ_j of the mean vector and the jth diagonal variance element σ_{jj} are estimated using all cases that are observed on the jth variable, disregarding their response status at the other measurement occasions. The (j, k)th element ($j \neq k$) of the covariance matrix is computed using all cases that are observed on both the jth and the kth variable.

This method is more efficient than the complete case method, since more information is used. The number of components of the outcome vector has no direct effect on the sample available for a particular mean or covariance component.

The method is valid only under MCAR. In this respect, it is no fundamental improvement over complete case analysis. An added disadvantage is that, although more information is used and a consistent estimator is obtained under MCAR, it is not guaranteed that the covariance matrix is positive semi-definite. Of course, this is only a small-sample problem and does not invalidate asymptotic results. However, for samples with a large number of variables or with fairly high correlations between pairs of outcomes, this nuisance feature is likely to occur.

Although a complete case analysis is possible for virtually every statistical method, and single imputation is also fairly generally applicable, extending an available case analysis beyond multivariate means and covariances can be tedious. This particular method has limited practical value.

EXAMPLE: Growth Data

We will focus on a straightforward but restrictive *available case* analysis from a frequentist perspective. Specifically, the parameters for the unstructured mean and covariance Model 1 will be estimated.

The estimated mean vector for girls is

$$(21.1818, 22.7857, 23.0909, 24.0909), b$$

whereas the vector for boys is

$$(22.8750, 24.1364, 25.7188, 27.4688).$$

The mean vector for girls is based on a sample of size 11, except for the second element, which is based on the seven complete observations. The corresponding sample sizes for boys are 16 and 11, respectively.

The estimated covariance matrix is

$$\begin{pmatrix} 5.4155 & 2.3155 & 3.9102 & 2.7102 \\ 2.3155 & 4.2763 & 2.0420 & 2.5741 \\ 3.9102 & 2.0420 & 6.4557 & 4.1307 \\ 2.7102 & 2.5741 & 4.1307 & 4.9857 \end{pmatrix}, \tag{5.17}$$

with the correlation matrix

$$\begin{pmatrix} 1.0000 & 0.4812 & 0.6613 & 0.5216 \\ 0.4812 & 1.0000 & 0.3886 & 0.5575 \\ 0.6613 & 0.3886 & 1.0000 & 0.7281 \\ 0.5216 & 0.5575 & 0.7281 & 1.0000 \end{pmatrix}.$$

The elements of the covariance matrix are computed as

$$\hat{\sigma}_{jk} = \frac{1}{25} \left\{ \sum_{i=1}^{11} (y_{ij}^g - \overline{y}_j^g)(y_{ik}^g - \overline{y}_k^g) + \sum_{i=1}^{16} (y_{ij}^b - \overline{y}_j^b)(y_{ik}^b - \overline{y}_k^b) \right\}, \; j, k \neq 2,$$

$$\hat{\sigma}_{j2} = \frac{1}{18} \left\{ \sum_{i=1}^{7} (y_{ij}^g - \overline{y}_j^g)(y_{i2}^g - \overline{y}_2^g) + \sum_{i=1}^{11} (y_{ij}^b - \overline{y}_j^b)(y_{i2}^b - \overline{y}_2^b) \right\}.$$

The superscripts g and b refer to girls and boys, respectively. It is assumed that, within each sex subgroup, the ordering is such that completers precede the incompletely measured children.

Looking at the available case procedure from the perspective of the individual observation, one might say that each observation contributes to the subvector of the parameter vector about which it contains information. For example, a complete observation in the GROWTH data set contributes to four (sex specific) mean components as well as to all 10 variance-covariance parameters. In an incomplete observation, there is information about three mean components and six variance-covariance parameters (excluding those with a subscript 2).

Whether or not there is nonrandom selection of the incomplete observations does not affect those parameters without a subscript 2. For the ones involving a subscript 2, potential differences between completers and noncompleters are not taken into account, and hence biased estimation may result when an MAR mechanism is operating. In fact, the estimates for the parameters with at least one subscript 2 equal their complete case analysis counterparts. Thus, MCAR is required. This observation is consistent with the theory in Rubin (1976), since the current available case method is frequentist rather than likelihood based.

5.7 Likelihood-Based Ignorable Analyses

As indicated in Section 5.3, likelihood-based inference is valid whenever the mechanism is MAR and provided the technical condition holds that the parameters describing the nonresponse mechanism are distinct from the measurement model parameters (Little and Rubin, 1987). In other words, the missing data process should be ignorable in the likelihood inference sense, because then the log-likelihood partitions into two functionally independent components. The practical implication is that a software module with likelihood estimation facilities and with the ability to handle incompletely observed subjects manipulates the correct likelihood, providing valid parameter estimates and likelihood ratio values.

EXAMPLE: Growth Data

As with the available case method of Section 5.6, a complete subject contributes to more parameters than an incomplete subject. Whereas these contributions were direct in terms of parameter vector components in Section 5.6, in the current framework subjects contribute information through their factor of the likelihood function. As such, this framework is consistent with likelihood inference and is valid under MAR. Hence, it ought to be the preferred standard mode of analysis. Moreover, in most software packages, such as the SAS procedure MIXED, this analysis is performed automatically, as will be discussed next.

Little and Rubin (1987) fitted the same eight models as Jennrich and Schluchter (1986) to the incomplete GROWTH data set. Whereas Little and Rubin made use of the EM algorithm, we set out to perform our analysis with direct maximization of the observed likelihood (with Fisher scoring or Newton-Raphson) in PROC MIXED. The results ought to coincide. Table 5.11 reproduces the findings of Little and Rubin. We added *p*-values.

Table 5.11 Growth data. Model fit summary for MAR analysis (Little and Rubin).

	Mean	Covar	par	-2ℓ	Ref	G^2	df	p
1	unstr.	unstr.	18	386.957				
2	$\neq$ slopes	unstr.	14	393.288	1	6.331	4	0.1758
3	= slopes	unstr.	13	397.400	2	4.112	1	0.0426
4	$\neq$ slopes	Toepl.	8	398.030	2	4.742	6	0.5773
5	$\neq$ slopes	AR(1)	6	409.523	2	16.235	8	0.0391
6	$\neq$ slopes	random	8	400.452	2	7.164	6	0.3059
7	$\neq$ slopes	CS	6	401.313	6	0.861	2	0.6502
					6	0.861	1:2	0.5018
8	$\neq$ slopes	simple	5	441.583	7	40.270	1	<0.0001
					7	40.270	0:1	<0.0001

The PROC MIXED programs, constructed in Section 5.4 to analyze the complete data set, will be applied to the incomplete GROWTHAV data set. The structure of this data set is given below. Although there would be four records for every subject in the complete data set, now there are nine subjects (e.g., subjects #3 and #27) with only three records.

Growth data. Extract of the incomplete data set

```
          OBS    IDNR   AGE    SEX    MEASURE

           1      1      8      2      21.0
           2      1     10      2      20.0
           3      1     12      2      21.5
           4      1     14      2      23.0
           5      2      8      2      21.0
           6      2     10      2      21.5
           7      2     12      2      24.0
           8      2     14      2      25.5
           9      3      8      2      20.5
          10      3     12      2      24.5
          11      3     14      2      26.0
          ...
          97     27      8      1      22.0
          98     27     12      1      23.5
          99     27     14      1      25.0
```

Applying the programs to the data yields some discrepancies, as seen from the model fit Table 5.12.

Let us take a close look at these discrepancies. Although most of the tests performed lead to the same conclusion, there is one fundamental difference. In Table 5.11, the AR(1) model is rejected, whereas it is not in Table 5.12. A puzzling difference is that the maximized log-likelihoods are different for Models 1 through 5, but not for Models 6 through 8. The same holds for the mean and covariance parameter estimates. To better understand this problem, let us consider the REPEATED statement (e.g., of Model 1):

```
repeated / type = un subject = idnr r rcorr;
```

This statement identifies the subject in terms of IDNR blocks but does not specify the ordering of the observations within a subject. Thus, PROC MIXED assumes the default ordering: 1, 2, 3, 4 for a complete subject and, erroneously, 1, 2, 3 for an incomplete one, whereas the correct incomplete ordering is 1, 2, 4. This means that, by default, dropout is assumed. Since this assumption is inadequate for the growth data, Models 1 through 5 in Table 5.12 are incorrect. However, in spite of the fact that Model 7 and 8 also use the REPEATED statement rather than the RANDOM statement, they give a correct answer.

Table 5.12 Growth data. Model fit summary with an inadequate MAR analysis (Little and Rubin).

	Mean	Covar	par	-2ℓ	Ref	G^2	df	p
1	unstr.	unstr.	18	394.309				
2	$\neq$ slopes	unstr.	14	397.862	1	3.553	4	0.4699
3	$=$ slopes	unstr.	13	401.935	2	4.073	1	0.0436
4	$\neq$ slopes	banded	8	400.981	2	3.119	6	0.7938
5	$\neq$ slopes	AR(1)	6	408.996	2	11.134	8	0.1942
6	$\neq$ slopes	random	8	400.452	2	2.590	6	0.8583
7	$\neq$ slopes	CS	6	401.312	6	0.860	2	0.6505
					6	0.860	1:2	0.5021
8	$\neq$ slopes	simple	5	441.582	7	40.270	1	<0.0001
					7	40.270	0:1	<0.0001

There are two equivalent ways to overcome this problem. The first is to adapt the data set slightly. An example is given below. The missing observations are indicated explicitly in the GROWTHAX data set.

Growth data. Extract of the incomplete data set. The missing observations are indicated explicitly.

OBS	IDNR	AGE	SEX	MEASURE
1	1	8	2	21.0
2	1	10	2	20.0
3	1	12	2	21.5
4	1	14	2	23.0
5	2	8	2	21.0
6	2	10	2	21.5
7	2	12	2	24.0
8	2	14	2	25.5
9	3	8	2	20.5
10	3	10	2	.
11	3	12	2	24.5
12	3	14	2	26.0

```
∿∿∿∿∿∿∿∿∿∿∿∿∿∿∿∿∿∿∿∿∿∿∿∿∿∿∿∿∿∿∿∿∿∿∿∿∿∿∿∿∿∿∿∿∿∿∿
...
   105     27      8    1      22.0
   106     27     10    1       .
   107     27     12    1      23.5
   108     27     14    1      25.0
```

The effect of using this data set is, of course, that incomplete records are deleted from the analysis, but that the relative positions are correctly passed on to PROC MIXED. Running Models 1 through 8 on this data set yields exactly the same results as in Table 5.11.

Alternatively, it is possible to use the data as presented before. Instead of passing on the position of the missing values through the data set, we then explicitly specify the ordering by coding it properly into the PROC MIXED program. For Model 1, the following code could be used:

```
proc mixed data = growthav method = ml;
    title 'Jennrich and Schluchter (MAR, Altern.), Model 1';
    class sex idnr age;
    model measure = sex age*sex / s;
    repeated age / type = un subject = idnr r rcorr;
    run;
```

The REPEATED statement now explicitly includes the ordering by means of the AGE variable. We consider it good practice to *always* include the time ordering variable of the measurements.

The corresponding Model 2 program would be the following:

```
proc mixed data = growthav method = ml;
    title 'Jennrich and Schluchter (MAR, Altern.), Model 2';
    class sex idnr;
    model measure = sex age*sex / s;
    repeated age / type = un subject = idnr r rcorr;
    run;
```

However, this program generates an error because the variables in the REPEATED statement have to be *categorical* variables, termed CLASS variables in PROC MIXED. One of the tricks to overcome this issue is by using the following program:

```
data help;
    set growthav;
    agec = age;
    run;

proc mixed data = help method = ml;
    title 'Jennrich and Schluchter (MAR, Altern.), Model 2';
    class sex idnr agec;
    model measure = sex age*sex / s;
    repeated agec / type = un subject = idnr r rcorr;
    run;
```

Thus, there are two identical copies of the variable AGE, only one of which is treated as a CLASS variable.

Let us now turn attention to the performance of the ignorable method of analysis and compare the results with the ones obtained earlier. First, the model comparisons performed in Tables 5.6 and 5.11 qualitatively yield the same conclusions. In both cases, linear profiles turn out to be consistent with the data, but parallel profiles do not. A Toeplitz correlation structure (Model 5) is acceptable, as well as a random intercepts and slopes model (Model 6). These models can be simplified further to compound symmetry (Model 7). The assumption of no correlation between repeated measures (Model 8) is untenable. This means that Model 7 is again the most parsimonious description of the data among the eight models considered. It has to be noted that the rejection of Models 3 and 5 is less compelling in the MAR analysis than it was in the complete data set. Of course, this is to be expected due to the reduction in the sample size, or rather in the number of available measurements. The likelihood ratio test statistic for a direct comparison of Model 5 to Model 4 is 11.494 on 2 degrees of freedom ($p = 0.0032$), which is, again, a clear indication of an unacceptable fit.

Figure 5.9 displays the fit of Models 1, 2, 3, and 7.

Figure 5.9 Growth data. Profiles for MAR analysis for a selected set of models. (The small dots are the observed group means for the complete data set. The large dots are the corresponding quantities for the incomplete data.)

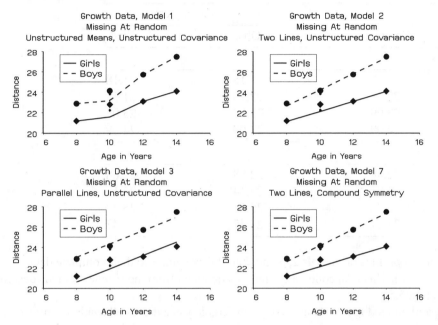

Let us consider the fit of Model 1 first. As mentioned earlier, the complete observations at age 10 are those with a higher measurement at age 8. Due to the within-subject correlation, they are the ones with a higher measurement at age 10 as well. This is seen by comparing the large dot with the corresponding small dot, reflecting the means for the complete data set and for those observed at age 10, respectively. Since the average of the observed measurements at age 10 is biased upward, the fitted profiles (least squares means) from the complete case analysis and from unconditional mean imputation were too high. Clearly, the average observed from the data is the same for the complete case analysis, the unconditional mean imputation, the available case analysis, and the present analysis. The most crucial difference is that the current Model 1, although saturated in the sense that there are eight mean parameters (one for each age-by-sex combination), does *not* let the (biased) observed and fitted averages at age 10 coincide, in contrast to the means at ages 8, 12 and 14. Indeed, if the model specification is correct, then an ignorable likelihood analysis produces a consistent estimator for the average profile, corresponding to the situation in which nobody would have dropped out. This is different from the observed data mean profile. For example, if patients with lower values typically drop out, then the complete data mean would be lower than the observed data mean. Of course, this effect might be blurred in relatively small data sets due to small-sample variability.

This discussion touches upon the key distinction between the frequentist available case analysis of Section 5.6 and the present likelihood-based available case analysis. The method of Section 5.6 constructs an estimate for the age 10 parameters, irrespective of the extra information available for the other parameters. The likelihood approach implicitly constructs a correction, based on (1) the fact that the measurements at ages 8, 12 and 14 differ between the subgroups of complete and incomplete observations and (2) the fairly strong correlation between the measurement at age 10 on the one hand and the measurements at ages 8, 12 and 14 on the other hand. A detailed treatment of likelihood estimation in incomplete multivariate normal samples is given in Little and Rubin (1987, Chapter 6). Clearly, this correction leads to an overshoot in the fairly small GROWTH data set, whence the predicted mean at age 10 is actually *smaller* than the one of the complete data set. The means are reproduced in Table 5.13. All means coincide for ages 8, 12 and 14. Irrespective of the small-sample behavior encountered here, the validity under MAR and the ease of implementation are good arguments that favor this ignorable analysis over other techniques.

Table 5.13 Growth data. Means under unstructured Model 1.

| Age | Complete | Incomplete | |
		Obs.	Pred.
	Girls		
8	21.18	21.18	21.18
10	22.23	22.79	21.58
12	23.09	23.09	23.09
14	24.09	24.09	24.09
	Boys		
8	22.88	22.88	22.88
10	23.81	24.14	23.17
12	25.72	25.72	25.72
14	27.47	27.47	27.47

The predicted mean profiles of Models 2, 3 and 7 are fairly similar to their complete data counterparts (not shown). This is in contrast to analyses obtained from the simple methods described and applied in Section 5.5.

In conclusion, a likelihood ignorable analysis is preferable since it uses all available information, without the need to delete or to impute measurements or entire subjects. It is theoretically justified whenever the missing data mechanism is MAR, which is a more relaxed assumption than the MCAR mechanism necessary for simple analyses (complete case, frequentist available case, and single-imputation based analyses, with the exception of Buck's method (Buck, 1960) of conditional mean imputation). There is no statistical information distortion, since observations are neither removed (such as in complete case analysis) nor added (such as in single imputation). There is no additional programming involved to perform an ignorable analysis in PROC MIXED, provided the order of the measurements is correctly specified. This can be done either by supplying records with missing data in the input data set or by properly indicating the order of the measurement in the REPEATED and/or RANDOM statements in PROC MIXED.

EXAMPLE: Depression Trial

Since no data manipulation is required for this likelihood analysis, the original DEPRESSION data set can be used, including the missing observations, which are denoted by dots. Again the fixed categorical effects of treatment, investigator, visit and treatment-by-visit, as well as the continuous fixed covariates of baseline score and baseline score-by-visit interaction are included.

Program 5.11 MAR analysis for the depression trial

```
proc mixed data=depression method=ml noitprint ic;
    class patient visit invest trt;
    model change = trt invest visit trt*visit basval basval*visit
```

```
              / solution ddfm=satterth;
    repeated visit / subject=patient type=un;
    run;
```

Output from Program 5.11

```
                    Covariance Parameter Estimates

                Cov Parm      Subject      Estimate

            *   UN(1,1)       PATIENT       17.1985
                UN(2,1)       PATIENT        8.2850
                UN(2,2)       PATIENT       26.8223
                UN(3,1)       PATIENT        6.6209
                UN(3,2)       PATIENT       16.6287
                UN(3,3)       PATIENT       38.8901
                UN(4,1)       PATIENT        5.7864
                UN(4,2)       PATIENT       14.7166
                UN(4,3)       PATIENT       23.1363
                UN(4,4)       PATIENT       34.1010
                UN(5,1)       PATIENT        3.4690
                UN(5,2)       PATIENT       10.8585
                UN(5,3)       PATIENT       18.8585
                UN(5,4)       PATIENT       26.9624
                UN(5,5)       PATIENT       40.2196


                          Fit Statistics

            -2 Log Likelihood                   4115.3
            AIC (smaller is better)             4207.3
            AICC (smaller is better)            4213.9
            BIC (smaller is better)             4351.6


                 Null Model Likelihood Ratio Test

                DF      Chi-Square      Pr > ChiSq

                14        209.54          <.0001


                      Information Criteria

Neg2LogLike    Parms      AIC       AICC       HQIC        BIC        CAIC

   4115.3       46      4207.3     4213.9     4265.8      4351.6     4397.6


                  Type 3 Tests of Fixed Effects

                         Num     Den
            Effect        DF      DF     F Value    Pr > F

            TRT            1      130     1.87       0.1744
            INVEST        16      168     4.89       <.0001
```

VISIT	4	133	1.18	0.3223
VISIT*TRT	4	134	1.70	0.1531
BASVAL	1	162	37.28	<.0001
BASVAL*VISIT	4	133	1.59	0.1817

The covariance matrix in this case is given by

$$\begin{pmatrix} 17.1985 & 8.2850 & 6.6209 & 5.7864 & 3.4690 \\ 8.2850 & 26.8223 & 16.6287 & 14.7166 & 10.8585 \\ 6.6209 & 16.6287 & 38.8901 & 23.1363 & 18.8585 \\ 5.7864 & 14.7166 & 23.1363 & 34.1010 & 26.9624 \\ 3.4690 & 10.8585 & 18.8585 & 26.9624 & 40.2196 \end{pmatrix}.$$

Again treatment ($p = 0.1744$) and treatment-by-visit interaction ($p = 0.1531$) are not significant.

5.8   Multiple Imputation

In the preceding section, we have suggested direct likelihood as a preferred mode for analyzing incomplete (longitudinal) data when the MAR assumption is deemed plausible. Two alternative methods are multiple imputation, discussed here, and the expectation-maximization algorithm, discussed in the next section.

Multiple imputation (MI) was formally introduced by Rubin (1978). Rubin (1987) provides a comprehensive treatment. Several other sources, such as Rubin and Schenker (1986), Little and Rubin (1987), Tanner and Wong (1987), and Schafer's (1997) book give excellent and easy-to-read descriptions of the technique.

The key idea of the multiple imputation procedure is to replace each missing value with a set of M plausible values, i.e., values "drawn" from the distribution of your data, that represent the uncertainty about the right value to impute. The imputed data sets are then analyzed by using standard procedures for complete data and combining the results from these analyses. Multiple imputation requires the missingness mechanism to be MAR.

An important question is when to use multiple imputation. Indeed, given the availability of PROC MIXED and related software tools, direct likelihood is within reach. We see at least three broad settings where MI can be of use. First, when there is a combination of missing covariates and missing outcomes, multiple imputation can be useful to deal with the missing covariates. A direct likelihood approach could then follow the imputation of covariates. Second, MI is useful when several mechanisms for missingness are postulated, and one would like to consider all of them. Then imputations could be drawn under all of these schemes and inferences could later be combined into a single one. Third, MI can be used as a tool to change nonmonotone missingness into monotone missingness. Often, nonmonotone missingness comes from a simpler mechanism on the one hand but tremendously complicates analysis on the other hand. After imputation to create monotone missingness, the monotonized data sets can then be analyzed with techniques for both MAR and MNAR missingness.

Clearly, multiple imputation involves three distinct phases:

- The missing values are filled in M times to generate M complete data sets.
- The M complete data sets are analyzed using standard procedures.
- The results from the M analyses are combined for the inference.

The SAS procedure PROC MI is a multiple imputation procedure that creates multiple imputed data sets for incomplete p-dimensional multivariate data. It uses methods that incorporate appropriate variability across the M imputations. Once the M complete data sets are analyzed using standard procedures, the procedure PROC MIANALYZE can be used to generate valid statistical inferences about these parameters by combining results for the M complete data sets.

5.8.1   Theoretical Justification

Suppose we have a sample of N, independent, identically distributed $n \times 1$ random vectors Y_i. Our interest lies in estimating some parameter vector θ of the distribution of Y_i. Multiple imputation fills in the missing data Y^m using the observed data Y^o several times, and then the completed data are used to estimate θ.

If we knew the distribution of $Y_i = (Y_i^o, Y_i^m)$, with parameter vector θ, then we could impute Y_i^m by drawing a value of Y_i^m from the conditional distribution

$$f(y_i^m | y_i^o, \theta).$$

The objective of the imputation process is to sample from this true predictive distribution. Since we do not know θ, we must estimate it from the data, say $\hat{\theta}$, and presumably use

$$f(y_i^m | y_i^o, \hat{\theta})$$

to impute the missing data. Frequentists sometimes favor incorporating uncertainty in θ in the multiple imputation scheme using bootstrap or other methods. However, in Bayesian terms, $\hat{\theta}$ is a random variable in which the distribution is a function of the data, so we must account for its uncertainty. The Bayesian approach relies on integrating out θ, which provides a more natural and unifying framework for accounting for the uncertainty in θ. Thus, θ is a random variable with mean equal to the estimated $\hat{\theta}$ from the data. Given this distribution, we use multiple imputation to first draw a random θ^* from the distribution of θ, and then put this θ^* in to draw a random Y_i^m from

$$f(y_i^m | y_i^o, \theta^*).$$

The imputation algorithm is as follows:

1. Draw θ^* from the distribution of θ.

2. Draw Y_i^{m*} from $f(y_i^m | y_i^o, \theta^*)$.

3. To estimate β, calculate the estimate of the parameter of interest, and its estimated variance, using the completed data, (Y^o, Y^{m*}):

$$\hat{\beta} = \hat{\beta}(Y) = \hat{\beta}(Y^o, Y^{m*}),$$

and the *within*-imputation variance is $U = \widehat{\text{Var}}(\hat{\beta})$.

4. Repeat steps 1, 2 and 3 a number of M times $\Rightarrow \hat{\beta}m$ and Um, for $m = 1, \ldots, M$.

Steps 1 and 2 are referred to as the *imputation task*. Step 3 is the *estimation task*.

5.8.2   Pooling Information

Of course, one wants to combine the M inferences into a single one. In this section, we will discuss parameter and precision estimation.

With no missing data, suppose that inference about the parameter β is made by

$$(\beta - \hat{\beta}) \sim N(0, U).$$

The M within-imputation estimates for β are pooled to give the multiple imputation estimate

$$\hat{\beta}* = \frac{\sum_{m=1}^{M} \hat{\beta}m}{M}.$$

Further, one can make normal-based inferences for β based upon

$$(\beta - \hat{\beta}*) \sim N(0, V),$$

where

$$V = W + \left(\frac{M+1}{M}\right) B,$$

$$W = \frac{\sum_{m=1}^{M} Um}{M}$$

is the average within-imputation variance, and

$$B = \frac{\sum_{m=1}^{M} (\hat{\beta}m - \hat{\beta}*)(\hat{\beta}m - \hat{\beta}*)'}{M-1}.$$

is the *between*-imputation variance (Rubin, 1987).

5.8.3 Hypothesis Testing

In case of multiple imputation, the asymptotic results and hence the χ^2 reference distributions do not depend only on the sample size N, but also on the number of imputations M. Therefore, Li, Raghunathan and Rubin (1991) propose the use of an F reference distribution. Precisely, to test the hypothesis $H_0 : \theta = \theta_0$, they advocate the following method to calculate p-values:

$$p = P(F_{k,w} > F),$$

where k is the length of the parameter vector θ, $F_{k,w}$ is an F random variable with k numerator and w denominator degrees of freedom, and

$$F = \frac{(\theta^* - \theta_0)' W^{-1} (\theta^* - \theta_0)}{k(1+r)},$$

$$w = 4 + (\tau - 4) \left[1 + \frac{(1 - 2\tau^{-1})}{r}\right]^2,$$

$$r = \frac{1}{k}\left(1 + \frac{1}{M}\right) \text{tr}(BW^{-1}),$$

$$\tau = k(M-1).$$

Here, r is the average relative increase in variance due to nonresponse across the components of θ. The limiting behavior of this F variable is that if $M \to \infty$, then the reference distribution of F approaches an $F_{k,\infty} = \chi^2/k$ distribution.

Clearly, this procedure is applicable not only when the full vector θ is the subject of hypothesis testing, but also when one component, a subvector, or a set of linear contrasts is the subject. In the case of a subvector, or as a special case one component, we use the corresponding submatrices of B and W in the formulas. For a set of linear contrasts $L\beta$, one should use the appropriately transformed covariance matrices: $\tilde{W} = LWL'$, $\tilde{B} = LBL'$, and $\tilde{V} = LVL'$.

5.8.4 Efficiency

Multiple imputation is attractive because it can be highly efficient even for small values of M. In many applications, merely three to five are sufficient to obtain excellent results. Rubin (1987, Page 114) shows that the efficiency of an estimate based on M imputations is approximately

$$\left(1 + \frac{\gamma}{M}\right)^{-1},$$

where γ is the fraction of missing information for the quantity being estimated. The fraction γ quantifies how much more precise the estimate might have been if no data had been missing. The

Table 5.14 Percent efficiency of multiple imputation estimation by number of imputations *M* and fraction of missing information γ.

m	γ 0.1	0.3	0.5	0.7	0.9
2	95	87	80	74	69
3	97	91	86	81	77
5	98	94	91	88	85
10	99	97	95	93	92
20	100	99	98	97	96

efficiencies achieved for various values of *M* and rates of missing information are shown in Table 5.14. This table shows that gains rapidly diminish after the first few imputations. In most situations there is little advantage to producing and analyzing more than a few imputed data sets.

5.8.5   Imputation Mechanisms

The method of choice to create the imputed data sets depends on the missing data pattern. A data set is said to have a monotone missing data pattern when the fact that an outcome Y_{ij} is missing for individual i implies that all subsequent variables $Y_{ik}, k > j$, are missing for individual i.

For monotone missing data patterns, either a parametric regression method that assumes multivariate normality or a nonparametric method that uses propensity scores is possible. For an arbitrary missing data pattern, a Markov chain Monte Carlo (MCMC) method (Schafer, 1997) that assumes multivariate normality can be used.

In the *regression method*, a regression model is fitted for each variable with missing values, with the previous variables as covariates. Based on the resulting model, a new regression model is then fitted and is used to impute the missing values for each variable (Rubin, 1987). Since the data set has a monotone missing data pattern, the process is repeated sequentially for variables with missing values.

The propensity score is the conditional probability of assignment to a particular treatment given a vector of observed covariates (Rosenbaum and Rubin, 1983). In the *propensity score method*, a propensity score is generated for each variable with missing values to indicate the probability of observations being missing. The observations are then grouped based on these propensity scores, and an approximate Bayesian bootstrap imputation (Rubin, 1987) is applied to each group. The propensity score method uses only the covariate information that is associated with whether the imputed variable values are missing. It does not use correlations among variables. It is effective for inferences about the distributions of individual imputed variables, but it is not appropriate for analyses involving the relationship among variables.

In statistical applications, MCMC is used to generate pseudo-random draws from multidimensional and otherwise intractable probability distributions via Markov chains. A Markov chain is a sequence of random variables in which the distribution of each element depends on the value of the previous one(s). In the *MCMC method*, one constructs a Markov chain long enough for the distribution of the elements to stabilize to a common distribution. This stationarity distribution is the one of interest. By repeatedly simulating steps of the chain, it simulates draws from the distribution of interest. In more detail, the MCMC method works as follows. We assume that the data are from a multivariate normal distribution. In the first step, we have to choose starting values. This can be done by computing a vector of means and a covariance matrix from the complete data. These are used to estimate the prior distribution, which means to estimate the parameters of the prior distributions for means and variances of the multivariate normal distribution with the informative prior option. The next step is called the imputation step: values for missing data items are simulated by randomly selecting a value from the available distribution of values—i.e., the predictive distribution of missing values given the observed values. In the posterior step, the posterior distribution of the mean and covariance parameters is updated by updating the parameters governing their distribution (e.g., the inverted Wishart distribution for the variance-covariance matrix and the normal distribution for the means). This is then followed by sampling from the posterior distribution of mean and covariance parameters, based on the updated parameters. The imputation and the posterior steps are iterated until the distribution is stationary. This means that the mean vector and covariance matrix are unchanged as we iterate. Finally, we use the imputations from the final iteration to form a data set that has no missing values.

5.8.6   SAS Procedures for Multiple Imputation

As mentioned before, PROC MI is used to generate the imputations. It creates M imputed data sets, physically stored in a single data set with indicator _IMPUTATION_ to separate the various imputed copies from each other. We will describe some options available in the PROC MI statement. The option SIMPLE displays simple descriptive statistics and pairwise correlations based on available cases in the input data set. The number of imputations is specified by NIMPUTE and is by default equal to 5. The option ROUND controls the number of decimal places in the imputed values (by default there is no rounding). If more than one number is specified, one should use a VAR statement, and the specified numbers must correspond to variables in the VAR statement. The SEED option specifies a positive integer, which is used by PROC MI to start the pseudo-random number generator. The default is a value generated from the time of day on the computer's clock. The imputation task is carried out separately for each level of the BY variables. In PROC MI, we can choose between one of the three imputation mechanisms we discussed in Section 5.8.5. For monotone missingness only, we use the MONOTONE statement. The parametric regression method (METHOD=REG) as well as the nonparametric propensity score method (METHOD=PROPENSITY) is available. For general patterns of missingness, we use the MCMC statement (the MCMC method is the default one). In all cases, several options are available to control the procedures; MCMC especially has a great deal of flexibility. For instance, NGROUPS specifies the number of groups based on propensity scores when the propensity scores method is used. For the MCMC method, we can give the initial mean and covariance estimates to begin the MCMC process by INITIAL. The PMM option in the MCMC statement uses the predictive mean matching method to impute an observed value that is closest to the predicted value in the MCMC method. The REGPMM option in the MONOTONE statement uses the predictive mean matching method to impute an observed value that is closest to the predicted value for data sets with monotone missingness. One can specify more than one method in the MONOTONE statement, and for each imputed variable the covariates can be specified separately. With INITIAL=EM (default), PROC MI uses the means and standard deviations from available cases as the initial estimates for the EM algorithm. The resulting estimates are used to begin the MCMC process. You can also specify INITIAL=*input SAS data set* to use a SAS data set with the initial estimates of the mean and covariance matrix for each imputation. Further, NITER specifies the number of iterations between imputations in a single chain (default is equal to 30).

The experimental CLASS statement is available since SAS 9.0 and is intended to specify categorical variables. Such classification variables are used as either covariates for imputed variables or as imputed variables for data sets with monotone missing patterns.

An important addition since SAS 9.0 are the experimental options LOGISTIC and DISCRIM in the MONOTONE statement, used to impute missing categorical variables by logistic and discriminant methods, respectively.

After the imputations have been generated, the imputed data sets are analyzed using a standard procedure. It is important to ensure that the BY statement is used to force an analysis for each of the imputed sets of data separately. Appropriate output (estimates and the precision thereof) is stored in output data sets.

Finally, PROC MIANALYZE combines the M inferences into a single one by making use of the theory laid out in Section 5.8.2. The options PARMS=. and COVB=., or their counterparts stemming from other standard procedures, name an input SAS data set that contains parameter estimates, and respectively covariance matrices of the parameter estimates, from the imputed data sets. The VAR statement lists the variables to be analyzed; they must be numeric. This statement is required.

This procedure is straightforward in a number of standard cases, such as PROC REG, PROC CORR, PROC GENMOD, PROC GLM, and PROC MIXED (for fixed effects in the cross-sectional case), but it is less straightforward in the PROC MIXED case when data are longitudinal or when interest is also in the variance components.

The experimental (since SAS 9.0) CLASS statement specifies categorical variables. PROC MIANALYZE reads and combines parameter estimates and covariance matrices for parameters with CLASS variables. The TEST statement allows testing of hypotheses about linear combinations of the parameters. The statement is based on Rubin (1987) and uses a *t* distribution that is the univariate version of the work by Li, Raghunathan and Rubin (1991), described in Section 5.8.3.

EXAMPLE: Growth Data

To begin, we show the standard, direct-likelihood-based MAR analysis using the PROC MIXED program for the GROWTH data set Model 7, which turned out to be the most parsimonious model (see Section 5.7).

Program 5.12 Direct-likelihood-based MAR analysis for Model 7

```
proc mixed data=growthax asycov covtest;
    title "Standard proc mixed analysis";
    class idnr age sex;
    model measure=age*sex / noint solution covb;
    repeated age / subject=idnr type=cs;
    run;
```

To perform this analysis using multiple imputation, the data need to be organized horizontally (one record per subject) rather than vertically. This can be done with the next program. A part of the horizontal data set obtained with this program is also given.

Program 5.13 Data manipulation for the imputation task

```
data hulp1;
    set growthax;
    meas8=measure;
    if age=8 then output;
    run;

data hulp2;
    set growthax;
    meas10=measure;
    if age=10 then output;
    run;

data hulp3;
    set growthax;
    meas12=measure;
    if age=12 then output;
    run;

data hulp4;
    set growthax;
    meas14=measure;
    if age=14 then output;
    run;

data growthmi;
    merge hulp1 hulp3 hulp4 hulp2;
    run;
```

```
proc sort data=growthmi;
    by sex;

proc print data=growthmi;
    title "Horizontal data set";
    run;
```

Horizontal data set

```
Obs   IDNR   INDIV   AGE   SEX   MEASURE   MEAS8   MEAS12   MEAS14   MEAS10

 1     12      1     10     1     25.0     26.0     29.0     31.0     25.0
 2     13      2     10     1       .      21.5     23.0     26.5       .
 3     14      3     10     1     22.5     23.0     24.0     27.5     22.5
 4     15      4     10     1     27.5     25.5     26.5     27.0     27.5
 5     16      5     10     1       .      20.0     22.5     26.0       .
. . .
```

The data are now ready for the so-called *imputation task*. This is done by PROC MI in the next program. Note that the measurement times are ordered as (8,12,14,10), since age 10 is incomplete. In this way, a monotone ordering is achieved. In line with the earlier analysis, we will use the monotone regression method.

Program 5.14 Imputation task

```
proc mi data=growthmi seed=459864 simple nimpute=10
        round=0.1 out=outmi;
    by sex;
    monotone method=reg;
    var meas8 meas12 meas14 meas10;
    run;
```

We show some output of the MI procedure for SEX=1. First, some pattern-specific information is given. Since we included the option SIMPLE, univariate statistics and pairwise correlations are calculated (not shown). Finally, multiple imputation variance information shows the total variance and the magnitudes of between and within variance.

Output from Program 5.14 (partial)

```
--------------------------------- SEX=1 ---------------------------------

                         Missing Data Patterns

    Group    MEAS8    MEAS12    MEAS14    MEAS10      Freq      Percent

      1       X         X         X         X          11       68.75
      2       X         X         X         .           5       31.25


                  ----------------------Group Means----------------------
    Group          MEAS8          MEAS12          MEAS14          MEAS10

      1          24.000000       26.590909       27.681818       24.136364
      2          20.400000       23.800000       27.000000           .
```

```
                    Multiple Imputation Variance Information
                    -----------------Variance----------------
        Variable           Between            Within          Total          DF

        MEAS10            0.191981          0.865816         1.076995       10.25


                                          Relative         Fraction
                                          Increase          Missing
                        Variable        in Variance       Information
                        MEAS10            0.243907          0.202863



                    Multiple Imputation Parameter Estimates

      Variable           Mean         Std Error      95% Confidence Limits        DF

      MEAS10           22.685000       1.037784      20.38028     24.98972      10.25


                                                                  t for H0:
      Variable        Minimum         Maximum        Mu0       Mean=Mu0     Pr > |t|

      MEAS10         21.743750       23.387500         0         21.86       <.0001
```

A selection of the imputed data set is shown below (first four observations, imputations 1 and 2). To prepare for a standard linear mixed model analysis (using PROC MIXED), a number of further data manipulation steps are conducted, including the construction of a vertical data set with one record per measurement and not one record per subject (i.e., back to the original format). Part of the imputed data set in vertical format is also given.

Portion of imputed data set in horizontal format

```
Obs _Imp_  IDNR  INDIV  AGE  SEX  MEASURE  MEAS8  MEAS12  MEAS14  MEAS10

  1    1      1     1    10    2    20.0    21.0   21.5    23.0    20.0
  2    1      2     2    10    2    21.5    21.0   24.0    25.5    21.5
  3    1      3     3    10    2     .      20.5   24.5    26.0    22.6
  4    1      4     4    10    2    24.5    23.5   25.0    26.5    24.5

 28    2      1     1    10    2    20.0    21.0   21.5    23.0    20.0
 29    2      2     2    10    2    21.5    21.0   24.0    25.5    21.5
 30    2      3     3    10    2     .      20.5   24.5    26.0    20.4
 31    2      4     4    10    2    24.5    23.5   25.0    26.5    24.5
```

Program 5.15 Data manipulation to use PROC MIXED

```
proc sort data=outmi;
    by_imputation_ idnr;
    run;

proc print data=outmi;
    title 'Horizontal imputed data set';
    run;
```

```
data outmi2;
    set outmi;
    array y (4) meas8 meas10 meas12 meas14;
    do j=1 to 4;
        measmi=y(j);
        age=6+2*j;
        output;
    end;
    run;

proc print data=outmi2;
    title "Vertical imputed data set";
    run;
```

Portion of imputed data set in vertical format

```
Obs _Imp_  IDNR INDIV AGE SEX MEASURE MEAS8 MEAS12 MEAS14 MEAS10 j measmi

  1    1     1     1    8   2    20.0  21.0  21.5   23.0   20.0  1  21.0
  2    1     1     1   10   2    20.0  21.0  21.5   23.0   20.0  2  20.0
  3    1     1     1   12   2    20.0  21.0  21.5   23.0   20.0  3  21.5
  4    1     1     1   14   2    20.0  21.0  21.5   23.0   20.0  4  23.0
  5    1     2     2    8   2    21.5  21.0  24.0   25.5   21.5  1  21.0
  6    1     2     2   10   2    21.5  21.0  24.0   25.5   21.5  2  21.5
  7    1     2     2   12   2    21.5  21.0  24.0   25.5   21.5  3  24.0
  8    1     2     2   14   2    21.5  21.0  24.0   25.5   21.5  4  25.5
  9    1     3     3    8   2      .   20.5  24.5   26.0   22.6  1  20.5
 10    1     3     3   10   2      .   20.5  24.5   26.0   22.6  2  22.6
 11    1     3     3   12   2      .   20.5  24.5   26.0   22.6  3  24.5
 12    1     3     3   14   2      .   20.5  24.5   26.0   22.6  4  26.0
```

After the imputation step and additional data manipulation, the imputed data sets can be analyzed using the MIXED procedure. Using the ODS statement, four sets of input for the inference task (i.e., the combination of all inferences into a single one) are preserved:

- parameter estimates of the fixed effects: MIXBETAP
- parameter estimates of the variance components: MIXALFAP
- covariance matrix of the fixed effects: MIXBETAV
- covariance matrix of the variance components: MIXALFAV.

Program 5.16 Analysis of imputed data sets using PROC MIXED

```
proc mixed data=outmi2 asycov;
    title "Multiple Imputation Call of PROC MIXED";
    class idnr age sex;
    model measmi=age*sex / noint solution covb;
    repeated age / subject=idnr type=cs;
    by_Imputation_;
    ods output solutionF=mixbetap covb=mixbetav
               covparms=mixalfap asycov=mixalfav;
    run;
```

```
proc print data=mixbetap;
    title "Fixed effects: parameter estimates";
    run;

proc print data=mixbetav;
    title "Fixed effects: variance-covariance matrix";
    run;

proc print data=mixalfav;
    title "Variance components: covariance parameters";
    run;

proc print data=mixalfap;
    title "Variance components: parameter estimates";
    run;
```

We show a selection of the output from the PROC MIXED call on imputation 1. We also show part of
the fixed effects estimates data set and part of the data set of the variance-covariance matrices of the
fixed effects (both imputations 1 and 2), as well as the estimates of the covariance parameters and their
covariance matrices. However, in order to call PROC MIANALYZE, one parameter vector and one
covariance matrix (per imputation) need to be passed on, *with the proper name*. This requires, once
again, some data manipulation.

Output from Program 5.16 (partial)

```
-------------------------- Imputation Number=1 --------------------------

                     Covariance Parameter Estimates

               Cov Parm      Subject      Estimate

               CS            IDNR          3.7019
               Residual                    2.1812


              Asymptotic Covariance Matrix of Estimates

          Row    Cov Parm         CovP1         CovP2

           1     CS              1.4510       -0.03172
           2     Residual       -0.03172       0.1269


                     Solution for Fixed Effects

                                   Standard
        Effect   AGE  SEX  Estimate   Error    DF   t Value   Pr > |t|

        AGE*SEX   8    1   22.8750   0.6064    73    37.72    <.0001
        AGE*SEX   8    2   21.0909   0.7313    73    28.84    <.0001
        AGE*SEX  10    1   23.3875   0.6064    73    38.57    <.0001
        AGE*SEX  10    2   22.1273   0.7313    73    30.26    <.0001
        AGE*SEX  12    1   25.7188   0.6064    73    42.41    <.0001
        AGE*SEX  12    2   22.6818   0.7313    73    31.01    <.0001
        AGE*SEX  14    1   27.4688   0.6064    73    45.30    <.0001
        AGE*SEX  14    2   24.0000   0.7313    73    32.82    <.0001
```

```
                        Covariance Matrix for Fixed Effects

    Row   Effect   AGE  SEX     Col1       Col2      Col3      Col4      Col5

     1   AGE*SEX    8    1     0.3677               0.2314              0.2314
     2   AGE*SEX    8    2               0.5348               0.3365
     3   AGE*SEX   10    1     0.2314               0.3677              0.2314
     4   AGE*SEX   10    2               0.3365               0.5348
     5   AGE*SEX   12    1     0.2314               0.2314              0.3677
     6   AGE*SEX   12    2               0.3365               0.3365
     7   AGE*SEX   14    1     0.2314               0.2314              0.2314
     8   AGE*SEX   14    2               0.3365               0.3365

                   Row       Col6        Col7       Col8

                    1                   0.2314
                    2      0.3365                   0.3365
                    3                   0.2314
                    4      0.3365                   0.3365
                    5                   0.2314
                    6      0.5348                   0.3365
                    7                   0.3677
                    8      0.3365                   0.5348


                     Type 3 Tests of Fixed Effects

                         Num    Den
               Effect     DF     DF    F Value    Pr > F

               AGE*SEX     8     73    469.91     <.0001
```

Part of the fixed effects estimates data set

```
Obs _Imputation_   Effect   AGE  SEX  Estimate   StdErr    DF   tValue   Probt

  1       1       AGE*SEX    8    1   22.8750    0.6064    73    37.72   <.0001
  2       1       AGE*SEX    8    2   21.0909    0.7313    73    28.84   <.0001
  3       1       AGE*SEX   10    1   23.3875    0.6064    73    38.57   <.0001
  4       1       AGE*SEX   10    2   22.1273    0.7313    73    30.26   <.0001
  5       1       AGE*SEX   12    1   25.7188    0.6064    73    42.41   <.0001
  6       1       AGE*SEX   12    2   22.6818    0.7313    73    31.01   <.0001
  7       1       AGE*SEX   14    1   27.4688    0.6064    73    45.30   <.0001
  8       1       AGE*SEX   14    2   24.0000    0.7313    73    32.82   <.0001
  9       2       AGE*SEX    8    1   22.8750    0.6509    73    35.15   <.0001
 10       2       AGE*SEX    8    2   21.0909    0.7850    73    26.87   <.0001
 11       2       AGE*SEX   10    1   22.7438    0.6509    73    34.94   <.0001
 12       2       AGE*SEX   10    2   21.8364    0.7850    73    27.82   <.0001
 13       2       AGE*SEX   12    1   25.7188    0.6509    73    39.52   <.0001
 14       2       AGE*SEX   12    2   22.6818    0.7850    73    28.90   <.0001
 15       2       AGE*SEX   14    1   27.4688    0.6509    73    42.20   <.0001
 16       2       AGE*SEX   14    2   24.0000    0.7850    73    30.57   <.0001
...
```

Part of the data set of the variance-covariance matrices of the fixed effects

Obs	_Imputation_	Row	Effect	AGE	SEX	Col1	Col2	Col3
1	1	1	AGE*SEX	8	1	0.3677	0	0.2314
2	1	2	AGE*SEX	8	2	0	0.5348	0
3	1	3	AGE*SEX	10	1	0.2314	0	0.3677
4	1	4	AGE*SEX	10	2	0	0.3365	0
5	1	5	AGE*SEX	12	1	0.2314	0	0.2314
6	1	6	AGE*SEX	12	2	0	0.3365	0
7	1	7	AGE*SEX	14	1	0.2314	0	0.2314
8	1	8	AGE*SEX	14	2	0	0.3365	0
9	2	1	AGE*SEX	8	1	0.4236	0	0.2504
10	2	2	AGE*SEX	8	2	0	0.6162	0
11	2	3	AGE*SEX	10	1	0.2504	0	0.4236
12	2	4	AGE*SEX	10	2	0	0.3642	0
13	2	5	AGE*SEX	12	1	0.2504	0	0.2504
14	2	6	AGE*SEX	12	2	0	0.3642	0
15	2	7	AGE*SEX	14	1	0.2504	0	0.2504
16	2	8	AGE*SEX	14	2	0	0.3642	0

...

Obs	Col4	Col5	Col6	Col7	Col8
1	0	0.2314	0	0.2314	0
2	0.3365	0	0.3365	0	0.3365
3	0	0.2314	0	0.2314	0
4	0.5348	0	0.3365	0	0.3365
5	0	0.3677	0	0.2314	0
6	0.3365	0	0.5348	0	0.3365
7	0	0.2314	0	0.3677	0
8	0.3365	0	0.3365	0	0.5348
9	0	0.2504	0	0.2504	0
10	0.3642	0	0.3642	0	0.3642
11	0	0.2504	0	0.2504	0
12	0.6162	0	0.3642	0	0.3642
13	0	0.4236	0	0.2504	0
14	0.3642	0	0.6162	0	0.3642
15	0	0.2504	0	0.4236	0
16	0.3642	0	0.3642	0	0.6162

...

Estimates of the covariance parameters in the original data set form

Obs	_Imputation_	CovParm	Subject	Estimate
1	1	CS	IDNR	3.7019
2	1	Residual		2.1812
3	2	CS	IDNR	4.0057
4	2	Residual		2.7721
5	3	CS	IDNR	4.5533
6	3	Residual		4.3697
7	4	CS	IDNR	4.0029
8	4	Residual		2.7910
9	5	CS	IDNR	4.1198
10	5	Residual		2.7918
11	6	CS	IDNR	4.0549

12	6	Residual		3.0254
13	7	CS	IDNR	3.9019
14	7	Residual		3.2477
15	8	CS	IDNR	4.3877
16	8	Residual		2.9076
17	9	CS	IDNR	4.0192
18	9	Residual		3.6492
19	10	CS	IDNR	3.8346
20	10	Residual		2.1826

Covariance matrices of the covariance parameters in the original data set form

Obs	_Imputation_	Row	CovParm	CovP1	CovP2
1	1	1	CS	1.4510	-0.03172
2	1	2	Residual	-0.03172	0.1269
3	2	1	CS	1.7790	-0.05123
4	2	2	Residual	-0.05123	0.2049
5	3	1	CS	2.5817	-0.1273
6	3	2	Residual	-0.1273	0.5092
7	4	1	CS	1.7807	-0.05193
8	4	2	Residual	-0.05193	0.2077
9	5	1	CS	1.8698	-0.05196
10	5	2	Residual	-0.05196	0.2078
11	6	1	CS	1.8671	-0.06102
12	6	2	Residual	-0.06102	0.2441
13	7	1	CS	1.7952	-0.07032
14	7	2	Residual	-0.07032	0.2813
15	8	1	CS	2.1068	-0.05636
16	8	2	Residual	-0.05636	0.2254
17	9	1	CS	1.9678	-0.08878
18	9	2	Residual	-0.08878	0.3551
19	10	1	CS	1.5429	-0.03176
20	10	2	Residual	-0.03176	0.1270

Program 5.17 Data manipulation for the inference task

```
data mixbetap0;
    set mixbetap;
    if age= 8 and sex=1 then effect='as081';
    if age=10 and sex=1 then effect='as101';
    if age=12 and sex=1 then effect='as121';
    if age=14 and sex=1 then effect='as141';
    if age= 8 and sex=2 then effect='as082';
    if age=10 and sex=2 then effect='as102';
    if age=12 and sex=2 then effect='as122';
    if age=14 and sex=2 then effect='as142';
    run;

data mixbetap0;
    set mixbetap0 (drop=age sex);
    run;

proc print data=mixbetap0;
    title "Fixed effects: parameter estimates (after manipulation)";
    run;
```

```
data mixbetav0;
    set mixbetav;
    if age= 8 and sex=1 then effect='as081';
    if age=10 and sex=1 then effect='as101';
    if age=12 and sex=1 then effect='as121';
    if age=14 and sex=1 then effect='as141';
    if age= 8 and sex=2 then effect='as082';
    if age=10 and sex=2 then effect='as102';
    if age=12 and sex=2 then effect='as122';
    if age=14 and sex=2 then effect='as142';
    run;

data mixbetav0;
    title "Fixed effects: variance-covariance matrix (after manipulation)";
    set mixbetav0 (drop=row age sex);
    run;

proc print data=mixbetav0;
    run;

data mixalfap0;
    set mixalfap;
    effect=covparm;
    run;

data mixalfav0;
    set mixalfav;
    effect=covparm;
    Col1=CovP1;
    Col2=CovP2;
    run;

proc print data=mixalfap0;
    title "Variance components: parameter estimates
            (after manipulation)";
    run;

proc print data=mixalfav0;
    title "Variance components: covariance parameters
             (after manipulation)";
    run;
```

The following outputs show parts of the data sets after this data manipulation.

Part of the fixed effects estimates data set after data manipulation

Obs	_Imputation_	Effect	Estimate	StdErr	DF	tValue	Probt
1	1	as081	22.8750	0.6064	73	37.72	<.0001
2	1	as082	21.0909	0.7313	73	28.84	<.0001
3	1	as101	23.3875	0.6064	73	38.57	<.0001
4	1	as102	22.1273	0.7313	73	30.26	<.0001
5	1	as121	25.7188	0.6064	73	42.41	<.0001
6	1	as122	22.6818	0.7313	73	31.01	<.0001
7	1	as141	27.4688	0.6064	73	45.30	<.0001
8	1	as142	24.0000	0.7313	73	32.82	<.0001

9	2	as081	22.8750	0.6509	73	35.15	<.0001
10	2	as082	21.0909	0.7850	73	26.87	<.0001
11	2	as101	22.7438	0.6509	73	34.94	<.0001
12	2	as102	21.8364	0.7850	73	27.82	<.0001
13	2	as121	25.7188	0.6509	73	39.52	<.0001
14	2	as122	22.6818	0.7850	73	28.90	<.0001
15	2	as141	27.4688	0.6509	73	42.20	<.0001
16	2	as142	24.0000	0.7850	73	30.57	<.0001

...

Part of the data set of the variance-covariance matrices of the fixed effects after data manipulation

Obs	_Imputation_	Effect	Col1	Col2	Col3
1	1	as081	0.3677	0	0.2314
2	1	as082	0	0.5348	0
3	1	as101	0.2314	0	0.3677
4	1	as102	0	0.3365	0
5	1	as121	0.2314	0	0.2314
6	1	as122	0	0.3365	0
7	1	as141	0.2314	0	0.2314
8	1	as142	0	0.3365	0
9	2	as081	0.4236	0	0.2504
10	2	as082	0	0.6162	0
11	2	as101	0.2504	0	0.4236
12	2	as102	0	0.3642	0
13	2	as121	0.2504	0	0.2504
14	2	as122	0	0.3642	0
15	2	as141	0.2504	0	0.2504
16	2	as142	0	0.3642	0

...

Obs	Col4	Col5	Col6	Col7	Col8
1	0	0.2314	0	0.2314	0
2	0.3365	0	0.3365	0	0.3365
3	0	0.2314	0	0.2314	0
4	0.5348	0	0.3365	0	0.3365
5	0	0.3677	0	0.2314	0
6	0.3365	0	0.5348	0	0.3365
7	0	0.2314	0	0.3677	0
8	0.3365	0	0.3365	0	0.5348
9	0	0.2504	0	0.2504	0
10	0.3642	0	0.3642	0	0.3642
11	0	0.2504	0	0.2504	0
12	0.6162	0	0.3642	0	0.3642
13	0	0.4236	0	0.2504	0
14	0.3642	0	0.6162	0	0.3642
15	0	0.2504	0	0.4236	0
16	0.3642	0	0.3642	0	0.6162

...

Estimates of the covariance parameters after manipulation, i.e., addition of an 'effect' column (identical to the 'CovParm' column)

Obs	_Imputation_	CovParm	Subject	Estimate	effect
1	1	CS	IDNR	3.7019	CS
2	1	Residual		2.1812	Residual
3	2	CS	IDNR	4.0057	CS
4	2	Residual		2.7721	Residual
5	3	CS	IDNR	4.5533	CS
6	3	Residual		4.3697	Residual
7	4	CS	IDNR	4.0029	CS
8	4	Residual		2.7910	Residual
9	5	CS	IDNR	4.1198	CS
10	5	Residual		2.7918	Residual
11	6	CS	IDNR	4.0549	CS
12	6	Residual		3.0254	Residual
13	7	CS	IDNR	3.9019	CS
14	7	Residual		3.2477	Residual
15	8	CS	IDNR	4.3877	CS
16	8	Residual		2.9076	Residual
17	9	CS	IDNR	4.0192	CS
18	9	Residual		3.6492	Residual
19	10	CS	IDNR	3.8346	CS
20	10	Residual		2.1826	Residual

Covariance matrices of the covariance parameters after manipulation, i.e., addition of an 'effect' column (identical to the 'CovParm' column)

Obs	_Imputation_	Row	CovParm	CovP1	CovP2	effect	Col1	Col2
1	1	1	CS	1.4510	-0.03172	CS	1.45103	-0.03172
2	1	2	Residual	-0.03172	0.1269	Residual	-0.03172	0.12688
3	2	1	CS	1.7790	-0.05123	CS	1.77903	-0.05123
4	2	2	Residual	-0.05123	0.2049	Residual	-0.05123	0.20492
5	3	1	CS	2.5817	-0.1273	CS	2.58173	-0.12729
6	3	2	Residual	-0.1273	0.5092	Residual	-0.12729	0.50918
7	4	1	CS	1.7807	-0.05193	CS	1.78066	-0.05193
8	4	2	Residual	-0.05193	0.2077	Residual	-0.05193	0.20772
9	5	1	CS	1.8698	-0.05196	CS	1.86981	-0.05196
10	5	2	Residual	-0.05196	0.2078	Residual	-0.05196	0.20784
11	6	1	CS	1.8671	-0.06102	CS	1.86710	-0.06102
12	6	2	Residual	-0.06102	0.2441	Residual	-0.06102	0.24409
13	7	1	CS	1.7952	-0.07032	CS	1.79518	-0.07032
14	7	2	Residual	-0.07032	0.2813	Residual	-0.07032	0.28127
15	8	1	CS	2.1068	-0.05636	CS	2.10683	-0.05636
16	8	2	Residual	-0.05636	0.2254	Residual	-0.05636	0.22544
17	9	1	CS	1.9678	-0.08878	CS	1.96778	-0.08878
18	9	2	Residual	-0.08878	0.3551	Residual	-0.08878	0.35510
19	10	1	CS	1.5429	-0.03176	CS	1.54287	-0.03176
20	10	2	Residual	-0.03176	0.1270	Residual	-0.03176	0.12703

Now, PROC MIANALYZE will be called, first for the fixed effects inferences, and then for the variance component inferences. The parameter estimates (MIXBETAP0) and the covariance matrix (MIXBETAV0) are the input for the fixed effects. Output is given following the program. For the fixed effects, there is only between-imputation variability for the age 10 measurement. However, for the variance components, we see that covariance parameters are influenced by missingness.

Program 5.18 Inference task using PROC MIANALYZE

```
proc mianalyze parms=mixbetap0 covb=mixbetav0;
    title "Multiple Imputation Analysis for Fixed Effects";
    var as081 as082 as101 as102 as121 as122 as141 as142;
    run;

proc mianalyze parms=mixalfap0 covb=mixalfav0;
    title "Multiple Imputation Analysis for Variance Components";
    var CS Residual;
    run;
```

Output from Program 5.18 (fixed effects)

```
                          Model Information
               PARMS Data Set           WORK.MIXBETAP0
               COVB Data Set            WORK.MIXBETAV0
               Number of Imputations    10


               Multiple Imputation Variance Information
               ----------------Variance----------------
     Parameter        Between        Within        Total        DF

       as081                0       0.440626     0.440626        .
       as082                0       0.640910     0.640910        .
       as101         0.191981       0.440626     0.651804    85.738
       as102         0.031781       0.640910     0.675868      3364
       as121                0       0.440626     0.440626        .
       as122                0       0.640910     0.640910        .
       as141                0       0.440626     0.440626        .
       as142                0       0.640910     0.640910        .


               Multiple Imputation Variance Information
                              Relative        Fraction
                              Increase         Missing
                Parameter   in Variance    Information
                as081                 0             .
                as082                 0             .
                as101          0.479271      0.339227
                as102          0.054545      0.052287
                as121                 0             .
                as122                 0             .
                as141                 0             .
                as142                 0             .
               Multiple Imputation Parameter Estimates


 Parameter      Estimate      Std Error    95% Confidence Limits       DF

 as081        22.875000       0.663796        .            .           .
 as082        21.090909       0.800568        .            .           .
 as101        22.685000       0.807344     21.07998     24.29002    85.738
 as102        22.073636       0.822112     20.46175     23.68553      3364
 as121        25.718750       0.663796        .            .           .
 as122        22.681818       0.800568        .            .           .
 as141        27.468750       0.663796        .            .           .
 as142        24.000000       0.800568        .            .           .
```

```
Multiple Imputation Parameter Estimates

        Parameter          Minimum          Maximum

        as081           22.875000        22.875000
        as082           21.090909        21.090909
        as101           21.743750        23.387500
        as102           21.836364        22.381818
        as121           25.718750        25.718750
        as122           22.681818        22.681818
        as141           27.468750        27.468750
        as142           24.000000        24.000000


        Multiple Imputation Parameter Estimates

                                            t for H0:
        Parameter      Theta0    Parameter=Theta0    Pr > |t|

        as081            0             .               .
        as082            0             .               .
        as101            0           28.10           <.0001
        as102            0           26.85           <.0001
        as121            0             .               .
        as122            0             .               .
        as141            0             .               .
        as142            0             .               .
```

Output from Program 5.18 (variance components)

```
                    Model Information
        PARMS Data Set           WORK.MIXALFAP0
        COVB Data Set            WORK.MIXALFAV0
        Number of Imputations    10


        Multiple Imputation Variance Information
        -----------------Variance----------------
Parameter        Between          Within          Total        DF

CS             0.062912        1.874201        1.943404      7097.8
Residual       0.427201        0.248947        0.718868      21.062

        Multiple Imputation Variance Information
                        Relative        Fraction
                        Increase        Missing
        Parameter     in Variance     Information
        CS             0.036924        0.035881
        Residual       1.887630        0.682480


        Multiple Imputation Parameter Estimates

Parameter     Estimate     Std Error     95% Confidence Limits         DF

CS            4.058178     1.394060     1.325404     6.790951      7097.8
Residual      2.991830     0.847861     1.228921     4.754740      21.062
```

```
          Multiple Imputation Parameter Estimates

          Parameter        Minimum        Maximum

          CS              3.701888       4.553271
          Residual        2.181247       4.369683


       Multiple Imputation Parameter Estimates

                                       t for H0:
          Parameter     Theta0    Parameter=Theta0   Pr > |t|

          CS               0              2.91        0.0036
          Residual         0              3.53        0.0020
```

It is clear that multiple imputation has an impact on the precision of the age 10 measurement, the only time at which incompleteness occurs. The manipulations are rather extensive, given that multiple imputation was used not only for fixed effects parameters, but also for variance components, in a genuinely longitudinal application. The main reason for the large amount of manipulation is to ensure input datasets have format and column headings in line with what is expected by PROC MIANALYZE. The take-home message is that, when one is prepared to undertake a bit of data manipulation, PROC MI and PROC MIANALYZE provide a valuable couple of procedures that enable multiple imputation in a wide variety of settings.

5.8.7 Creating Monotone Missingness

When missingness is nonmonotone, one might think of several mechanisms operating simultaneously: e.g., a simple (MCAR or MAR) mechanism for the intermediate missing values and a more complex (MNAR) mechanism for the missing data past the moment of dropout. However, analyzing such data is complicated because many model strategies, especially those under the assumption of MNAR, have been developed for dropout only. Therefore, a solution might be to generate multiple imputations that render the data sets monotone missing by including the following statement in PROC MI:

```
mcmc impute = monotone;
```

and then applying a method of choice to the multiple sets of data that are thus completed. Note that this is different from the monotone method in PROC MI, intended to fully complete already monotone sets of data.

5.9 The EM Algorithm

This section deals with the expectation-maximization algorithm, popularly known as the EM algorithm. It is an alternative to direct likelihood in settings where the observed-data likelihood is complicated and/or difficult to access. Note that direct likelihood is within reach for many settings, including Gaussian longitudinal data, as outlined in Section 5.7.

The EM algorithm is a general-purpose iterative algorithm to find maximum likelihood estimates in parametric models for incomplete data. Within each iteration of the EM algorithm, there are two steps, called the expectation step, or E-step, and the maximization step, or M-step. The name EM algorithm was given by Dempster, Laird and Rubin (1977), who provided a general formulation of the EM algorithm, its basic properties, and many examples and applications of it. The books by Little and Rubin (1987), Schafer (1997), and McLachlan and Krishnan (1997) provide detailed descriptions and applications of the EM algorithm.

The basic idea of the EM algorithm is to associate with the given incomplete data problem a complete data problem for which maximum likelihood estimation is computationally more tractable. Starting from suitable initial parameter values, the E- and M-steps are repeated until convergence. Given a set of parameter estimates—such as the mean vector and covariance matrix for a multivariate normal setting—the E-step calculates the conditional expectation of the complete data log-likelihood given the observed data and the parameter estimates. This step is often reduced to simple sufficient statistics. Given the complete data log-likelihood, the M-step then finds the parameter estimates to maximize the complete data log-likelihood from the E-step.

An initial criticism was that the EM algorithm did not produce estimates of the covariance matrix of the maximum likelihood estimators. However, developments have provided methods for such estimation that can be integrated into the EM computational procedures. Another issue is the slow convergence in certain cases. This has resulted in the development of modified versions of the algorithm as well as many simulated-based methods and other extensions of it (McLachlan and Krishnan, 1997).

The condition for the EM algorithm to be valid, in its basic form, is ignorability and hence MAR.

5.9.1 The Algorithm

The Initial Step

Let $\theta^{(0)}$ be an initial parameter vector, which can be found, for example, from a complete case analysis, an available case analysis, or a simple method of imputation.

The E-Step

Given current values $\theta^{(t)}$ for the parameters, the E-step computes the objective function, which in the case of the missing data problem is equal to the expected value of the observed-data log-likelihood, given the observed data and the current parameters

$$Q(\theta|\theta^{(t)}) = \int \ell(\theta, Y) f(Y^m|Y^o, \theta^{(t)}) \, dY^m$$

$$= E\left[\ell(\theta|Y)|Y^o, \theta^{(t)}\right],$$

i.e., substituting the expected value of Y^m, given Y^o and $\theta^{(t)}$. In some cases, this substitution can take place directly at the level of the data, but often it is sufficient to substitute only the function of Y^m appearing in the complete-data log-likelihood. For exponential families, the E-step reduces to the computation of complete-data sufficient statistics.

The M-Step

The M-step determines $\theta^{(t+1)}$, the parameter vector maximizing the log-likelihood of the imputed data (or the imputed log-likelihood). Formally, $\theta^{(t+1)}$ satisfies

$$Q(\theta^{(t+1)}|\theta^{(t)}) \geq Q(\theta|\theta^{(t)}), \text{ for all } \theta.$$

One can show that the likelihood increases at every step. Since the log-likelihood is bounded from above, convergence is forced to apply.

The fact that the EM algorithm is guaranteed of convergence to a possibly local maximum is a great advantage. However, a disadvantage is that this convergence is slow (linear or superlinear), and that precision estimates are not automatically provided.

5.9.2 Missing Information

We will now turn attention to the principle of missing information. We use obvious notation for the observed and expected information matrices for the complete and observed data. Let

$$I(\theta, Y^o) = \frac{\partial^2 \ln \ell(\theta)}{\partial \theta \partial \theta'}$$

be the matrix of the negative of the second-order partial derivatives of the incomplete-data log-likelihood function with respect to the elements of θ, i.e., the observed information matrix for the observed data model. The expected information matrix for observed data model is termed $\mathcal{I}(\theta, Y^o)$. In analogy with the complete data $Y = (Y^o, Y^m)$, we let $I_c(\theta, Y)$ and $\mathcal{I}_c(\theta, Y)$ be the observed and expected information matrices for the complete data model, respectively. Now, both likelihoods are connected via

$$\ell(\theta) = \ell_c(\theta) - \ln \frac{f_c(y^0, y^m|\theta)}{f_c(y^0|\theta)} = \ell_c(\theta) - \ln f(y^m|y^o, \theta).$$

This equality carries over onto the information matrices:

$$I(\theta, Y^o) = I_c(\theta, Y) + \frac{\partial^2 \ln f(y^m|y^o, \theta)}{\partial\theta\partial\theta'}.$$

Taking expectation over $Y|Y^o = y^o$ leads to

$$I(\theta, y^o) = \mathcal{I}_c(\theta, y^o) - \mathcal{I}_m(\theta, y^o),$$

where $\mathcal{I}_m(\theta, y^o)$ is the expected information matrix for θ based on Y^m when conditioned on Y^o. This information can be viewed as the "missing information," resulting from observing Y^o only and not also Y^m. This leads to the *missing information principle*

$$\mathcal{I}_c(\theta, y) = I(\theta, y) + \mathcal{I}_m(\theta, y),$$

which has the following interpretation: the (conditional expected) complete information equals the observed information plus the missing information.

5.9.3 Rate of Convergence

The notion that the rate at which the EM algorithm converges depends upon the amount of missing information in the incomplete data compared to the hypothetical complete data will be made explicit by deriving results regarding the rate of convergence in terms of information matrices.

Under regularity conditions, the EM algorithm will converge linearly. By using a Taylor series expansion we can write

$$\theta^{(t+1)} - \theta^* \simeq J(\theta^*)[\theta^{(t)} - \theta^*].$$

Thus, in a neighborhood of θ^*, the EM algorithm is essentially a linear iteration with rate matrix $J(\theta^*)$, since $J(\theta^*)$ is typically nonzero. For this reason, $J(\theta^*)$ is often referred to as the matrix rate of convergence, or simply the rate of convergence. For vector θ^*, a measure of the actual observed convergence rate is the global rate of convergence, which can be assessed by

$$r = \lim_{t\to\infty} \frac{||\theta^{(t+1)} - \theta^*||}{||\theta^{(t)} - \theta^*||},$$

where $|| \cdot ||$ is any norm on d-dimensional Euclidean space $\mathbb{R}^d$, and d is the number of missing values. In practice, during the process of convergence, r is typically assessed as

$$r = \lim_{t\to\infty} \frac{||\theta^{(t+1)} - \theta^{(t)}||}{||\theta^{(t)} - \theta^{(t-1)}||}.$$

Under regularity conditions, it can be shown that r is the largest eigenvalue of the $d \times d$ rate matrix $J(\theta^*)$.

Now, $J(\theta^*)$ can be expressed in terms of the observed and missing information:

$$J(\theta^*) = I_d - \mathcal{I}_c(\theta^*, Y^o)^{-1}I(\theta^*, Y^o) = \mathcal{I}_c(\theta^*, Y^o)^{-1}\mathcal{I}_m(\theta^*, Y^o).$$

This means the rate of convergence of the EM algorithm is given by the largest eigenvalue of the information ratio matrix $\mathcal{I}_c(\theta, Y^o)^{-1}\mathcal{I}_m(\theta, Y^o)$, which measures the proportion of information about θ that is missing as a result of not also observing Y^m in addition to Y^o. The greater the proportion of missing information, the slower the rate of convergence. The fraction of information loss may vary across different components of θ, suggesting that certain components of θ may approach θ^* rapidly using the EM algorithm, while other components may require a large number of iterations. Further, exceptions to the convergence of the EM algorithm to a local maximum of the likelihood function occur if $J(\theta^*)$ has eigenvalues exceeding unity.

5.9.4   EM Acceleration

Using the concept of rate matrix

$$\theta^{(t+1)} - \theta^* \simeq J(\theta^*)[\theta^{(t)} - \theta^*],$$

we can solve this for θ^*, to yield

$$\widetilde{\theta^*} = (I_d - J)^{-1}(\theta^{(t+1)} - J\theta^{(t)}).$$

The J matrix can be determined empirically, using a sequence of subsequent iterations. It also follows from the observed and complete or, equivalently, missing information:

$$J = I_d - \mathcal{I}_c(\theta^*, Y)^{-1}I(\theta^*, Y).$$

Here, $\widetilde{\theta^*}$ can then be seen as an accelerated iteration.

5.9.5   Calculation of Precision Estimates

The observed information matrix is not directly accessible. It has been shown by Louis (1982) that

$$\mathcal{I}_m(\theta, Y^o) = E[S_c(\theta, Y)S_c(\theta, Y)'|y^o] - S(\theta, Y^o)S(\theta, Y^o)'.$$

This leads to an expression for the observed information matrix in terms of quantities that are available (McLachlan and Krishnan, 1997):

$$I(\theta, Y) = \mathcal{I}_m(\theta, Y) - E[S_c(\theta, Z)S_c(\theta, Z)'|y] + S(\theta, Y)S(\theta, Y)'.$$

From this equation, the observed information matrix can be computed as

$$I(\hat{\theta}, Y) = \mathcal{I}_m(\hat{\theta}, Y) - E[S_c(\hat{\theta}, Z)S_c(\hat{\theta}, Z)'|y],$$

where $\hat{\theta}$ is the maximum likelihood estimator.

5.9.6   EM Algorithm Using SAS

A version of the EM algorithm for both multivariate normal and categorical data can be conducted using the MI procedure in SAS. Indeed, with the MCMC imputation method (for general nonmonotone settings), the MCMC chain is started using EM-based starting values. It is possible to suppress the actual MCMC-based multiple imputation, thus restricting action of PROC MI to the EM algorithm.

The NIMPUTE option in the MI procedure should be set equal to zero. This means the multiple imputation will be skipped, and only tables of model information, missing data patterns, descriptive statistics (in case the SIMPLE option is given) and the MLE from the EM algorithm (EM statement) are displayed.

We have to specify the EM statement so that the EM algorithm is used to compute the maximum likelihood estimate (MLE) of the data with missing values, assuming a multivariate normal distribution for the data. The following five options are available with the EM statement. The option CONVERGE=.

sets the convergence criterion. The value must be between 0 and 1. The iterations are considered to have converged when the maximum change in the parameter estimates between iteration steps is less than the value specified. The change is a relative change if the parameter is greater than 0.01 in absolute value; otherwise it is an absolute change. By default, CONVERGE=1E-4. The iteration history in the EM algorithm is printed if the option ITPRINT is given. The maximum number of iterations used in the EM algorithm is specified with the MAXITER=. option. The default is MAXITER=200. The option OUTEM=. creates an output SAS data set containing the MLE of the parameter vector (μ, Σ), computed with the EM algorithm. Finally, OUTITER=. creates an output SAS data set containing parameters for each iteration. The data set includes a variable named _ITERATION_ to identify the iteration number.

PROC MI uses the means and standard deviations from the available cases as the initial estimates for the EM algorithm. The correlations are set equal to zero.

EXAMPLE: Growth Data

Using the horizontal version of the GROWTH data set created in Section 5.8, we can use the following program:

Program 5.19 The EM algorithm using PROC MI

```
proc mi data=growthmi seed=495838 simple nimpute=0;
    em itprint outem=growthem1;
    var meas8 meas12 meas14 meas10;
    by sex;
    run;
```

Part of the output generated by this program (for SEX=1) is given below. The procedure displays the initial parameter estimates for EM, the iteration history (because option ITPRINT is given), and the EM parameter estimates, i.e., the maximum likelihood estimates for μ and Σ from the incomplete GROWTH data set.

Output from Program 5.19 (SEX=1 group)

```
------------------------------- SEX=1 -----------------------------------

                   Initial Parameter Estimates for EM

_TYPE_ _NAME_           MEAS8          MEAS12          MEAS14          MEAS10


  MEAN                22.875000       25.718750       27.468750       24.136364
  COV     MEAS8        6.016667               0               0               0
  COV     MEAS12              0        7.032292               0               0
  COV     MEAS14              0               0        4.348958               0
  COV     MEAS10              0               0               0        5.954545



                   EM (MLE) Iteration History


            _Iteration_          -2 Log L          MEAS10


                      0        158.065422       24.136364
                      1        139.345763       24.136364
                      2        138.197324       23.951784
                      3        137.589135       23.821184
                      4        137.184304       23.721865
                      5        136.891453       23.641983
```

```
                          .
                          .
                          .
           42        136.070697        23.195650
           43        136.070694        23.195453
           44        136.070693        23.195285
           45        136.070692        23.195141
           46        136.070691        23.195018
           47        136.070690        23.194913


                   EM (MLE) Parameter Estimates
```

TYPE	_NAME_	MEAS8	MEAS12	MEAS14	MEAS10
MEAN		22.875000	25.718750	27.468750	23.194913
COV	MEAS8	5.640625	3.402344	1.511719	5.106543
COV	MEAS12	3.402344	6.592773	3.038086	2.555289
COV	MEAS14	1.511719	3.038086	4.077148	1.937547
COV	MEAS10	5.106543	2.555289	1.937547	7.288687

```
                   EM (Posterior Mode) Estimates
```

TYPE	_NAME_	MEAS8	MEAS12	MEAS14	MEAS10
MEAN		22.875000	25.718750	27.468750	23.194535
COV	MEAS8	4.297619	2.592262	1.151786	3.891806
COV	MEAS12	2.592262	5.023065	2.314732	1.947220
COV	MEAS14	1.151786	2.314732	3.106399	1.476056
COV	MEAS10	3.891806	1.947220	1.476056	5.379946

One can also output the EM parameter estimates into an output data set with the OUTEM=. option. A printout of the GROWTHEM1 data set produces a handy summary for both sexes:

Summary for both sex groups

Obs	SEX	_TYPE_	_NAME_	MEAS8	MEAS12	MEAS14	MEAS10
1	1	MEAN		22.8750	25.7188	27.4688	23.1949
2	1	COV	MEAS8	5.6406	3.4023	1.5117	5.1065
3	1	COV	MEAS12	3.4023	6.5928	3.0381	2.5553
4	1	COV	MEAS14	1.5117	3.0381	4.0771	1.9375
5	1	COV	MEAS10	5.1065	2.5553	1.9375	7.2887
6	2	MEAN		21.0909	22.6818	24.0000	22.0733
7	2	COV	MEAS8	4.1281	5.0744	4.3636	2.9920
8	2	COV	MEAS12	5.0744	7.5579	6.6591	3.9260
9	2	COV	MEAS14	4.3636	6.6591	6.6364	3.1666
10	2	COV	MEAS10	2.9920	3.9260	3.1666	2.9133

Should we want to combine this program with genuine multiple imputation, then the program can be augmented as follows (using the MCMC default):

Program 5.20 Combining EM algorithm and multiple imputation

```
proc mi data=growthmi seed=495838 simple nimpute=5 out=growthmi2;
    em itprint outem=growthem2;
    var meas8 meas12 meas14 meas10;
    by sex;
    run;
```

5.10 Categorical Data

The non-Gaussian setting is different in the sense that there is no generally accepted counterpart to the linear mixed effects model. We therefore first sketch a general taxonomy for longitudinal models in this context, including marginal, random effects (or subject-specific), and conditional models. We then argue that marginal and random effects models both have their merit in the analysis of longitudinal clinical trial data and focus on two important representatives: the generalized estimating equations (GEE) approach within the marginal family and the generalized linear mixed effects model (GLMM) within the random effects family. We highlight important similarities and differences between these model families. While GLMM parameters can be fitted using maximum likelihood, the same is not true for the frequentist GEE method. Therefore, Robins, Rotnitzky and Zhao (1995) have devised so-called weighted generalized estimating equations (WGEE), valid under MAR but requiring the specification of a dropout model in terms of observed outcomes and/or covariates in order to specify the weights.

5.10.1 Discrete Repeated Measures

We distinguish between several generally nonequivalent extensions of univariate models. In a *marginal model*, marginal distributions are used to describe the outcome vector Y, given a set X of predictor variables. The correlation among the components of Y can then be captured either by adopting a fully parametric approach or by means of working assumptions, such as in the semiparametric approach of Liang and Zeger (1986). Alternatively, in a *random effects model*, the predictor variables X are supplemented with a vector θ of random effects, conditional upon which the components of Y are usually assumed to be independent. This does not preclude that more elaborate models are possible if residual dependence is detected (Longford, 1993). Finally, a *conditional model* describes the distribution of the components of Y, conditional on X but also conditional on a subset of the other components of Y. Well-known members of this class of models are log-linear models (Gilula and Haberman, 1994).

Marginal and random effects models are two important subfamilies of models for repeated measures. Several authors, such as Diggle et al. (2002) and Aerts et al. (2002) distinguish between three such families. Still focusing on continuous outcomes, a marginal model is characterized by the specification of a marginal mean function

$$E(Y_{ij}|x_{ij}) = x'_{ij}\beta, \tag{5.18}$$

whereas in a random effects model we focus on the expectation, conditional upon the random effects vector:

$$E(Y_{ij}|b_i, x_{ij}) = x'_{ij}\beta + z'_{ij}b_i. \tag{5.19}$$

Finally, a third family of models conditions a particular outcome on the other responses or a subset thereof. In particular, a simple first-order stationary transition model focuses on expectations of the form

$$E(Y_{ij}|Y_{i,j-1}, \ldots, Y_{i1}, x_{ij}) = x'_{ij}\beta + \alpha Y_{i,j-1}. \tag{5.20}$$

In the linear mixed model case, random effects models imply a simple marginal model. This is due to the elegant properties of the multivariate normal distribution. In particular, the expectation described in equation (5.18) follows from equation (5.19) by either (a) marginalizing over the random effects or by (b) conditioning upon the random effects vector $b_i = 0$. Hence, the fixed effects parameters β have both a marginal as well as a hierarchical model interpretation. Finally, when a conditional model is expressed in terms of residuals rather than outcomes directly, it also leads to particular forms of the general linear mixed effects model.

Such a close connection between the model families does not exist when outcomes are of a nonnormal type, such as binary, categorical, or discrete. We will consider each of the model families in turn and then point to some particular issues arising within them or when comparisons are made between them.

5.10.2   Marginal Models

In marginal models, the parameters characterize the marginal probabilities of a subset of the outcomes without conditioning on the other outcomes. Advantages and disadvantages of conditional and marginal modeling have been discussed in Diggle et al. (2002) and Fahrmeir and Tutz (2002). The specific context of clustered binary data has received treatment in Aerts et al. (2002). Apart from full likelihood approaches, nonlikelihood approaches, such as generalized estimating equations (Liang and Zeger, 1986) or pseudo-likelihood (le Cessie and van Houwelingen, 1994; Geys, Molenberghs and Lipsitz, 1998) have been considered.

Bahadur (1961) proposed a marginal model, accounting for the association via marginal correlations. Ekholm (1991) proposed a so-called success probabilities approach. George and Bowman (1995) proposed a model for the particular case of exchangeable binary data. Ashford and Sowden (1970) considered the multivariate probit model for repeated ordinal data, thereby extending univariate probit regression. Molenberghs and Lesaffre (1994) and Lang and Agresti (1994) have proposed models which parameterize the association in terms of marginal odds ratios. Dale (1986) defined the bivariate global odds ratio model, based on a bivariate Plackett distribution (Plackett, 1965). Molenberghs and Lesaffre (1994, 1999) extended this model to multivariate ordinal outcomes. They generalize the bivariate Plackett distribution in order to establish the multivariate cell probabilities. Their 1994 method involves solving polynomials of high degree and computing the derivatives thereof, while in 1999 generalized linear models theory is exploited, together with the use of an adaption of the iterative proportional fitting algorithm. Lang and Agresti (1994) exploit the equivalence between direct modeling and imposing restrictions on the multinomial probabilities, using undetermined Lagrange multipliers. Alternatively, the cell probabilities can be fitted using a Newton iteration scheme, as suggested by Glonek and McCullagh (1995). We will consider generalized estimating equations (GEE) and weighted generalized estimating equations (WGEE) in turn.

Generalized Estimating Equations

The main issue with full likelihood approaches is the computational complexity they entail. When we are mainly interested in first-order marginal mean parameters and pairwise association parameters—i.e., second-order moments—a full likelihood procedure can be replaced by quasi-likelihood methods (McCullagh and Nelder, 1989). In quasi-likelihood, the mean response is expressed as a parametric function of covariates; the variance is assumed to be a function of the mean up to possibly unknown scale parameters. Wedderburn (1974) first noted that likelihood and quasi-likelihood theories coincide for exponential families and that the quasi-likelihood estimating equations provide consistent estimates of the regression parameters β in any generalized linear model, even for choices of link and variance functions that do not correspond to exponential families.

For clustered and repeated data, Liang and Zeger (1986) proposed so-called *generalized estimating equations* (GEE or GEE1) which require only the correct specification of the univariate marginal distributions provided one is willing to adopt working assumptions about the association structure. They estimate the parameters associated with the expected value of an individual's vector of binary responses and phrase the working assumptions about the association between pairs of outcomes in terms of marginal correlations. The method combines estimating equations for the regression parameters β with moment-based estimating for the correlation parameters entering the working assumptions.

Prentice (1988) extended their results to allow joint estimation of probabilities and pairwise correlations. Lipsitz, Laird and Harrington (1991) modified the estimating equations of Prentice to allow modeling of the association through marginal odds ratios rather than marginal correlations. When adopting GEE1 one does not use information of the association structure to estimate the main effect parameters. As a result, it can be shown that GEE1 yields consistent main effect estimators, even when the association structure is misspecified. However, severe misspecification may seriously affect the efficiency of the GEE1 estimators. In addition, GEE1 should be avoided when some scientific interest is placed on the association parameters.

A second order extension of these estimating equations (GEE2) that includes the marginal pairwise association as well has been studied by Liang, Zeger and Qaqish (1992). They note that GEE2 is nearly fully efficient, though bias may occur in the estimation of the main effect parameters when the association structure is misspecified.

Usually, when confronted with the analysis of clustered or otherwise correlated data, conclusions based on mean parameters (e.g., dose effect) are of primary interest. When inferences for the parameters in the mean model $E(y_i)$ are based on classical maximum likelihood theory, full specification of the joint distribution for the vector y_i of repeated measurements within each unit i is necessary. For discrete data, this implies specification of the first-order moments as well as all higher-order moments and, depending on whether marginal or random effects models are used, assumptions are either explicitly made or implicit in the random effects structure. For Gaussian data, full-model specification reduces to modeling the first- and second-order moments only. However, even then inappropriate covariance models can seriously invalidate inferences for the mean structure. Thus, a drawback of a fully parametric model is that incorrect specification of nuisance characteristics can lead to invalid conclusions about key features of the model.

After this short overview of the GEE approach, the GEE methodology, which is based on two principles, will now be explained a little further. First, the score equations to be solved when computing maximum likelihood estimates under a marginal normal model $y_i \sim N(X_i\beta, V_i)$ are given by

$$\sum_{i=1}^{N} X_i'(A_i^{1/2} R_i A_i^{1/2})^{-1}(y_i - X_i\beta) = 0, \tag{5.21}$$

in which the marginal covariance matrix V_i has been decomposed in the form $A_i^{1/2} R_i A_i^{1/2}$, with A_i the matrix with the marginal variances on the main diagonal and zeros elsewhere, and with R_i equal to the marginal correlation matrix. Second, the score equations to be solved when computing maximum likelihood estimates under the marginal generalized linear model (5.18), assuming independence of the responses within units (i.e., ignoring the repeated measures structure), are given by

$$\sum_{i=1}^{N} \frac{\partial\mu_i}{\partial\beta'}(A_i^{1/2} I_{n_i} A_i^{1/2})^{-1}(y_i - \mu_i) = 0, \tag{5.22}$$

where A_i is again the diagonal matrix with the marginal variances on the main diagonal.

Note that expression (5.21) has the same form as expression (5.22) but with the correlations between repeated measures taken into account. A straightforward extension of expression (5.22) that accounts for the correlation structure is

$$S(\beta) = \sum_{i=1}^{N} \frac{\partial\mu_i}{\partial\beta'}(A_i^{1/2} R_i A_i^{1/2})^{-1}(y_i - \mu_i) = 0, \tag{5.23}$$

which is obtained from replacing the identity matrix I_{n_i} with a correlation matrix $R_i = R_i(\alpha)$, often referred to as the *working* correlation matrix. Usually, the marginal covariance matrix $V_i = A_i^{1/2} R_i A_i^{1/2}$ contains a vector α of unknown parameters which is replaced for practical purposes by a consistent estimate.

Assuming that the marginal mean μ_i has been correctly specified as $h(\mu_i) = X_i\beta$, it can be shown that, under mild regularity conditions, the estimator $\hat{\beta}$ obtained from solving expression (5.23) is asymptotically normally distributed with mean β and with covariance matrix

$$I_0^{-1} I_1 I_0^{-1}, \tag{5.24}$$

where

$$I_0 = \left(\sum_{i=1}^{N} \frac{\partial \mu_i'}{\partial \beta} V_i^{-1} \frac{\partial \mu_i}{\partial \beta'} \right),$$

$$I_1 = \left(\sum_{i=1}^{N} \frac{\partial \mu_i'}{\partial \beta} V_i^{-1} \text{Var}(y_i) V_i^{-1} \frac{\partial \mu_i}{\partial \beta'} \right).$$

In practice, $\text{Var}(y_i)$ in the matrix (5.24) is replaced by $(y_i - \mu_i)(y_i - \mu_i)'$, which is unbiased on the sole condition that the mean was again correctly specified.

Note that valid inferences can now be obtained for the mean structure, only assuming that the model assumptions with respect to the first-order moments are correct. Note also that, although arising from a likelihood approach, the GEE equations in expression (5.23) cannot be interpreted as score equations corresponding to some full likelihood for the data vector y_i.

Liang and Zeger (1986) proposed moment-based estimates for the working correlation. To this end, first define deviations

$$e_{ij} = \frac{y_{ij} - \mu_{ij}}{\sqrt{v(\mu_{ij})}}$$

and decompose the variance slightly more generally as above in the following way:

$$V_i = \phi A_i^{1/2} R_i A_i^{1/2},$$

where ϕ is an overdispersion parameter.

Some of the more popular choices for the working correlations are independence $(\text{Corr}(Y_{ij}, Y_{ik}) = 0, \ j \neq k)$, exchangeability $(\text{Corr}(Y_{ij}, Y_{ik}) = \alpha, \ j \neq k)$, AR(1) $(\text{Corr}(Y_{ij}, Y_{i,j+t}) = \alpha^t, t = 0, 1, \ldots, n_i - j)$, and unstructured $(\text{Corr}(Y_{ij}, Y_{ik}) = \alpha_{jk}, \ j \neq k)$. Typically, moment-based estimation methods are used to estimate these parameters, as part of an integrated iterative estimation procedure (Aerts et al., 2002). The overdispersion parameter is approached in a similar fashion. The standard iterative procedure to fit GEE, based on Liang and Zeger (1986), is then as follows: (1) compute initial estimates for β, using a univariate GLM (i.e., assuming independence); (2) compute the quantities needed in the estimating equation: b_i; (3) compute Pearson residuals e_{ij}; (4) compute estimates for α; (5) compute $R_i(\alpha)$; (6) compute an estimate for ϕ; (7) compute $V_i(\beta, \alpha) = \phi A_i^{1/2}(\beta) R_i(\alpha) A_i^{1/2}(\beta)$. (8) update the estimate for β:

$$\beta^{(t+1)} = \beta^{(t)} - \left[\sum_{i=1}^{N} \frac{\partial \mu_i'}{\partial \beta} V_i^{-1} \frac{\partial \mu_i}{\partial \beta} \right]^{-1} \left[\sum_{i=1}^{N} \frac{\partial \mu_i'}{\partial \beta} V_i^{-1} (y_i - \mu_i) \right].$$

Steps (2) through (8) are iterated until convergence.

Weighted Generalized Estimating Equations

The problem of dealing with missing values is common throughout statistical work and is almost always present in the analysis of longitudinal or repeated measurements. For categorical outcomes, as we have seen before, the GEE approach could be adapted. However, as Liang and Zeger (1986) pointed out, inferences with the GEE are valid only under the strong assumption that the data are missing completely at random (MCAR). To allow the data to be missing at random (MAR), Robins, Rotnitzky and Zhao (1995) proposed a class of weighted estimating equations. They can be viewed as an extension of generalized estimating equations.

The idea is to weight each subject's measurements in the GEEs by the inverse probability that a subject drops out at that particular measurement occasion. This can be calculated as

$$v_{it} \equiv P[D_i = t] = \prod_{k=2}^{t-1}(1 - P[R_{ik} = 0 | R_{i2} = \ldots = R_{i,k-1} = 1]) \times$$

$$P[R_{it} = 0 | R_{i2} = \ldots = R_{i,t-1} = 1]^{I\{t \leq T\}}$$

if dropout occurs by time t or we reach the end of the measurement sequence, and

$$v_{it} \equiv P[D_i = t] = \prod_{k=2}^{t}(1 - P[R_{ik} = 0 | R_{i2} = \ldots = R_{i,k-1} = 1])$$

otherwise. Recall that we partitioned Y_i into the unobserved components Y_i^m and the observed components Y_i^o. Similarly, we can make the exact same partition of μ_i into μ_i^m and μ_i^o. In the weighted GEE approach, which is proposed to reduce possible bias of $\hat{\beta}$, the score equations to be solved when taking into account the correlation structure are:

$$S(\beta) = \sum_{i=1}^{N} \frac{1}{v_i} \frac{\partial \mu_i}{\partial \beta'}(A_i^{1/2} R_i A_i^{1/2})^{-1}(y_i - \mu_i) = 0$$

or

$$S(\beta) = \sum_{i=1}^{N} \sum_{d=2}^{n+1} \frac{I(D_i = d)}{v_{id}} \frac{\partial \mu_i}{\partial \beta'}(d)(A_i^{1/2} R_i A_i^{1/2})^{-1}(d)(y_i(d) - \mu_i(d)) = 0,$$

where $y_i(d)$ and $\mu_i(d)$ are the first $d - 1$ elements of y_i and μ_i respectively. We define $\frac{\partial \mu_i}{\partial \beta'}(d)$ and $(A_i^{1/2} R_i A_i^{1/2})^{-1}(d)$ analogously, in line with the definition of Robins, Rotnitzky and Zhao (1995).

5.10.3   Random Effects Models

Models with subject-specific parameters are differentiated from population-averaged models by the inclusion of parameters which are specific to the cluster. Unlike for correlated Gaussian outcomes, the parameters of the random effects and population-averaged models for correlated binary data describe different types of effects of the covariates on the response probabilities (Neuhaus, 1992).

The choice between population-averaged and random effects strategies should heavily depend on the scientific goals. Population-averaged models evaluate the overall risk as a function of covariates. With a subject-specific approach, the response rates are modeled as a function of covariates and parameters, specific to a subject. In such models, interpretation of fixed effects parameters is conditional on a constant level of the random effects parameter. Population-averaged comparisons, on the other hand, make no use of within-cluster comparisons for cluster-varying covariates and are therefore not useful to assess within-subject effects (Neuhaus, Kalbfleisch and Hauck, 1991).

Whereas the linear mixed model is unequivocally the most popular choice in the case of normally distributed response variables, there are more options in the case of nonnormal outcomes. Stiratelli, Laird and Ware (1984) assume the parameter vector to be normally distributed. This idea has been carried further in the work on so-called *generalized linear mixed models* (Breslow and Clayton, 1993), which is closely related to linear and nonlinear mixed models. Alternatively, Skellam (1948) introduced the beta-binomial model, in which the response probability of any response of a particular subject comes from a beta distribution. Hence, this model can also be viewed as a random effects model. We will consider generalized linear mixed models.

Generalized Linear Mixed Models

Perhaps the most commonly encountered subject-specific (or random effects) model is the generalized linear mixed model. A general framework for mixed effects models can be expressed as follows. Assume that Y_i (possibly appropriately transformed) satisfies

$$Y_i | b_i \sim F_i(\theta, b_i), \tag{5.25}$$

i.e., conditional on b_i, Y_i follows a prespecified distribution F_i, possibly depending on covariates, and is parameterized through a vector θ of unknown parameters common to all subjects. Further, b_i is a q-dimensional vector of subject-specific parameters, called random effects, assumed to follow a so-called mixing distribution G which may depend on a vector ψ of unknown parameters, i.e., $b_i \sim G(\psi)$. The term b_i reflects the between-unit heterogeneity in the population with respect to the distribution of Y_i. In the presence of random effects, conditional independence is often assumed, under which the components Y_{ij} in Y_i are independent, conditional on b_i. The distribution function F_i in equation (5.25) then becomes a product over the n_i independent elements in Y_i.

In general, unless a fully Bayesian approach is followed, inference is based on the marginal model for Y_i which is obtained from integrating out the random effects, over their distribution $G(\psi)$. Let $f_i(y_i | b_i)$ and $g(b_i)$ denote the density functions corresponding to the distributions F_i and G, respectively. The marginal density function of Y_i equals

$$f_i(y_i) = \int f_i(y_i | b_i) g(b_i) db_i, \tag{5.26}$$

which depends on the unknown parameters θ and ψ. Assuming independence of the units, estimates of $\hat{\theta}$ and $\hat{\psi}$ can be obtained from maximizing the likelihood function built from equation (5.26), and inferences immediately follow from classical maximum likelihood theory.

It is important to realize that the random effects distribution G is crucial in the calculation of the marginal model (5.26). One often assumes G to be of a specific parametric form, such as a (multivariate) normal. Depending on F_i and G, the integration in equation (5.26) may or may not be possible analytically. Proposed solutions are based on Taylor series expansions of $f_i(y_i | b_i)$ or on numerical approximations of the integral, such as (adaptive) Gaussian quadrature.

Note that there is an important difference with respect to the interpretation of the fixed effects β. Under the classical linear mixed model (Verbeke and Molenberghs, 2000), we have that $E(Y_i)$ equals $X_i \beta$, such that the fixed effects have a subject-specific as well as a population-averaged interpretation. Under nonlinear mixed models, however, this no longer holds in general. The fixed effects now only reflect the conditional effect of covariates, and the marginal effect is not easily obtained anymore, as $E(Y_i)$ is given by

$$E(Y_i) = \int y_i \int f_i(y_i | b_i) g(b_i) db_i dy_i.$$

However, in a biopharmaceutical context, one is often primarily interested in hypothesis testing and the random effects framework can be used to this effect.

The generalized linear mixed model (GLMM) is the most frequently used random effects model for discrete outcomes. A general formulation is as follows. Conditionally on random effects b_i, it assumes that the elements Y_{ij} of Y_i are independent, with the density function usually based on a classical exponential family formulation. This implies that the mean equals $E(Y_{ij} | b_i) = a'(\eta_{ij}) = \mu_{ij}(b_i)$, with variance $\text{Var}(Y_{ij} | b_i) = \phi a''(\eta_{ij})$. One needs a link function h (e.g., the logit link for binary data or the Poisson link for counts) and typically uses a linear regression model with parameters β and b_i for the mean, i.e., $h(\mu_i(b_i)) = X_i \beta + Z_i b_i$. Note that the linear mixed model is a special case, with an identity link function. The random effects b_i are again assumed to be sampled from a multivariate normal distribution with mean 0 and covariance matrix D. Usually, the canonical link function is used; i.e., $h = a'^{-1}$, such that $\eta_i = X_i \beta + Z_i b_i$. When the link function is chosen to be of the logit form and the random effects are assumed to be normally distributed, the familiar logistic-linear GLMM follows.

EXAMPLE: Depression Trial

Let us now analyze the clinical depression trial introduced in Section 5.2. The binary outcome of interest is 1 if the HAMD17 score is larger than 7, and 0 otherwise. We added this variable, called YBIN, to the DEPRESSION data set. The primary null hypothesis will be tested using both GEE and WGEE, as well as GLMM. We include the fixed categorical effects of treatment, visit, and treatment-by-visit interaction, as well as the continuous, fixed covariates of baseline score and baseline score-by-visit interaction. A random intercept will be included when considering the random effect models. Analyses will be implemented using PROC GENMOD and PROC NLMIXED.

Program 5.21 Creation of binary outcome

```
data depression;
   set depression;
   if y<=7 then ybin=0;
   else ybin=1;
   run;
```

Partial listing of the binary depression data

Obs	PATIENT	VISIT	Y	ybin	CHANGE	TRT	BASVAL	INVEST
1	1501	4	18	1	-7	1	25	6
2	1501	5	11	1	-14	1	25	6
3	1501	6	11	1	-14	1	25	6
4	1501	7	8	1	-17	1	25	6
5	1501	8	6	0	-19	1	25	6
6	1502	4	16	1	-1	4	17	6
7	1502	5	13	1	-4	4	17	6
8	1502	6	13	1	-4	4	17	6
9	1502	7	12	1	-5	4	17	6
10	1502	8	9	1	-8	4	17	6
11	1504	4	21	1	9	4	12	6
12	1504	5	17	1	5	4	12	6
13	1504	6	31	1	19	4	12	6
14	1504	7	.	.	.	4	12	6
15	1504	8	.	.	.	4	12	6
16	1510	4	21	1	3	1	18	6
17	1510	5	23	1	5	1	18	6
18	1510	6	18	1	0	1	18	6
19	1510	7	9	1	-9	1	18	6
20	1510	8	9	1	-9	1	18	6
...								
836	4801	4	17	1	5	4	12	999
837	4801	5	6	0	-6	4	12	999
838	4801	6	5	0	-7	4	12	999
839	4801	7	3	0	-9	4	12	999
840	4801	8	2	0	-10	4	12	999
841	4803	4	10	1	-6	1	16	999
842	4803	5	8	1	-8	1	16	999
843	4803	6	8	1	-8	1	16	999
844	4803	7	6	0	-10	1	16	999
845	4803	8	.	.	.	1	16	999
846	4901	4	11	1	2	1	9	999
847	4901	5	3	0	-6	1	9	999
848	4901	6	.	.	.	1	9	999

```
849      4901    7    .    .      .    1    9    999
850      4901    8    .    .      .    1    9    999
```

Marginal Models

First, let us consider the GEE approach. In the PROC GENMOD statement, the option DESCENDING is used to require modeling of $P(YBIN_{ij} = 1)$ rather than $P(YBIN_{ij} = 0)$. The CLASS statement specifies which variables should be considered as factors. Such classification variables can be either character or numeric. Internally, each of these factors will correspond to a set of dummy variables.

The MODEL statement specifies the response, or dependent variable, and the effects, or explanatory variables. If one omits the explanatory variables, the procedure fits an intercept-only model. An intercept term is included in the model by default. The intercept can be removed with the NOINT option. The DIST=. option specifies the built-in probability distribution to use in the model. If the DIST=. option is specified and a user-defined link function is omitted, the default link function is chosen. For the binomial distribution, the logit link is the default.

The REPEATED statement specifies the covariance structure of multivariate responses for fitting the GEE model in the GENMOD procedure, and hence turns an otherwise cross-sectional procedure into one for repeated measures. SUBJECT=*subject-effect* identifies subjects in the input data set. The *subject-effect* can be a single variable, an interaction effect, a nested effect, or a combination. Each distinct value, or level, of the effect identifies a different subject or cluster. Responses from different subjects are assumed to be statistically independent, and responses within subjects are assumed to be correlated. A *subject-effect* must be specified, and variables used in defining the *subject-effect* must be listed in the CLASS statement. The WITHINSUBJECT=. option defines the order of measurements within subjects. Each distinct level of the within-subject-effect defines a different response from the same subject. If the data are in proper order within each subject, one does not need to specify this option. The TYPE=. option specifies the structure of the working correlation matrix used to model the correlation of the responses from subjects. The following table shows an overview of the correlation structure keywords and the corresponding correlation structures. The default working correlation type is independence.

Table 5.15 Correlation structure types

Keyword	Correlation Matrix Type
AR | AR(1)	autoregressive(1)
EXCH | CS	exchangeable
IND	independent
MDEP(NUMBER)	*m*-dependent with *m*=number
UNSTR | UN	unstructured
USER | FIXED (MATRIX)	fixed, user-specified correlation matrix

We use the exchangeable working correlation matrix. The CORRW option displays the estimated working correlation matrix. The MODELSE option gives an analysis of parameter estimates table using model-based standard errors. By default, an "Analysis of Parameter Estimates" table, based on empirical standard errors is displayed.

Program 5.22 Standard GEE code

```
proc genmod data=depression descending;
    class patient visit trt;
    model ybin = trt visit trt*visit basval basval*visit / dist=binomial type3;
    repeated subject=patient / withinsubject=visit type=cs corrw modelse;
    contrast 'endpoint' trt 1 -1 visit*trt 0 0 0 0 0 0 0 1 -1;
    contrast 'main' trt 1 -1;
    run;
```

Output from Program 5.22

```
              Analysis Of Initial Parameter Estimates

                                 Standard       Wald 95%        Chi-
Parameter          DF  Estimate   Error   Confidence Limits   Square
Intercept           1   -1.3970   0.8121   -2.9885   0.1946    2.96
TRT        1        1   -0.6153   0.3989   -1.3972   0.1665    2.38
TRT        4        0    0.0000   0.0000    0.0000   0.0000     .
VISIT      4        1    0.8316   1.2671   -1.6519   3.3151    0.43
VISIT      5        1   -0.3176   1.1291   -2.5306   1.8953    0.08
VISIT      6        1   -0.0094   1.0859   -2.1377   2.1189    0.00
VISIT      7        1   -0.3596   1.1283   -2.5710   1.8519    0.10
VISIT      8        0    0.0000   0.0000    0.0000   0.0000     .
...
Scale               0    1.0000   0.0000    1.0000   1.0000


                     Analysis Of Initial
                      Parameter Estimates

           Parameter          Pr > ChiSq

           Intercept            0.0854
           TRT        1         0.1229
           TRT        4          .
           VISIT      4         0.5116
           VISIT      5         0.7785
           VISIT      6         0.9931
           VISIT      7         0.7500
           VISIT      8          .
           ...
           Scale
NOTE: The scale parameter was held fixed.



                     GEE Model Information
        Correlation Structure             Exchangeable
        Within-Subject Effect        VISIT (5 levels)
        Subject Effect            PATIENT (170 levels)
        Number of Clusters                       170
        Clusters With Missing Values              61
        Correlation Matrix Dimension               5
        Maximum Cluster Size                       5
        Minimum Cluster Size                       1

Algorithm converged.



                  Working Correlation Matrix

            Col1       Col2       Col3       Col4       Col5

     Row1  1.0000     0.3701     0.3701     0.3701     0.3701
     Row2  0.3701     1.0000     0.3701     0.3701     0.3701
```

Row3	0.3701	0.3701	1.0000	0.3701	0.3701
Row4	0.3701	0.3701	0.3701	1.0000	0.3701
Row5	0.3701	0.3701	0.3701	0.3701	1.0000

Analysis Of GEE Parameter Estimates
Empirical Standard Error Estimates

| | | | Standard | 95% Confidence | | | |
Parameter		Estimate	Error	Limits		Z	Pr > |Z|
Intercept		-1.2158	0.7870	-2.7583	0.3268	-1.54	0.1224
TRT	1	-0.7072	0.3808	-1.4536	0.0392	-1.86	0.0633
TRT	4	0.0000	0.0000	0.0000	0.0000	.	.
VISIT	4	0.4251	1.2188	-1.9637	2.8138	0.35	0.7273
VISIT	5	-0.4772	1.2304	-2.8887	1.9344	-0.39	0.6982
VISIT	6	0.0559	1.0289	-1.9607	2.0725	0.05	0.9567
VISIT	7	-0.2446	0.9053	-2.0190	1.5298	-0.27	0.7870
VISIT	8	0.0000	0.0000	0.0000	0.0000	.	.

...

Analysis Of GEE Parameter Estimates
Model-Based Standard Error Estimates

| | | | Standard | 95% Confidence | | | |
Parameter		Estimate	Error	Limits		Z	Pr > |Z|
Intercept		-1.2158	0.7675	-2.7201	0.2885	-1.58	0.1132
TRT	1	-0.7072	0.3800	-1.4521	0.0377	-1.86	0.0628
TRT	4	0.0000	0.0000	0.0000	0.0000	.	.
VISIT	4	0.4251	1.0466	-1.6262	2.4763	0.41	0.6846
VISIT	5	-0.4772	0.9141	-2.2688	1.3145	-0.52	0.6017
VISIT	6	0.0559	0.8621	-1.6338	1.7456	0.06	0.9483
VISIT	7	-0.2446	0.8881	-1.9853	1.4961	-0.28	0.7830
VISIT	8	0.0000	0.0000	0.0000	0.0000	.	.
...							
Scale		1.0000					

NOTE: The scale parameter was held fixed.

Score Statistics For Type 3 GEE Analysis

| | | Chi- | |
Source	DF	Square	Pr > ChiSq
TRT	1	0.89	0.3467
VISIT	4	1.37	0.8493
VISIT*TRT	4	4.97	0.2905
BASVAL	1	20.76	<.0001
BASVAL*VISIT	4	6.44	0.1683

Contrast Results for GEE Analysis

| | | Chi- | | |
Contrast	DF	Square	Pr > ChiSq	Type
endpoint	1	3.38	0.0658	Score
main	1	0.89	0.3467	Score

Note first that we did not show full output; results of interaction terms are often excluded.

The output starts off with the initial parameter estimates. These estimates result from fitting the model while ignoring the correlation structure—i.e., from fitting a classical GLM to the data, using PROC GENMOD. This is equivalent to a classical logistic regression in this case. The reported log-likelihood also corresponds to this model, and therefore should not be interpreted. The reported initial parameter estimates are used as starting values in the iterative estimation procedure for fitting GEE.

Next, bookkeeping information about the longitudinal nature of the data is provided. The number of clusters (subjects) and cluster sizes (more specific, boundaries for n_i) are given. There are 170 subjects (clusters) and each patient has five observations (minimum cluster size = maximum cluster size = 5), even though some are incomplete due to missingness. Hence the minimum cluster size is 1.

The estimated working correlation matrix is printed as a result of the CORRW option in the REPEATED statement. The constant correlation between two repeated measurements is estimated to be 0.3701. Note that this is a working assumption parameter only and should not be made the subject of statistical inference.

Then, parameter estimates and inference based on estimated sandwich standard errors (empirical, robust) and on model-based estimated standard errors (naive) are listed in turn. Note that the model-based and empirical parameter estimates are identical. Indeed, the choice between naive and empirical only affects the estimation of the covariance matrix of the regression parameters in β. On the other hand, between model-based and robust inferences there is a difference. In many cases, the model-based standard errors are much too small, because they are based on the assumption that all observations in the data set are independent. They therefore overestimate the amount of available information and the precision of the estimates. This especially holds true when the correct correlation structure differs considerably from the posited working correlation structure. When we use the independence working correlation, the estimated regression parameters are identical to the initial estimates.

Further, we included two CONTRAST statements to the program. A first one, ENDPOINT, is used to obtain comparisons at the last scheduled visit. Note that the test for TRT in the "Analysis of GEE Parameter Estimates" section in the output is also a test of the treatment difference at the last scheduled visit, since the last visit is the reference. The second contrast MAIN tests for the overall treatment effect, which is the same as the Type III test for treatment.

On the other hand, WGEE is applied to perform an ignorable MAR analysis. Fitting this type of model to the data is a little more complicated but is an important equivalent to a likelihood-based ignorable analysis. The complication stems from the fact that GEE is a frequentist (or sampling-based) procedure, ignorable only under the stringent MCAR condition.

We will explain this important procedure step by step.

To compute the weights, we first have to fit the dropout model, using logistic regression. The outcome DROPOUT is binary and indicating whether dropout occurs at a given time, yes or no, from the start of the measurement sequence until the time of dropout or the end of the sequence. Covariates in the model are the outcomes at previous occasions (variable PREV), supplemented with genuine covariate information. The %DROPOUT macro is used to construct the variables DROPOUT and PREV.

Program 5.23 Macro to create DROPOUT and PREV variables

```
%macro dropout(data=,id=,time=,response=,out=);
%if %bquote(&data)= %then %let data=&syslast;
proc freq data=&data noprint;
    tables &id /out=freqid;
    tables &time / out=freqtime;
    run;
proc iml;
    reset noprint;
    use freqid;
```

```
      read all var {&id};
      nsub = nrow(&id);
   use freqtime;
      read all var {&time};
      ntime = nrow(&time);
      time = &time;
   use &data;
      read all var {&id &time &response};
      n = nrow(&response);
   dropout = j(n,1,0);
   ind = 1;
   do while (ind <= nsub);
      j=1;
      if (&response[(ind-1)*ntime+j]=.)
         then print "First Measurement is Missing";
      if (&response[(ind-1)*ntime+j]^=.) then
        do;
           j = ntime;
           do until (j=2);
              if (&response[(ind-1)*ntime+j]=.) then
                do;
                   dropout[(ind-1)*ntime+j]=1;
                   j = j-1;
                end;
                else j = 2;
           end;
        end;
      ind = ind+1;
   end;
   prev = j(n,1,1);
   prev[2:n] = &response[1:n-1];
   i=1;
   do while (i<=n);
      if &time[i]=time[1] then prev[i]=.;
      i = i+1;
   end;
   create help var {&id &time &response dropout prev};
   append;
   quit;
data &out;
   merge &data help;
   run;
%mend;

%dropout(data=depression,id=patient,time=visit,response=ybin,out=dropout)
```

Fitting an appropriate logistic regression model is done with PROC GENMOD. Previous HAMD17 score and treatment are the covariates included in this model. The PREDICTED or PRED option in the MODEL statement requests that predicted values, the linear predictor, its standard error, and the Hessian weight be displayed. In the OUTPUT statement, a data set PRED is created with all statistics produced by the PRED option.

Program 5.24 WGEE: dropout model

```
proc genmod data=dropout descending;
    class trt;
    model dropout = prev trt / pred dist=b;
    output out=pred p=pred;
    run;
```

Next, the predicted probabilities of dropping out need to be translated into weights. These weights are defined at the individual measurement level:

- At the first occasion, the weight is $w = 1$.
- At other than the last occasion, the weight is the already accumulated weight, multiplied by $1-$the predicted probability of dropping out.
- At the last occasion *within a sequence where dropout occurs* the weight is multiplied by the predicted probability of dropping out.
- At the end of the process, the weight is inverted.

This process can be performed using the data manipulations shown next.

Program 5.25 WGEE: data manipulation to prepare for analysis

```
data studdrop;
    merge pred dropout;
    if (pred=.) then delete;
    run;

data wgt (keep=patient wi);
    set studdrop;
    by patient;
    retain wi;
    if first.patient then wi=1;
    if not last.patient then wi=wi*(1-pred);
    if last.patient then do;
      if visit<8 then wi=wi*pred;   /* DROPOUT BEFORE LAST OBSERVATION */
      else wi=wi*(1-pred);          /* NO DROPOUT */
      wi=1/wi;
      output;
    end;
    run;

data total;
    merge dropout wgt;
    by patient;
    run;
```

After this preparatory endeavor, we merely need to include the weights by means of the WEIGHT (or SCWGT) statement within the GENMOD procedure. This statement identifies a variable in the input data set to be used as the weight for the exponential family dispersion parameter for each observation. The exponential family dispersion parameter is divided by the WEIGHT variable value for each observation. Together with the use of the REPEATED statement, weighted GEE are then obtained. The code is given below. Also here the exchangeable working correlation matrix is used.

Program 5.26 WGEE: GENMOD program

```
proc genmod data=total descending;
    weight wi;
    class patient visit trt;
    model ybin = trt visit trt*visit basval basval*visit / dist=bin type3;
    repeated subject=patient / withinsubject=visit type=cs corrw modelse;
    contrast 'endpoint' trt 1 -1 visit*trt 0 0 0 0 0 0 0 1 -1;
    contrast 'main' trt 1 -1;
    run;
```

Output from Program 5.26

```
                 Analysis Of Initial Parameter Estimates

                             Standard      Wald 95%           Chi-
Parameter       DF  Estimate   Error   Confidence Limits     Square
Intercept        1   -1.3710   0.6955   -2.7342   -0.0078      3.89
TRT        1     1   -0.6170   0.3416   -1.2865    0.0525      3.26
TRT        4     0    0.0000   0.0000    0.0000    0.0000       .
VISIT      4     1    0.4730   0.9697   -1.4275    2.3736      0.24
VISIT      5     1    0.4317   0.7869   -1.1105    1.9740      0.30
VISIT      6     1    0.4172   0.8196   -1.1892    2.0235      0.26
VISIT      7     1   -0.3656   0.9667   -2.2603    1.5292      0.14
VISIT      8     0    0.0000   0.0000    0.0000    0.0000       .
...
Scale            0    1.0000   0.0000    1.0000    1.0000
```

```
                    Analysis Of Initial
                    Parameter Estimates

            Parameter            Pr > ChiSq

            Intercept              0.0487
            TRT         1          0.0709
            TRT         4             .
            VISIT       4          0.6257
            VISIT       5          0.5832
            VISIT       6          0.6108
            VISIT       7          0.7053
            VISIT       8             .
            ...
            Scale
NOTE: The scale parameter was held fixed.
```

```
                    GEE Model Information
        Correlation Structure              Exchangeable
        Within-Subject Effect           VISIT (5 levels)
        Subject Effect              PATIENT (170 levels)
        Number of Clusters                        170
        Clusters With Missing Values               61
        Correlation Matrix Dimension                5
        Maximum Cluster Size                        5
        Minimum Cluster Size                        1


Algorithm converged.
```

```
                        Working Correlation Matrix

              Col1        Col2        Col3        Col4        Col5

   Row1     1.0000      0.3133      0.3133      0.3133      0.3133
   Row2     0.3133      1.0000      0.3133      0.3133      0.3133
   Row3     0.3133      0.3133      1.0000      0.3133      0.3133
   Row4     0.3133      0.3133      0.3133      1.0000      0.3133
   Row5     0.3133      0.3133      0.3133      0.3133      1.0000


                   Analysis Of GEE Parameter Estimates
                   Empirical Standard Error Estimates

                           Standard   95% Confidence
   Parameter       Estimate   Error      Limits          Z  Pr > |Z|

   Intercept        -0.5596   0.9056  -2.3345   1.2153  -0.62  0.5366
   TRT        1     -0.9049   0.4088  -1.7061  -0.1037  -2.21  0.0268
   TRT        4      0.0000   0.0000   0.0000   0.0000    .      .
   VISIT      4     -0.1489   1.9040  -3.8806   3.5829  -0.08  0.9377
   VISIT      5     -0.2296   1.5357  -3.2396   2.7803  -0.15  0.8811
   VISIT      6      0.1510   1.1293  -2.0625   2.3645   0.13  0.8936
   VISIT      7     -0.2692   0.8847  -2.0032   1.4648  -0.30  0.7609
   VISIT      8      0.0000   0.0000   0.0000   0.0000    .      .
   ...


                   Analysis Of GEE Parameter Estimates
                   Model-Based Standard Error Estimates

                           Standard   95% Confidence
   Parameter       Estimate   Error      Limits          Z  Pr > |Z|

   Intercept        -0.5596   0.6259  -1.7863   0.6672  -0.89  0.3713
   TRT        1     -0.9049   0.3166  -1.5255  -0.2844  -2.86  0.0043
   TRT        4      0.0000   0.0000   0.0000   0.0000    .      .
   VISIT      4     -0.1489   0.8512  -1.8172   1.5194  -0.17  0.8612
   VISIT      5     -0.2296   0.6758  -1.5542   1.0949  -0.34  0.7340
   VISIT      6      0.1510   0.6908  -1.2029   1.5049   0.22  0.8269
   VISIT      7     -0.2692   0.7826  -1.8030   1.2646  -0.34  0.7309
   VISIT      8      0.0000   0.0000   0.0000   0.0000    .      .
   ...
   Scale             1.0000     .         .         .      .      .
NOTE: The scale parameter was held fixed.
                Score Statistics For Type 3 GEE Analysis
                                       Chi-
                   Source       DF    Square   Pr > ChiSq

                   TRT           1     3.05      0.0809
                   VISIT         4     1.41      0.8429
                   VISIT*TRT     4     5.95      0.2032
                   BASVAL        1     8.99      0.0027
                   BASVAL*VISIT  4     4.41      0.3535
```

```
              Contrast Results for GEE Analysis
                             Chi-
         Contrast      DF    Square   Pr > ChiSq   Type

         endpoint       1     4.78     0.0289      Score
         main           1     3.05     0.0809      Score
```

Comparing the above output to the one obtained under ordinary GEE, we observe a number of differences in both parameter estimates as well as standard errors. The difference in standard errors (often, but not always, larger under WGEE) are explained by the fact that additional sources of uncertainty, due to missingness, come into play. However, point estimates tend to differ as well. The resulting inferences can be different. For example, TRT 1 is nonsignificant with GEE, whereas a significant difference is found under the correct WGEE analysis. Also the result of both contrasts changes a lot when performing a WGEE instead of a GEE analysis. Thus, one may fail to detect such important effects as treatment differences when GEE is used rather than the admittedly more laborious WGEE.

Random Effects Models

To fit generalized linear mixed models, we use the SAS procedure NLMIXED, which allows fitting a wide class of linear, generalized linear, and nonlinear mixed models. PROC NLMIXED enables the user to specify a conditional distribution for the data (given the random effects) having either a standard form (normal, binomial, or Poisson) or a general distribution that is coded using SAS programming statements. It relies on numerical integration. Different integral approximations are available, the principal one being (adaptive) Gaussian quadrature. The procedure also includes a number of optimization algorithms. A detailed discussion of the procedure is beyond the scope of this work. We will restrict ourselves to the options most relevant for our purposes.

The procedure performs adaptive or nonadaptive Gaussian quadrature. The option NOAD in the NLMIXED statement requests nonadaptive Gaussian quadrature; i.e., the quadrature points are centered at zero for each of the random effects and the current random effects covariance matrix is used as the scale matrix, the other one being the default. The number of quadrature points can be specified with the option QPOINTS=m. By default, the number of quadrature points is selected adaptively by evaluating the log-likelihood function at the starting values of the parameters until two successive evaluations show sufficiently small relative change. By specifying the option TECHNIQUE=*newrap*, the procedure can maximize the marginal likelihood using the Newton-Raphson algorithm instead of the default Quasi-Newton algorithm.

In the PARMS statement starting values for parameters in the model are given. By default, parameters not listed in the PARMS statement are given an initial value of 1.

The conditional distribution of the data, given the random effects, is specified in the MODEL statement. Valid distributions are:

- NORMAL(m, v): Normal with mean m and variance v
- BINARY(p): Bernoulli with probability p
- BINOMIAL(n, p): Binomial with count n and probability p
- GAMMA(a, b): Gamma with shape a and scale b
- NEGBIN(n, p): Negative binomial with count n and probability p
- POISSON(m): Poisson with mean m
- GENERAL($\ell\ell$): General model with log-likelihood $\ell\ell$.

The RANDOM statement defines the random effects and their distribution. The procedure requires the data to be ordered by subject.

The models used in PROC NLMIXED have two limitations. First, only a single level of hierarchy in random effects is allowed, and second, PROC NLMIXED may not allow the incorporation of serial correlation of responses in the model.

Since no factors can be defined in the NLMIXED procedure, explicit creation of dummy variables is required. In the next program, we make dummies for the variables representing treatment and visit.

Program 5.27 Creating dummy variables in preparation of NLMIXED call

```
data dummy;
   set depression;
   if trt=1 then treat=1;
   else treat=0;
   visit_4=0;
   visit_5=0;
   visit_6=0;
   visit_7=0;
   if visit=4 then visit_4=1;
   if visit=5 then visit_5=1;
   if visit=6 then visit_6=1;
   if visit=7 then visit_7=1;
   run;
```

We will compare the results using Gaussian versus adaptive Gaussian quadrature and the Newton-Raphson algorithm versus the default algorithm in SAS. Throughout, we assume MAR. Since our procedure is likelihood based, ignorability applies, exactly as when the linear mixed model is used for Gaussian data (see Section 5.7).

First, we consider Gaussian quadrature and the default algorithm (i.e., Quasi-Newton). We take 0.5 as starting value for each parameter, and let the procedure decide on the number of quadrature points. The SAS code is given in Program 5.28. The estimates thereof will be used as starting values for the next three programs.

Program 5.28 GLMM code

```
proc nlmixed data=dummy noad;
   parms intercept=0.5 trt=0.5 basvalue=0.5
      vis4=0.5 vis5=0.5 vis6=0.5 vis7=0.5 trtvis4=0.5
      trtvis5=0.5 trtvis6=0.5 trtvis7=0.5 basvis4=0.5 basvis5=0.5
      basvis6=0.5 basvis7=0.5 sigma=0.5;
   teta = b + intercept + basvalue*BASVAL + trt*TREAT
    + vis4*VISIT_4 + vis5*VISIT_5 + vis6*VISIT_6 + vis7*VISIT_7
    + trtvis4*TREAT*VISIT_4 + trtvis5*TREAT*VISIT_5
    + trtvis6*TREAT*VISIT_6 + trtvis7*TREAT*VISIT_7
    + basvis4*BASVAL*VISIT_4 + basvis5*BASVAL*VISIT_5
    + basvis6*BASVAL*VISIT_6 + basvis7*BASVAL*VISIT_7;
   expteta=exp(teta);
   p=expteta/(1+expteta);
   model ybin ~ binary(p);
   random b ~ normal(0,sigma**2) subject=patient;
   run;
```

Output from Program 5.28

	Dimensions
Observations Used	700
Observations Not Used	150
Total Observations	850
Subjects	170

```
                     Max Obs Per Subject        5
                     Parameters                16
                     Quadrature Points          7
```

```
                            Parameters

intercept      TRT     basvalue       vis4       vis5       vis6
vis7

     0.5        0.5        0.5         0.5        0.5        0.5        0.5
```

```
                            Parameters

 trtvis4     trtvis5     trtvis6     trtvis7     basvis4     basvis5     basvis6

   0.5         0.5         0.5         0.5         0.5         0.5         0.5
```

```
                            Parameters

           basvis7        sigma      NegLogLike

             0.5           0.5       3480.03956
```

```
                        Iteration History

     Iter     Calls     NegLogLike        Diff      MaxGrad       Slope

       1         4      1501.64067     1978.399     6515.154      -167969
       2         6       656.936841     844.7038    1280.283     -5024.85
       3         7       566.431993      90.50485    410.2825     -135.178
       4         9       535.112938      31.31905   1220.039      -40.3054
       5        11       452.689732      82.42321    438.6939      -47.1849
     ...
      41        81       314.697481       0.000015     0.154422    -0.00001
      42        84       314.696451       0.00103      1.493996    -0.00002
      43        87       314.658342       0.038109     1.376788    -0.00197
      44        89       314.655269       0.003073     0.101871    -0.00555
      45        91       314.655261       7.317E-6     0.103042    -0.00001
      46        93       314.655137       0.000124     0.332802    -2.39E-6
        NOTE: GCONV convergence criterion satisfied.
```

```
                          Fit Statistics

         -2 Log Likelihood                    629.3
         AIC (smaller is better)              661.3
         AICC (smaller is better)             662.1
         BIC (smaller is better)              711.5
```

```
〜〜〜〜〜〜〜〜〜〜〜〜〜〜〜〜〜〜〜〜〜〜〜〜〜〜〜〜〜〜〜〜〜〜〜〜〜〜〜
                        Parameter Estimates


                  Standard
Parameter  Estimate   Error    DF  t Value  Pr > |t|  Alpha    Lower

intercept   -2.6113   1.2338   169  -2.12    0.0358    0.05   -5.0469
trt         -0.8769   0.7273   169  -1.21    0.2297    0.05   -2.3127
basvalue     0.1494   0.06879  169   2.17    0.0312    0.05    0.01363
vis4         0.6438   1.7768   169   0.36    0.7176    0.05   -2.8637
vis5        -0.9406   1.4956   169  -0.63    0.5302    0.05   -3.8930
vis6         0.1439   1.4144   169   0.10    0.9191    0.05   -2.6484
vis7        -0.3019   1.4292   169  -0.21    0.8329    0.05   -3.1233
trtvis4      0.5629   0.9645   169   0.58    0.5603    0.05   -1.3411
trtvis5      0.9815   0.8138   169   1.21    0.2295    0.05   -0.6250
trtvis6      1.6249   0.7711   169   2.11    0.0366    0.05    0.1026
trtvis7      0.5433   0.7665   169   0.71    0.4794    0.05   -0.9698
basvis4      0.2183   0.1124   169   1.94    0.0539    0.05   -0.00369
basvis5      0.1815   0.08909  169   2.04    0.0432    0.05    0.005601
basvis6      0.01497  0.07842  169   0.19    0.8488    0.05   -0.1398
basvis7      0.03718  0.07963  169   0.47    0.6412    0.05   -0.1200
sigma        2.3736   0.3070   169   7.73    <.0001    0.05    1.7675


                        Parameter Estimates

              Parameter    Upper    Gradient

              intercept   -0.1756   -0.00724
              trt          0.5590   -0.02275
              basvalue     0.2852   -0.3328
              vis4         4.1513   -0.00432
              vis5         2.0117   -0.07675
              vis6         2.9362    0.035626
              vis7         2.5194   -0.01581
              trtvis4      2.4668    0.009434
              trtvis5      2.5879   -0.10719
              trtvis6      3.1472    0.005033
              trtvis7      2.0565    0.032709
              basvis4      0.4403   -0.02261
              basvis5      0.3573   -0.06662
              basvis6      0.1698    0.208574
              basvis7      0.1944   -0.24876
              sigma        2.9798    0.000794
```

In the first part of the output, we observe that the number of quadrature points is seven. Next, an analysis of the initial parameters is given and the iteration history is listed. 'Diff' equals the change in negative log-likelihood from the previous step. The other statistics in the iteration history are specific to the selected numerical maximization algorithm.

The value for minus twice the maximized log-likelihood, as well as the values for associated information criteria, are printed under "Fit Statistics." Finally, parameter estimates, standard errors, approximate *t*-tests and confidence intervals are given.

To investigate the accuracy of the numerical integration method, we refit the model three times. The first one uses again the Gaussian quadrature and the default maximization algorithm (Quasi-Newton). The second one considers adaptive Gaussian quadrature and the Quasi-Newton algorithm, whereas the last one also makes use of the adaptive Gaussian quadrature and the Newton-Raphson algorithm. We look at these three programs for five different numbers of quadrature points (3, 5, 10, 20 and 50). Results are given in Table 5.16.

All three cases reveal that parameter estimates stabilize with an increasing number of quadrature points. However, the Gaussian quadrature method obviously needs more quadrature points than the

Table 5.16 Results of GLMM in the depression trial (interaction terms are not shown)

| | Gaussian quadrature, Quasi-Newton algorithm | | | | | | | | | |
| | Q=3 | | Q=5 | | Q=10 | | Q=20 | | Q=50 | |
	Est.	(S.E.)	Est.	(S.E.)	Est.	(S.E.)	Est.	(S.E.)	Est.	(S.E.)
intercept	−2.97	(1.20)	−2.78	(1.22)	−2.03	(1.27)	−2.33	(1.39)	−2.32	(1.34)
treatment	−0.56	(0.67)	−0.70	(0.71)	−1.29	(0.72)	−1.16	(0.72)	−1.16	(0.72)
baseline	0.16	(0.06)	0.15	(0.07)	0.14	(0.07)	0.15	(0.08)	0.15	(0.07)
visit 4	0.44	(1.79)	0.65	(1.80)	0.68	(1.73)	0.65	(1.75)	0.65	(1.75)
visit 5	−1.01	(1.48)	−0.96	(1.50)	−0.73	(1.50)	−0.79	(1.51)	−0.79	(1.51)
visit 6	0.13	(1.41)	0.09	(1.42)	0.26	(1.41)	0.21	(1.42)	0.21	(1.41)
visit 7	−0.25	(1.42)	−0.31	(1.43)	−0.20	(1.42)	−0.26	(1.43)	−0.25	(1.43)
σ	1.98	(0.24)	2.27	(0.28)	2.39	(0.32)	2.39	(0.31)	2.39	(0.32)
-2ℓ	639.5		630.9		629.6		629.4		629.4	

| | Adaptive Gaussian quadrature, Quasi-Newton algorithm | | | | | | | | | |
| | Q=3 | | Q=5 | | Q=10 | | Q=20 | | Q=50 | |
	Est.	(S.E.)	Est.	(S.E.)	Est.	(S.E.)	Est.	(S.E.)	Est.	(S.E.)
intercept	−2.27	(1.31)	−2.30	(1.33)	−2.32	(1.34)	−2.32	(1.34)	−2.32	(1.34)
treatment	−1.14	(0.70)	−1.16	(0.71)	−1.17	(0.72)	−1.16	(0.72)	−1.16	(0.72)
baseline	0.14	(0.07)	0.14	(0.07)	0.15	(0.07)	0.15	(0.07)	0.15	(0.07)
visit 4	0.67	(1.72)	0.67	(1.74)	0.65	(1.75)	0.65	(1.75)	0.65	(1.75)
visit 5	−0.77	(1.49)	−0.78	(1.50)	−0.79	(1.51)	−0.79	(1.51)	−0.79	(1.51)
visit 6	0.21	(1.41)	0.21	(1.41)	0.21	(1.41)	0.21	(1.41)	0.21	(1.41)
visit 7	−0.25	(1.42)	−0.25	(1.43)	−0.25	(1.43)	−0.25	(1.43)	−0.25	(1.43)
σ	2.27	(0.29)	2.34	(0.30)	2.39	(0.31)	2.39	(0.32)	2.39	(0.32)
-2ℓ	632.4		629.9		629.4		629.4		629.4	

| | Adaptive Gaussian quadrature, Newton-Raphson algorithm | | | | | | | | | |
| | Q=3 | | Q=5 | | Q=10 | | Q=20 | | Q=50 | |
	Est.	(S.E.)	Est.	(S.E.)	Est.	(S.E.)	Est.	(S.E.)	Est.	(S.E.)
intercept	−2.26	(1.31)	−2.29	(1.33)	−2.31	(1.34)	−2.31	(1.34)	−2.31	(1.34)
treatment	−1.17	(0.70)	−1.19	(0.71)	−1.20	(0.72)	−1.20	(0.72)	−1.20	(0.72)
baseline	0.14	(0.07)	0.14	(0.07)	0.15	(0.07)	0.15	(0.07)	0.15	(0.07)
visit 4	0.65	(1.72)	0.66	(1.74)	0.64	(1.75)	0.64	(1.75)	0.64	(1.75)
visit 5	−0.75	(1.49)	−0.77	(1.50)	−0.78	(1.51)	−0.78	(1.51)	−0.78	(1.51)
visit 6	0.18	(1.41)	0.18	(1.41)	0.19	(1.42)	0.19	(1.41)	0.19	(1.41)
visit 7	−0.28	(1.42)	−0.27	(1.43)	−0.27	(1.43)	−0.27	(1.43)	−0.27	(1.43)
σ	2.27	(0.29)	2.35	(0.30)	2.39	(0.31)	2.39	(0.32)	2.39	(0.32)
-2ℓ	632.4		629.9		629.4		629.40		629.40	

adaptive Gaussian quadrature. Focusing on the last column ($Q = 50$), we see that the parameter estimates for the first and the second version are almost equal. On the other hand, the parameter estimates of the third one are somewhat different. Another remarkable point is that the likelihood is the same in these three cases. A reason that the default and Newton-Raphson methods give other estimates could be that we are dealing with fairly flat likelihood. To confirm this idea, we ran the three programs again, but using the parameter estimates of the third one as starting values. This led to parameter estimates almost exactly equal in all cases.

Note that both WGEE and GLMM are valid under MAR, with the extra condition that the model for weights in WGEE has been specified correctly. Nevertheless, the parameter estimates between the two are rather different. This is because GEE and WGEE parameters have a marginal intepretation describing average longitudinal profiles, whereas GLMM parameters describe a longitudinal profile conditional upon the value of the random effects.

The following paragraphs provide an overview of the differences between marginal and random effects models for non-Gaussian outcomes. A detailed discussion can be found in Molenberghs and Verbeke (2003).

The interpretation of the parameters in both types of model (marginal or random effects) is completely different. A schematic display is given in Figure 5.10. Depending on the model family (marginal or random effects), one is led to either marginal or hierarchical inference. It is important to realize that in the general case the parameter β^M resulting from a marginal model is different from the parameter β^{RE}, even when the latter is estimated using marginal inference. Some of the confusion surrounding this issue may result from the equality of these parameters in the very special linear mixed model case. When a random effects model is considered, the marginal mean profile can be derived, but it will generally not produce a simple parametric form. In Figure 5.10 this is indicated by putting the corresponding parameter between quotes.

Figure 5.10 Representation of model families and corresponding inference. A superscript 'M' stands for marginal, 'RE' for random effects. A parameter between quotes indicates that marginal functions but no direct marginal parameters are obtained, since they result from integrating out the random effects from the fitted hierarchical model.

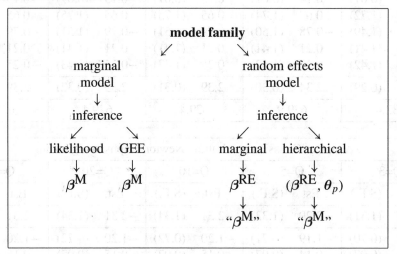

As an important example, consider our GLMM with logit link function, where the only random effects are intercepts b_i. It can then be shown that the marginal mean $\mu_i = E(Y_{ij})$ satisfies $h(\mu_i) \approx X_i \beta^M$ with

$$\frac{\beta^{RE}}{\beta^M} = \sqrt{c^2 \sigma^2 + 1} > 1, \tag{5.27}$$

in which c equals $16\sqrt{3}/15\pi$. Hence, although the parameters β^{RE} in the generalized linear mixed model have no marginal interpretation, they do show a strong relation to their marginal counterparts. Note that, as a consequence of this relation, larger covariate effects are obtained under the random effects model in comparison to the marginal model.

After this longitudinal analysis, we can also restrict attention to the last planned occasion. However, the very nature of MAR implies that one still explicitly wants to consider the incomplete profiles for use in the correct estimation of effects when incompleteness occurs. Thus, one has to consider the full longitudinal model. The analyses considered before will therefore be the basis.

Let α_i be the effect of treatment arm i at the last measurement occasion, where i can be A1 or C. We want to test whether at the last measurement occasion the effects of therapy A1 and the nonexperimental drug C are the same. This means $\alpha_{A1} = \alpha_C$, or similarly $\alpha_{A1} - \alpha_C = 0$. Using the parameter names as they are used in the SAS code (where C is the reference treatment), this translates to TRT. This hypothesis can easily be tested using the CONTRAST statement. The CONTRAST statement enables one to conduct a statistical test that several expressions simultaneously equal zero. The expressions are typically contrasts—that is, differences whose expected values equal zero under the hypothesis of interest. In the CONTRAST statement you must provide a quoted string to identify the contrast and then a list of valid SAS expressions separated by commas. Multiple CONTRAST statements are permitted, and results from all statements are listed in a common table. PROC NLMIXED constructs approximate F tests for each statement using the delta method to approximate the variance-covariance matrix of the constituent expressions.

In the NLMIXED procedure, we add only the following statement to Program 5.28:

```
contrast 'last visit' trt;
```

Note that the same result is found by looking at the ouput of TRT in the "Parameter Estimates" section.

Output from Program 5.28 with CONTRAST statement added

	Contrasts			
Label	Num DF	Den DF	F Value	Pr > F
last visit	1	169	2.81	0.0954

Since $p = 0.0954$, we retain a nonsignificant result.

5.11 MNAR and Sensitivity Analysis

Even though the assumption of likelihood ignorability encompasses both MAR and the more stringent and often implausible MCAR mechanisms, it is difficult to exclude the option of a more general missingness mechanism. One solution is to fit an MNAR model as proposed by Diggle and Kenward (1994), who fitted models to the full data using the simplex algorithm (Nelder and Mead, 1965). However, as pointed out by several authors in discussion of Diggle and Kenward (1994), one has to be extremely careful with interpreting evidence for or against MNAR using only the data under analysis. See also Verbeke and Molenberghs (2000, Chapter 18).

A sensible compromise between blindly shifting to MNAR models or ignoring them altogether is to make them a component of a sensitivity analysis. In that sense, it is important to consider the effect on key parameters such as treatment effect or evolution over time. One such route for sensitivity analysis is to consider pattern-mixture models as a complement to selection models (Thijs et al., 2002; Michiels et al., 2002). Further routes to explore sensitivity are based on global and local influence methods (Verbeke et al., 2001; Molenberghs et al., 2001). Robins, Rotnitzky and Scharfstein (1998) discuss sensitivity analysis in a semiparametric context.

The same considerations can be made when compliance data are available. In such a case, arguably, a definitive analysis would not be possible and it might be sensible to resort to sensitivity analysis ideas (Cowles, Carlin and Connett, 1996).

A full treatment of sensitivity analysis is beyond the scope of this chapter.

5.12 Summary

We have indicated that analyzing incomplete (longitudinal) data, both of a Gaussian as well as of a non-Gaussian nature, can easily be conducted under the relatively relaxed assumption of missingness at random (MAR) using standard statistical software tools. Likelihood-based methods include the linear mixed model (e.g., implemented in the SAS procedure MIXED) and generalized linear mixed models (e.g., implemented in the SAS procedure NLMIXED). In addition, weighted generalized estimating equations (WGEE) can be used as a relatively straightforward alteration of ordinary generalized estimating equations (GEE) so that also this technique is valid under MAR. Both theoretical considerations as well as illustrations using two case studies have been given. These methods are highly useful when inferential focus is on the entire longitudinal profile or aspects thereof, as well as when one is interested in a single measurement occasion only, e.g., the last planned one.

Alternative methods which allow ignoring the missing data mechanism under MAR include multiple imputation (MI) and the expectation-maximization (EM) algorithm.

All of this implies that traditionally popular but much more restricted modes of analysis, including complete case (CC) analysis, last observation carried forward (LOCF), or other simple imputation methods, ought to be abandoned, given the highly restrictive assumptions on which they are based.

Appendix

Chapter 1
%MinRisk Macro: Minimum Risk Test for Stratified Binary Data

```
%macro MinRisk(dataset);
/*
Inputs:

DATASET  = Input data set with event rates observed in each stratum.
           The input data set must include variables named EVENT1 (number
           of events of interest in Treatment group 1), EVENT2 (number of
           events of interest in Treatment group 2), NOEVENT1 (number of
           non-events in Treatment group 1), NOEVENT2 (number of non-events
           in Treatment group 2) with one record per stratum.
*/
proc iml;
    use &dataset;
    read all var {event1 noevent1 event2 noevent2} into data;
    m=nrow(data);
    p=j(m,2,0); n=j(m,2,0);
    n[,1]=data[,1]+data[,2];
    n[,2]=data[,3]+data[,4];
    total=sum(n);
    p[,1]=data[,1]/n[,1];
    p[,2]=data[,3]/n[,2];
    delta=p[,1]-p[,2];
    v=p[,1]#(1-p[,1])/n[,1]+p[,2]#(1-p[,2])/n[,2];
    pave=(p[,1]#n[,1]+p[,2]#n[,2])/(n[,1]+n[,2]);
    v0=pave#(1-pave)#(1/n[,1]+1/n[,2]);
    alpha=delta*sum(1/v)-sum(delta/v);
    c=1+alpha*sum((n[,1]+n[,2])#delta/total);
    h=diag(v*sum(1/v))+alpha*delta`;
    wmr=inv(h)*c;
    dmr=wmr`*delta;
    zmr1=abs(dmr)-3/(16*sum(n[,1]#n[,2]/(n[,1]+n[,2])));
    zmr2=sqrt(sum(wmr#wmr#v0));
    zmr=zmr1/zmr2;
    pmr=2*(1-probnorm(zmr));
    title={"Estimate", "Statistic", "P-value"};
    minrisk=dmr||zmr||pmr;
    print minrisk [colname=title format=best6.];
    win=(1/v)/sum(1/v);
```

```
        din=win'*delta;
        zin=abs(din)/sqrt(sum(win#win#v0));
        pin=2*(1-probnorm(zin));
        invar=din||zin||pin;
        print invar [colname=title format=best6.];
        wss=(n[,1]#n[,2]/(n[,1]+n[,2]))/sum(n[,1]#n[,2]/(n[,1]+n[,2]));
        dss=wss'*delta;
        zss=abs(dss)/sqrt(sum(wss#wss#v0));
        pss=2*(1-probnorm(zss));
        ssize=dss||zss||pss;
        print ssize [colname=title format=best6.];
        quit;
%mend MinRisk;
```

%GailSimon Macro: Gail-Simon Test for Qualitative Interaction

```
%macro GailSimon(dataset,est,stderr,testtype);
/*
Inputs:

DATASET  = Data set with test statistics and associated standard
           errors for each stratum.

EST      = Name of the variable containing the test statistics.

STDERR   = Name of the variable containing the standard errors.

TESTTYPE = P, N, T to carry out the one-sided Gail-Simon test
           for positive or negative differences or the two-sided
           Gail-Simon test, respectively.
*/
data pvalue;
    set &dataset nobs=m;
    format stat 6.3 p 6.4;
    retain qminus 0 qplus 0;
    qminus=qminus+(&est>0)*(&est/&stderr)**2;
    qplus=qplus+(&est<0)*(&est/&stderr)**2;
    if _n_=m then do;
        if upcase(&testtype)="P" then do; stat=qplus; df=m+1; end;
        if upcase(&testtype)="N" then do; stat=qminus; df=m+1; end;
        if upcase(&testtype)="T" then do; stat=min(qminus,qplus); df=m; end;
        p=0;
        do i=1 to df-1;
            p=p+pdf("binomial",i,0.5,df-1)*(1-probchi(stat,i));
        end;
    end;
    label stat="Test statistic" p="P-value";
    if _n_=m;
    keep stat p;
proc print data=pvalue noobs label;
    %if %upcase(&testtype)="P" %then %do;
        title "One-sided Gail-Simon test for positive differences"; %end;
    %if %upcase(&testtype)="N" %then %do;
        title "One-sided Gail-Simon test for negative differences"; %end;
    %if %upcase(&testtype)="T" %then %do;
        title "Two-sided Gail-Simon test"; %end;
```

```
        run;
%mend GailSimon;
```

%Pushback Macro: Pushback Test for Qualitative Interaction

```
%macro pushback(dataset,est,stderr,n,testtype,outdata);
/*
Inputs:

DATASET  = Data set with test statistics, associated standard
           errors and numbers of patients for each strata.

EST      = Name of the variable containing the test statistics.

STDERR   = Name of the variable containing the standard errors.

N        = Name of the variable containing the numbers of patients.

TESTTYPE = N, T to carry out the pushback test using the order
           statistics from a normal or t distribution, respectively.
*/
proc univariate data=&dataset noprint;
    var &est;
    weight &n;
    output out=med median=med;
data stand;
    set &dataset;
    if _n_=1 then set med;
    tau=(&est-med)/&stderr;
proc sort data=stand;
    by tau;
data &outdata;
    set stand nobs=m;
    ordstr=_n_;
    if upcase(&testtype)="N" then do;
        t=probit((3*ordstr-1)/(3*m+1));
    end;
    if upcase(&testtype)="T" then do;
        if ordstr<=m/2 then t=tinv(betainv(0.1,ordstr,m-ordstr+1),&n-2);
        if ordstr>m/2 then t=tinv(betainv(0.9,ordstr,m-ordstr+1),&n-2);
        if ordstr=(m+1)/2 then t=0;
    end;
    if tau*(tau-t)>0 then rho=tau-t;
    if tau*(tau-t)<=0 then rho=0;
    dstar=&stderr*rho+med;
    run;
%mend pushback;
```

Chapter 2

%GlobTest Macro: Global Tests for Multiple Endpoints

```
%macro GlobTest(dataset,group,ngroups,varlist,test);
/*
Inputs:
```

```
       DATASET = Data set to be analyzed

       GROUP   = Name of the group variable in the data set

       NGROUPS = Number of groups in the data set

       VARLIST = List of variable names corresponding to multiple endpoints

       TEST    = OLS, GLS, MGLS or RS, for OLS test, GLS test,
                 modified GLS test or rank-sum test, respectively
*/
%if &test="RS" %then %do;
proc rank data=&dataset out=ranks;
    var &varlist;
data comp;
    set ranks;
    array endp{*} &varlist;
    comp=0;
    do i=1 to dim(endp);
        comp=comp+endp{i};
    end;
proc mixed data=comp;
    class &group;
    model comp=&group;
    ods output tests3=pval;
data pval;
    set pval;
    format fvalue 5.2 ndf 3.0 ddf 3.0 adjp 6.4;
    ndf=numdf;
    ddf=dendf;
    adjp=probf;
    label fvalue="F-value" adjp="Global p-value";
    keep ndf ddf fvalue adjp;
%end;
%else %do;
%let m=1;
%let word=%scan(&varlist,&m);
%do %while (&word ne);
    %let m=%eval(&m+1);
    %let word=%scan(&varlist,&m);
%end;
%let m=%eval(&m-1);
data stand;
%do i=1 %to &m;
    %let var=%scan(&varlist,&i);
    proc glm data=&dataset;
        class &group;
        model &var=&group;
        ods output FitStatistics=est(keep=rootmse depmean);
    data stand;
        set stand est;
%end;
data stand;
    set stand;
    if rootmse^=.;
data _null_;
    set &dataset nobs=m;
```

```
        call symput("n",trim(put(m,5.0)));
proc corr data=&dataset outp=corr(where=(_type_="CORR"))
    noprint;
    var &varlist;
proc iml;
    use &dataset var{&varlist};
    read all into data;
    use stand var{depmean};

    read all into mean;
    meanmat=j(nrow(data),ncol(data),1)*diag(mean);
    use stand var{rootmse};
    read all into pooledsd;
    sdmat=inv(diag(pooledsd));
    use corr var{&varlist};
    read all into r;
    stand=(data-meanmat)*sdmat;
    rinv=inv(r);
    if &test="OLS" then comp=stand*j(&m,1);
    if &test="GLS" then comp=stand*rinv*j(&m,1);
    if &test="MGLS" then comp=stand*sqrt(diag(rinv))*j(&m,1);
    create comp from comp;
    append from comp;
data comp;
    merge comp &dataset;
    comp=col1;
    drop col1;
proc mixed data=comp;
    class &group;
    model comp=&group;
    ods output tests3=pval;
data pval;
    set pval;
    format fvalue 5.2 ndf 3.0 ddf 3.0 adjp 6.4;
    ndf=&ngroups-1;
    ddf=&n-&m*&ngroups;
    adjp=1-probf(fvalue,ndf,ddf);
    label fvalue="F-value" adjp="Global p-value";
    keep ndf ddf fvalue adjp;
%end;
proc print data=pval noobs label;
    run;
%mend GlobTest;
```

%GateKeeper Macro: Gatekeeping Procedures Based on Marginal Multiple Tests

```
%macro GateKeeper(dataset,test,outdata);
/*
Inputs:

DATASET = Data set with information about sequential families
          of hypotheses (testing type, weights, relative importance of
          gatekeeper hypotheses and raw p-values).

TEST    = B, MB, or S for Bonferroni, modified Bonferroni
          or Simes gatekeeping procedure, respectively.
```

```
            OUTDATA = Output data set with adjusted p-values.
        */
        proc iml;
            use &dataset;
            read all var {family serial weight relimp raw_p} into data;
            data=t(data);
            nhyps=ncol(data); nfams=data[1,ncol(data)]; nints=2**nhyps-1;
            h=j(nints,nhyps,0);

            do i=1 to nhyps;
                do j=0 to nints-1;
                    k=floor(j/2**(nhyps-i));
                    if k/2=floor(k/2) then h[j+1,i]=1;
                end;
            end;
            v=j(nints,nhyps,0); modv=j(nints,nhyps,0);
            hyp=j(nints,nhyps,0); adjp=j(nhyps,1,0);
            do i=1 to nints;
                r=1; tempv=j(1,nhyps,0); tempmodv=j(1,nhyps,0);
                do j=1 to nfams;
                    window=(data[1,]=j);
                    sumw=sum(window#data[3,]#h[i,]);
                    serial=sum(window#data[2,]);
                    if (serial=0 & j<nfams) & sumw>0 then do;
                        tempv=r#window#data[3,]#h[i,]#
                            ((1-data[4,])+data[4,]/sumw);
                        if sum(h[i,]#(data[1,]>j))=0 then
                        tempmodv=r#window#data[3,]#h[i,]/sumw;
                        else tempmodv=tempv;
                    end;
                    if (serial>0 | j=nfams) & sumw>0 then do;
                        tempv=r#window#data[3,]#h[i,]/sumw;
                        tempmodv=tempv;
                    end;
                    if sumw>0 then do;
                        r=r-sum(tempv); v[i,]=v[i,]+tempv;
                        modv[i,]=modv[i,]+tempmodv;
                    end;
                end;
                if &test="B" then hyp[i,]=h[i,]*
                    min(data[5,loc(v[i,])]/v[i,loc(v[i,])]);
                if &test="MB" then hyp[i,]=h[i,]*
                    min(data[5,loc(modv[i,])]/modv[i,loc(modv[i,])]);
                if &test="S" then do;
                    comb=data[5,loc(modv[i,])]//modv[i,loc(modv[i,])];
                    temp=comb;
                    comb[,rank(data[5,loc(modv[i,])])]=temp;
                    hyp[i,]=h[i,]*min(comb[1,]/cusum(comb[2,]));
                end;
            end;
            do i=1 to nhyps; adjp[i]=max(hyp[,i]); end;
            create adjp from adjp[colname={adjp}];
            append from adjp;
            quit;
        data &outdata;
            merge &dataset adjp;
```

```
        run;
%mend GateKeeper;
```

%ResamGate Macro: Resampling-Based Gatekeeping Procedures

```
%macro ResamGate(dataset,resp,test,outdata);
/*
Inputs:

DATASET = Data set with information about sequential families of hypotheses (testing type,
          weights, relative importance of gatekeeper hypotheses and raw p-values).

RESP    = Data set with p-values obtained via resampling.

TEST    = B, MB, or S for Bonferroni, modified Bonferroni
          or Simes gatekeeping procedure, respectively.

OUTDATA = Output data set with adjusted p-values.
*/
proc iml;
    use &dataset;
    read all var {family serial weight relimp raw_p} into data;
    data=t(data);
    use &resp;
    read all var _all_ into resp;
    nhyps=ncol(data); nfams=data[1,ncol(data)];
    nints=2**nhyps-1; nsims=nrow(resp);
    h=j(nints,nhyps,0);
    do i=1 to nhyps;
        do j=0 to nints-1;
            k=floor(j/2**(nhyps-i));
            if k/2=floor(k/2) then h[j+1,i]=1;
        end;
    end;
    v=j(nints,nhyps,0); modv=j(nints,nhyps,0);
    hyp=j(nints,nhyps,0); adjp=j(nhyps,1,0);
    start bonf(p,w);
        bonfp=min(p[loc(w)]/w[loc(w)]);
        return(bonfp);
    finish bonf;
    start simes(p,w);
        comb=t(p[loc(w)])//t(w[loc(w)]); temp=comb;
        comb[,rank(p[loc(w)])]=temp;
        simesp=min(comb[1,]/cusum(comb[2,]));
        return(simesp);
    finish simes;
    do i=1 to nints;
        r=1; tempv=j(1,nhyps,0); tempmodv=j(1,nhyps,0);
        do j=1 to nfams;
            window=(data[1,]=j);
            sumw=sum(window#data[3,]#h[i,]);
            serial=sum(window#data[2,]);
            if (serial=0 & j<nfams) & sumw>0 then do;
                tempv=r#window#data[3,]#h[i,]#
                    ((1-data[4,])+data[4,]/sumw);
                if sum(h[i,]#(data[1,]>j))=0 then
                tempmodv=r#window#data[3,]#h[i,]/sumw;
                else tempmodv=tempv;
```

```
            end;
            if (serial>0 | j=nfams) & sumw>0 then do;
                tempv=r#window#data[3,]#h[i,]/sumw;
                tempmodv=tempv;
            end;
            if sumw>0 then do;
                r=r-sum(tempv); v[i,]=v[i,]+tempv;
                modv[i,]=modv[i,]+tempmodv;
            end;
        end;
        if &test="B" then samp=bonf(data[5,],v[i,]);
        if &test="MB" then samp=bonf(data[5,],modv[i,]);
        if &test="S" then samp=simes(data[5,],modv[i,]);
        do j=1 to nsims;
            if &test="B" then resamp=bonf(resp[j,],v[i,]);
            if &test="MB" then resamp=bonf(resp[j,],modv[i,]);
            if &test="S" then resamp=simes(resp[j,],modv[i,]);
            hyp[i,]=hyp[i,]+h[i,]*(resamp<samp)/nsims;
        end;
    end;
    do i=1 to nhyps; adjp[i]=max(hyp[,i]); end;
    create adjp from adjp[colname={adjp}];
    append from adjp;
    quit;
data &outdata;
    merge &dataset adjp;
    run;
%mend ResamGate;
```

Chapter 3

QTCCONC Data Set (Change in the QTc Interval and Plasma Drug Concentration)

```
data qtcconc;
    input qtcchange conc @@;
    datalines;
-11 0.0 -12 0.0   0 0.0 -14 0.0 -11 0.0 -30 0.0  -8 0.0 -14 0.0   3 0.0
 11 0.0 -25 0.0   8 0.0  10 0.0 -29 0.1  10 0.1  -2 0.1  10 0.2   4 0.2
  0 0.2  12 0.2 -10 0.3 -11 0.3  -3 0.3  -4 0.3   2 0.3  -4 0.4  11 0.4
  1 0.4 -12 0.4   1 0.4   3 0.4  -8 0.4  24 0.5  -3 0.5   8 0.5  -1 0.5
 -1 0.6 -18 0.6   9 0.6  -5 0.6 -18 0.6   5 0.6  -8 0.6  11 0.6 -29 0.7
 21 0.7  -6 0.7 -23 0.7  11 0.8 -25 0.8   3 0.8   0 0.8   7 0.8  10 0.8
-13 0.9   8 0.9 -30 0.9   5 0.9   3 1.0   0 1.0   6 1.0  -8 1.0   3 1.0
 10 1.0   0 1.0   5 1.0 -15 1.0   6 1.0  -3 1.0  12 1.1  -7 1.1  12 1.2
 -4 1.2  11 1.2 -11 1.2   9 1.2   5 1.2   8 1.2  -1 1.2   1 1.2   2 1.2
 10 1.2  12 1.2   6 1.2 -16 1.2  16 1.3   7 1.3  10 1.3   2 1.3   3 1.3
  1 1.3  -4 1.4   8 1.4  10 1.5  10 1.5  -6 1.5  14 1.5  15 1.5   0 1.5
-18 1.5  -3 1.6   9 1.6 -25 1.6   5 1.6 -10 1.6 -20 1.6   0 1.6   5 1.6
 11 1.7 -28 1.7   9 1.7  -8 1.7 -18 1.8  11 1.8  14 1.8  16 1.8  12 1.8
 -2 1.8   6 1.9   7 1.9 -14 1.9 -22 1.9 -25 1.9  -6 1.9  -5 1.9  -6 1.9
 30 1.9   0 1.9 -25 2.0 -21 2.0   4 2.0  -5 2.0  10 2.0   3 2.0  -9 2.0
-25 2.0   6 2.0   1 2.0 -17 2.1  -9 2.1  20 2.1   7 2.1   2 2.1  21 2.1
-16 2.1   8 2.1   9 2.2  16 2.2  22 2.2   8 2.2  -4 2.2  -6 2.2  12 2.2
-14 2.2  12 2.2   0 2.3  21 2.3  -5 2.3  11 2.3  -8 2.3  -9 2.4 -13 2.4
  1 2.4 -11 2.4 -20 2.4 -12 2.5 -11 2.5   2 2.5  15 2.5   9 2.5 -27 2.5
```

```
    1 2.6    3 2.6    1 2.7   -3 2.7  -11 2.7    8 2.7   11 2.7    1 2.8   -4 2.8
   -8 2.8  -10 2.8   18 2.8    7 2.8   20 2.9   -5 3.0   24 3.0   -2 3.0    0 3.0
  -11 3.1  -11 3.1   14 3.1    5 3.2   17 3.3   22 3.3  -11 3.3   34 3.4    5 3.4
  -11 3.5   -1 3.5   10 3.5    2 3.7  -11 3.8    7 3.9  -10 3.9   -6 4.0  -11 4.0
  -11 4.0   17 4.0    0 4.0  -12 4.0  -24 4.0  -10 4.1   -3 4.1   18 4.1   -9 4.1
   -2 4.2    0 4.3   16 4.3  -12 4.3   -8 4.3    8 4.3   -6 4.4   -6 4.4   14 4.5
   11 4.5   -7 4.6   -1 4.6    5 4.6   22 4.7   18 4.7  -11 4.7    6 4.7    4 4.7
    2 4.8   22 4.8   12 4.8   12 4.8  -23 4.8    2 4.9   30 4.9   -7 4.9    8 4.9
  -11 4.9   15 4.9    0 4.9    3 4.9   13 5.0   -6 5.0   -8 5.0  -21 5.0   -9 5.1
   12 5.1  -12 5.1   -5 5.1   -2 5.1   -5 5.2  -15 5.2   -3 5.2   -4 5.2   19 5.2
   -9 5.3    8 5.4    0 5.4   18 5.4    0 5.4    9 5.4
   ;
```

RACOUNT Data Set (Patient Pain Assessment, Tender and Swollen Joints in a Rheumatoid Arthritis Trial)

```
data racount;
    input ptpain tjcount sjcount @@;
    datalines;
68 25 23   66 23 23   50 16 18   75 23 20   67 26 25   50 22 18   39 18 21
50 18 10   41  8  7   29 11  9   60 20 21   55 17 12   18  7  3   46 13 16
37  9 17   59 11 13   68 18 24   96 27 27   47 16 12   64 24 13   72 18 17
51 10  8   43 14 12   55 12 20   51 14 12   80 13 19   77 24 18   80 23  9
42 12 12   11 12 14   42  8  9   26 16 24   60  8  8   77 12  6   45 16 10
16  7  6   58  9  4   53 12 10   90 10 10   63 12 14   57 18 15   69 27 19
78 13 12   76 14 17   18  8 10   49 12 15   17  8 10   70 23 22   84 16 20
46 16 19   46  7 13   50  7 11   58  9 13   18  8 10   73 14 10   75 15 13
69 20 13   75 21 19   61 16 17   64 12 15   16  2 20   37  9 11   58 11 12
68 23 24   60  8 11   34 12 20   54 19 18   70 12 17   94 10  5   46 17 16
49 23 22   82 13 16   55 10 13   67 22 20   56 17 13   38 11  8   68 12 10
48 15 12   47 11  8   81 16 15   34 12  7   52 14 19   58 24 22   69 16 10
51  5  6   64 19 21   15 15 12   22 10 11   45 10 11   49 19 10   83 18 20
70 17  9   33 10 11   15 10  4   17 13  9   52 17 17   48  7  5   47  5  7
47 16 12   20  9  9   38 10  9   39 12 12   45 14 12   52 11  8   37  7 12
60 13 13   69 20  7   34 12 20   82 15 15   60  8  7   15  8  6   69 12 16
59 10 10   70 13  5   35 12 16   32  8 14   59  5 15   88 23 10   67 28 25
75 12 21   85 13 21   53 16 12   83 12 17   64 11 15   36  7 10  100 26 21
91 13 24   55 12 11   64 17 14   56 14 13   49  8 10   71 10 13   65 21 19
75 18 17   85 26 21   79 14 18   50 10 14   74 26 21   46 15 13   65 19 15
50 17 11   34  9  6   30 14  9   55 23 12   61 19 14   66  9  6   82 20 12
70 16 11   83 28 20   17 14 13   59 11 12   58  9  6   54 12  8   59  7  6
55  9  4   83 26 12   18 12 11   51 10 12   65 22 11   23 24 11   51 22 15
50 26 15   49 13 12   49  8  6   50  9  5   29  9  9   39 15 11   26 10 19
65 14 14   36 12 11   88 25 25   42  8 15   66 20 18   73 16 16   80 24 24
53 25 12   82 21 21   73 16 13   89 25 14   86 24 13   37 20 16   39 10  9
31  6  4   50 11  6   25  6  4   18  9  7   18 12 14   46 13  5   39  8 14
60 19 19   58 21 15   68 12 16   56  6  6   50 16 20   56 10  5   31 12  9
70 16 14   77 12 15   54 11  7   53 24 20   68 16  9   77 18 14   42 16 12
67 26 25   76 26 14   51 16 10   20 26 24   92 14  7   60 18 11   48 25 23
71 17 13   66 13 11   74  9 11   75 14 13   66 18 14   44 13 12   41 10  9
34 23 18   50 24 21   41  9 12   57 18 10   64 15 13   67 15 14   47 17 15
61 19 17   64 24 18   58 11 11   42 14 12   16  7  6   39 23 20   23 11 10
64 18  6   85 12  7   68  9  9   51 15  5    9 10  7   41 17  8   80 22 18
78 18 15   69  8  6   19 13  9   60 23 16   47  9  4   38 14 14   77 19 10
68 14 11   87 24 17   60 22 21   82 24 23   31 21 21   77  7  8
    ;
```

%GlobalQSmooth Macro: A Polynomial Approximation to the Conditional Quantile Function

```
/**********************************************************
Inputs:

DATASET = Data set to be analyzed

GRID    = Data set with grid points (X variable)

GAMMA   = Quantile of the conditional distribution function

P       = Degree of the polynomial approximation

OUTDATA = Output data set containing the polynomial (POLY variable),
          its first derivative (FIRSTDER variable) and second derivative
          (SECDER variable) evaluated at the grid points
**********************************************************/

%macro GlobalQSmooth(dataset,grid,gamma,p,outdata);
data variable;
    set &dataset;
    array cov{*} cov1-cov&p;
    do i=1 to &p; cov{i}=x**i; end;
proc mixed data=variable;
    model y=cov1-cov&p/s;
    ods output SolutionF=param;
data equation;
    set param nobs=m;
    retain c0-c&p;
    if effect="Intercept" then c0=estimate;
    call symput("c0",compress(put(c0,best8.)));
    %do i=1 %to &p;
        if effect="cov&i" then c&i=estimate;
        call symput("c&i",compress(put(c&i,best8.)));
    %end;
    if _n_=m;
    run;
proc nlin data=variable nohalve maxiter=500 converge=0.0005;
    parms c0=&c0 %do i=1 %to &p; c&i=&&c&i %end;;
    model y=c0 %do i=1 %to &p; +c&i*cov&i %end;;
    der.c0=1;
    %do i=1 %to &p; der.c&i=cov&i; %end;
    resid=y-model.y;
    if resid>0 then _weight_=&gamma/resid;
    if resid<0 then _weight_=(&gamma-1)/resid;
    if resid=0 then _weight_=0;
    ods output ParameterEstimates=est;
data coef;
    set est nobs=m;
    retain d0-d&p;
    %do i=0 %to &p;
        if parameter="c&i" then d&i=estimate;
    %end;
    if _n_=m;
data &outdata;
    set &grid;
```

```
    if _n_=1 then set coef;
    array d{*} d1-d&p;
    poly=d0; firstder=d1;
    if &p>=2 then secder=2*d2; else secder=0;
    do i=1 to &p;
        poly=poly+d{i}*x**i;
        if i>=2 then firstder=firstder+i*d{i}*x**(i-1);
        if i>=3 then secder=secder+(i-1)*i*d{i}*x**(i-2);
    end;
    run;
%mend GlobalQSmooth;
```

%LocalQSmooth Macro: A Local Linear Approximation to the Conditional Quantile Function

```
/*************************************************************
Inputs:

DATASET = Data set to be analyzed

GAMMA   = Quantile of the conditional distribution function

INITIAL = Data set with the grid points (X variable),
          initial values of the intercept and slope
          of the local linear model (POLY and FIRSTDER variables)
          and the bandwidth parameter (H variable)

OUTDATA = Output data set containing the local estimates
          of the quantile function evaluated at the grid points
          (ESTIMATE variable)
*************************************************************/
%macro LocalQSmooth(dataset,gamma,initial,outdata);
data quantile;
data _null_;
    set &initial nobs=m;
    call symput("n",m);
run;
%do i=1 %to &n;
data _null_;
    set &initial;
    if _n_=&i then do;
        call symput("x",x);
        call symput("inita",poly);
        call symput("initb",firstder);
        call symput("h",h);
    end;
    run;
proc nlin data=&dataset nohalve noitprint maxiter=300 converge=0.001;
    parms a=&inita b=&initb;
    model y=a+b*(x-&x);
    der.a=1; der.b=x-&x; resid=y-model.y;
    if resid>0 then w1=&gamma/resid;
    if resid<0 then w1=(&gamma-1)/resid;
    if resid=0 then w1=0;
    w2=pdf("normal",(x-&x)/&h)/&h; _weight_=w1*w2;
    ods output ParameterEstimates=est(where=(parameter="a"));
data result;
```

```
    set est;
    x=&x;
data quantile;
    set quantile result;
    keep x estimate;
%end;
data &outdata;
    set quantile;
    where x^=.;
    run;
%mend LocalQSmooth;
```

%TolLimit Macro: Computation of Two-Sided and One-Sided Tolerance Intervals

```
/********************************************************
Inputs:

DATASET = Data set to be analyzed

VAR     = Variable for which tolerance limits will be computed

GAMMA   = Content of the tolerance interval

BETA    = Confidence of the tolerance interval

OUTDATA = Data set with one-sided and two-sided tolerance limits

********************************************************/
%macro TolLimit(dataset,var,gamma,beta,outdata);
data _null_;
    set &dataset nobs=m;
    call symput("n",compress(put(m,6.0)));
    run;
data _null_;
    prev1=probbeta(&gamma,&n,1);
    do s=2 to &n;
        next1=probbeta(&gamma,&n-s+1,s);
        if prev1<=1-&beta and next1>1-&beta then
            call symput("rank1",compress(put(s-1,6.0)));
        prev1=next1;
    end;
prev2=probbeta(&gamma,&n-1,2);
    do s=2 to &n/2;
        next2=probbeta(&gamma,&n-2*s+1,2*s);
        if prev2<=1-&beta and next2>1-&beta then
            call symput("rank2",compress(put(s-1,6.0)));
        prev2=next2;
    end;
    run;
proc rank data=&dataset out=ranks;
    var &var;
    ranks ranky;
proc sort data=ranks;
    by ranky;
```

```
data upper1;
    set ranks;
    if ranky>&n-&rank1+1 then delete;
data _null_;
    set upper1 nobs=m;
    if _n_=m then call symput("upper1",compress(put(&var,best8.)));
data upper2;
    set ranks;
    if ranky>&n-&rank2+1 then delete;
data _null_;
    set upper2 nobs=m;
    if _n_=m then call symput("upper2",compress(put(&var,best8.)));
data lower2;
    set ranks;
    if ranky>&rank2 then delete;
data _null_;
    set lower2 nobs=m;
    if _n_=m then call symput("lower2",compress(put(&var,best8.)));
    run;
data &outdata;
    upper1=&upper1; lower2=&lower2; upper2=&upper2;
    label upper1="Upper one-sided tolerance limit"
          upper2="Upper two-sided tolerance limit"
          lower2="Lower two-sided tolerance limit";
    run;
%mend TolLimit;
```

%VarPlot Macro: Examination of Trends and Variability in Data Sets with Bivariate Measurements

```
/***********************************************************
Inputs:

DATASET = Data set to be analyzed

GRID    = Data set with the grid points (X variable)

Q1, Q2, Q3
        = Low, middle and upper quantiles to be estimated

H       = Bandwidth parameter for local smoothing

OUTDATA = Output data set containing the local estimates
          of the three quantile functions evaluated at the grid points
          (ESTIMATE variable) as well as the raw data points
***********************************************************/
%macro VarPlot(dataset,grid,q1,q2,q3,h,outdata);
%GlobalQSmooth(dataset=&dataset,grid=&grid,gamma=&q1,p=5,outdata=upper);
%GlobalQSmooth(dataset=&dataset,grid=&grid,gamma=&q2,p=5,outdata=mid);
%GlobalQSmooth(dataset=&dataset,grid=&grid,gamma=&q3,p=5,outdata=lower);
data initial;
    set upper; h=&h;
%LocalQSmooth(dataset=&dataset,gamma=&q1,initial=initial,outdata=q1);
data initial;
    set mid; h=&h;
%LocalQSmooth(dataset=&dataset,gamma=&q2,initial=initial,outdata=q2);
```

```
data initial;
    set lower; h=&h;
%LocalQSmooth(dataset=&dataset,gamma=&q3,initial=initial,outdata=q3);
data q1;
    set q1;
    quantile=1;
data q2;
    set q2;
    quantile=2;
data q3;
    set q3;
    quantile=3;
data rawdata;
    set &dataset;
    quantile=0;
    estimate=y;
data &outdata;
    set q1 q2 q3 rawdata;
%mend VarPlot;
```

Chapter 4
%EffDesign Macro: Design of Group Sequential Trials for Efficacy Testing

```
%macro EffDesign(fraction, effsize, power, alpha, rho, boundary, sizepower);
/***********************************************************
Inputs:
FRACTION = Input data set that contains fractions of the total sample
           size accrued at successive analyses

EFFSIZE  = True effect size

POWER    = Power

ALPHA    = One-sided Type I error probability

RHO      = Shape parameter of stopping boundary

           (0.5 if Pocock boundary and 0 if O'Brien-Fleming boundary)

BOUNDARY = Output data set that contains stopping probabilities at scheduled
           looks

SIZEPOWER= Output data set that contains average sample number and power for
           selected effect sizes

***********************************************************/
proc iml;
    start DriftSearch(d) global(m,critvalue,stfract,inc,infinity);
        upper=critvalue*stfract##&rho;
        adjustment=d*stfract;
        boundary=infinity//(upper-adjustment);
        call seq(p,boundary) eps=1e-8 tscale=inc;
        diff=abs(1-&power-(p[2,]-p[1,])[m]);
        return(diff);
    finish;
```

```
use &fraction;
read all var _all_ into fraction;
m=nrow(fraction);
fract=t(fraction);
stfract=fract/fract[1];
inc=j(1,m-1,0);
do i=1 to m-1;
    inc[i]=(fract[i+1]-fract[i])/fract[1];
end;
infinity=repeat(.m,1,m);
upper=stfract##&rho;
boundary=infinity//upper;
call seqscale(prob,critvalue,boundary,1-&alpha) eps=1e-8 tscale=inc;
upper=critvalue*stfract##&rho;
boundary=infinity//upper;
stopz=critvalue*stfract##(&rho-0.5);
stopp=1-probnorm(stopz);
call seq(prob0,boundary) eps=1e-8 tscale=inc;
nfixed=2*((probit(&power)+probit(1-&alpha))/&effsize)**2;
start=&effsize*sqrt(nfixed*fract[1]/2);
tc=repeat(.,1,12);
tc[1]=100;
tc[3]=1e-5;
call nlpdd(rc,drift,"DriftSearch",start) tc=tc;
max=2*(drift/&effsize)*(drift/&effsize)/fract[1];
upper=critvalue*stfract##&rho;
adjustment=drift*stfract;
boundary=infinity//(upper-adjustment);
call seq(prob1,boundary) eps=1e-8 tscale=inc;
&boundary=j(m,8,0);
&boundary[,1]=t(1:m);
&boundary[,2]=ceil(cusum(fraction)*max);
&boundary[,3]=t(stopz);
&boundary[,4]=t(stopp);
&boundary[,5]=t(prob0[3,]-prob0[2,]+prob0[1,]);
&boundary[,6]=t(cusum(prob0[3,]-prob0[2,]+prob0[1,]));
&boundary[,7]=t(prob1[3,]-prob1[2,]+prob1[1,]);
&boundary[,8]=t(cusum(prob1[3,]-prob1[2,]+prob1[1,]));
varnames={"Analysis", "Size", "TestStBoundary", "PValBoundary", "ProbH0",
    "CumProbH0", "ProbH1", "CumProbH1"};
create &boundary from &boundary[colname=varnames];
append from &boundary;
&sizepower=j(21,3,0);
do i=0 to 20;
    upper=critvalue*stfract##&rho;
    adjustment=i*&effsize*sqrt(max*fract[1]/2)*stfract/10;
    boundary=infinity//(upper-adjustment);
    call seq(prob2,boundary) eps=1e-8 tscale=inc;
    stop=prob2[3,]-prob2[2,]+prob2[1,];
    &sizepower[i+1,1]=i*&effsize/10;
    &sizepower[i+1,2]=ceil(max*(1-(1-fract)*stop`));
    &sizepower[i+1,3]=1-(prob2[2,]-prob2[1,])[m];
end;
varnames={"EffSize", "AveSize", "Power"};
create &sizepower from &sizepower[colname=varnames];
append from &sizepower;
summary=j(1,4,0);
```

```
        summary[1]=ceil(max); summary[2]=&sizepower[1,2];
        summary[3]=&sizepower[11,2];
        summary[4]=ceil(nfixed);
        create summary from summary;
        append from summary;
        quit;
data summary;
        set summary;
        format value best6.;
        length par $50;
        par="One-sided Type I error probability";
            value=&alpha; output;
        par="Power"; value=&power; output;
        par="True effect size"; value=&effsize; output;
        par="Stopping boundary parameter"; value=&rho; output;
        par="Maximum sample size per group"; value=col1; output;
        par="Average sample size per group under H0"; value=col2; output;
        par="Average sample size per group under H1"; value=col3; output;
        par="Fixed sample size per group"; value=col4; output;
        label par="Summary" value="Value";
        keep par value;
proc print data=summary noobs label;
        var par value;
data &boundary;
        set &boundary;
        format TestStBoundary PValBoundary ProbH0 CumProbH0 ProbH1 CumProbH1 6.4
            Analysis Size 4.0;
        label Analysis="Analysis"
              Size="Sample size per group"
              TestStBoundary="Stopping boundary (test statistic scale)"
              PValBoundary="Stopping boundary (p-value scale)"
              ProbH0="Stopping probability under H0"
              CumProbH0="Cumulative stopping probability under H0"
              ProbH1="Stopping probability under H1"
              CumProbH1="Cumulative stopping probability under H1";
data &sizepower;
        set &sizepower;
        format EffSize best6. AveSize 5.0;
        label EffSize="True effect size"
              AveSize="Average sample size per group"
              Power="Power";
        run;
%mend EffDesign;
```

%EffFutDesign Macro: Design of Group Sequential Trials for Simultaneous Efficacy and Futility Testing

```
%macro EffFutDesign(fraction, effsize, power, alpha, rhoeff, rhofut,
boundary, sizepower);
/***********************************************************
Inputs:
FRACTION = Input data set that contains fractions of the total sample
           size accrued at successive analyses

EFFSIZE  = True effect size
```

```
POWER     = Power

ALPHA     = One-sided Type I error probability

RHOEFF    = Shape parameter of upper (efficacy) stopping boundary
            (0.5 if Pocock boundary and 0 if O'Brien-Fleming boundary)

RHOFUT    = Shape parameter of lower (futility) stopping boundary
            (0.5 if Pocock boundary and 0 if O'Brien-Fleming boundary)

BOUNDARY = Output data set that contains stopping probabilities at scheduled
            looks

SIZEPOWER= Output data set that contains average sample number and power for
            selected effect sizes

*********************************************************/
proc iml;
    start ParSearch(c) global(m,lastlook,stfract,inc);
        drift=(c[1]*lastlook##&rhoeff+c[2]*lastlook##&rhofut)/lastlook;
        upper=c[1]*stfract##&rhoeff;
        lower=drift*stfract-c[2]*stfract##&rhofut;
        lower[m]=lower[m]-1e-5;
        boundary=lower//upper;
        call seq(p,boundary) eps=1e-8 tscale=inc;
        crossh0=sum(p[3,]-p[2,])-&alpha;
        adjustment=drift*stfract;
        boundary=(lower-adjustment)//(upper-adjustment);
        call seq(p,boundary) eps=1e-8 tscale=inc;
        crossh1=sum(p[3,]-p[2,])-&power;
        diff=abs(crossh0)+abs(crossh1);
        return(diff);
    finish;
    use &fraction;
    read all var _all_ into fraction;
    m=nrow(fraction);
    fract=t(fraction);
    stfract=fract/fract[1];
    inc=j(1,m-1,0);
    do i=1 to m-1;
        inc[i]=(fract[i+1]-fract[i])/fract[1];
    end;
    lastlook=stfract[m];
    nfixed=2*((probit(&power)+probit(1-&alpha))/&effsize)**2;
    start={1 1};
    tc=repeat(.,1,12);
    tc[1]=100;
    tc[3]=1e-5;
    call nlpdd(rc,c,"ParSearch",start) tc=tc;
    drift=(c[1]*lastlook##&rhoeff+c[2]*lastlook##&rhofut)/lastlook;
    upper=c[1]*stfract##&rhoeff;
    lower=drift*stfract-c[2]*stfract##&rhofut;
    lower[m]=lower[m]-1e-5;
    boundary=lower//upper;
    call seq(prob0,boundary) eps=1e-8 tscale=inc;
    adjustment=drift*stfract;
```

```
        boundary=(lower-adjustment)//(upper-adjustment);
        call seq(prob1,boundary) eps=1e-8 tscale=inc;
        upperz=(stfract##(-0.5))#upper;
        lowerz=(stfract##(-0.5))#lower;
        upperp=1-probnorm(upperz);
        lowerp=1-probnorm(lowerz);
        max=2*(drift/&effsize)*(drift/&effsize)/fract[1];
        boundary=j(m,10,0);
        boundary[,1]=t(1:m);
        boundary[,2]=ceil(cusum(fraction)*max);
        boundary[,3]=t(lowerz);
        boundary[,4]=t(upperz);
        boundary[,5]=t(lowerp);
        boundary[,6]=t(upperp);
        boundary[,7]=t(prob0[3,]-prob0[2,]+prob0[1,]);
        boundary[,8]=t(cusum(prob0[3,]-prob0[2,]+prob0[1,]));
        boundary[,9]=t(prob1[3,]-prob1[2,]+prob1[1,]);
        boundary[,10]=t(cusum(prob1[3,]-prob1[2,]+prob1[1,]));
        varnames={"Analysis", "Size", "LowerTestStBoundary", "UpperTestStBoundary",
            "LowerPValBoundary", "UpperPValBoundary",
            "ProbH0", "CumProbH0", "ProbH1", "CumProbH1"};
        create &boundary from boundary[colname=varnames];
        append from boundary;
        sizepower=j(21,3,0);
        do i=0 to 20;
            adjustment=i*drift*stfract/10;
            boundary=(lower-adjustment)//(upper-adjustment);
            call seq(prob2,boundary) eps=1e-8 tscale=inc;
            stop=prob2[3,]-prob2[2,]+prob2[1,];
            sizepower[i+1,1]=i*&effsize/10;
            sizepower[i+1,2]=ceil(max*(1-(1-fract)*stop`));
            sizepower[i+1,3]=sum(prob2[3,]-prob2[2,]);*1-(prob2[2,]-prob2[1,])[m];
        end;
        varnames={"EffSize", "AveSize", "Power"};
        create &sizepower from sizepower[colname=varnames];
        append from sizepower;
        summary=j(1,4,0);
        summary[1]=ceil(max); summary[2]=sizepower[1,2]; summary[3]=sizepower[11,2];
        summary[4]=ceil(nfixed);
        create summary from summary;
        append from summary;
        quit;
data summary;
        set summary;
        format value best6.;
        length par $50;
        par="One-sided Type I error probability"; value=&alpha; output;
        par="Power"; value=&power; output;
        par="True effect size"; value=&effsize; output;
        par="Shape parameter of upper boundary"; value=&rhoeff; output;
        par="Shape parameter of lower boundary"; value=&rhofut; output;
        par="Maximum sample size per group"; value=col1; output;
        par="Average sample size per group under H0"; value=col2; output;
        par="Average sample size per group under H1"; value=col3; output;
        par="Fixed sample size per group"; value=col4; output;
        label par="Summary" value="Value";
        keep par value;
```

```
proc print data=summary noobs label;
    var par value;
data &boundary;
    set &boundary;
    format LowerTestStBoundary UpperTestStBoundary LowerPValBoundary
        UpperPValBoundary ProbH0 CumProbH0 ProbH1 CumProbH1 6.4
        Analysis Size 4.0;
    label Analysis="Analysis"
        Size="Sample size per group"
        LowerTestStBoundary="Lower stopping boundary (test statistic scale)"
        UpperTestStBoundary="Upper stopping boundary (test statistic scale)"
        LowerPValBoundary="Lower stopping boundary (p-value scale)"
        UpperPValBoundary="Upper stopping boundary (p-value scale)"
        ProbH0="Stopping probability under H0"
        CumProbH0="Cumulative stopping probability under H0"
        ProbH1="Stopping probability under H1"
        CumProbH1="Cumulative stopping probability under H1";
data &sizepower;
    set &sizepower;
    format EffSize best6. AveSize 5.0;
    label EffSize="True effect size"
        AveSize="Average sample size per group"
        Power="Power";
    run;
%mend EffFutDesign;
```

%EffMonitor Macro: Efficacy Monitoring of Group Sequential Trials

```
%macro EffMonitor(fraction, data, effsize, power, alpha, rho, spfunction,
sprho, decision, inference);
/**********************************************************
Inputs:
FRACTION  = Input data set that contains fractions of the total sample
            size accrued at successive analyses.

DATA      = Input data set containing summary statistics computed at each
            analysis. The data set must include the following two variables:
            N is the number of patients in each treatment group (or the
            average of the numbers of patients if they are not the same)
            and STAT is the value of a normally distributed test statistic.

EFFSIZE   = True effect size.

POWER     = Power.

ALPHA     = One-sided Type I error probability.

RHO       = Shape parameter of stopping boundary
            (0.5 if Pocock boundary and 0 if O'Brien-Fleming boundary).

SPFUNCTION= Error spending function code (1, design-based function;
            2, ten-look function; 3, a function the Lan-DeMets family;
            4, a function from the Jennison-Turnbull family;
            5, a function from the Hwang-Shih-DeCani family).

SPRHO     = Shape parameter of the error spending function.
```

```
DECISION  = Output data set that contains stopping boundaries and
            probabilities as well as one-sided repeated confidence
            intervals for treatment difference at each interim look.

INFERENCE = Output data set containing bias-adjusted estimate of treatment
            effect with a one-sided confidence interval computed at the
            last look.


*************************************************************/
proc iml;
    start DriftSearch(d) global(m,critvalue,stfract,inc,infinity);
        upper=critvalue*stfract##&rho;
        adjustment=d*stfract;
        boundary=infinity//(upper-adjustment);
        call seq(p,boundary) eps=1e-8 tscale=inc;
        diff=abs(1-&power-(p[2,]-p[1,])[m]);
        return(diff);
    finish;
    start BoundSearch(new) global(stage,alpha,adjbound,sinf,infinc);
        alphainc=alpha[stage]-alpha[stage-1];
        tempb=t(adjbound[1:stage]#sqrt(sinf[1:stage]));
        tempb[stage]=new*sqrt(sinf[stage]);
        tempinf=repeat(.m,1,stage);
        tempinc=t(infinc[1:stage-1]);
        boundary=tempinf//tempb;
        call seq(p,boundary) eps=1e-8 tscale=tempinc;
        diff=abs(p[3,stage]-p[2,stage]-alphainc);
        return(diff);
    finish;
    start AdjQuant(est) global(quantile,sall,observed,tempinc,infinity);
        adjustment=est*sall;
        upper=observed#(sall##0.5);
        boundary=infinity//(upper-adjustment);
        call seq(prob,boundary) eps=1e-8 tscale=tempinc;
        sss=sum(prob[3,]-prob[2,]);
        diff=abs(quantile-sss);
        return(diff);
    finish;
    use &fraction;
    read all var _all_ into fraction;
    m=nrow(fraction);
    fract=t(fraction);
    stfract=fract/fract[1];
    inc=j(1,m-1,0);
    do i=1 to m-1;
        inc[i]=(fract[i+1]-fract[i])/fract[1];
    end;
    infinity=repeat(.m,1,m);
    upper=stfract##&rho;
    boundary=infinity//upper;
    call seqscale(prob,critvalue,boundary,1-&alpha) eps=1e-8 tscale=inc;
    upper=critvalue*stfract##&rho;
    boundary=infinity//upper;
    call seq(prob1,boundary) eps=1e-8 tscale=inc;
    spend1=cusum(prob1[3,]-prob1[2,]+prob1[1,]);
    beta=1-&power;
    nfixed=2*((probit(&power)+probit(1-&alpha))/&effsize)**2;
```

```
start=&effsize*sqrt(nfixed*fract[1]/2);
tc=repeat(.,1,12);
tc[1]=100;
tc[3]=1e-5;
call nlpdd(rc,drift,"DriftSearch",start) tc=tc;
max=2*(drift/&effsize)*(drift/&effsize)/fract[1];
use &data;
read all var {n stat} into mon;
n=nrow(mon);
ss=mon[,1];
infofrac=ss/max;
statistic=mon[,2];
pvalue=1-probnorm(mon[,2]);
sinf=infofrac/infofrac[1];
if n>1 then do;
    infinc=j(1,n-1,0);
    do i=1 to n-1;
        infinc[i]=sinf[i+1]-sinf[i];
    end;
end;
else infinc=j(1,1,1);
alpha=j(n,1,0);
level=j(n,1,0);
adjbound=j(n,1,0);
tc=repeat(.,1,12);
tc[1]=200;
tc[3]=1e-6;
* Design-based error spending function;
if &spfunction=1 then
do;
    t=0 || fract;
    s=0 || spend1;
    do stage=1 to n;
        x=infofrac[stage];
        do i=1 to m;
            if t[i]<=x & x<t[i+1] then
                alpha[stage]=(s[i+1]*(x-t[i])+s[i]*(t[i+1]-x))/

        (t[i+1]-t[i]);
         end;
         if x>=1 then alpha[stage]=&alpha;
    end;
end;
* Ten-look error spending function;
if &spfunction=2 then
do;
    k=10;
    infinity=repeat(.m,1,k);
    upper=(1:k)###&rho;
    boundary=infinity//upper;
    call seqscale(prob,critvalue,boundary,1-&alpha) eps=1e-8;
    upper=critvalue*(1:k)###&rho;
    boundary=infinity//upper;
    call seq(prob0,boundary) eps=1e-8;
    spend=t(cusum(prob0[3,]-prob0[2,]+prob0[1,]));
    do stage=1 to n;
        x=infofrac[stage];
```

```
            if x<1 then do;
                l=floor(k*x); u=floor(k*x)+1;
                alpha[stage]=spend[l]+(k*x-1)*(spend[u]-spend[l])/(u-1);
            end;
            if x>=1 then alpha[stage]=&alpha;
        end;
end;
* Lan-DeMets error spending function;
if &spfunction=3 then
do;
    do stage=1 to n;
        x=infofrac[stage];
        if x<1 & &sprho=0 then alpha[stage]=2-
            2*probnorm(probit(1-&alpha/2)/sqrt(x));
        if x<1 & &sprho=0.5 then alpha[stage]=&alpha*log(1+(exp(1)-1)*x);
        if x>=1 then alpha[stage]=&alpha;
    end;
end;
* Jennison-Turnbull error spending function;
if &spfunction=4 then
do;
    do stage=1 to n;
        x=infofrac[stage];
        if x<1 then alpha[stage]=&alpha*(x**&sprho);
        if x>=1 then alpha[stage]=&alpha;
    end;
end;
* Hwang-Shih-DeCani error spending function;
if &spfunction=5 then
do;
    do stage=1 to n;
        x=infofrac[stage];
        if x<1 & &sprho^=0 then alpha[stage]=
            &alpha*(1-exp(-&sprho*x))/(1-exp(-&sprho));
        if x<1 & &sprho=0 then alpha[stage]=&alpha*x;
        if x>=1 then alpha[stage]=&alpha;
    end;
end;
do stage=1 to n;
    if stage=1 then do;
        adjbound[1]=probit(1-alpha[1]);
        level[1]=alpha[1];
    end;
    if stage>1 then do;
        new=probit(1-alpha[stage]);
        call nlpdd(rc,adj,"BoundSearch",new) tc=tc;
        adjbound[stage]=adj;
        level[stage]=1-probnorm(adj);
    end;
end;
lowercl=(statistic-adjbound)#sqrt(2/ss);
reject=(statistic>adjbound);
stop=0;
do i=1 to n;
    if reject[i]=1 & stop=0 then stop=i;
end;
if stop=0 then last=n; else last=stop;
```

```
observed=t(adjbound[1:last]);
observed[last]=statistic[last];
tall=t(ss[1:last]);
k=ncol(tall);
tall=tall/tall[k];
sall=tall/tall[1];
tempinc=j(1,k-1,0);
do i=1 to k-1;
    tempinc[i]=sall[i+1]-sall[i];
end;
infinity=repeat(.m,1,k);
tc=repeat(.,1,12);
tc[1]=100;
tc[3]=1e-5;
inference=j(2,1,.);
quantile=0.5;
est=statistic[last];
call nlpdd(rc,qest,"AdjQuant",est) tc=tc;
qest=&effsize*qest/drift;
inference[1]=qest;
quantile=&alpha;
est=((statistic-probit(1-&alpha))#sqrt(2/ss))[last];
est=est*drift/&effsize;
call nlpdd(rc,qest,"AdjQuant",est) tc=tc;
qest=&effsize*qest/drift;
inference[2]=qest;
create &inference from inference;
append from inference;
&decision=j(last,9,0);
&decision[,1]=t(1:last);
&decision[,2]=ss[1:last];
&decision[,3]=infofrac[1:last];
&decision[,4]=statistic[1:last];
&decision[,5]=pvalue[1:last];
&decision[,6]=adjbound[1:last];
&decision[,7]=level[1:last];
&decision[,8]=lowercl[1:last];
&decision[,9]=reject[1:last];
varnames={"Analysis", "Size", "Fraction", "TestStatistic", "PValue",
    "TestStBoundary", "PValBoundary", "LowerLimit", "Reject"};
create &decision from &decision[colname=varnames];
append from &decision;
quit;
%let conf=%sysevalf(100*(1-&alpha));
data &inference;
    set &inference;
    length par $50;
    format value best6.;
    if _n_=1 then par="Median unbiased estimate"; value=col1;
    if _n_=2 then par="Lower &conf.% confidence limit"; value=col1;
    label par="Parameter" value="Value";
    keep par value;
data &decision;
    set &decision;
    format TestStatistic PValue TestStBoundary PValBoundary LowerLimit
        Fraction 6.4 Analysis Size 4.0;
    length Decision $10.;
```

```
      label Analysis="Analysis"
            Size="Sample size per group"
            Fraction="Sample size fraction"
            TestStatistic="Test statistic"
            PValue="P-value"
            TestStBoundary="Stopping boundary (test statistic scale)"
            PValBoundary="Stopping boundary (p-value scale)"
            LowerLimit="Lower &conf.% repeated confidence limit"
            Decision="Decision";
      if reject=0 then decision="Continue"; else decision="Reject H0";
      drop reject;
      run;
%mend EffMonitor;
```

%EffFutMonitor Macro: Efficacy and Futility Monitoring of Group Sequential Trials

```
%macro EffFutMonitor(fraction,data,effsize,power,alpha,rhoeff,rhofut,
    spfunction,sprho,decision,inference);
/*
Inputs:
FRACTION  = Input data set that contains fractions of the total sample
            size accrued at successive analyses.

DATA      = Input data set containing summary statistics computed at each analysis.
            The data set must include the following two variables: N is the number of
            patients in each treatment group (or the average of the numbers of
            patients if they are not the same) and STAT is the value of a normally
            distributed test statistic.

EFFSIZE   = True effect size.

POWER     = Power.

ALPHA     = One-sided Type I error probability.

RHOEFF    = Shape parameter of upper (efficacy) stopping boundary
            (0.5 if Pocock boundary and 0 if O'Brien-Fleming boundary)

RHOFUT    = Shape parameter of lower (futility) stopping boundary
            (0.5 if Pocock boundary and 0 if O'Brien-Fleming boundary)

SPFUNCTION= Error spending function code (1, design-based function; 2, ten-look function;
            3, a function the Lan-DeMets family; 4, a function from the Jennison-Turnbull
            family; 5, a function from the Hwang-Shih-DeCani family).

SPRHO     = Shape parameter of the error spending function.

DECISION  = Output data set that contains stopping boundaries and probabilities as well as
            one-sided repeated confidence intervals for treatment difference at each interim
            look.

INFERENCE = Output data set containing bias-adjusted estimate of treatment effect
            with a one-sided confidence interval computed at the last look.
*/
```

```
proc iml;
    start ParSearch(c) global(lastlook,scf,scale);
        drift=(c[1]*lastlook##&rhoeff+c[2]*lastlook##&rhofut)/lastlook;
        upper=c[1]*scf##&rhoeff;
        lower=drift*scf-c[2]*scf##&rhofut;
        length=ncol(lower);
        lower[length]=lower[length]-1e-5;
        boundary=lower//upper;
        call seq(p,boundary) eps=1e-8 tscale=scale;
        crossh0=sum(p[3,]-p[2,])-&alpha;
        adjustment=drift*scf;
        boundary=(lower-adjustment)//(upper-adjustment);
        call seq(p,boundary) eps=1e-8 tscale=scale;
        crossh1=sum(p[3,]-p[2,])-&power;
        diff=abs(crossh0)+abs(crossh1);
        return(diff);
    finish;
    start BoundSearch(guess) global(stage,alpha,beta,adjlower,adjupper,
        ss,sinf,infinc);
        if guess[1]>guess[2] then do;
            alphainc=alpha[stage]-alpha[stage-1];
            betainc=beta[stage]-beta[stage-1];
            tempupp=t(adjupper[1:stage]#sqrt(sinf[1:stage]));
            templow=t(adjlower[1:stage]#sqrt(sinf[1:stage]));
            tempinc=t(infinc[1:stage-1]);
            tempupp[stage]=guess[1]*sqrt(sinf[stage]);
            templow[stage]=guess[2]*sqrt(sinf[stage]);
            boundary=templow//tempupp;
            call seq(p,boundary) eps=1e-8 tscale=tempinc;
            crossh0=p[3,stage]-p[2,stage]-alphainc;
            adjustment=&effsize*t(sqrt(ss[1:stage]#sinf[1:stage]/2));
            boundary=(templow-adjustment)//(tempupp-adjustment);
            call seq(p,boundary) eps=1e-8 tscale=tempinc;
            crossh1=p[1,stage]-betainc;
            diff=abs(crossh0)+abs(crossh1);
            return(diff);
        end;
        if guess[1]<=guess[2] then do;
            diff=1;
            return(diff);
        end;
    finish;
    start AdjQuant(est) global(quantile,sall,observed,tempinc,infinity);
        adjustment=est*sall;
        upper=observed#(sall##0.5);
        boundary=infinity//(upper-adjustment);
        call seq(prob,boundary) eps=1e-8 tscale=tempinc;
        sss=sum(prob[3,]-prob[2,]);
        diff=abs(quantile-sss);
        return(diff);
    finish;
    use &fraction;
    read all var _all_ into fraction;
    m=nrow(fraction);
    fract=t(fraction);
    stfract=fract/fract[1];
    inc=j(1,m-1,0);
```

```
do i=1 to m-1;
    inc[i]=(fract[i+1]-fract[i])/fract[1];
end;
nfixed=2*((probit(&power)+probit(1-&alpha))/&effsize)**2;
start={1 1};
tc=repeat(.,1,12);
tc[1]=100;
tc[3]=1e-5;
lastlook=stfract[m];
scf=stfract;
scale=inc;
call nlpdd(rc,c,"ParSearch",start) tc=tc;
drift=(c[1]*lastlook##&rhoeff+c[2]*lastlook##&rhofut)/lastlook;
max=2*(drift/&effsize)*(drift/&effsize)/fract[1];
upper=c[1]*stfract##&rhoeff;
lower=drift*stfract-c[2]*stfract##&rhofut;
lower[m]=lower[m]-1e-5;
boundary=lower//upper;
call seq(prob0,boundary) eps=1e-8 tscale=inc;
alspend=cusum(prob0[3,]-prob0[2,]);
adjustment=drift*stfract;
boundary=(lower-adjustment)//(upper-adjustment);
call seq(prob1,boundary) eps=1e-8 tscale=inc;
bespend=cusum(prob1[1,]);
use &data;
read all var {n stat} into mon;
n=nrow(mon);
ss=mon[,1];
infofrac=ss/max;
statistic=mon[,2];
pvalue=1-probnorm(statistic);
sinf=infofrac/infofrac[1];
infinc=j(1,n-1,0);
do i=1 to n-1;
    infinc[i]=sinf[i+1]-sinf[i];
end;
alpha=j(n,1,0);
beta=j(n,1,0);
* Design-based error spending function;
if &spfunction=1 then
do;
    t=0 || fract;
    a=0 || alspend;
    b=0 || bespend;
    do stage=1 to n;
        x=infofrac[stage];
        do i=1 to m;
            if t[i]<=x & x<t[i+1] then do;
                alpha[stage]=(a[i+1]*(x-t[i])+a[i]*(t[i+1]-x))/

    (t[i+1]-t[i]);
                beta[stage]=(b[i+1]*(x-t[i])+b[i]*(t[i+1]-x))/

    (t[i+1]-t[i]);
            end;
        end;
        if x>=1 then do;
```

```
            alpha[stage]=&alpha;
            beta[stage]=1-&power;
        end;
    end;
end;
* Ten-look error spending function;
if &spfunction=2 then
do;
    k=10;
    t=repeat(0.1,1,10);
    cf=cusum(t);
    scf=cf/cf[1];
    in=j(1,k-1,0);
    do i=1 to k-1;
        in[i]=t[i+1]/t[1];
    end;
    start={1 1};
    tc=repeat(.,1,12);
    tc[1]=100;
    tc[3]=1e-5;
    lastlook=k;
    scale=in;
    call nlpdd(rc,c,"ParSearch",start) tc=tc;
    drift=(c[1]*lastlook##&rhoeff+c[2]*lastlook##&rhofut)/lastlook;
    upper=c[1]*scf##&rhoeff;
    lower=drift*scf-c[2]*scf##&rhofut;
    boundary=lower//upper;
    call seq(prob0,boundary) eps=1e-8 tscale=in;
    als=cusum(prob0[3,]-prob0[2,]);
    adjustment=drift*scf;
    boundary=(lower-adjustment)//(upper-adjustment);
    call seq(prob1,boundary) eps=1e-8 tscale=in;
    bes=cusum(prob1[1,]);
    do stage=1 to n;
        x=infofrac[stage];
        if x<1 then do;
            l=floor(k*x); u=floor(k*x)+1;
            alpha[stage]=als[l]+(k*x-l)*(als[u]-als[l])/(u-l);
            beta[stage]=bes[l]+(k*x-l)*(bes[u]-bes[l])/(u-l);
        end;
        if x>=1 then do;
            alpha[stage]=&alpha;
            beta[stage]=1-&power;
        end;
    end;
end;
* Lan-DeMets error spending function;
if &spfunction=3 then
do;
    do stage=1 to n;
        x=infofrac[stage];
        if x<1 & &sprho=0 then alpha[stage]=2-
            2*probnorm(probit(1-&alpha/2)/sqrt(x));
        if x<1 & &sprho=0.5 then alpha[stage]=&alpha*log(1+(exp(1)-1)*x);
        if x>=1 then alpha[stage]=&alpha;
    end;
end;
```

```
* Jennison-Turnbull error spending function;
if &spfunction=4 then
do;
    do stage=1 to n;
        x=infofrac[stage];
        if x<1 then alpha[stage]=&alpha*(x**&sprho);
        if x>=1 then alpha[stage]=&alpha;
    end;
end;
* Hwang-Shih-DeCani error spending function;
if &spfunction=5 then
do;
    do stage=1 to n;
        x=infofrac[stage];
        if x<1 & &sprho^=0 then alpha[stage]=
            &alpha*(1-exp(-&sprho*x))/(1-exp(-&sprho));
        if x<1 & &sprho=0 then alpha[stage]=&alpha*x;
        if x>=1 then alpha[stage]=&alpha;
    end;
end;
adjlower=j(n,1,0);
adjupper=j(n,1,0);
adjlowp=j(n,1,0);
adjuppp=j(n,1,0);
reject=j(n,1,0);
guess=j(1,2,0);
tc=repeat(.,1,12);
tc[1]=100;
tc[3]=1e-5;
do stage=1 to n;
    if stage=1 then do;
        adjupper[1]=probit(1-alpha[1]);
        stdelta=&effsize*sqrt(ss[1]/2);
        adjlower[1]=stdelta+probit(beta[1]);
        adjuppp[1]=alpha[1];
        adjlowp[1]=1-probnorm(adjlower[1]);
    end;
    if stage>1 then do;
        guess[1]=probit(1-alpha[stage]);
        stdelta=&effsize*sqrt(ss[stage]/2);
        guess[2]=stdelta+probit(beta[stage]);
        call nlpdd(rc,adj,"BoundSearch",guess) tc=tc;
        adjupper[stage]=adj[1];
        adjlower[stage]=adj[2];
        adjuppp[stage]=1-probnorm(adj[1]);
        adjlowp[stage]=1-probnorm(adj[2]);
    end;
end;
lowercl=(statistic-adjupper)#sqrt(2/ss);
reject=(statistic>adjupper)-(statistic<adjlower);
stop=0;
do i=1 to n;
    if reject[i]^=0 & stop=0 then stop=i;
end;
if stop=0 then last=n; else last=stop;
observed=t(adjupper[1:last]);
observed[last]=statistic[last];
```

```
            tall=t(ss[1:last]);
            k=ncol(tall);
            tall=tall/tall[k];
            sall=tall/tall[1];
            tempinc=j(1,k-1,0);
            do i=1 to k-1;
                tempinc[i]=sall[i+1]-sall[i];
            end;
            infinity=repeat(.m,1,k);
            tc=repeat(.,1,12);
            tc[1]=100;
            tc[3]=1e-5;
            inference=j(2,1,.);
            quantile=0.5;
            est=statistic[last];
            call nlpdd(rc,qest,"AdjQuant",est) tc=tc;
            qest=&effsize*qest/drift;
            inference[1]=qest;
            quantile=&alpha;
            est=((statistic-probit(1-&alpha))#sqrt(2/ss))[last];
            est=est*drift/&effsize;
            call nlpdd(rc,qest,"AdjQuant",est) tc=tc;
            qest=&effsize*qest/drift;
            inference[2]=qest;
            create &inference from inference;
            append from inference;
            &decision=j(last,11,0);
            &decision[,1]=t(1:last);
            &decision[,2]=ss[1:last];
            &decision[,3]=infofrac[1:last];
            &decision[,4]=statistic[1:last];
            &decision[,5]=pvalue[1:last];
            &decision[,6]=adjupper[1:last];
            &decision[,7]=adjlower[1:last];
            &decision[,8]=adjuppp[1:last];
            &decision[,9]=adjlowp[1:last];
            &decision[,10]=lowercl[1:last];
            &decision[,11]=reject[1:last];
            varnames={"Analysis", "Size", "Fraction", "TestStatistic", "PValue",
                "UpperTestStBoundary", "LowerTestStBoundary", "UpperPValBoundary",
                "LowerPValBoundary", "LowerLimit", "Reject"};
            create &decision from &decision[colname=varnames];
            append from &decision;
            quit;
%let conf=%sysevalf(100*(1-&alpha));
data &inference;
    set &inference;
    length par $50;
    format value best6.;
    if _n_=1 then par="Median unbiased estimate"; value=col1;
    if _n_=2 then par="Lower &conf.% confidence limit"; value=col1;
    label par='Parameter' value='Value';
    keep par value;
data &decision;
    set &decision;
    format TestStatistic PValue UpperTestStBoundary LowerTestStBoundary
        UpperPValBoundary LowerPValBoundary LowerLimit Fraction 6.4 Analysis Size 4.0;
```

```
    length Decision $10.;
    label Analysis='Analysis'
        Size='Sample size per group'
        Fraction='Sample size fraction'
        TestStatistic='Test statistic'
        PValue='P-value'
        UpperTestStBoundary='Upper stopping boundary (test statistic scale)'
        LowerTestStBoundary='Lower stopping boundary (test statistic scale)'
        UpperPValBoundary='Upper stopping boundary (p-value scale)'
        LowerPValBoundary='Lower stopping boundary (p-value scale)'
        LowerLimit="Lower &conf.% repeated confidence limit"
        Decision='Decision';
    if reject=0 then decision='Continue';
    if reject=1 then decision='Reject H0';
    if reject=-1 then decision='Reject H1';
    drop reject;
    run;
%mend EffFutMonitor;
```

%CondPowerLSH Macro: Lan-Simon-Halperin Conditional Power Test

```
%macro CondPowerLSH(data,effsize,alpha,gamma,nn,prob,boundary);
/**********************************************************
Inputs:
DATA    = Data set to be analyzed (includes number of patients per
          group and test statistic at each interim look)

EFFSIZE = Hypothesized effect size

ALPHA   = One-sided Type I error probability of the significance
          test carried out at the end of the trial

GAMMA   = Futility index

NN      = Projected number of patients per treatment group

PROB    = Name of an output data set containing conditional power
          at each interim look

BOUNDARY= Name of an output data set containing stopping boundary
          of the conditional power test

**********************************************************/
proc iml;
    use &data;
    read all var {n teststat} into data;
    m=nrow(data);
    n=data[,1];
    teststat=data[,2];
    prob=j(m,4,0);
    prob[,1]=t(1:m);
    prob[,2]=n/&nn;
    prob[,3]=teststat;
    prob[,4]=1-probnorm((sqrt(&nn)*probit(1-&alpha)-sqrt(n)#teststat
        -(&nn-n)*&effsize/sqrt(2))/sqrt(&nn-n));
    varnames={"Analysis" "Fraction" "TestStat" "CondPower"};
```

```
       create &prob from prob[colname=varnames];
       append from prob;
       bound=j(50,2,0);
       frac=(1:50)*&nn/50;
       bound[,1]=t(frac/&nn);
       bound[,2]=t(sqrt(&nn/frac)*probit(1-&alpha)+sqrt((&nn-frac)/frac)
               *probit(1-&gamma)-&effsize*(&nn-frac)/sqrt(2*frac));
       varnames={"Fraction" "StopBoundary"};
       create &boundary from bound[colname=varnames];
       append from bound;
       quit;
data &prob;
       set &prob;
       format Fraction 4.2 TestStat 7.4 CondPower 6.4;
       label Fraction="Fraction of total sample size"
             TestStat="Test statistic"
             CondPower="Conditional power";
%mend CondPowerLSH;
```

%CondPowerPAB Macro: Pepe-Anderson-Betensky Conditional Power Test

```
%macro CondPowerPAB(data,alpha,gamma,c,nn,prob,boundary);
/********************************************************
Inputs:
DATA     = Data set to be analyzed (includes number of patients per
           group and test statistic at each interim look)

ALPHA    = One-sided Type I error probability of the significance
           test carried out at the end of the trial

GAMMA    = Futility index

C        = Parameter determining the shape of the stopping boundary
           (Pepe and Anderson (1992) set C to 1 and Betensky (1997)
           recommended to set C to 2.326)

NN       = Projected number of patients per treatment group

PROB     = Name of an output data set containing conditional power
           at each interim look

BOUNDARY= Name of an output data set containing stopping boundary
          of the conditional power test

********************************************************/
proc iml;
     use &data;
     read all var {n teststat} into data;
     m=nrow(data);
     n=data[,1];
     teststat=data[,2];
     prob=j(m,4,0);
     prob[,1]=t(1:m);
     prob[,2]=n/&nn;
```

```
        prob[,3]=teststat;
        prob[,4]=1-probnorm((sqrt(&nn)*probit(1-&alpha)-sqrt(n)#teststat
            -(&nn-n)#(teststat+&c)/sqrt(n))/sqrt(&nn-n));
        varnames={"Analysis" "Fraction" "TestStat" "CondPower"};
        create &prob from prob[colname=varnames];
        append from prob;
        bound=j(50,2,0);
        frac=(1:50)*&nn/50;
        bound[,1]=t(frac/&nn);
        bound[,2]=t(sqrt(frac/&nn)*probit(1-&alpha)+sqrt(frac#(&nn-frac)/
            (&nn*&nn))*probit(1-&gamma)-&c*(&nn-frac)/&nn);
        varnames={"Fraction" "StopBoundary"};
        create &boundary from bound[colname=varnames];
        append from bound;
        quit;
data &prob;
    set &prob;
    format Fraction 4.2 TestStat 7.4 CondPower 6.4;
    label Fraction="Fraction of total sample size"
          TestStat="Test statistic"
          CondPower="Conditional power";
%mend CondPowerPAB;
```

%BayesFutilityCont Macro: Predictive Power and Predictive Probability Tests for Continuous, Normally Distributed Endpoints

```
%macro BayesFutilityCont(data,par,delta,eta,alpha,prob);
/***********************************************************
Inputs:
DATA    = Data set to be analyzed (includes number of patients,
          estimated mean treatment effects and sample standard
          deviations in two treatment groups at each interim look)

PAR     = Name of an input data set with projected sample size in
          each treatment group and parameters of prior distributions

DELTA   = Clinically significant difference (required by Bayesian
          predictive probability method and ignored by predictive
          power method)

ETA     = Confidence level of Bayesian predictive probability method
          (required by Bayesian predictive probability method and
          ignored by predictive power method)

ALPHA   = One-sided Type I error probability of the significance
          test carried out at the end of the trial (required by
          predictive power method and ignored by Bayesian predictive
          probability method

PROB    = Name of an output data set containing predictive power and
          predictive probability at each interim look

***********************************************************/
proc iml;
    use &data;
```

```
    read all var {n1 mean1 sd1 n2 mean2 sd2} into data;
    n=(data[,1]+data[,4])/2;
    s=sqrt(((data[,1]-1)#data[,3]#data[,3]+(data[,4]-1)
        #data[,6]#data[,6])/(data[,1]+data[,4]-2));
    z=(data[,2]-data[,5])/(s#sqrt(1/data[,1]+1/data[,4]));
    m=nrow(data);
    use &par;
    read all var {nn1 nn2 mu1 mu2 sigma} into par;
    nn=(par[,1]+par[,2])/2;
    sigma=par[,5];
    a1=(n-nn)/nn+(nn-n)/(nn#(1+(s/sigma)#(s/sigma)/n));
    b1=sqrt(n/(2*nn))#(nn-n)#(par[,3]-par[,4])/(1+n#(sigma/s)
        #(sigma/s));
    c1=1/(1+n#(sigma/s)#(sigma/s));
    output=j(m,4,0);
    output[,1]=t(1:m);
    output[,2]=n/nn;
    num1=sqrt(nn)#z#(1+a1)+b1/s-sqrt(n)*probit(1-&alpha);
    den1=sqrt((nn-n)#((nn-n)#(1-c1)+n)/nn);
    output[,3]=probnorm(num1/den1);
    an=1/(1+n#(sigma/s)#(sigma/s));
    ann=1/(1+nn#(sigma/s)#(sigma/s));
    b2=sqrt(n#nn/2)#(par[,3]-par[,4])/(1+n#(sigma/s)#(sigma/s));
    c2=1-1/sqrt(1+(s/sigma)#(s/sigma)/nn);
    num2=sqrt(nn)#z#(1-an)+b2/s-(&delta/s)#sqrt(n#nn/2)-sqrt(n)
        #(1-c2)*probit(&eta);
    den2=sqrt((1-ann)#(1-ann)#(nn-n)#((nn-n)#(1-an)+n)/nn);
    output[,4]=probnorm(num2/den2);
    varnames={"Analysis", "Fraction", "PredPower", "PredProb"};
    create &prob from output[colname=varnames];
    append from output;
    quit;
data &prob;
    set &prob;
    format Fraction 4.2 PredPower PredProb 6.4;
    label Fraction="Fraction of total sample size"
        PredPower="Predictive power"
        PredProb="Predictive probability";
%mend BayesFutilityCont;
```

%BayesFutilityBin Macro: Predictive Power and Predictive Probability Tests for Binary Endpoints

```
%macro BayesFutilityBin(data,par,delta,eta,alpha,prob);
/*********************************************************
Inputs:
DATA    = Data set to be analyzed (includes number of patients and
          observed event counts in two treatment groups at each
          interim look)

PAR     = Name of an input data set with projected sample size in
          each treatment group and parameters of prior distributions

DELTA   = Clinically significant difference (required by Bayesian
          predictive probability method and ignored by predictive
```

```
                         power method)

    ETA      = Confidence level of Bayesian predictive probability method
               (required by Bayesian predictive probability method and
               ignored by predictive power method)

    ALPHA    = One-sided Type I error probability of the significance
               test carried out at the end of the trial (required by
               predictive power method and ignored by Bayesian predictive
               probability method

    PROB     = Name of an output data set containing predictive power and
               predictive probability at each interim look

*********************************************************/
proc iml;
    start integral(p) global(ast,bst);
        i=p**(ast[1]-1)*(1-p)**(bst[1]-1)*
            probbeta(p-&delta,ast[2],bst[2]);
        return(i);
    finish;
    start beta(a,b);
        beta=exp(lgamma(a)+lgamma(b)-lgamma(a+b));
        return(beta);
    finish;
    use &data;
    read all var {n1 count1 n2 count2} into data;
    n=data[,1]||data[,3];
    s=data[,2]||data[,4];
    m=nrow(n);
    use &par;
    read all var {nn1 nn2 alpha1 alpha2 beta1 beta2} into par;
    nn=t(par[1:2]);
    a=t(par[3:4]);
    b=t(par[5:6]);
    t=j(1,2,0);
    output=j(m,4,0);
    range=j(1,2,0);
    range[1]=&delta; range[2]=1;
    do i=1 to m;
    output[i,1]=i;
    output[i,2]=(n[i,1]+n[i,2])/(nn[1]+nn[2]);
    do t1=0 to nn[1]-n[i,1];
    do t2=0 to nn[2]-n[i,2];
        t[1]=t1; t[2]=t2;
        ast=s[i,]+t+a;
        bst=nn-s[i,]-t+b;
        b1=beta(ast,bst);
        b2=exp(lgamma(nn-n[i,]+1)-lgamma(nn-n[i,]-t+1)-lgamma(t+1));
        b3=beta(s[i,]+a,n[i,]-s[i,]+b);
        pr=(b1#b2)/b3;
        mult=pr[1]*pr[2];
        p=(s[i,]+t)/nn;
        ave=(p[1]+p[2])/2;
        aven=(nn[1]+nn[2])/2;
        teststat=(p[1]-p[2])/sqrt(2*ave*(1-ave)/aven);
        output[i,3]=output[i,3]+(teststat>probit(1-&alpha))*mult;
```

```
              call quad(value,"integral",range) eps=1e-8;
              output[i,4]=output[i,4]+(value/beta(ast[1],bst[1])>&eta)*mult;
      end;
      end;
      end;
      varnames={"Analysis", "Fraction", "PredPower", "PredProb"};
      create &prob from output[colname=varnames];
      append from output;
      quit;
data &prob;
      set &prob;
      format Fraction 4.2 PredPower PredProb 6.4;
      label Fraction="Fraction of total sample size"
            PredPower="Predictive power"
            PredProb="Predictive probability";
%mend BayesFutilityBin;
```

References

Aerts, M., Geys, H., Molenberghs, G., Ryan, L.M. (2002). *Topics in Modeling of Clustered Data*. London: Chapman and Hall.

Afifi, A., Elashoff, R. (1966). Missing observations in multivariate statistics I: Review of the literature. *Journal of the American Statistical Association* 61, 595–604.

Agresti, A. (2001). Exact inference for categorical data: Recent advances and continuing controversies. *Statistics in Medicine* 20, 2709–2722.

Agresti, A. (2002). *Categorical Data Analysis*. 2nd ed. New York: Wiley.

Agresti, A., Hartzel, J. (2000). Strategies for comparing treatments on a binary response with multi-centre data. *Statistics in Medicine* 19, 1115–1139.

Allison, P.D. (1995). *Survival Analysis Using the SAS System*. Cary, NC: SAS Institute Inc.

Altham, P.M.E. (1984). Improving the precision of estimation by fitting a model. *Journal of the Royal Statistical Society, Series B* 46, 118–119.

Andersen, P.K., Klein, J.P., Zhang, M. (1999). Testing for centre effects in multi-centre survival studies: A Monte Carlo comparison of fixed and random effects tests. *Statistics in Medicine* 18, 1489–1500.

Armitage, P., McPherson, C.K., Rowe, B.C. (1969). Repeated significance tests on accumulating data. *Journal of the Royal Statistical Society, Series A* 132, 235–244.

Ashford, J.R., Sowden, R.R. (1970). Multivariate probit analysis. *Biometrics* 26, 535–546.

Azzalini, A., Cox, D.R. (1984). Two new tests associated with analysis of variance. *Journal of the Royal Statistical Society, Series B* 46, 335–343.

Bahadur, R.R. (1961). A representation of the joint distribution of responses to *n* dichotomous items. *Studies in Item Analysis and Prediction*. Solomon, H. (editor). Stanford Mathematical Studies in the Social Sciences VI. Stanford, CA: Stanford University Press.

Bancroft, T.A. (1968). *Topics in Intermediate Statistical Methods*. Ames, Iowa: Iowa State University Press.

Bauer, P. (1991). Multiple testings in clinical trials. *Statistics in Medicine* 10, 871–890.

Bauer, P., Röhmel, J., Maurer, W., Hothorn, L. (1998). Testing strategies in multi-dose experiments including active control. *Statistics in Medicine* 17, 2133–2146.

Beach, M.L., Meier, P. (1989). Choosing covariates in the analysis of clinical trials. *Controlled Clinical Trials* 10, 161S–175S.

Benjamini, Y., Hochberg, Y. (1995). Controlling the false discovery rate: A new and powerful approach to multiple testing. *Journal of the Royal Statistical Society, Series B* 57, 1289–1300.

Benjamini, Y., Hochberg, Y. (1997). Multiple hypothesis-testing and weights. *Scandinavian Journal of Statistics* 24, 407–418.

Berger, R.L. (1982). Multiparameter hypothesis-testing and acceptance sampling. *Technometrics* 24, 295–300.

Berger, R.L. (1997). Likelihood ratio tests and intersection-union tests. *Advances in Statistical Decision Theory and Applications*. Panchepakesan, S., Balakrishnan, N. (editors). Boston: Birkhauser.

Berkey, C. S., Dockery, D. W., Wang, X., Wypij, D., Ferris, B. (1993). Longitudinal height velocity standards for U.S. adolescents. *Statistics in Medicine* 12, 403–414.

Bernardo, M.V.P., Ibrahim, J.G. (2000). Group sequential designs for cure rate models with early stopping in favour of the null hypothesis. *Statistics in Medicine* 19, 3023–3035.

Betensky, R.A. (1997). Early stopping to accept H_0 based on conditional power: Approximations and comparisons. *Biometrics* 53, 794–806.

Birch, M.W. (1964). The detection of partial association I. *Journal of the Royal Statistical Society, Series B* 26, 313–324.

Bonney, G.E. (1987). Logistic regression for dependent binary observations. *Biometrics* 43, 951–973.

Breiman, L., Friedman, J.H., Olshen, R.A., Stone, C.J. (1984). *Classification and Regression Trees.* Belmont, CA: Wadsworth.

Breslow, N. (1970). A generalized Kruskal-Wallis test for comparing K samples subject to unequal patterns of censorship. *Biometrika* 57, 579–594.

Breslow, N. (1974). Covariance analysis of censored survival data. *Biometrics* 30, 89–99.

Breslow, N. (1981). Odds ratio estimators when the data are sparse. *Biometrika* 68, 73–84.

Breslow, N.E., Clayton, D.G. (1993). Approximate inference in generalized linear mixed models. *Journal of the American Statistical Association* 88, 9–25.

Breslow, N.E., Day, N.E. (1980). *Statistical Methods in Cancer Research. Volume 1: The Analysis of Case-Control Studies.* Lyon: International Agency for Research on Cancer.

Brown, B.W., Russell, K. (1997). Methods correcting for multiple testing: Operating characteristics. *Statistics in Medicine* 16, 2511–2528.

Buck, S.F. (1960). A method of estimation of missing values in multivariate data suitable for use with an electronic computer. *Journal of the Royal Statistical Society, Series B* 22, 302–306.

Cantor, A. (1997). *Extending SAS Survival Analysis Techniques for Medical Research.* Cary, NC: SAS Institute Inc.

Chakravorti, S.R., Grizzle, J.E. (1975). Analysis of data from multiclinic experiments. *Biometrics* 31, 325–338.

Chang, W.H., Chuang-Stein, C. (2004). Type I error and power in trials with one interim futility analysis. *Pharmaceutical Statistics* 3, 51–59.

Chi, E.M., Reinsel, G.C. (1989). Models for longitudinal data with random effects and AR(1) errors. *Journal of the American Statistical Association* 84, 452–459.

Chi, G.Y.H. (1998). Multiple testings: Multiple comparisons and multiple endpoints. *Drug Information Journal* 32, 1347S–1362S.

Chinchilli, V.M., Bortey, E.B. (1991). Testing for consistency in a single multicenter trial. *Journal of Biopharmaceutical Statistics* 1, 67–80.

Chuang-Stein, C. (1998). Safety analysis in controlled clinical trials. *Drug Information Journal* 32, 1363S–1372S.

Chuang-Stein, C., Tong, D.M. (1995). Multiple comparisons procedures for comparing several treatments with a control based on binary data. *Statistics in Medicine* 14, 2509–2522.

Ciminera, J.L., Heyse, J.F., Nguyen, H.H., Tukey, J.W. (1993). Tests for qualitative treatment-by-centre interaction using a "pushback" procedure. *Statistics in Medicine* 12, 1033–1045.

Cochran, W.G. (1954a). The combination of estimates from different experiments. *Biometrics* 10, 101–129.

Cochran, W.G. (1954b). Some methods for strengthening the common χ^2 tests. *Biometrics* 10, 417–451.

Cochran, W.G. (1983). *Planning and Analysis of Observational Studies.* New York: Wiley.

Coe, P.R., Tamhane, A.C. (1993). Small sample confidence intervals for the difference, ratio, and odds ratio of two success probabilities. *Communications in Statistics (Simulation and Computation)* 22, 925–938.

Collett, D. (1994). *Modelling Survival Data in Medical Research.* London: Chapman and Hall.

Cowles, M.K., Carlin, B.P., Connett, J.E. (1996). Bayesian tobit modeling of longitudinal ordinal clinical trial compliance data with nonignorable missingness. *Journal of the American Statistical Association* 91, 86–98.

Cox, D.R. (1958). Two further applications of a model for binary regression. *Biometrika* 45, 562–565.

Cox, D.R. (1972). Regression models and life-tables. *Journal of the Royal Statistical Society, Series B* 34, 187–220.

Cox, D.R., Oakes, D.O. (1984). *Analysis of Survival Data*. London: Chapman and Hall.

D'Agostino, R.B. (2000). Controlling alpha in clinical trials: The case for secondary endpoints. *Statistics in Medicine* 19, 763–766.

Dale, J.R. (1986). Global cross-ratio models for bivariate, discrete, ordered responses. *Biometrics* 42, 909–917.

Davis, B.R., Hardy, R.J. (1990). Upper bounds for type I and type II error rates in conditional power calculations. *Communications in Statistics, Part A* 19, 3571–3584.

Day, N.E., Byar, D.P. (1979). Testing hypotheses in case-control studies: Equivalence of Mantel-Haenszel statistics and logit score tests. *Biometrics* 35, 623–630.

DeMets, D.L., Lan, K.K.G. (1984). An overview of sequential methods and their application in clinical trials. *Communications in Statistics, Part A* 13, 2315–2338.

DeMets, D.L., Ware, J.H. (1980). Group sequential methods for clinical trials with a one-sided hypothesis. *Biometrika* 67, 651–660.

Dempster, A.P., Laird, N.M., Rubin, D.B. (1977). Maximum likelihood from incomplete data via the EM algorithm (with discussion). *Journal of the Royal Statistical Society, Series B* 39, 1–38.

Dempster, A.P., Rubin, D.B. (1983). Overview. *Incomplete Data in Sample Surveys, Vol. II: Theory and Annotated Bibliography*. Madow, W.G., Olkin, I., Rubin, D.B. (editors). New York: Academic Press.

Denne, J.S., Koch, G.G. (2002). A sequential procedure for studies comparing multiple doses. *Pharmaceutical Statistics* 1, 107–118.

Diggle, P.J. (1988). An approach to the analysis of repeated measures. *Biometrics* 44, 959–971.

Diggle, P.J., Heagerty, P.J., Liang, K.-Y., Zeger, S.L. (2002). *Analysis of Longitudinal Data*. 2nd ed. Oxford: Oxford University Press.

Diggle, P.J., Kenward, M.G. (1994). Informative drop-out in longitudinal data analysis (with discussion). *Applied Statistics* 43, 49–93.

Diggle, P.J., Liang, K.-Y., Zeger, S.L. (1994). *Analysis of Longitudinal Data*. Oxford: Clarendon Press.

Dmitrienko, A. (2003a). Covariate-adjusted reference intervals for diagnostic data. *Journal of Biopharmaceutical Statistics* 13, 191–208.

Dmitrienko, A. (2003b). Modeling paired categorical outcomes in clinical trials. *Pharmaceutical Statistics* 2, 279–289.

Dmitrienko, A., Govindarajulu, Z. (2000). Sequential confidence regions for maximum likelihood estimates. *Annals of Statistics* 28, 1472–1501.

Dmitrienko, A., Offen, W., Westfall, P.H. (2003). Gatekeeping strategies for clinical trials that do not require all primary effects to be significant. *Statistics in Medicine* 22, 2387–2400.

Dmitrienko, A., Sides, G., Winters, K., Kovacs, R., Eisenberg, P., Groh, W. (2004). Electrocardiogram reference ranges derived from a standardized clinical trial population. *Journal of Cardiovascular Electrophysiology*. Forthcoming.

Dmitrienko, A., Smith, B. (2002). Analysis of QT interval in clinical trials. *Drug Information Journal* 36, 269–279.

Dmitrienko, A., Wang, M.D. (2004). Bayesian predictive approach to interim monitoring in clinical trials. Unpublished manuscript.

Dunnett, C.W. (1955). A multiple comparison procedure for comparing several treatments with a control. *Journal of the American Statistical Association* 50, 1096–1121.

Dunnett, C.W., Tamhane, A.C. (1992). A step-up multiple test procedure. *Journal of the American Statistical Association* 87, 162–170.

Dunnett, C.W., Tamhane, A.C. (1995). Step-up multiple testing of parameters with unequally correlated estimates. *Biometrics* 51, 217–227.

Efron, B. (1977). The efficiency of Cox's likelihood function for censored data. *Journal of the American Statistical Association* 72, 557–565.

Efron, B. (1979). Bootstrap methods: Another look at the jackknife. *Annals of Statistics* 7, 1–26.

Efron, B., Tibshirani, R. (1993). *An Introduction to the Bootstrap*. New York: Chapman and Hall.

Ekholm, A. (1991). Algorithms versus models for analyzing data that contain misclassification errors. *Biometrics* 47, 1171–1182.

Ellenberg, S.S., Fleming, T.R., DeMets, D.L. (2002). *Data Monitoring Committees in Clinical Trials: A Practical Perspective.* New York: Wiley.

Emerson, S.S., Fleming, T.R. (1989). Symmetric group sequential test designs. *Biometrics* 45, 905–923.

Emerson, S.S., Fleming, T.R. (1990). Parameter estimation following group sequential hypothesis testing. *Biometrica* 77, 875–892.

Enas G.G., Dornseif B.E., Sampson C.B., Rockhold F.W., Wuu J. (1989). Monitoring versus interim analysis of clinical trials: Perspective from the pharmaceutical industry. *Controlled Clinical Trials* 10, 57–70.

Fahrmeir, L., Tutz, G. (2002). *Multivariate Statistical Modeling Based on Generalized Linear Models.* 2nd ed. Springer Series in Statistics. New York: Springer-Verlag.

Fan, J., Hu, T.C., Truong, Y.K. (1994). Robust nonparametric function estimation. *Scandinavian Journal of Statistics* 21, 433–446.

Faries, D., Herrera, J., Rayamajhi, J., DeBrota, D., Demitrack, M., Potter, W.Z. (2000). The responsiveness of the Hamilton depression rating scale. *Journal of Psychiatric Research* 34, 3–10.

Felson, D.T., Anderson, J.J., Boers, M., Bombardier, C., Furst, D., Goldsmith, C., Katz, L.N., Lightfoot, R. Jr., Paulus, H., Strand, V., Tugwell, P., Weinblatt, M., Williams, H.J., Wolfe, F., Kieszak, S. (1995). American College of Rheumatology preliminary definition of improvement in rheumatoid arthritis. *Arthritis and Rheumatology* 38, 727–735.

Fleiss, J.L. (1981). *Statistical Methods for Rates and Proportions.* 2nd ed. New York: Wiley.

Fleiss, J.L. (1986). Analysis of data from multiclinic trials. *Controlled Clinical Trials* 7, 267–275.

Fleiss, J.L. (1986). *The Design and Analysis of Clinical Experiments.* New York: Wiley.

Follmann, D. (1995). Multivariate tests for multiple endpoints in clinical trials. *Statistics in Medicine* 14, 1163–1175.

Follmann, D. (1996). A simple multivariate test for one-sided alternatives. *Journal of the American Statistical Association* 91, 854–861.

Ford, I., Norrie, J., Ahmadi, S. (1995). Model inconsistency, illustrated by the Cox proportional hazards model. *Statistics in Medicine* 14, 735–746.

Freedman, L.S., Spiegelhalter, D.J. (1983). The assessment of the subjective opinion and its use in relation to stopping rules for clinical trials. *The Statistician* 32, 153–160.

Friedman, L.M., Furberg, C.D., DeMets, D.L. (1996). *Fundamentals of Clinical Trials.* St. Louis: Mosby-Year Book.

Gail, M.H., Lubin, J.H., Rubinstein, L.V. (1981). Likelihood calculations for matched case-control studies and survival studies with tied death times. *Biometrika* 68, 703–707.

Gail, M.H., Simon, R. (1985). Testing for qualitative interactions between treatment effects and patient subsets. *Biometrics* 41, 361–372.

Gail, M.H., Tan, W.Y., Piantadosi, S. (1988). Tests for no treatment effect in randomized clinical trials. *Biometrika* 75, 57–64.

Gail, M.H., Wieand, S., Piantadosi, S. (1984). Biased estimates of treatment effect in randomized experiments with nonlinear regressions and omitted covariates. *Biometrika* 71, 431–444.

Gallo, P.P. (2000). Center-weighting issues in multicenter clinical trials. *Journal of Biopharmaceutical Statistics* 10, 145–163.

Gastwirth, J.L. (1985). The use of maximin efficiency robust tests in combining contingency tables and survival analysis. *Journal of the American Statistical Association* 80, 380–384.

Gehan, E.A. (1965). A generalized Wilcoxon test for comparing arbitrary singly censored samples. *Biometrika* 52, 203–223.

Geisser, S. (1992). On the curtailment of sampling. *Canadian Journal of Statistics* 20, 297–309.

Geisser, S., Johnson, W. (1994). Interim analysis for normally distributed observables. In *Multivariate Analysis and Its Applications. IMS Lecture Notes*, 263–279.

George, E.O., Bowman, D. (1995). A full likelihood procedure for analysing exchangeable binary data. *Biometrics* 51, 512–523.

Geys, H., Molenberghs, G., Lipsitz, S.R. (1998). A note on the comparison of pseudo-likelihood and generalized estimating equations for marginal odds ratio models. *Journal of Statistical Computation and Simulation* 62, 45–72.

Gilula, Z., Haberman, S. (1994). Conditional log-linear models for analyzing categorical panel data. *Journal of the American Statistical Association* 89, 645–656.

Glonek, G.F.V., McCullagh, P. (1995). Multivariate logistic models. *Journal of the Royal Statistical Society, Series B* 81, 477–482.

Goldberg, J.D., Koury, K.J. (1990). Design and analysis of multicenter trials. *Statistical Methodology in the Pharmaceutical Sciences*. Berry, D.A. (editor). New York: Marcel Dekker.

Gönen, M., Westfall, P.H., Johnson, W.O. (2003). Bayesian multiple testing for two-sample multivariate endpoints. *Biometrics* 59, 76–82.

Gould, A.L. (1998). Multi-center trial analysis revisited. *Statistics in Medicine* 17, 1779–1797.

Greenland, S., Robins, J.M. (1985). Estimation of a common effect parameter from sparse follow-up data. *Biometrics* 41, 55–68.

Hájek, J., Šidák, Z. (1967). *Theory of Rank Tests*. New York: Academic Press.

Halperin, M., Lan, K.K.G., Ware, J.H., Johnson, N.J., DeMets, D.L. (1982). An aid to data monitoring in long-term clinical trials. *Controlled Clinical Trials* 3, 311–323.

Hamilton, M. (1967). Development of a rating scale for primary depressive illness. *British Journal of Clinical Psychology* 6, 278–296.

Harrington, D.P., Fleming, T.R. (1982). A class of rank test procedures for censored survival data. *Biometrika* 69, 553–566.

Hartley, H.O., Hocking, R. (1971). The analysis of incomplete data. *Biometrics* 27, 7783–7808.

Hartley, H.O., Rao, J.N.K. (1967). Maximum-likelihood estimation for the mixed analysis of variance model. *Biometrika* 54, 93–108.

Hastie, T., Tibshirani, R. (1990). *Generalized Additive Models*. New York: Chapman and Hall.

Herson, J. (1979). Predictive probability early termination plans for Phase II clinical trials. *Biometrics* 35, 775–783.

Heyting, A., Tolboom, J., Essers, J. (1992). Statistical handling of dropouts in longitudinal clinical trials. *Statistics in Medicine* 11, 2043–2061.

Hochberg, Y. (1988). A sharper Bonferroni procedure for multiple significance testing. *Biometrika* 75, 800–802.

Hochberg, Y., Benjamini, Y. (1990). More powerful procedures for multiple significance testing. *Statistics in Medicine* 9, 811–818.

Hochberg, Y., Rom, D. (1995). Extensions of multiple testing procedures based on Simes' test. *Journal of Statistical Planning and Inference* 48, 141–152.

Hochberg, Y., Tamhane, A.C. (1987). *Multiple Comparison Procedures*. New York: Wiley.

Holland, B.S., Copenhaver, M.D. (1987). An improved sequentially rejective Bonferroni test procedure. *Biometrics* 43, 417–423. Correction in *Biometrics* 43, 737.

Holland, P.W., Welsch, R.E. (1977). Robust regression using iteratively reweighted least-squares. *Communications in Statistics Series A* 6, 813–828.

Hollander, M., Wolfe, D.A. (1999). *Nonparametric Statistical Method*. 2nd ed. New York: Wiley.

Holm, S. (1979). A simple sequentially rejective multiple test procedure. *Scandinavian Journal of Statistics* 6, 65–70.

Hommel, G. (1983). Test of the overall hypothesis for arbitrary dependence structures. *Biometrical Journal* 25, 423–430.

Hommel, G. (1986). Multiple test procedures for arbitrary dependence structures. *Metrika* 33, 321–336.

Hommel, G. (1988). A stagewise rejective multiple procedure based on a modified Bonferroni test. *Biometrika* 75, 383–386.

Hommel, G. (1989). A comparison of two modified Bonferroni procedures. *Biometrika* 76, 624–625.

Hosmane, B., Shu, V., Morris, D. (1994). Finite sample properties of van Elteren test. *ASA Proceedings of the Biopharmaceutical Section*, 430–434.

Hsu, J.C. (1996). *Multiple Comparisons: Theory and Methods*. London: Chapman and Hall.

Hsu, J.C., Berger, R.L. (1999). Stepwise confidence intervals without multiplicity adjustment for dose-response and toxicity studies. *Journal of the American Statistical Association* 94, 468–482.

Huque, M. F., Sankoh, A. J. (1997). A reviewer's perspective on multiple endpoint issues in clinical trials. *Journal of Biopharmaceutical Statistics* 7, 545–564.

Hwang, I.K., Shih, W.J., DeCani, J.S. (1990). Group sequential designs using a family of type I error probability spending functions. *Statistics in Medicine* 9, 1439–1445.

Jennison, C., Turnbull, B.W. (1989). Interim analysis: The repeated confidence interval approach. *Journal of the Royal Statistical Society, Series B* 51, 305–361.

Jennison, C., Turnbull, B.W. (1990). Statistical approaches to interim monitoring of medical trials: A review and commentary. *Statistical Science* 5, 299–317.

Jennison, C., Turnbull, B.W. (2000). *Group Sequential Methods with Applications to Clinical Trials*. Boca Raton: Chapman and Hall/CRC.

Jennrich, R.I., Schluchter, M.D. (1986). Unbalanced repeated measures models with structured covariance matrices. *Biometrics* 42, 805–820.

Johns, D., Anderson, J.S. (1999). Use of predictive probabilities in Phase II and Phase III clinical trials. *Journal of Biopharmaceutical Statistics* 9, 67–79.

Jones, B., Teather, D., Wang, J., Lewis, J.A. (1998). A comparison of various estimators of a treatment difference for a multi-centre clinical trial. *Statistics in Medicine* 17, 1767–1777.

Kalbfleisch, J.D., Prentice, R.L. (1973). Marginal likelihoods based on Cox's regression and life model. *Biometrika* 60, 267–278.

Kalbfleisch, J.D., Prentice, R.L. (1980). *The Statistical Analysis of Failure Time Data*. New York: Wiley.

Kallen, A. (1997). Treatment-by-center interaction: What is the issue? *Drug Information Journal* 31, 927–936.

Kenward, M.G., Molenberghs, G. (1998). Likelihood-based frequentist inference when data are missing at random. *Statistical Science* 12, 236–247.

Kim, K., DeMets, D.L. (1987). Design and analysis of group sequential tests based on the type I error spending rate function. *Biometrika* 74, 149–154.

Kling, Y., Benjamini, Y. (2002). A cost-based approach to multiplicity control. Unpublished manuscript.

Knaus, W.A., Draper, E.A., Wagner, D.P., Zimmerman, J.E. (1985). APACHE II: A severity of disease classification system. *Critical Care Medicine* 13, 818–829.

Koch, G.G., Amara, I.A., Davis, G.W., Gillings, D.B. (1982). A review of some statistical methods for covariance analysis of categorical data. *Biometrics* 38, 563–595.

Koch, G.G., Carr, G.J., Amara, I.A., Stokes, M.E., Uryniak, T.J. (1990). Categorical data analysis. *Statistical Methodology in the Pharmaceutical Sciences*. Berry, D.A. (editor). New York: Marcel Dekker.

Koch, G.G., Edwards, S. (1988). Clinical efficacy with categorical data. *Biopharmaceutical Statistics for Drug Development*. Peace, K.K. (editor). New York: Marcel Dekker.

Koch, G.G., Gansky, S.A. (1996). Statistical considerations for multiplicity in confirmatory protocols. *Drug Information Journal* 30, 523–534.

Koenker, R., Bassett, G. (1978). Regression quantiles. *Econometrica* 46, 33–50.

Lachin, J.M. (2000). *Biostatistics Methods: The Assessment of Relative Risks*. New York: Wiley.

Lagakos, S.W., Schoenfeld, D.A. (1984). Properties of proportional hazards score tests under misspecified regression models. *Biometrics* 40, 1037–1048.

Laird, N.M., Ware, J.H. (1982). Random effects models for longitudinal data. *Biometrics* 38, 963–974.

Lan, K.K.G., DeMets, D.L. (1983). Discrete sequential boundaries for clinical trials. *Biometrika* 70, 659–663.

Lan, K.K.G., DeMets, D.L. (1989). Changing frequency of interim analysis in sequential monitoring. *Biometrics* 45, 1017–1020.

Lan, K.K.G., Lachin, J.M., Bautista, O.M. (2003). Over-ruling a group sequential boundary—a stopping rule versus a guideline. *Statistics in Medicine* 22, 3347–3355.

Lan, K.K.G., Simon, R., Halperin, M. (1982). Stochastically curtailed tests in long-term clinical trials. *Communications in Statistics. Sequential Analysis* 1, 207–219.

Lan, K.K.G., Wittes, J. (1988). The B-Value: A tool for monitoring data. *Biometrics* 44, 579–585.

Lang, J.B., Agresti, A. (1994). Simultaneously modeling joint and marginal distributions of multivariate categorical responses. *Journal of the American Statistical Association* 89, 625–632.

Laska, E.M., Meisner, M.J. (1989). Testing whether an identified treatment is best. *Biometrics* 45, 1139–1151.

Läuter, J. (1996). Exact *t* and *F* tests for analyzing studies with multiple endpoints. *Biometrics* 52, 964–970.

Lavori, P.W., Dawson, R., Shera, D. (1995). A multiple imputation strategy for clinical trials with truncation of patient data. *Statistics in Medicine* 14, 1913–1925.

le Cessie, S., van Houwelingen, J.C. (1991). A goodness-of-fit test for binary regression models, based on smoothing methods. *Biometrics* 47, 1267–1282.

Lee, E.T., Desu, M.M., Gehan, E.A. (1975). A Monte Carlo study of the power of some two-sample tests. *Biometrika* 62, 425–432.

Lee, J.W. (1994). Group sequential testing in clinical trials with multivariate observations: A review. *Statistics in Medicine* 13, 101–111.

Lehmacher, W., Wassmer, G., Reitmeir, P. (1991). Procedures for two-sample comparisons with multiple endpoints controlling the experimentwise error rate. *Biometrics* 47, 511–521.

Lehmann, E.L. (1975). *Nonparametrics: Statistical Methods Based on Ranks*. San Francisco: Holden-Day.

Leung, H.M., O'Neill, R.T. (1986). Statistical assessment of combination drugs: A regulatory view. *ASA Proceedings of the Biopharmaceutical Section*, 33–36.

Li, K.H., Raghunathan, T.E., Rubin, D.B. (1991). Large-sample significance levels from multiply imputed data using moment-based statistics and an *F* reference distribution. *Journal of the American Statistical Association* 86, 1065–1073.

Liang, K.-Y., Zeger, S.L. (1986). Longitudinal data analysis using generalized linear models. *Biometrika* 73, 13–22.

Liang, K.-Y., Zeger, S.L., Qaqish, B. (1992). Multivariate regression analyses for categorical data. *Journal of the Royal Statistical Society, Series B* 54, 3–40.

Lin, Z. (1999). An issue of statistical analysis in controlled multicentre studies: How shall we weight the centers? *Statistics in Medicine* 18, 365–373.

Lindsey, J.K. (1999). *Models for Repeated Measurements*. 2nd ed. Oxford: Clarendon Press.

Lindsey, J.K., Lambert, P. (1998). On the appropriateness of marginal models for repeated measurements in clinical trials. *Statistics in Medicine* 17, 447–469.

Lipsitz, S.R., Kim, K., Zhao, L. (1994). Analysis of repeated categorical data using generalized estimating equations. *Statistics in Medicine* 13, 1149–1163.

Lipsitz, S.R., Laird, N.M., Harrington, D.P. (1991). Generalized estimating equations for correlated binary data: Using the odds ratio as a measure of association. *Biometrika* 78, 153–160.

Littell, R.C., Freund, R.J., Spector, P.C. (1991). *SAS System for Linear Models*. 3rd ed. Cary, NC: SAS Institute Inc.

Littell, R.C., Milliken, G.A., Stroup, W.W., Wolfinger, R.D. (1996). *SAS System for Mixed Models*. Cary, NC: SAS Institute Inc.

Little, R.J.A. (1993). Pattern-mixture models for multivariate incomplete data. *Journal of the American Statistical Association* 88, 125–134.

Little, R.J.A. (1994). A class of pattern-mixture models for normal incomplete data. *Biometrika* 81, 471–483.

Little, R.J.A., Rubin, D.B. (1987). *Statistical Analysis with Missing Data*. New York: Wiley.

Liu, Q., Pierce, D.A. (1994). A note on Gauss-Hermite quadrature. *Biometrika* 81, 624–629.

Liu, W. (1996). Multiple tests of a non-hierarchical finite family of hypotheses. *Journal of the Royal Statistical Society, Series B* 58, 455–461.

Longford, N.T. (1993). *Random Coefficient Models*. Oxford: Oxford University Press.

Louis, T.A. (1982). Finding the observed information matrix when using the EM algorithm. *Journal of the Royal Statistical Society, Series B* 44, 226–233.

Mallinckrodt, C.H., Clark, W.S., Carroll, R.J., Molenberghs, G. (2003a). Assessing response profiles from incomplete longitudinal clinical trial data under regulatory considerations. *Journal of Biopharmaceutical Statistics* 13, 179–190.

Mallinckrodt, C.H., Clark, W.S., Stacy R.D. (2001a). Type I error rates from mixed effects model repeated measures versus fixed effects analysis of variance with missing values imputed via last observation carried forward. *Drug Information Journal* 35 (4), 1215–1225.

Mallinckrodt, C.H., Clark, W.S., Stacy R.D. (2001b). Accounting for dropout bias using mixed effects models. *Journal of Biopharmaceutical Statistics* 11 (1 & 2), 9–21.

Mallinckrodt, C.H., Sanger, T.M., Dube, S., Debrota, D.J., Molenberghs, G., Carroll, R.J., Zeigler Potter, W.M., Tollefson, G.D. (2003b). Assessing and interpreting treatment effects in longitudinal clinical trials with missing data. *Biological Psychiatry* 53, 754–760.

Mallows, C.L. (1973). Some comments on C_p. *Technometrics* 15, 661–675.

Mantel, N. (1966). Evaluation of survival data and two new rank order statistics arising in its consideration. *Cancer Chemo Reports* 50, 163–170.

Mantel, N., Fleiss, J.L. (1980). Minimum expected cell size requirements for the Mantel-Haenszel one-degree-of-freedom chi-square test and a related rapid procedure. *American Journal of Epidemiology* 112, 129–134.

Mantel, N., Haenszel, W. (1959). Statistical aspects of the analysis of data from retrospective studies of disease. *Journal of the National Cancer Institute* 22, 719–748.

Marcus, R., Peritz, E., Gabriel, K.R. (1976). On closed testing procedures with special reference to ordered analysis of variance. *Biometrika* 63, 655–660.

McCullagh, P. (1978). A class of parametric models for the analysis of square contingency tables with ordered categories. *Biometrika* 65, 413–418.

McCullagh, P., Nelder, J.A. (1989). *Generalized Linear Models*. 2nd ed. London: Chapman and Hall.

McCulloch, C.E., Searle, S.R. (2001). *Generalized, Linear and Mixed Models*. New York: Wiley.

McLachlan, G.J., Krishnan, T. (1997). *The EM Algorithm and Extensions*. New York: Wiley.

Mehrotra, D.V. (2001). Stratification issues with binary endpoints. *Drug Information Journal* 35, 1343–1350.

Mehrotra, D.V., Heyse, J.F. (2001). Multiplicity considerations in clinical safety analyses. *Proceedings of the Annual Meeting of the American Statistical Association*.

Mehrotra, D.V., Railkar, R. (2000). Minimum risk weights for comparing treatments in stratified binomial trials. *Statistics in Medicine* 19, 811–825.

Mehta, C.R., Patel, N.R. (1985). Exact logistic regression: Theory and examples. *Statistics in Medicine* 14, 2143–2160.

Meinert, C.L. (1986). *Clinical Trials: Design, Conduct and Analysis*. New York: Oxford University Press.

Michiels, B., Molenberghs, G., Bijnens, L., Vangeneugden, T., Thijs, H. (2002). Selection models and pattern-mixture models to analyze longitudinal quality of life data subject to dropout. *Statistics in Medicine* 21, 1023–1041.

Milliken, G.A., Johnson, D.E. (1984). *Analysis of Messy Data: Designed Experiments*. London: Chapman and Hall.

Molenberghs, G., Lesaffre, E. (1994). Marginal modeling of correlated ordinal data using a multivariate Plackett distribution. *Journal of the American Statistical Association* 89, 633–644.

Molenberghs, G., Lesaffre, E. (1999). Marginal modeling of multivariate categorical data. *Statistics in Medicine* 18, 2237–2255.

Molenberghs, G., Thijs, H., Jansen, I., Beunckens, C., Kenward, M.G., Mallinckrodt, C., Carroll, R.J. (2003). Analyzing incomplete longitudinal clinical trial data. Submitted for publication.

Molenberghs, G., Verbeke, G. (2003). Meaningful statistical model formulations. *Statistica Sinica* 14, 989–1020.

Molenberghs, G., Verbeke, G., Thijs, H., Lesaffre, E., Kenward, M.G. (2001). Mastitis in dairy cattle: Influence analysis to assess sensitivity of the dropout process. *Computational Statistics and Data Analysis* 37, 93–113.

Morrell, C.H., Pearson, J.D., Brant, L.J. (1997). Linear transformations of linear mixed effects models. *The American Statistician* 51, 338–343.

Moyé, L.A. (2000). Alpha calculus in clinical trials: Considerations and commentary for the new millennium. *Statistics in Medicine* 19, 767–779.

National Committee for Clinical Laboratory Standards (1995). *How to define and determine reference intervals in the clinical laboratory. Approved guideline.* Document C28-A (http://www.nccls.org/).

Nelder, J. (1977). A reformulation of linear models. *Journal of the Royal Statistical Society, Series A* 140, 48–76.

Nelder, J.A. (1994). The statistics of linear models: Back to basics. *Statistics and Computing* 4, 221–234.

Nelder, J.A., Mead, R. (1965). A simplex method for function minimisation. *The Computer Journal* 7, 303–313.

Nelder, J.A., Wedderburn, R.W.M. (1972). Generalized linear models. *Journal of the Royal Statistical Society, Series A* 135, 370–384.

Neuhaus, J.M. (1992). Statistical methods for longitudinal and clustered designs with binary responses. *Statistical Methods in Medical Research* 1, 249-273.

Neuhaus, J.M., Kalbfleisch, J.D., Hauck, W.W. (1991). A comparison of cluster-specific and population-averaged approaches for analyzing correlated binary data. *International Statistical Review* 59, 25–35.

Nickens, D.J. (1998). Using tolerance limits to evaluate laboratory data. *Drug Information Journal* 32, 261–269.

O'Brien, P.C. (1984). Procedures for comparing samples with multiple endpoints. *Biometrics* 40, 1079–1087.

O'Brien, P.C. (1990). Group sequential methods in clinical trials. *Statistical Methodology in the Pharmaceutical Sciences*, 291–311.

O'Brien, P.C., Fleming, T.R. (1979). A multiple testing procedure for clinical trials. *Biometrics* 35, 549–556.

O'Neill, R.T. (1997). Secondary endpoints cannot be validly analyzed if the primary endpoint does not demonstrate clear statistical significance. *Controlled Clinical Trials* 18, 550–556.

Pampallona, S., Tsiatis, A.A. (1994). Group sequential designs for one-sided and two-sided hypothesis testing with provision for early stopping in favour of the null hypothesis. *Journal of Statistical Planning and Inference* 42, 19–35.

Pampallona, S., Tsiatis, A.A., Kim, K. (2001). Interim monitoring of group sequential trials using spending functions for the type I and type II error probabilities. *Drug Information Journal* 35, 1113–1121.

Peixoto, J.L. (1987). Hierarchical variable selection in polynomial regression models. *The American Statistician* 41, 311–313.

Peixoto, J.L. (1990). A property of well-formulated polynomial regression models. *The American Statistician* 44, 26–30.

Pepe, M.S., Anderson, G.L. (1992). Two-stage experimental designs: Early stopping with a negative result. *Applied Statistics* 41, 181–190.

Perlman, M.D. (1969). One-sided testing problems in multivariate analysis. *Annals of Mathematical Statistics* 40, 549–567.

Peto, R. (1982). Statistical aspects of cancer trials. *Treatment of Cancer.* Halnan, K.E. (editor). London: Chapman and Hall.

Peto, R., Peto, J. (1972). Asymptotically efficient rank invariant test procedures. *Journal of the Royal Statistical Society, Series A* 135, 185–206.

Phillips, A., Ebbutt, A., France, L., Morgan, D. (2000). The International Conference on Harmonization guideline "Statistical principles for clinical trials": Issues in applying the guideline in practice. *Drug Information Journal* 34, 337–348.

Piantadosi, S. (1997). *Clinical Trials: A Methodologic Perspective.* New York: Wiley.

Pinheiro, J., Bates, D. M. (2000). *Mixed-Effects Models in S and S-Plus.* New York: Springer-Verlag.

Plackett, R.L. (1965). A class of bivariate distributions. *Journal of the American Statistical Association* 60, 516–522.

Pocock, S.J. (1977). Group sequential methods in the design and analysis of clinical trials. *Biometrika* 64, 191–199.

Pocock, S.J. (1983). *Clinical Trials: A Practical Approach.* New York: Wiley.

Pocock, S.J., Geller, N. L., Tsiatis, A.A. (1987). The analysis of multiple endpoints in clinical trials. *Biometrics* 43, 487–493.

Potthoff, R.F., Roy, S.N. (1964). A generalized multivariate analysis of variance model useful especially for growth curve problems. *Biometrika* 51, 313–326.

Prentice, R.L. (1978). Linear rank tests with right censored data. *Biometrika* 65, 167–180.

Prentice, R.L. (1988). Correlated binary regression with covariates specific to each binary observation. *Biometrics* 44, 1033-1048.

Prentice, R.L., Marek, P. (1979). A qualitative discrepancy between censored data rank. *Biometrics* 35, 861–867.

Proschan, M.A., Follman, D.A., Waclawiw, M.A. (1992). Effects of assumption violations on type I error rate in group sequential monitoring. *Biometrics* 48, 1131–1143.

Radhakrishna, S. (1965). Combination of results from several 2×2 contingency tables. *Biometrics* 21, 86–98.

Rao, C.R. (1973). *Linear Statistical Inference and Its Application*. 2nd ed. New York: Wiley.

Rasch, G. (1961). On general laws and the meaning of measurement in psychology. *Proceedings of the Fourth Berkeley Symposium on Mathematical Statistics and Probability* 4, 321–333.

Rautaharju, P.M., Zhou, S.H., Wong, S., Calhoun, H.P., Berenson, G.S., Prineas, R., Davignon, A. (1992). Sex differences in the evolution of the electrocardiographic QT interval with age. *Canadian Journal of Cardiology* 8, 690–695.

Robins, J.M., Rotnitzky, A., Scharfstein, D.O. (1998). Semiparametric regression for repeated outcomes with nonignorable nonresponse. *Journal of the American Statistical Association* 93, 1321–1339.

Robins, J.M., Rotnitzky, A., Zhao, L.P. (1995). Analysis of semiparametric regression models for repeated outcomes in the presence of missing data. *Journal of the American Statistical Association* 90, 106–121.

Robinson, L.D., Jewell, N.P. (1991). Some surprising results about covariate adjustment in logistic regression models. *International Statistical Review* 58, 227–240.

Rodriguez, R., Tobias, R., Wolfinger, R. (1995). Comments on J.A. Nelder 'The Statistics of Linear Models: Back to Basics.' *Statistics and Computing* 5, 97–101.

Rom, D.M., Costello, R.J., Connell, L.T. (1994). On closed test procedures for dose-response analysis. *Statistics in Medicine* 13, 1583–1596.

Rosenbaum, P.R., Rubin, D.B. (1983). The central role of the propensity score method in observational studies for causal effects. *Biometrika* 70, 41–55.

Rubin, D.B. (1976). Inference and missing data. *Biometrika* 63, 581–592.

Rubin, D.B. (1978). Multiple imputations in sample surveys—A phenomenological Bayesian approach to nonresponse. *Imputation and Editing of Faulty or Missing Survey Data*. Washington, DC: U.S. Department of Commerce.

Rubin, D.B. (1987). *Multiple Imputation for Nonresponse in Surveys*. New York: Wiley.

Rubin, D.B., Schenker, N. (1986). Multiple imputation for interval estimation from simple random samples with ignorable nonresponse. *Journal of the American Statistical Association* 81, 366–374.

Rüger, B. (1978). Das maximale Signifikanzniveau des Tests "Lehne H_0 ab, wenn k unter n gegebenen Tests zur Ablehnungführen." *Metrika* 25, 171–178.

Sankoh, A. J., Huque, M. F., Dubey, S. D. (1997). Some comments on frequently used multiple endpoint adjustment methods in clinical trials. *Statistics in Medicine* 16, 2529–2542.

Sarkar, S., Chang, C.K. (1997). Simes' method for multiple hypothesis-testing with positively dependent test statistics. *Journal of the American Statistical Association* 92, 1601–1608.

Schafer J.L. (1997). *Analysis of Incomplete Multivariate Data*. London: Chapman & Hall.

Scheffe, H. (1953). A method for judging all contrasts in the analysis of variance. *Biometrika* 40, 87–104.

Scheffe, H. (1959). *The Analysis of Variance*. New York: Wiley.

Searle, S.R. (1971). *Linear Models*. New York: Wiley.

Searle, S.R. (1976). Comments on ANOVA calculations for messy data. *SAS Users Group International Conference I*, 298–308.

Searle, S.R. (1992). *Variance Components*. New York: Wiley.

Self, S.G., Liang, K.-Y. (1987). Asymptotic properties of maximum likelihood estimators and likelihood ratio tests under nonstandard conditions. *Journal of the American Statistical Association* 82, 605–610.

Senn, S. (1997). *Statistical Issues in Drug Development*. New York and Chichester: Wiley.

Senn, S.J. (1997). *Statistical Issues in Drug Development*. Chichester: John Wiley.

Senn, S. (1998). Some controversies in planning and analyzing multicenter trials. *Statistics in Medicine* 17, 1753–1765.

Senn, S. (2000). The many modes of meta. *Drug Information Journal* 34, 535–549.

Shaffer, J.P. (1986). Modified sequentially rejective multiple test procedures. *Journal of the American Statistical Association* 81, 826–831.

Šidák, Z. (1967). Rectangular confidence regions for the means of multivariate normal distributions. *Journal of the American Statistical Association* 62, 626–633.

Siddiqui, O., Ali, M.W. (1998). A comparison of the random effects pattern mixture model with last observation carried forward (LOCF) analysis in longitudinal clinical trials with dropouts. *Journal of Biopharmaceutical Statistics* 8, 545–563.

Siegel, J.N. (1999). Development of an FDA guidance document for clinical trials in SLE. *Lupus* 8, 581–585.

Siegmund, D. (1978). Estimation following sequential tests. *Biometrika* 65, 341–349.

Simes, R.J. (1986). An improved Bonferroni procedure for multiple tests of significance. *Biometrika* 63, 655–660.

Skellam, J.G. (1948). A probability distribution derived from the binomial distribution by regarding the probability of success as variable between the sets of trials. *Journal of the Royal Statistical Society, Series B* 10, 257–261.

Solberg, H.E. (1987). International Federation of Clinical Chemistry: Approved recommendations on the theory of reference values. *Journal of Clinical Chemistry and Clinical Biochemistry* 25, 337–342.

Speed, F.M., Hocking, R.R. (1976). The use of $R()$ notation with unbalanced data. *American Statistician* 30, 30–33.

Speed, F.M., Hocking, R.R. (1980). A characterization of the GLM sums of squares. *SAS Users Group International Conference V*, 215–223.

Speed, F.M., Hocking, R.R., Hackney, O.P. (1978). Methods of analysis of linear models with unbalanced data. *Journal of the American Statistical Association* 73, 105–112.

Spiegelhalter, D.J., Freedman, L.S., Blackburn, P.R. (1986). Monitoring clinical trials: Conditional or predictive power? *Controlled Clinical Trials* 7, 8–17.

Steel, R.G.D. (1959). A multiple comparison rank sum test: Treatments versus control. *Biometrics* 15, 560–572.

Stiratelli, R., Laird, N.M., Ware, J.H. (1984). Random effects models for serial observations with binary response. *Biometrics* 40, 961–971.

Stokes, M.E., Davis, C.S., Koch, G.G. (2000). *Categorical Data Analysis Using the SAS System*. 2nd ed. Cary, NC: SAS Institute Inc.

Stram, D.O., Lee, J.W. (1994). Variance components testing in the longitudinal mixed effects model. *Biometrics* 50, 1171–1177.

Stram, D.O., Lee, J.W. (1995). Correction to: Variance components testing in the longitudinal mixed effects model. *Biometrics* 51, 1196.

Tang, D.I., Geller, N.L., Pocock, S.J. (1993). On the design and analysis of randomized clinical trials with multiple endpoints. *Biometrics* 49, 23–30.

Tang, D.I., Gnecco, C., Geller, N.L. (1989a). An approximate likelihood ratio test for a normal mean vector with nonnegative components with application to clinical trials. *Biometrika* 76, 751–754.

Tang, D.I., Gnecco, C., Geller, N.L. (1989b). Design of group sequential trials with multiple endpoints. *Journal of the American Statistical Association* 84, 776–779.

Tanner, M.A., Wong, W.H. (1987). The calculation of posterior distributions by data augmentation. *Journal of the American Statistical Association* 82, 528–550.

Tarone, R.E., Ware, J. (1977). On distribution-free tests for equality of survival distribution. *Biometrika* 64, 156–160.

Taylor, I.K., O'Shaughnessy, K.M., Fuller, R.W., Dollery, C.T. (1991). Effect of cysteinyl-leukotreine receptor antagonist ICI 204.219 on allergen-induced bronchoconstriction and airway hyperreactivity in atopic subjects. *Lancet* 337, 690–693.

Thijs, H., Molenberghs, G., Michiels, B., Verbeke, G., Curran, D. (2002). Strategies to fit pattern-mixture models. *Biostatistics* 3, 245–265.

Troendle, J.F., Legler, J.M. (1998). A comparison of one-sided methods to identify significant individual outcomes in a multiple outcome setting: Stepwise tests or global tests with closed testing. *Statistics in Medicine* 17, 1245–1260.

Tsiatis, A.A. (1981). A large sample study of Cox's regression model. *Annals of Statistics* 9, 93–108.

Tsiatis, A.A., Rosner, G.L., Mehta, C.R. (1984). Exact confidence intervals following a group sequential test. *Biometrics* 40, 797–803.

Tukey, J.W. (1947). Nonparametric estimation. Statistically equivalent blocks and tolerance regions: The continuous case. *Annals of Mathematical Statistics* 18, 529–539.

Van Den Berghe, G., Wouters, P., Weekers, F., Verwaest, C., Bruyninckx, F., Schetz, I., Vlasselaers, D., Ferdinande, P., Lauwers, P., Bouillon, R. (2001). Intensive insulin therapy in critically ill patients. *The New England Journal of Medicine* 345, 1359–1367.

van Elteren, P.H. (1960). On the combination of independent two-sample tests of Wilcoxon. *Bulletin of the International Statistical Institute* 37, 351–361.

Verbeke, G., Lesaffre, E., Brant L.J. (1998). The detection of residual serial correlation in linear mixed models. *Statistics in Medicine* 17, 1391–1402.

Verbeke, G., Molenberghs, G. (1997). *Linear Mixed Models in Practice: A SAS-Oriented Approach*. Lecture Notes in Statistics 126. New York: Springer-Verlag.

Verbeke, G., Molenberghs, G. (2000). *Linear Mixed Models for Longitudinal Data*. New York: Springer-Verlag.

Verbeke, G., Molenberghs, G., Thijs, H., Lesaffre, E., Kenward, M.G. (2001). Sensitivity analysis for nonrandom dropout: A local influence approach. *Biometrics* 57, 7–14.

Wade, A.M., Ades, A.E. (1998). Incorporating correlations between measurements into the estimation of age-related reference ranges. *Statistics in Medicine* 17, 1989–2002.

Wang, S.K., Tsiatis, A.A. (1987). Approximately optimal one-parameter boundaries for group sequential trials. *Biometrics* 43, 193–199.

Ware, J.H., Muller, J.E., Braunwald, E. (1985). The futility index: An approach to the cost-effective termination of randomized clinical trials. *American Journal of Medicine* 78, 635–643.

Wassmer, G., Reitmeir, P., Kieser, M., Lehmacher, W. (1999). Procedures for testing multiple endpoints in clinical trials: An overview. *Journal of Statistical Planning and Inference* 82, 69–81.

Wedderburn, R.W.M. (1974). Quasi-likelihood functions, generalized linear models, and the Gauss-Newton method. *Biometrika* 61, 439–447.

Westfall, P.H., Krishen, A. (2001). Optimally weighted, fixed sequence, and gatekeeping multiple testing procedures. *Journal of Statistical Planning and Inference* 99, 25–40.

Westfall, P.H., Tobias, R.D. (2000). *Multiple Comparisons and Multiple Tests Using the SAS System Workbook*. Cary, NC: SAS Institute Inc.

Westfall, P.H., Tobias, R.D., Rom, D., Wolfinger, R.D., Hochberg, Y. (1999). *Multiple Comparisons and Multiple Tests Using the SAS System*. Cary, NC: SAS Institute Inc.

Westfall, P.H., Wolfinger, R.D. (2000). Closed multiple testing procedures and PROC MULTTEST. *Observations: Technical Journal for SAS Software Users* 23 (available at http://support.sas.com/documentation/periodical/obs/obswww23).

Westfall, P.H., Young, S.S. (1989). *P*-value adjustments for multiple tests in multivariate binomial models. *Journal of the American Statistical Association* 84, 780–786.

Westfall, P.H., Young, S.S. (1993). *Resampling-Based Multiple Testing: Examples and Methods for P-Value Adjustment*. New York: Wiley.

Whitehead, J. (1986). On the bias of maximum likelihood estimation following a sequential test. *Biometrika* 73, 573–581.

Whitehead, J. (1997). *The Design and Analysis of Sequential Clinical Trials*. 2nd ed. Chichester: Wiley.

Whitehead, J. (1999). A unified theory for sequential clinical trials. *Statistics in Medicine* 18, 2271–2286.

Whitehead, J., Stratton, I. (1983). Group sequential clinical trials with triangular continuation regions. *Biometrics* 39, 227–236.

Wilks, S.S. (1941). Determination of sample sizes for setting tolerance limits. *Annals of Mathematical Statistics* 12, 91–96.

Wilson, M.G. (2000). Lilly reference ranges. *Encyclopedia of Pharmaceutical Statistics*. New York: Marcel Dekker.

Yamaguchi, T., Ohashi, Y. (1999). Investigating centre effects in a multi-centre clinical trial of superficial bladder cancer. *Statistics in Medicine* 18, 1961–1971.

Yates, F. (1934). The analysis of multiple classifications with unequal numbers in the different classes. *Journal of the American Statistical Association* 29, 51–66.

Yu, K., Jones, M.C. (1998). Local linear quantile regression. *Journal of the American Statistical Association* 93, 228–237.

Zeger, S.L., Liang, K.-Y. (1986). Longitudinal data analysis for discrete and continuous outcomes. *Biometrics* 42, 121–130.

Zeger, S.L., Liang, K.-Y., Albert, P.S. (1988). Models for longitudinal data: A generalized estimating equations approach. *Biometrics* 44, 1049–1060.

Zhao, L.P., Prentice, R.L. (1990). Correlated binary regression using a quadratic exponential model. *Biometrika* 77, 642–648.

Index

Numbers

Symbols

Books Available from SAS Press

Advanced Log-Linear Models Using SAS®
by **Daniel Zelterman**................................ Order No. A57496

Analysis of Clinical Trials Using SAS®: A Practical Guide
by **Alex Dmitrienko, Walter Offen, Christy Chuang-Stein,**
and **Geert Molenbergs** .... Order No. A59390

Annotate: Simply the Basics
by **Art Carpenter**...................................... Order No. A57320

*Applied Multivariate Statistics with SAS® Software,
Second Edition*
by **Ravindra Khattree**
and **Dayanand N. Naik** .... Order No. A56903

*Applied Statistics and the SAS® Programming Language,
Fourth Edition*
by **Ronald P. Cody**
and **Jeffrey K. Smith**................................ Order No. A55984

An Array of Challenges — Test Your SAS® Skills
by **Robert Virgile**...................................... Order No. A55625

*Carpenter's Complete Guide to the SAS® Macro Language,
Second Edition*
by **Art Carpenter**...................................... Order No. A59224

The Cartoon Guide to Statistics
by **Larry Gonick**
and **Woollcott Smith**................................ Order No. A55153

*Categorical Data Analysis Using the SAS® System,
Second Edition*
by **Maura E. Stokes, Charles S. Davis,**
and **Gary G. Koch** .... Order No. A57998

Cody's Data Cleaning Techniques Using SAS® Software
by **Ron Cody** ....Order No. A57198

*Common Statistical Methods for Clinical Research with
SAS® Examples, Second Edition*
by **Glenn A. Walker**................................. Order No. A58086

*Debugging SAS® Programs: A Handbook of Tools
and Techniques*
by **Michele M. Burlew** .... Order No. A57743

*Efficiency: Improving the Performance of Your
SAS® Applications*
by **Robert Virgile**...................................... Order No. A55960

*The Essential PROC SQL Handbook for
SAS® Users*
by **Katherine Prairie** .... Order No. A58546

*Fixed Effects Regression Methods for Longitudinal Data
Using SAS®*
by **Paul D. Allisoin** .... Order No. A58348

Genetic Analysis of Complex Traits Using SAS®
Edited by **Arnold M. Saxton** .... Order No. A59454

*A Handbook of Statistical Analyses Using SAS®,
Second Edition*
by **B.S. Everitt**
and **G. Der** .... Order No. A58679

Health Care Data and the SAS® System
by **Marge Scerbo, Craig Dickstein,**
and **Alan Wilson**...................................... Order No. A57638

The How-To Book for SAS/GRAPH® Software
by **Thomas Miron** .... Order No. A55203

*In the Know ... SAS® Tips and Techniques From
Around the Globe*
by **Phil Mason** .... Order No. A55513

*Instant ODS: Style Templates for the Output
Delivery System*
by **Bernadette Johnson** .... Order No. A58824

*Integrating Results through Meta-Analytic Review Using
SAS® Software*
by **Morgan C. Wang**
and **Brad J. Bushman** .... Order No. A55810

Learning SAS® in the Computer Lab, Second Edition
by **Rebecca J. Elliott**.............................. Order No. A57739

The Little SAS® Book: A Primer
by **Lora D. Delwiche**
and **Susan J. Slaughter** .... Order No. A55200

The Little SAS® Book: A Primer, Second Edition
by **Lora D. Delwiche**
and **Susan J. Slaughter** .... Order No. A56649
(updated to include Version 7 features)

The Little SAS® Book: A Primer, Third Edition
by **Lora D. Delwiche**
and **Susan J. Slaughter** .... Order No. A59216
(updated to include SAS 9.1 features)

*Logistic Regression Using the SAS® System:
Theory and Application*
by **Paul D. Allison** .... Order No. A55770

Longitudinal Data and SAS®: A Programmer's Guide
by **Ron Cody** .... Order No. A58176

Survival Analysis Using the SAS® System:
A Practical Guide
by **Paul D. Allison** .... Order No. A55233

Tuning SAS® Applications in the OS/390 and z/OS
Environments, Second Edition
by **Michael A. Raithel** .... Order No. A58172

Univariate and Multivariate General Linear Models:
Theory and Applications Using SAS® Software
by **Neil H. Timm**
and **Tammy A. Mieczkowski** .... Order No. A55809

Using SAS® in Financial Research
by **Ekkehart Boehmer, John Paul Broussard,**
and **Juha-Pekka Kallunki** .... Order No. A57601

Using the SAS® Windowing Environment: A Quick Tutorial
by **Larry Hatcher** .... Order No. A57201

Visualizing Categorical Data
by **Michael Friendly** .... Order No. A56571

Web Development with SAS® by Example
by **Frederick Pratter** .... Order No. A58694

Your Guide to Survey Research Using the SAS® System
by **Archer Gravely** .... Order No. A55688

JMP® Books

JMP® for Basic Univariate and Multivariate Statistics: A Step-by-
Step Guide
by **Ann Lehman, Norm O'Rourke, Larry Hatcher,**
and **Edward J. Stepanski** .... Order No. A59814

JMP® Start Statistics, Third Edition
by **John Sall, Ann Lehman,**
and **Lee Creighton** .... Order No. A58166

Regression Using JMP®
by **Rudolf J. Freund, Ramon C. Littell,**
and **Lee Creighton** .... Order No. A58789